Athletic Training
Exam Review

Athletic Training
Exam Review

Barbara H. Long, MS, VATL, ATC

Chair, Health and Exercise Science
Director, Athletic Training Program
Assistant Professor, Health and Exercise Science
Bridgewater College
Bridgewater, Virginia

Charles W. Hale IV, MSEd, VATL, ATC

Assistant Professor, Health and Exercise Science
Assistant Athletic Trainer
Bridgewater College
Bridgewater, Virginia

 Wolters Kluwer | Lippincott Williams & Wilkins
Health

Philadelphia • Baltimore • New York • London
Buenos Aires • Hong Kong • Sydney • Tokyo

Acquisitions Editor: Emily Lupash
Managing Editor: Andrea M. Klingler
Marketing Manager: Christen Murphy
Manufacturing Coordinator: Margie Orzech-Zeranko
Project Manager: Nicole Walz
Designer: Steve Druding
Compositor: Laserwords Private Limited, Chennai, India

© 2010 by **LIPPINCOTT WILLIAMS & WILKINS, a WOLTERS KLUWER business**

351 West Camden Street 530 Walnut Street
Baltimore, MD 21201   Philadelphia, PA 19106

Printed in the United States of America

Library of Congress Cataloging-in-Publication Data

Long, Barbara H.
  Athletic training exam review / Barbara H. Long, Charles W. Hale IV.
    p. ; cm.
  Includes bibliographical references and index.
  ISBN-13: 978-0-7817-8052-0
  ISBN-10: 0-7817-8052-7
  1. Sports medicine–Examinations, questions, etc. 2. Athletic trainers–Examinations, questions, etc. I. Hale, Charles W. II. Title.
  [DNLM: 1. Sports Medicine–methods–Examination Questions. 2. Physical Education and Training–methods–Examination Questions. QT 18.2 L848a 2010]
  RC1213.L66 2010
  617.1'027076–dc22

                                                          2008045929

Care has been taken to confirm the accuracy of the information presented and to describe generally accepted practices. However, the authors, editors, and publisher are not responsible for errors or omissions or for any consequences from application of the information in this book and make no warranty, expressed or implied, with respect to the currency, completeness, or accuracy of the contents of the publication. Application of this information in a particular situation remains the professional responsibility of the practitioner.

The authors, editors, and publisher have exerted every effort to ensure that drug selection and dosage set forth in this text are in accordance with current recommendations and practice at the time of publication. However, in view of ongoing research, changes in government regulations, and the constant flow of information relating to drug therapy and drug reactions, the reader is urged to check the package insert for each drug for any change in indications and dosage and for added warnings and precautions. This is particularly important when the recommended agent is a new or infrequently employed drug.

Some drugs and medical devices presented in this publication have Food and Drug Administration (FDA) clearance for limited use in restricted research settings. It is the responsibility of health care providers to ascertain the FDA status of each drug or device planned for use in their clinical practice.

To purchase additional copies of this book, call our customer service department at (800) 638-3030 or fax orders to (301) 223-2320. International customers should call (301) 223-2300.

Visit Lippincott Williams & Wilkins on the Internet: at LWW.com. Lippincott Williams & Wilkins customer service representatives are available from 8:30 AM to 6 PM, EST.

                                                          10 9 8 7 6

———————

To our parents, Carroll and Dorothy Hottle and Bill and Glenna Hale, for showing us what is important, how to finish what we start, and for loving us unconditionally.

———————

Preface

This book has been compiled as a way to focus the athletic training student during their preparation for the Board of Certification (BOC) examination. Education of the athletic training student is an extensive process—one that cannot be adequately summarized in one text. This material is intended to provide a framework for the student to begin the certification examination preparation. As with all educational materials, this text is a subset of larger reservoirs of information. Students should use this *Athletic Training Exam Review* to help focus their study rather than being used exclusively as a preparation program. Reviewing the material within the book should help the student identify content areas that are less familiar. Through the process, students may then refer back to other texts or coursework notes to reinforce the unfamiliar concepts.

Throughout the writing process, we have determined that the book may also be useful to focus the clinical education program for students. Athletic training education requires that each student be enrolled in clinical affiliations with varying populations, levels of risk, as well as medical conditions. These affiliation sites are selected by program directors or clinical education coordinators based on the experiences that students receive and the clinical instructor with whom they will work. Every institution has the autonomy to assess clinical proficiencies in whatever way meets the standards associated with educational accreditation. Utilizing this text and online ancillaries will formulate a framework of materials associated with each affiliation, yet provide that material in smaller, digestible subsections for the athletic training student. Online quiz and video clip capabilities will assist the clinical educator in integrating the athletic training student's learning from competency based material to the ability to initiate clinical judgment.

TEXT ORGANIZATION

As faculty within a Commission on Accreditation of Athletic Training Education accredited program, the authors have been preparing students for the BOC examination since 1999. In that time frame, it has become apparent that students rarely focus their study for the examination until about a month (or less) before the exam. The authors have formulated and used items from this text within their curriculum. Students comment that this outline format helps them focus by removing the narrative portion of texts. When they find content areas that are more unfamiliar, the student can then return to text, course notes, or ask questions of their faculty for assistance.

The outline format text begins with a section titled Fundamental Knowledge. It is imperative to include the Fundamental Knowledge section because this content is often given to students very early in their academic careers. In many instances, the student has not matured intellectually to the degree required to properly use the knowledge instructed in courses like Human Anatomy, Human Physiology, and Kinesiology. Studying for each classroom test seems to be the mantra early—get a grade, which will assure entrance into the Athletic Training Educational Program (ATEP). There is rarely connection between content and application such as understanding muscle function and manual muscle testing, at least initially. Reviewing foundational information is another way to reinforce the importance of the early knowledge and to promote a synthesis or integration of this knowledge in order to make the student proficient as entry-level athletic trainers.

Text and ancillary layout acknowledges multiple learning styles in an attempt to reduce content boredom and more efficiently engage the reader. Combinations of pictures, tables, and ancillary material should actively entice the reader to use and thereby recall the material. There are more than 150 tables and images within the book. Each section has numerous facts and test taking tips boxes to break the visual monotony of a heavy text laden project. Ancillaries add an interactive multimedia component to the material including the option to practice taking tests online with some similar features found on the current BOC examination.

Finally, at the end of the text, there is a section entitled Flash Box. This section is a single "at a glance" informational page consisting of major regions of the body. Content will include a box layout incorporating information regarding each joint (e.g., range of motion, special test names, proprioceptive neuromuscular facilitation [PNF] patterns, etc.) onto a single page. Students will have the ability to use these pages as quick recall or memory "joggers" for the material.

TEXT FEATURES

- Test Taking Information
- Test Taking Tips
- Section Overview
- Fundamental Knowledge Section
- Sections involving the 12 Educational Competency Content Areas
- National Athletic Trainers' Association (NATA) Educational Competency 4th Edition Proficiency List
- Outline/Bulleted Lists of Information
- Quick Facts
- Medical Terms

- Tables (43 dispersed throughout the book)
- Figures (116 dispersed throughout the book)
- Practice Questions and Answers (1,180 questions in the text)
- Flash Box (Joint information "at a glance")
- Study Check List
- Suggested Readings
- Ancillaries

ANCILLARIES

Each section has specific additional information for the ancillary portion of the project. The ancillaries include extensive quiz questions with the capability for identification, drag and drop, multiple choice, true and false, matching, and scenario-type formats. These online questions more closely mimic the evolution of the BOC examination. Components of the ancillaries include:

- Approximately 1,000 additional practice examination questions in varied formats for the student to practice computer-based testing situations
- Auditory pronunciation of key terms (approximately 900 medical terms)

- Full-color pictures including those of skin disorders, manual muscle testing, and goniometric measurements
- Web links to position statements and key resources
- 31 "How to . . ." items that identify the key steps to measuring Q-angle; auscultating the heart and lungs, and so on.
- More than 300 muscle origin, insertion, action, innervation, and arterial supply flash cards
- Advanced manual muscle testing, special test, and goniometry techniques
- General medical conditions and injury pathology (identification, etiology, signs/symptoms, and management)
- More than 120 video clips of special tests and joint mobilization techniques
- Dictionary of key terms from the text
- 120 question "Challenge" game that allows the student(s) to test their knowledge in specific content areas.

Barbara Long

Charles Hale

Acknowledgment

It has been said that "it takes a village to raise a child." In fact, we believe that it takes a village to develop a textbook. Throughout the process, so many people have contributed ideas, encouragements, and critiques to the development of our academic child—this book. Our heartfelt gratitude and admiration is expressed to everyone who supported us throughout this process.

We thank the many Bridgewater College Athletic Training students who have taught us throughout the years (especially those who endured our shenanigans during the 2007–2008 academic year). Your guidance has clearly defined this book and its need.

We thank the certified athletic training staff at Bridgewater College: Chris Horschel, Ellen Hicks, and Sarah Cook, you always filled in the gaps while we were off on a deadline—thanks seems such a small tribute to your contributions.

Thank you Dr. Paula Maxwell, you believed in the project and us throughout the entire process. We cannot describe how important it was to have your encouragement, feedback, and late-night caffeine runs!

Finally, to our families: Stuart, Tyler, and Cassie Long; and Ada, Charlie, and Stella Hale, you each sacrificed so that we might reach for this dream. Thank you for supporting us during the upswings and challenges of writing this book, we are so proud of each of you and love you all very much.

Reviewers

Contents

Preface vi

Acknowledgment viii

Reviewers ix

Taking the Test xii

SECTION 1
FUNDAMENTAL KNOWLEDGE 1

PART 1 Systemic Anatomy and Physiology 2
PART 2 Anatomy of the Head, Neck, Spine, and Thorax 38
PART 3 Anatomy of the Upper Extremity 51
PART 4 Anatomy of the Lower Extremity 64
PART 5 Kinesiology 84
SECTION 1 EXAMINATION 90

SECTION 2
RISK MANAGEMENT AND INJURY PREVENTION 99

PART 1 Risk Factors for Activity 101
PART 2 Preparticipation Examinations 101
PART 3 Protective Devices and Procedures 103
PART 4 Environmental Factors 105
SECTION 2 EXAMINATION 109

SECTION 3
PATHOLOGY OF INJURIES AND ILLNESSES 119

PART 1 Human Cell Function and Dysfunction 120
PART 2 Inflammation and Infection 124
PART 3 Circulation and Homeostasis 129
PART 4 Exercise and Illness, Injury, or Disease 132
PART 5 Common Injuries 136
SECTION 3 EXAMINATION 143

SECTION 4
ORTHOPAEDIC CLINICAL EXAMINATION AND DIAGNOSIS 151

PART 1 Principles of Clinical Examination 152
PART 2 Examination of the Head, Neck, Spine, and Thorax 158
PART 3 Examination of the Upper Extremity 163
PART 4 Examination of the Lower Extremity 172
SECTION 4 EXAMINATION 180

SECTION 5
MEDICAL CONDITIONS AND DISABILITIES 189

PART 1 General Medical Assessment 190
PART 2 Medical Conditions 198
SECTION 5 EXAMINATION 204

SECTION 6
ACUTE CARE OF INJURIES AND ILLNESSES 213

PART 1 Responding to Emergencies 215
PART 2 Skin and Musculoskeletal Injuries 221
PART 3 Head, Face, Spine, and Thorax Injuries 222
PART 4 Respiratory and Cardiac Emergencies 228
PART 5 Environmental Injuries and Illnesses 230
PART 6 Other Medical Emergencies 231
PART 7 Ambulation and Moving Patients 233
SECTION 6 EXAMINATION 235

SECTION 7
THERAPEUTIC MODALITIES 245

PART 1 Science of Modalities 246
PART 2 Pain 248
PART 3 Modalities 250
SECTION 7 EXAMINATION 259

SECTION 8
CONDITIONING AND REHABILITATIVE EXERCISE 267

PART 1 General Exercise and Rehabilitation Parameters 269
PART 2 Joint Mobilizations 275
PART 3 Proprioceptive Neuromuscular Facilitation (PNF) 279
PART 4 Aquatic Exercise 281
SECTION 8 EXAMINATION 284

SECTION 9
PHARMACOLOGY 293

PART 1 Administrative and Legal Issues 294
PART 2 Science of Chemical Agents 297
SECTION 9 EXAMINATION 302

SECTION 10

PSYCHOSOCIAL INTERVENTION AND REFERRAL 311

PART 1   Mental Health and Illnesses 313

PART 2   Psychosocial Interactions 315

Section 10 Examination 318

SECTION 11

NUTRITIONAL ASPECTS OF INJURIES AND ILLNESSES 323

PART 1   Healthy and Pathologic Nutrition 325

PART 2   Nutrition and Athletic Performance 330

PART 3   Weight Management and Eating Disorders 332

PART 4   Dietary Supplements and Ergogenic Aids 335

Section 11 Examination 337

SECTION 12

HEALTH CARE ADMINISTRATION 345

PART 1   Monitoring Systems 346

PART 2   Risk Management 346

PART 3   Resource Management 348

PART 4   Third-Party Reimbursement 349

PART 5   Federal Statutes 351

PART 6   Documentation 352

PART 7   Administrative Concepts 353

Section 12 Examination 355

SECTION 13

PROFESSIONAL DEVELOPMENT AND RESPONSIBILITY 363

PART 1   Professional History, Governance, and Standards 364

PART 2   Research and Evidence-Based Practice 365

Section 13 Examination 367

SECTION 14

FLASH BOXES 371

Appendix: Examination Answers 379

Index 387

Taking the Test

Every year students take the BOC examination and invariably raise their stress levels to monumental proportions. After at least 2 years in an accredited ATEP, you are taking the plunge into an entry-level position as an athletic trainer. There is just one step between you and that position—the BOC examination. It can be daunting to know that all of your clinical experiences, classes, late-night study sessions, and college tuition are held accountable by this one test.

Stop! That thought will get into your psyche and freeze your efforts. Reframe that thought and believe that those same experiences have paved the way for you to be successful on a minimum-competency examination. Do you feel minimally competent to tape an ankle? Do you feel minimally competent to rehabilitate a knee sprain or fit a football helmet? I doubt your ATEP program director would feel you are incompetent, or she or he would not sign the affidavit assuring that you are ready for the test. From this moment forward you can only think positively; you have the basic knowledge but probably need to brush up on the specific details. You can't lament over the impossibility of the BOC examination but you can't take it lightly either.

Prepare yourself! Remember that first day you walked into the athletic training room and had absolutely no idea what to do with an athlete having muscle cramps? Now you know the steps. Better yet, you have performed the steps and reinforced the knowledge into something usable: clinical judgment. Approach the BOC examination with that same work ethic and use the knowledge; reinforce the knowledge by teaching it and your clinical judgment will grow.

The BOC examination is undoubtedly tough but your preparations make *you* tougher. It is certainly true that nearly two thirds of those taking the examination don't pass it the first time. Yet again, a negative mindset will force you to think about whether you are good enough to take the examination. Notice we didn't say good enough to be an athletic trainer!

This book is about making you feel prepared for the BOC examination and will help guide you through the process; however, it is not a passive process. You must work hard to review much of the material. When you stumble with some of the content, go back to your course notes, textbooks, and faculty for help. Even your faculty has to review material when they have not used it in a while. For example, osmosis, saltatory conduction, or the sliding filament theory may not have been in the forefront of your mind for several semesters. Review and share the information with others (teaching it to someone else will help reinforce it in you). Fitting football equipment or

assessing general medical conditions may be your focus this semester so you may not need to spend as much time reviewing that material.

Place yourself in the position to be successful by beginning the preparation for the BOC examination *now*! That process is defined by when *now* is in the continuum toward certification. Are you beginning your senior year or is it the last month before the examination? Either way, the *Athletic Training Exam Review* can help with the process.

TEST-TAKING STRATEGIES

The best test-taking strategy is to begin preparing when, as an athletic training student, you are not at a level at which you think you should be. Think about this comment: "Are you proficient at everything you attempt?" For example, when evaluating an ankle, can you palpate the navicular, calculate the amount of rearfoot varus, apply a peroneal assist tape job, and assess the dermatomes associated with the ankle? If you can do all of those things well, move on to other skills within the ankle or another part of the body. Don't spend time working on things you have already mastered. Challenge yourself each day as you prepare for the examination. Trying something and failing will help you grow as a professional, but trying nothing will make you stagnant. In a life-long learning profession like athletic training, inactivity is absolutely more dangerous than activity. Make a pact to grow and progress every day in your journey toward certification.

Prepare for the new test format. The BOC examination is not the examination your faculty took to become certified. This is a computer-based examination that is evolving. Practice taking computer-based test questions like the ones accompanying this text. A baseball player doesn't show up for the game without having practiced throwing the ball or swinging the bat. You need to dedicate time to your practice, not just have it occur by chance.

Help those around you understand how important these next few months or weeks will be to your future. Specific time and locations for study will help you reach your goal. Always keep the goal of becoming certified in the forefront of your mind and don't let distractions derail your efforts.

Finally, when stumped by a test question, use your intuition and clinical decision-making skills. Ask yourself, what would I do with this information if faced with it in the field? Students often second guess themselves or try to read more into a question than is presented. Read the question for what it says, don't think about how the scenario or question could change given other parameters. If the question says:

> As the athletic trainer at a high school football game, you run onto the field when seeing an apparently unconscious football player on the ground. What would you do?

Your first response is not to activate emergency medical services (EMS)—you wouldn't do that clinically, yet many answer this way each year when faced with similar questions on the BOC examination. As an athletic training student ready to take the BOC examination, you have synthesized your knowledge into something usable, so don't forget that just because you are about to take an examination. Trust your faculty and your efforts and use your clinical decision-making skills. The new BOC examination is waiting for students to use their higher learning skills, not just regurgitate the knowledge they have obtained.

BEFORE TAKING THE BOARD OF CERTIFICATION EXAMINATION

The new BOC examination allows for a computer-based registration process. This process will be initiated by your ATEP program director by submitting the names of students eligible to take the examination. After confirmation of eligibility, the BOC will recognize you and allow the online registration process to begin. Although there are many testing sites throughout the country, some may only have four or five seats available during a specific testing period. Assure that you have a shot at the location you want by starting the registration process as early as possible. Make sure that you have secured your ATEP program director's endorsement, transcripts, current cardiopulmonary resuscitation/automatic external defibrillator (CPR/AED) certification (American Red Cross Professional Rescuer or similar), and complete the appropriate online forms (including payment for the test). Your registration will conclude once all online components are completed and you have mailed the specified documents to the BOC (e.g., transcripts and CPR/AED card copy). The BOC will send a confirmation e-mail to you, which you need to keep and bring with you to the test site on test day.

WHAT TO EXPECT ON BOARD OF CERTIFICATION TEST DAY

On the test day, you should arrive early to the test site. In fact, it would be a good idea to drive by the site the day before to assure you know the location. You will be apprehensive on test day, but if you control the things you can, you will be less antsy. Remember, you are ready for this big day...have a bit of swagger going into the test. You will not be able to bring anything with you into the test site. Make sure that you eat and drink something before the test. Don't get distracted by a grumbling belly when trying to determine the function of cranial nerve IV. You will need official photo identification (e.g., driver's license), a BOC password, and, for back-up, the aforementioned BOC

confirmation e-mail. Four hours now separate you from the end of this whole process—well, 4 hours and 15 minutes if you read the examination tutorial.

You must read the examination tutorial. Make sure that you understand all of the features of the BOC examination. Don't assume that you know how to use all of the features of the computer-based examination. You will complete 125 multiple choice questions and 4 hybrid questions. The multiple choice questions have a single correct item and four items that are distracters (incorrect). The hybrid questions are a combination of the old written simulation and practical portions of the examination. You may be asked to perform a given task, like wound care or mark certain structures like the dermatome for C6. Most likely, this type of test is not easily reproducible in a normal classroom and therefore not the most familiar to you. We have attempted to help with that by providing the online ancillary examination questions. Practice them often. There are nearly 1,000 questions from which you may learn. The BOC examination continues to evolve so the exact question numbers and styles may vary a bit over time, but that variety doesn't matter so much. What really matters is your confidence, preparation, and skills.

Invariably, you will start the examination and find questions that you aren't sure of the answer. While answering the multiple-choice portion, you can mark the questions and come back to them. If you have a total brain blank, mark several questions until you find one that you are certain the answer. Build the confidence; don't allow the examination to chip it away. If you need to, take a break, you will be asked to sign-out during that time. Hopefully, a good night's sleep the night before and a good meal the day of the test will limit the need for much break time away from the computer.

Finally, you're done! There will be a mixture of feelings. Some leave the examination feeling completely confident while others leave feeling like failures. The truth is that most leave exhausted. Don't take your feelings, good or bad, as an indication of success or failure. Just leave knowing that you've done the best you can on the test at that particular time.

HINTS FROM YOUR PEERS

We asked past and present BOC examination participants if they had any hints or strategies for taking the BOC examination. Enlisted below are a few of their comments:
- Think of the answer to the question before looking at the answer options.
- "Don't be freaked if you don't know an answer."
- Don't read into the question—only look at what is asked by the question.
- Use the provided scrap paper and pencil to problem-solve. This gives your eyes a break from the computer screen.
- Don't be fearful if a scenario ends and the computer asks about things you didn't do in the scenario. (This is not an indication that you have gotten the question wrong, you have to answer every assigned question either before or after the scenario. Just use your clinical judgment in every case.)

- Don't be surprised by an abrupt ending to the hybrid questions. You have no way of knowing when the end is coming, like you will with the multiple choice questions.
- Take lots of deep breaths and back away from the computer occasionally to clear your brain.
- Study early to alleviate stress.
- Don't do anything athletic-training oriented (especially studying) the day before the test.

TEST-TAKING TIPS

And finally, given below are some test-taking tips to help you as you prepare for the big day!
- Prepare, prepare, prepare...nothing substitutes for preparation!
- Use practice questions often.
- Do not study late the day before the examination. In fact, don't study *at all* the day before the examination. Let your mind relax. Have a good dinner, go to a movie, or do something fun with a nonathletic training friend.
- Arrive at the test center early to alleviate the stress of possibly being late. You may want to drive by the location the day before to ensure you know the route.
- Use mnemonics to remember key concepts.
- Read directions thoroughly.
- Be confident! Have a little swagger when you go into the test. You have invested *many* hours and *many* dollars into your education. Trust your ATEP faculty and yourself. *You are ready!*
- *Visualize success!* Imagine the feeling you will have when you open the computer file saying, "Congratulations, the Board of Certification is pleased to inform you...."

- Arrive relaxed, stay relaxed, and leave relaxed! On examination day you can't do anything more to be successful.
- Dress comfortably.
- When reading the question, don't look at the solutions. Devise your own answer beforehand and go with it.
- Read every question carefully before answering.
- Eliminate obviously wrong choices or distracters from the possible answer list.
- Don't waiver—make a decision and stick with it.
- Pay attention to key words and qualifiers like usually, always, sometimes, and never.
- Remember, this is an examination to assure *minimum* competency, not maximum competency. Answer the questions as if you are treating the injury on the lacrosse field. What would you do if...?
- When studying for the examination, try teaching the material to a younger athletic training student so that you might engage with the material in a more comprehensive way.
- If you are taking the examination, your program director is saying that if her or his son were face down on the football field with an injury, you can handle it. She or he has confidence in you!
- *Study light!* The earlier you begin the BOC examination preparation, the smaller chunks you can take. Start small by beginning early and build from there. Remember, 15 minutes a day is better than nothing.

SECTION
1
Fundamental Knowledge

Part 1   Systemic Anatomy and Physiology

Part 2   Anatomy of the Head, Neck, Spine, and Thorax

Part 3   Anatomy of the Upper Extremity

Part 4   Anatomy of the Lower Extremity

Part 5   Kinesiology

Section 1 Examination

OVERVIEW

There are certain fundamental or foundational knowledge items required to adequately understand the field of athletic training. Often, students have human anatomy and physiology courses early in their academic careers and then forget the importance of such courses. This section of the study preparation guide is designed to provide a reminder of those foundational courses. Parts within this section provide an outline of critical information in the areas of anatomy, physiology, and kinesiology. The student should review the material and investigate further where recall is more difficult.

CLINICAL PROFICIENCIES

There are no proficiencies assigned by the *Athletic Training Educational Competencies*, 4th edition for this section.

Systemic Anatomy and Physiology

KEY TERMS

- Abdominal aorta
- Acetylcholine
- Acidosis
- Actin filament
- Action potential
- Adenohypophysis
- Adenosine 5′-diphosphate (ADP)
- Adenosine 5′-triphosphate (ATP)
- Afferent fibers
- Alkalosis
- Anaerobic power
- Anaerobic respiration
- Anaerobic threshold
- Analgesia
- Anatomic position
- Antecubital
- Apnea
- Aponeurosis, aponeuroses
- Apophysis, apophyses
- Arteriole
- Articular cartilage
- Bile
- Bipartite
- Broca center
- Bursa, bursae
- Capillary
- Caudal
- Cephalad
- Cervical rib
- Chondroclast
- Chondrocyte
- Chordae tendineae of heart
- Clonus
- Conjunctiva, conjunctivae
- Decussate
- Deoxyribonucleic acid (DNA)
- Diffusion
- Ectomorph
- Effector
- Electrolyte
- Endocardium, endocardia

- Endogenous
- Endomorph
- Endomysium
- Epimysium
- Etiology
- Expiratory reserve volume (ERV)
- Fascia, fasciae
- Fascicle
- Femoral triangle
- Functional residual capacity (FRC)
- Gap junction
- Glucagon
- Glucose
- Glycogenesis
- Glycogenolysis
- Glycolysis
- Gustation
- Gynecomastia, gynecomasty
- Halitosis
- H band
- Hematopoietic system
- Homeostasis
- Hormone
- I band
- Idiopathic
- Immediate energy system
- Insufficiency
- Intrafusal fibers
- Ischemia
- Jaundice
- Joint
- Joint capsule
- Juxtaposition
- Latent period
- Ligament
- Limbic system
- Line of pull
- Lipid
- Lipolysis
- Livid
- Long-term memory (LTM)
- Luteal phase

- Mastication
- Mesomorph
- Metabolic acidosis
- Metabolic alkalosis
- Metabolic equivalent (MET)
- Metabolism
- Metabolite
- Microfilament
- Mineralocorticoid
- Mitochondrion
- Mixed nerve
- Monocyte
- Motor cortex
- Motor point
- Myelin sheath
- Myofascial
- Myofibril
- Myofilaments
- Nerve conduction
- Olfaction
- Oligodendroglia
- Ossification
- Osteoblast
- Osteoclast
- Osteocyte
- Papillary muscle
- Perilymph
- Perimysium, perimysia
- Periosteum, periostea
- Peripheral nervous system
- Permeable
- Postsynaptic membrane
- Potable
- Presynaptic membrane
- Progesterone
- Propagate
- Pyramidal decussation
- Pyramidal tract
- Ranvier node
- Raphe nuclei
- Reflex
- Reflex arc
- Regeneration
- Regurgitate
- Relapse
- Residual volume (RV)
- Respiratory acidosis
- Respiratory alkalosis

- Saltatory conduction
- Sarcomere
- Sarcoplasm
- Sarcoplasmic reticulum
- Sclerotome
- Slow-twitch fibers
- Somatic
- Spasticity
- Spinal ganglion
- Stem cell
- Summation
- Supine
- Synapse, synapses
- Synthesis, syntheses
- Tendinosis
- Tendon
- Unmyelinated fibers
- Uptake
- Vaginate
- Vital capacity (VC)
- Wolff law
- Z filament
- Z line

MUSCULOSKELETAL SYSTEM

Skeletal System

- Approximately 206 bones (exact number may vary)
- Divisions
  - Axial skeleton (80 bones)
  - Appendicular skeleton (126 bones)

 Quick fact Supernumerary bones are bones that exceed the standard number of 206. An example of this is an eighth cervical rib.

Skeletal System Divisions

- Axial skeleton
  - Skull, spinal column, ribs, and sternum
- Appendicular skeleton
  - Upper extremities, shoulder/pectoral girdle (scapula and clavicle), lower extremities, and pelvic girdle (ilium, ischium, and pubis)

 Use the DVD or visit the website at http://thePoint.lww.com/Long for additional materials about *bone markings*.

Quick fact
> Some sources classify the sternum as being part of the shoulder girdle, and therefore part of the appendicular skeleton.
> Some sources classify the sacrum and coccyx of the spinal column as being part of the pelvic girdle, and therefore part of the appendicular skeleton.

Roles of the Skeletal System
- Supports body weight
- Transfers body weight
- Body movement
- Muscle and ligament attachment
- Organ protection
- Bone marrow storage
- Mineral storage

Bone Classification by Shape
- Long (see Fig. 1.1)
  - Long cylindrical shaft (diaphysis)
  - Protruding ends (epiphyses)
  - Function as levers
  - Example—humerus and fibula
- Short
  - Short and relatively symmetrical
  - No diaphysis
  - Example—carpals and tarsals
- Flat
  - Flat or curved surface
  - Example—scapula and ilium
- Irregular
  - Irregular-shaped bones
  - Example—maxilla and vertebra
- Sesamoid
  - Round (sesame seed shaped)
  - Embedded within a tendon
  - Provide protection and leverage/mechanical advantage
  - Example—patella and sesamoid bones of great toe
- Wormian
  - Tiny bones found in the suture joints of the cranium

Quick fact
> Some sources classify sesamoid bones as being irregular, therefore not having a classification of its own.

Anatomy of Long Bones
- Diaphysis (shaft) (see Fig. 1.2)
  - Cylinder shaped
  - Wall (cortex) is composed of cortical (compact) bone tissue
  - Inner surface is lined with cancellous (spongy or trabecular) bone
  - Contains the medullary (marrow) cavity
- Epiphyseal (growth) plates
  - Cartilaginous
  - Separate epiphysis and diaphysis early in life
  - Both ends of the bone grow from this plate
  - Replaced by bone ("close") as skeleton matures
  - Some do not completely "close" until age 25
- Epiphyses
  - Proximal and distal ends of a long bone
  - Composed primarily of cancellous (spongy or trabecular) bone that is surrounded by a layer of cortical bone
  - Wider surface area increases joint stability
  - Articular (hyaline) cartilage covers the articular surface of the epiphyses
- Articular (hyaline) cartilage
  - Covers articular surfaces of bones
  - Protects from joint "wear and tear"
  - Provides shock absorption
  - Poor blood supply
- Periosteum
  - Fibrous membrane that surrounds the diaphysis
  - Attachment site for tendons and ligaments
  - Contains bone forming/repairing cells and blood vessels
- Endosteum
  - Fibrous membrane that lines the walls of the medullary (marrow) cavity
  - Contains bone forming/repairing cells
- Medullary (marrow) cavity
  - Tube-like space located within the diaphysis
  - Contains bone marrow

Quick fact
> The epiphyses bones articulate with each other to form joints.

Skeleton Formation
- Skeletal formation
  - Endochondral ossification
  - Intramembranous ossification
- Endochondral ossification
  - Develops from hyaline cartilage
  - Most common
- Intramembranous ossification
  - Occurs within a membrane
  - Example—flat bones of the cranium

Bone Tissue
- Composed of bone cells and matrix
- Types of bone cells
  - Osteoblasts—build bone tissue
  - Osteoclasts—breakdown or resorb bone tissue
  - Osteocytes—located within lacunae (small cavities within a bone)

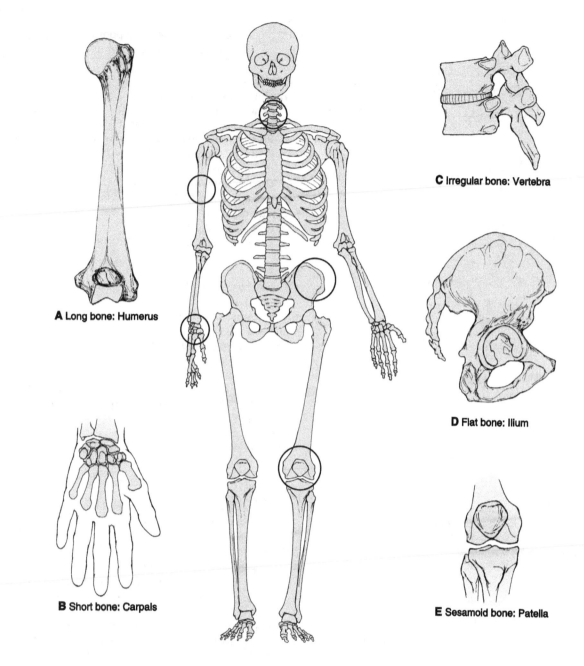

A Long bone: Humerus

B Short bone: Carpals

C Irregular bone: Vertebra

D Flat bone: Ilium

E Sesamoid bone: Patella

Figure 1.1 Bone Classification by Shape. (From Premkumar K. *The massage connection anatomy and physiology*. Baltimore: Lippincott Williams & Wilkins; 2004.)

- Types of matrix
  - Organic matrix—composed primarily of collagen fibers
  - Inorganic matrix—composed primarily of mineral salts and calcium

Types of Bone Tissue

- Cortical (compact) bone
  - Ordered and dense arrangement
  - Found primarily in shaft of long bones
  - Osteon—structural unit of compact bone

- Cancellous (trabecular or spongy) bone
  - Irregular and sponge-like arrangement
  - Found primarily in epiphyses of long bones
  - Trabeculae—form the "latticework" of spongy bone

Quick fact Osteons contain a Haversian canal, in which a blood vessel is located.

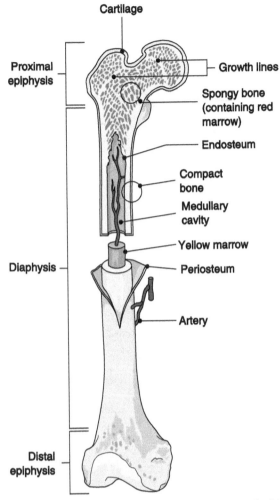

Figure 1.2 Anatomy of a Long Bone. (Reprinted with permission from Cohen BJ, Wood DL. *Memmler's the human body in health and disease*, 9th ed. Philadelphia: Lippincott Williams & Wilkins; 2000.)

Principles of Physical Stress on Bone

- The Wolff law—bone responds to the physical demands that are placed on it
  - Increased stress → greater bone mass
  - Decreased stress → lesser bone mass
  - Excessive stress → bone pathology (i.e., stress fracture)

Cartilage

- Connective tissue
- Composed of cartilage cells and matrix
- Cartilage cells
  - Chondroblasts—cartilage "builders"
  - Chondrocytes—mature chondroblasts
- Cartilage matrix
  - Collagen (provides tensile strength) and elastin (provides elasticity)
  - Ground substance (proteoglycans—glucosamine and chondroitin sulfate)

> **Quick fact** Cartilage tissue has a poor blood supply, and therefore it does not heal well.

Cartilage Types

- Hyaline (articular) cartilage
  - Articular surfaces of bones
  - Allows for smooth movement
  - Protects from joint "wear and tear"
  - Provides shock absorption
- Fibrocartilage
  - Greater amount of collagen fibers
  - Example—interpubic disc and menisci
- Elastic cartilage
  - Collagen and elastin fibers
  - Example—epiglottis and outer ear

Menisci

- Crescent-shaped fibrocartilage (semilunar cartilage) (see Fig. 1.3)
- The medial and lateral menisci are located on the tibial plateau
- The inner edges are thinner than the outer edges
- The outer edges are connected to the tibial plateau via the coronary ligaments
- Vacularity declines as you move toward inner edges
- Medial meniscus is attached to the medial collateral ligament (MCL)
- Increase area of articular surface
- Provide shock absorption and stability

> **Quick fact** The menisci are supplied by the genicular arteries around the knee.

Labrum

- A ring-shaped fibrocartilage
- Glenoid labrum—shoulder (attached to glenoid fossa)
- Long head of the biceps brachii tendon attaches to the superior portion of glenoid labrum
- Acetabular labrum—hip (attached to acetabulum)
- Deepens articular surface of glenohumeral joint
- Provides shock absorption and stability

Articular Discs

- Disc-shaped fibrocartilage
- Increase area of articular surface
- Provide shock absorption and stability
- Example—pubic symphysis and sternoclavicular joint

Ligaments

- Dense fibrous connective tissue
- Composed primarily of collagen with some elastin fibers
- Strong tensile strength
- Connect bone to bone
- Facilitate or limit movement
- Provide static joint stability
- Intracapsular ligaments—located inside of joint capsule

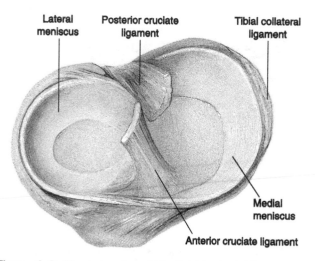

Figure 1.3 The Lateral and Medial Menisci. (Asset provided by Anatomical Chart Co.)

- Extracapsular ligaments—located outside of joint capsule
- Poor blood supply
- Example—MCL and acromioclavicular (AC) ligament

Quick fact Ligaments may blend in with the fibrous capsule of a joint.

Joint Capsules

- Surround synovial joints
- Two layers
  - Fibrous—outer layer
  - Synovial membrane—inner layer that secretes synovial fluid
- Example—glenohumeral joint capsule

Bursae

- Synovial fluid-filled sacs (see Fig. 1.4)
- Commonly found between tendon and bone or skin and bone
- Cushion and reduce friction
- Example—olecranon bursa and prepatellar bursa

Tendons

- Dense fibrous connective tissue
- Cord-like shape
- Primarily composed of collagen with some elastin fibers

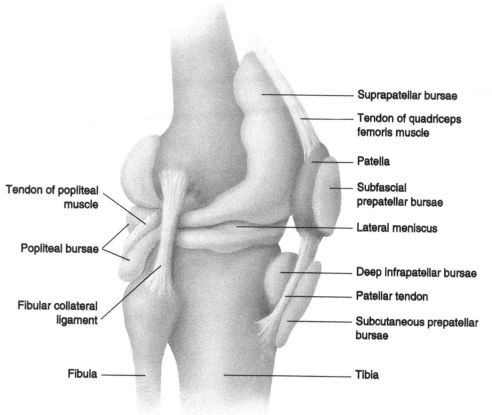

Figure 1.4 Bursae of the Knee. (Asset provided by Anatomical Chart Co.)

- Strong tensile strength
- Connect muscle to bone
- Transmit force from muscle to bone to create movement
- Surrounded by peritendinous or synovial tendon sheath
- Bound down by sheets retinaculum (e.g., superior peroneal retinaculum)
- Poor blood supply

> **Quick fact** Tendons are attached to bone by structures known as *Sharpey fibers*.

Properties of Skeletal Connective Tissues

- Excitability (irritability)—responsive to mechanical, electrical, or chemical stimuli
- Contractility—develops tension (unique to muscular tissue)
- Extensibility (stretch)—lengthen
- Elasticity (viscoelasticity)—returns to resting length after being stretched
- Plasticity (viscoplasticity)—shape can change, and then retain original shape
- Creep—gradual change in tissue shape when a slow and sustained force is applied
- Tensile strength—able to withstand tension forces
- Weight bearing—sustains compressive forces due to body weight

Types of Muscle Tissue

- Skeletal (striated) (see Fig. 1.5)
  - Voluntary
  - Comprises skeletal muscle
- Cardiac
  - Involuntary
  - Comprises the heart
- Smooth
  - Involuntary
  - Comprises the walls of blood vessels and hollow organs

Skeletal Muscle Tissue

- Voluntary
- Striated appearance
  - Alternating A bands (dark) and I bands (light)
- Contains two types of tissue—(a) skeletal muscle tissue and (b) fibrous fascia
- Skeletal muscle tissue
  - Skeletal muscle (fibers) cells—primary structural and functional units
- Fibrous fascia
  - Surrounds the entire muscle
  - Continues to form tendons

> **Quick fact** Skeletal muscle tissue may be named by its characteristics (i.e., shape, size, and fiber direction).

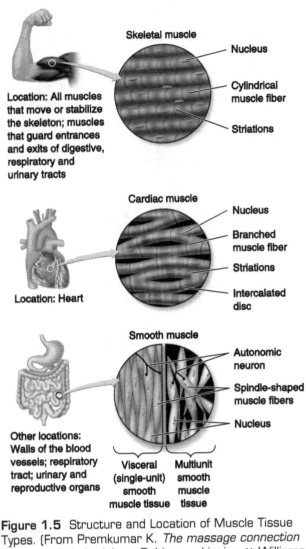

Figure 1.5 Structure and Location of Muscle Tissue Types. (From Premkumar K. *The massage connection anatomy and physiology*. Baltimore: Lippincott Williams & Wilkins; 2004.)

Forms of Skeletal Muscle

- Parallel (Longitudinal) muscles
  - Fibers arranged in parallel manner
- Pennate muscles
  - Fibers arranged in oblique manner from a central tendon

Parallel (Longitudinal) Muscles

- Flat (see Fig. 1.6)
  - Thin and broad
  - Example—rectus abdominis
- Fusiform (spindle)
  - Spindle shaped
  - Example—brachioradialis
- Triangular (radiate)
  - Fan shaped
  - Example—trapezius
- Strap
  - Long parallel manner
  - Example—sartorius

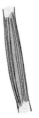

Parallel

Figure 1.6 Parallel (Longitudinal) Muscle. (Adapted from Premkumar K. *The massage connection anatomy and physiology*. Baltimore: Lippincott Williams & Wilkins; 2004.)

- Sphincter (circular)
  ○ Around a body opening
  ○ Example—orbicularis occuli
- Spiral
  ○ Arranged around long axis
  ○ Example—latissimus dorsi

Pennate Muscles
- Unipennate (see Fig. 1.7)
  ○ Diagonally arranged fibers from a central tendon on one side only
  ○ Example—brachialis
- Bipennate
  ○ Diagonally arranged fibers from a central tendon on both sides
  ○ Example—biceps femoris
- Multipennate
  ○ Diagonally arranged fibers from multiple tendons
  ○ Example—deltoid

Structure of Skeletal Muscle

Skeletal Muscle (Cells) Fibers
- Cylindrical shape (see Figs. 1.8 and 1.9)
- Multinucleate

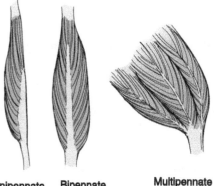

Unipennate   Bipennate   Multipennate

Figure 1.7 Types of Pennate Muscles. (Adapted from Premkumar K. *The massage connection anatomy and physiology*. Baltimore: Lippincott Williams & Wilkins; 2004.)

- Rich in mitochondria
- Contain myoglobin (oxygen-binding molecule)
- Comprise multiple muscle fibers (arrangement varies)

 Use the DVD or visit the website at http://thePoint.lww.com/Long for additional material about *skeletal muscle (cells) fibers.*

Primary Types of Skeletal Muscle Fibers
- Type I (slow twitch)
  ○ Slow oxidative
  ○ Small in diameter
  ○ Red in color
  ○ High myoglobin content
  ○ Slow speed of contraction
  ○ Slow rate of fatigue
- Type IIA (intermediate)
  ○ Fast oxidative glycolytic
  ○ Intermediate in diameter
  ○ Red in color
  ○ Intermediate myoglobin content
  ○ Fast speed of contraction
  ○ Intermediate rate of fatigue
- Type IIB (fast twitch)
  ○ Fast glycolytic
  ○ Large in diameter
  ○ White in color
  ○ Low myoglobin content
  ○ Fast speed of contraction
  ○ Fast rate of fatigue

Roles of Muscles
- Agonist
  ○ Muscle that contracts
- Antagonist
  ○ Action opposite of agonist
  ○ Muscle that lengthens
- Synergist
  ○ Assists agonist
  ○ Increases movement efficiency
  ○ Prevents unnessary movement
- Fixators
  ○ Stops unwanted action at fixed attachment point of a muscle
- Neutralizers
  ○ Stops unwanted action at mobile attachment point of a muscle

Muscle Contractions (Actions)
- Contraction (action)—development of muscle tension
- Roles of muscle contractions
- Primary types of muscle contractions—(a) isometric and (b) isotonic
  ○ Isometric (static) contraction—tension is developed within a muscle, but no joint movement occurs
  ○ Isotonic (dynamic) contraction—tension is developed within a muscle that causes or controls movement of a joint

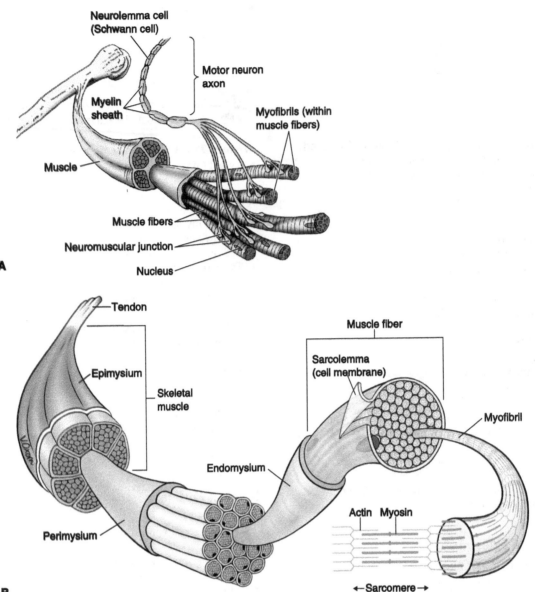

Figure 1.8 Structure of Skeletal Muscle. **A:** Motor Unit. **B:** Muscle Components. (From Moore KL, Agur A. *Essential clinical anatomy*, 2nd ed. Philadelphia: Lippincott Williams & Wilkins; 2002.)

- Types of isotonic muscle contractions
  - Concentric (positive) contraction—tension is developed as muscle lengthens
  - Eccentric (negative) contraction—tension is developed as muscle shortens

> **Quick fact** Muscle contractions cause, control, and prevent joint movements.

> **Quick fact** An agonist muscle is also known as a *mover*.

Sliding Filament (Mechanism) Theory

- Physiological process of sarcomere shortening (muscle contraction) (see Fig. 1.10)
- Energy source = adenosine triphosphate (ATP)
- Sliding filament mechanism process
  - Action potential (AP) to muscle
  - Sarcoplasmic reticulum releases calcium ions into the sarcoplasm
  - Calcium ions attach to troponin molecules of actin filaments
  - Troponin moves tropomyosin out of the way, which exposes actin-binding sites
  - Myosin heads attach to actin-binding sites that create cross bridges between myosin and actin

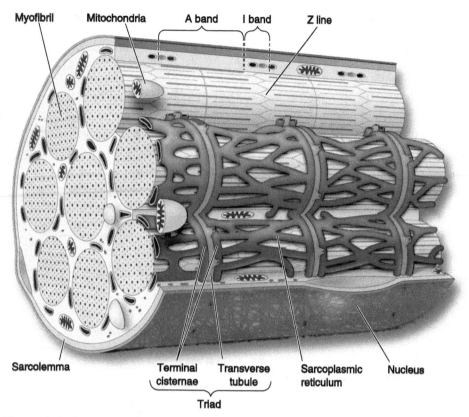

Figure 1.9 Structure of a Skeletal Muscle Fiber. (From McArdle WD, Katch FI, Katch VL. *Essentials of exercise physiology*, 2nd ed. Baltimore: Lippincott Williams & Wilkins; 2000.)

- Each myosin cross bridge pulls actin toward the center of the sarcomere
- Cross bridges break
- Then reattach and continue as APs dictate

Quick **fact** The sliding filament (mechanism) theory is also known as the *ratchet theory*.

INTEGUMENTARY (SKIN) SYSTEM

Integumentary System Components
- Skin
- Blood vessels
- Nerves
- Glands
- Sensory organs
- Hair
- Nails

Skin Functions
- Prevents dehydration
- Prevents infection
- Regulates body temperature
- Provides sensory information

- Absorbs substances for example, medications
- Manufacture vitamin D
- Excretion (e.g., electrolytes)

Skin Structure
- Epidermis (see Fig. 1.11)
- Dermis
- Subcutaneous (hypodermis)
- Accessory structures
  - Sebaceous (oil) glands
  - Meibomian (tarsal) glands
  - Sudoriferous (sweat) glands
  - Hair
  - Nails

Quick **fact** Meibomian glands are a type of sebaceous gland that are found at the eyelids.

Epidermis
- Outermost portion
- Epithelial cells
- Epidermal cells cytoplasm replaced with keratin
- No blood vessels
- Nourished by capillaries in the dermis
- Layers of epidermis

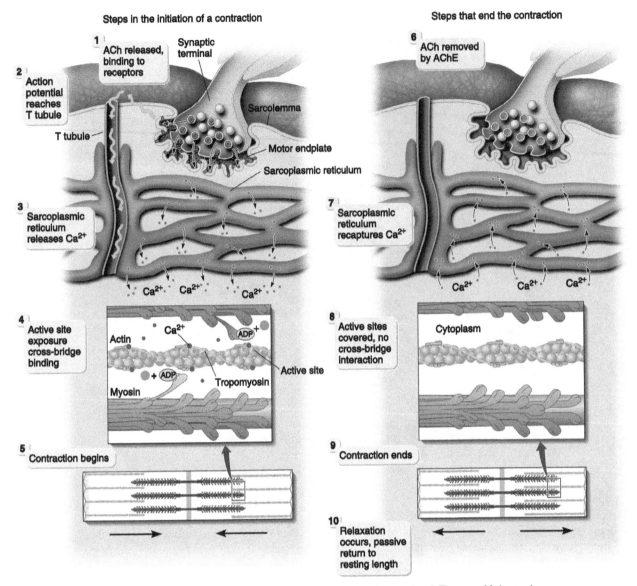

Figure 1.10 The Process of the Sliding Filament (Mechanism) Theory. (Adapted from Premkumar K. *The massage connection anatomy and physiology*. Baltimore: Lippincott Williams & Wilkins; 2004.)

- ○ Stratum basale (stratum germinativum)—closest to the dermis (produces new epidermal cells)
- ○ Stratum corneum—outer layer of epidermis
- ○ Stratum lucidum—found in thick skin (another layer that resists abrasion)

Dermis
- • "True skin"
- • Under the epidermis
- • Ability to stretch extensively
- • Composition
  - ○ Elastic connective tissue
  - ○ Blood vessels
  - ○ Nerves
- • Accessory structures found in this layer
- • Dermal papillae—areas where dermis projects toward surface of epidermis (finger and foot prints)

Subcutaneous Layer (Hypodermis)
- • Below the dermis
- • Connects skin to the superficial muscles
- • Composition
  - ○ Adipose tissue
  - ○ Loose connective tissue
  - ○ Blood vessels
  - ○ Nerves
  - ○ Nerve endings

Accessory Integumentary Structures
- • Sebaceous (oil) glands
  - ○ Sac-like structures
  - ○ Open to hair follicles
  - ○ Used for lubrication of skin/hair (prevents dryness)
  - ○ Meibomian glands—lubricate eyes

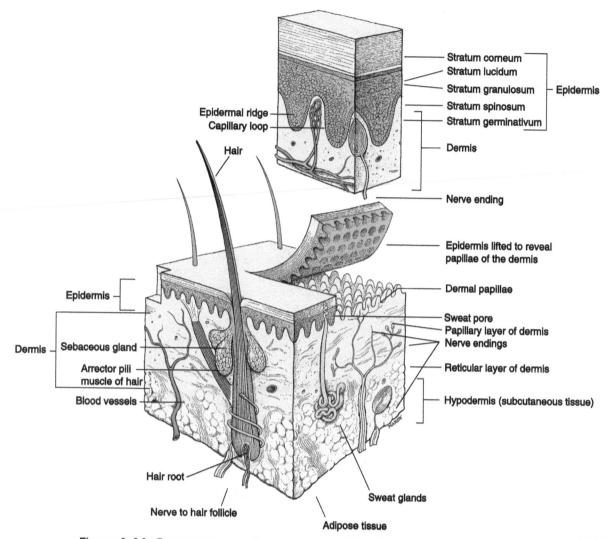

Figure 1.11 Components and Structure of the Skin. (From *Stedman's Medical Dictionary*, 27th ed. Baltimore: Lippincott Williams & Wilkins; 2000.)

- ○ Sebaceous cysts—blocked sebaceous gland with associated sebum accumulation
- Sudoriferous (sweat) glands
  - ○ Function to cool the body
  - ○ Two primary types of sweat glands—
    (a) eccrine—secretes sweat and
    (b) apocrine—axillae and groin (small number of sweat glands)
  - ○ Modified sweat glands—(a) mammary glands,
    (b) ceruminous glands (produce ear wax), and
    (c) ciliary glands (eyelids)
- Hair
  - ○ Hair follicle—epithelial cells and connective tissue that encloses hair
  - ○ Hair is not living (mostly keratin)
  - ○ Melanocytes—pigments that color hair
  - ○ Hair root—portion of hair below the skin
  - ○ Erector (arrector) pili—thin band of involuntary muscle
- Nails
  - ○ Hard keratin produced in stratum corneum

- ○ Nail root—proximal end of nail
- ○ Nail matrix—nail growth region
- ○ Lunala ("little moon")—proximal nail over thickest portion of growth region
- ○ Cuticle—seals space between skin and nail plate

Determining Skin Color

- Pigmentation (melanin production)
- Quality of circulating blood
- Substances in the blood

 Quick fact Melanocytes produce melanin, which determine skin color.

Quick fact Erector pili are the structures responsible for causing "goose bumps."

Quick fact Blackheads are a combination of keratin and dried sebum.

NEUROLOGIC SYSTEM

Structural Divisions of the Nervous System

- Central nervous system (CNS)—brain and spinal cord
- Peripheral nervous system (PNS)—all nerves outside CNS

Functional Divisions of the Nervous System

- Somatic nervous system
- Autonomic nervous system (ANS)

Somatic Nervous System

- Voluntary
- Effector—skeletal muscle
- Motor nerve travels from spinal cord to skeletal muscle

Autonomic Nervous System

- Involuntary
- Effector—glands, cardiac muscle, and smooth muscle
- Subdivisions
  - Sympathetic nervous system
  - Parasympathetic nervous system

Neuron Structure

- Dendrites (see Fig. 1.12)
  - "Tree-like" appearance
  - Impulse to cell body
  - Receptors receive stimulus
- Axon
  - Impulse away from cell body
  - Single fiber with end branches
- Myelin sheath
  - Insulation around some nerves
  - Produced by Schwann cells in the PNS
  - Fatty material
  - Speeds up conduction of APs

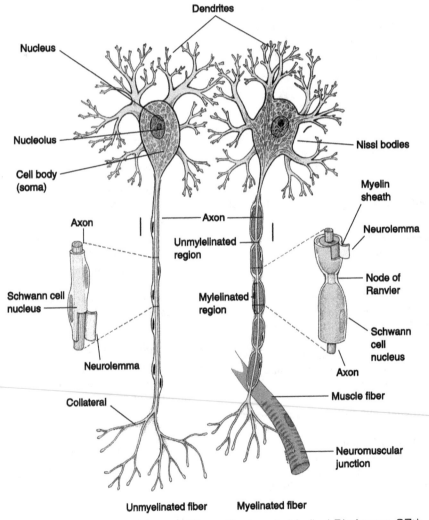

Figure 1.12 Structure of a Neuron. (From *Stedman's Medical Dictionary*, 27th ed. Baltimore: Lippincott Williams & Wilkins; 2000.)

- ○ AP jumps from node to node instead of traveling entire nerve length
  - ○ Small spaces (nodes of Ranvier)
- Neurilemma
  - ○ Outer membranes of Schwann cells
  - ○ Not found in CNS cells

> **Quick fact** Myelin sheath is also known as *white color, white matter,* or *white fiber.*

Types of Neurons
- Afferent (sensory) neurons—toward CNS
- Efferent (motor) neurons—away from CNS
- Interneurons (central or association neurons)—within CNS

Neuroglia
- *Glial* cells
- Found in CNS and PNS
- Nonconducting cells
- Multiply throughout life
- Specialized functions
  - ○ Help repair cells
  - ○ Protect the nervous systems
  - ○ Phagocytes
  - ○ Regulate fluid composition around the cells
  - ○ Scaffolding or support system for the nervous system
- Schwann cells—example of neuroglia in the PNS
- Astrocytes—example of neuroglia in CNS
- Brain tumors are usually caused by neuroglia

> **Quick fact** *Glial* is a Greek term meaning glue.

Neuroglia of the Central Nervous System
- Astrocytes (macroglia)
  - ○ Star shaped
  - ○ Twist around nerve cells to support CNS
  - ○ Attach neurons to capillaries
  - ○ Protect brain from harm
- Microglia
  - ○ Small in size
  - ○ Grow from monocytes
  - ○ Act as brain macrophages
  - ○ Engulf and destroy pathogens
- Oligodendrocytes (oligodendroglia)
  - ○ Produce myelin sheath around CNS axons
  - ○ Provide support in CNS

> **Quick fact** Oligodendrocytes are similar in shape to astrocytes except that they have fewer and shorter projections.

Nerve Impulse
- Resting potential—ionic charge along the plasma membrane of an unstimulated nerve
  - ○ Inside membrane—resting potential is negative
  - ○ Outside membrane—resting potential is positive
- Nerve impulse—reverses membrane potential because of reversal of ion concentrations
- AP—sudden electrical change in ion concentrations of a nerve
  - ○ AP = nerve impulse = salutatory conduction
- Resting state—more Na^+ outside and more K^+ inside
- Depolarization—energy allows diffusion of Na^+ into cell membrane; increases charge inside to more positive
  - ○ Electrical
  - ○ Chemical
  - ○ Mechanical
- Repolarization—membrane electrical charge returns to resting potential
  - ○ K^+ channels open causing K^+ to leave the cell
  - ○ Simultaneously, cell uses active transport to move Na^+ and K^+ back to original concentrations called *Na^+/K^+ pump*

Types of Synapses
- Chemical (gap) synapse (see Fig. 1.13)
  - ○ Axon of presynaptic cell to dendrite of postsynaptic cell
  - ○ Axon stores neurotransmitters in end bulbs
  - ○ AP causes end bulbs to fuse with dendrite and release neurotransmitters into synaptic cleft
  - ○ Neurotransmitter acts as a chemical signal generating AP of postsynaptic cell
- Electrical synapse
  - ○ CNS, cardiac, and smooth muscle
  - ○ The membranes of presynaptic and postsynaptic cells are close enough for electrical charge to spread

Neurotransmitters
- Stimulate or inhibit postsynaptic cells
- Most common neurotransmitters
  - ○ Epinephrine (adrenaline)
  - ○ Norepinephrine (noradrenaline)
  - ○ Acetylcholine (ACh)—neuromuscular junction

 Use the DVD or visit the website at http://thePoint.lww.com/Long for additional material about *neurotransmitters*.

Spinal Cord
- Ends between L1 and L2 vertebrae (adults) (see Fig. 1.14)
- *Cauda equina*
- Gray matter—unmyelinated tissue
- White matter—myelinated tissue
- White matter surrounds gray matter
- Gray commissure—bridge right and left horns
- Central canal—center of gray commissure containing cerebrospinal fluid (CSF)

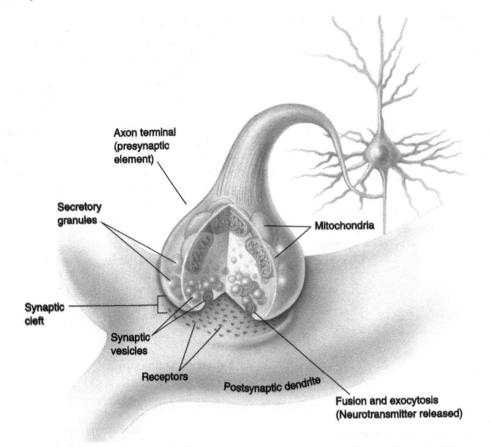

Figure 1.13 Structure of a Chemical (Gap) Synapse. (From Bear M, Connor B, Paradiso M. *Neuroscience: Exploring the brain*, 2nd ed. Baltimore: Lippincott Williams & Wilkins; 2000.)

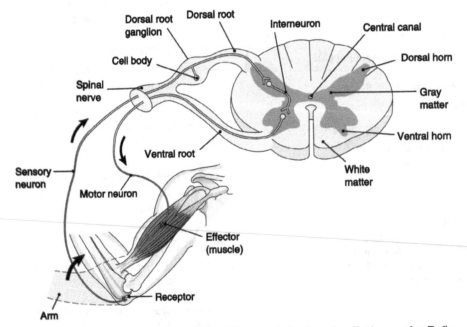

Figure 1.14 Cross Section of the Spinal Cord and the Impulse Pathway of a Reflex Arc. (From Cohen BJ. *Medical terminology*, 4th ed. Philadelphia: Lippincott Williams & Wilkins; 2003.)

- Ascending tracts—afferent (sensory)
  - White matter tracts carrying information toward the brain
- Descending tracts—efferent (motor)
  - Carry information toward the PNS
- Sensory information enters CNS through dorsal horn
- Motor information leaves CNS through ventral horn

> **Quick fact**
> Gray matter looks like the letter H or a butterfly because of the shape of the dorsal and ventral horns.

Reflex Arc

- Receptor—detects stimulus
- Afferent neuron—transmits impulse toward CNS
- CNS—interprets and organizes response
- Efferent neuron—transmits impulse from CNS to PNS
- Effector—response unit (muscle or gland)

Simplest Reflex

- Stretch reflex and spinal reflex (e.g., knee jerk reflex)
- Does not involve brain, therefore termed *spinal reflex*
- Predictable and reliable assessment of nervous system function
- 1. Receptor → 2. Sensory neuron → 3. Dorsal horn → 4. Interneuron → 5. Ventral horn → 6. Motor neuron → 7. Effector

Spinal Nerves

- 31 pairs
- Attached to spinal cord by two roots
  - Dorsal root—sensory
  - Ventral root—motor
- Dorsal root has ganglion—sensory gray matter outside CNS
- All spinal nerves are mixed (sensory and motor)

Primary Plexuses in the Body (Four)

- Cervical plexus
- Brachial plexus
- Lumbar plexus
- Sacral plexus

Cervical Plexus

- Sensory impulses from neck and back of head
- Motor impulses to muscles of the neck
- C1-4 with some C5 contribution
- Contains cranial nerves XI and XII
- Superficial nerve branches
  - Lesser occipital (C2-3)
  - Greater auricular (C2-3)
  - Transverse cervical (C2-3)
  - Supraclavicular (C3-4)
- Deep nerve branches
  - Ansa cervicalis—inferior/superior root (C1-4)
  - Phrenic nerve innervates the diaphragm (C3-5)
  - Segmental branches (C1-5)

Brachial Plexus

- Upper extremity and shoulder region
- Nerve roots → trunks → divisions → peripheral nerve
- C5-T1 with some distribution from C4 to T2
- C5-6 → superior trunk
- C7 → middle trunk
- C8-T1 → inferior trunk
- Each trunk turns into an anterior and posterior division
- Divisions unite to form cords
- Posterior cord → posterior divisions of the superior, middle, and inferior trunks
- Medial cord → anterior division of the inferior trunk
- Lateral cord → anterior divisions of the superior and middle trunk
- Root nerves
  - Dorsal scapular (C5)
  - Long thoracic (C5-7)
- Trunk nerves
  - Subclavius (C5-6)
  - Suprascapular (C5-6)
- Posterior cord nerves
  - Upper subscapular (C5-6)
  - Thoracodorsal (C6-8)
  - Lower subscapular (C5-6)
  - Axillary (C5-6)
  - Radial (C5-T1)
- Medial cord nerves
  - Medial pectoral (C8-T1)
  - Medial brachial cutaneous (C8-T1)
  - Medial antebrachial cutaneous (C8-T1)
  - Median (middle head) (C5-T1)
  - Ulnar (C8-T1)
- Lateral cord nerves
  - Musculocutaneous (C5-7)
  - Median (lateral head) (C5-7)
  - Lateral pectoral (C5-7)

Lumbar Plexus

- Supplies anterolateral abdominal wall, external genitalia, and part of the lower extremity
- L1-4
- Roots → anterior and posterior divisions
- Anterior division nerves
  - Ilioinguinal (L1)
  - Genitofemoral (L1-2)
  - Obtrurator (L2-4)
- Posterior division nerves
  - Iliohypogastric (T12-L1)
  - Lateral femoral cutaneous (L2-3)
  - Femoral (L2-4)

Sacral Plexus

- Supplies buttocks, perineum, and lower extremity
- L4-S4
- Roots → anterior and posterior divisions
- Sciatic nerve—largest nerve in the body arising from sacral plexus
- Anterior division nerves
  - Nerve to quadratus femoris and inferior gemellus (L4-S1)
  - Nerve to obturator internus and superior gemellus (L5-S2)

- ◦ Perforating cutaneous (S2-3)
- ◦ Tibial (L4-S3)
- ◦ Pudendal (S2-4)
- Posterior division nerves
  - ◦ Superior gluteal (L4-S1)
  - ◦ Inferior gluteal (L5-S2)
  - ◦ Piriformis (S1-2)
  - ◦ Posterior cutaneous (S1-3)
  - ◦ Common peroneal (L4-S2)

Autonomic Nervous System

- Regulates actions of glands, smooth muscles of hollow organs and vessels, and cardiac muscle
- Automatic—no conscious awareness
- ANS divisions
  - ◦ Sympathetic nervous system
  - ◦ Parasympathetic nervous system

Use the DVD or visit the website at http://thePoint.lww.com/Long for additional material about the *autonomic nervous system*.

Quick fact The autonomic nervous system is also known as the *visceral system*.

Sympathetic Nervous System

- Fight or flight stress response
- Thoracic and lumbar spinal areas (T1-L2)
- Adrenergic actions—activated by adrenaline
- Mostly uses epinephrine and norepinephrine as neurotransmitter
- Sympathetic chains
  - ◦ Two cord-like strands of ganglia
  - ◦ Both sides of spinal column
  - ◦ Lower neck to upper abdomen
- Acts as an accelerator of organ function
- Fight or flight response
  - ◦ Increases rate and force of heart contractions
  - ◦ Increases blood pressure (BP)
  - ◦ Increases basal metabolic rate (BMR)
  - ◦ Decreases urinary and digestive systems
  - ◦ Dilates pupils, bronchial tubes, and skeletal blood vessels

Use the DVD or visit the website at http://thePoint.lww.com/Long for additional materials about *sympathetic nervous system*.

Parasympathetic Nervous System

- Reverses the fight or flight stress response
- Craniosacral region—brainstem (midbrain and medulla) and sacrum
- Cholinergic actions—activated by ACh
- Acts as a depressor or decelerator of organ functions

Table 1.1 Cranial Nerve Function

Name	Type	Function
I. Olfactory	Sensory	Smell
II. Optic	Sensory	Vision
III. Oculomotor	Motor	Effect on pupillary reaction and size Elevation of upper eyelid Eye adduction and downward rolling
IV. Trochlear	Motor	Upward eye rolling
V. Trigeminal	Mixed	Sensory: sensation of nose, forehead, temple, scalp, lips, tongue, and lower jaw Motor: muscles of mastication
VI. Abducens	Motor	Lateral eye movement
VII. Facial	Mixed	Sensory: taste Motor: muscles of expression
VIII. Vestibulocochlear (Acoustic or Auditory)	Sensory	Hearing and equilibrium
IX. Glossopharyngeal	Mixed	Sensory: taste Motor: pharyngeal muscles
X. Vagus	Mixed	Sensory: gag reflex Motor: muscles of pharynx and larynx
XI. Accessory	Motor	Trapezius and sternocleidomastoid muscles
XII. Hypoglossal	Motor	Tongue movement

Cranial Nerves

- 12 pairs identified as Roman numerals I to XII (see Table 1.1)
- Named for position anterior to posterior
- Cranial nerves III to XII arise from brainstem
- Four categories of cranial nerve information
  - ◦ Special sensory impulses—smell, taste, hearing, and vision
  - ◦ General sensory impulses—pain, touch, temperature, pressure, vibration, and deep muscle sensation
  - ◦ Somatic motor impulses—voluntary control of skeletal muscles
  - ◦ Visceral motor impulses—involuntary control of cardiac/smooth muscle, glands, and parasympathetic system

BRAIN

Neural Tube Forms Brain

- Prosencephalon (forebrain)
  - ◦ Telencephalon—cerebral hemispheres
  - ◦ Diencephalon—thalamus and hypothalamus
- Mesencephalon (midbrain)
- Rhombencephalon (hindbrain)
  - ◦ Metencephalon—pons and cerebellum
  - ◦ Myelencephalon—medulla oblongata

Areas of the Brain

- Cerebrum (see Fig. 1.15)
- Diencephalon
- Brainstem
- Cerebellum

Cerebrum

- Five paired lobes
- Largest portion
- Two convoluted hemispheres
- Corpus callosum connects right and left hemispheres
- Cerebral cortex—outer layer

> **Quick fact** The cerebrum accounts for 80% of the brain's mass.

Diencephalon

- Between cerebrum and brainstem
- Thalamus and hypothalamus
- Thalamus sorts and redirects sensory inputs
- Hypothalamus is responsible for homeostasis, ANS control, and pituitary gland control

Brainstem

- Below the cerebrum
- Connects cerebrum with spinal cord and diencephalon
- Three parts of the brainstem
  - Midbrain
    - Vision and hearing
    - Connects lower portion of brain to cerebrum
    - Cranial nerves III and IV originate
  - Pons
    - Helps regulate respiration
    - Mostly myelinated nerves
    - Bridges cerebrum, cerebellum, and brainstem
    - Cranial nerves V to VIII originate
  - Medulla oblongata
    - Connects brain with spinal cord
    - Controls vital functions (e.g., heart beat, respiration)
    - Highly myelinated
    - Motor fibers decussate
    - Three centers
      - Respiratory
      - Cardiac
      - Vasomotor
    - Cranial nerves IX to XII originate

Cerebellum

- Coordinates voluntary muscles
- Balance and muscle tone maintenance
- Outer covering—gray matter
- Inner area—white matter

> **Quick fact** The cerebellum is also known as the *little brain*.

Lobes of the Cerebrum (Five)

- Frontal lobe
  - Primary motor control area
  - Speech centers (written and motor)
  - Conscious control of skeletal muscle
- Parietal lobe
  - Primary sensory area
  - Somatesthetic sensation—sensation arising from cutaneous, muscle, tendon, and joint receptors
  - Temperature interpretion
  - Distance, size, and shape interpretation
- Temporal lobe
  - Auditory centers including interpretation and association of auditory information
  - Olfactory area
- Occipital lobe
  - Vision and coordination of eye movements
  - Visual receiving and association areas
  - Read with understanding
- Insula
  - Memory
  - Integration of other cerebral activities
  - Deep within each hemisphere

Basal Nuclei (Basal Ganglia)

- Masses of gray matter composed of neuron cell bodies
- Located deep within the white matter of the cerebrum
- Function to control voluntary movements
- Secrete dopamine

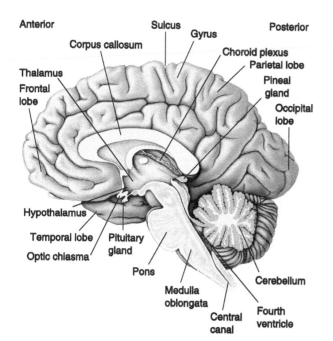

Anterior • Sulcus • Gyrus • Posterior
Corpus callosum • Choroid plexus • Parietal lobe
Thalamus • Pineal gland
Frontal lobe • Occipital lobe
Hypothalamus
Temporal lobe • Pituitary gland
Optic chiasma
Pons
Medulla oblongata
Central canal • Fourth ventricle • Cerebellum

Figure 1.15 Areas of the Brain. (From Bear M, Connor B, Paradiso M. *Neuroscience: Exploring the brain*, 2nd ed. Baltimore: Lippincott Williams & Wilkins; 2000.)

Cerebral Cortex

- Outer 2 to 4 mm covering of the cerebrum
- Conscious thought, memory, reasoning, and abstract mental functions
- Thought processes (e.g., association, judgment, and discrimination)
- Voluntary actions
- Gray matter with underlying white matter
- Folds and grooves are called *convolutions*
- Elevated folds are called *gyri*
- Depressed grooves are called *sulci*
- Left hemisphere of the cerebral cortex is the language area
  - Broca area
    - Frontal lobe
    - Motor aphasia
  - Wernicke area
    - Speech comprehension center
    - Found in temporal lobe

> **Quick fact** People with Broca aphasia comprehend speech perfectly but cannot speak unimpaired.

> **Quick fact** Persons with Wernicke aphasia speak perfectly but are unable to comprehend speech.

Corpus Callosum

- Band of white matter
- Bridge permitting impulses to cross between cerebral hemispheres

Cerebrospinal Fluid

- Formed in the ventricles of the brain
- Supports nervous tissue
- Shock absorber
- Carries nutrients and waste
- Arachnoid villi in dural sinuses

> **Quick fact** Cerebrospinal fluid returns to the blood through the dural sinuses in subarachnoid space.

Limbic System

- Part of the brain that controls the emotional state (with the hypothalamus)
  - Fear, pleasure, aggression, feeding, sex, and goal-directed behavior
- Nuclei and fibers that form a ring around the brainstem
- Stimulates the reticular formation
- Hippocampus—long-term memory (LTM) and learning

> **Quick fact** The limbic system was once called the *rhinencephalon* or *smell brain* because of its olfactory processing.

Reticular Formation

- Network along brainstem
- Influences sleep and wakefulness

Meninges

- Dura mater (see Fig. 1.16)
  - Outermost layer

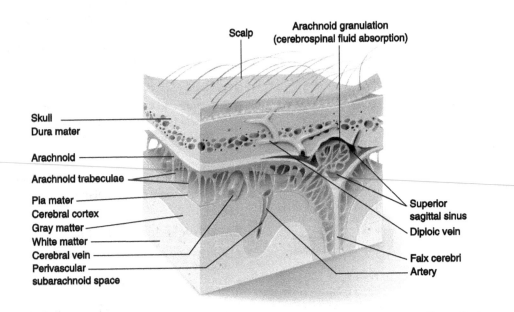

Figure 1.16 The Layers of the Meninges. (Asset provided by Anatomical Chart Co.)

- ○ Thickest and toughest
- ○ Two layers to this meninge
  - Outer layer to cranium
  - Some separation forming dural sinuses
- Arachnoid
  - ○ Middle layer
  - ○ Web-like
  - ○ Allows CSF to flow between dura and arachnoid
- Pia mater
  - ○ Innermost layer
  - ○ Attached to CNS nervous tissue
  - ○ Follows contours of CNS structures
  - ○ Holds blood vessels supplying oxygen and nutrition to CNS

Rhombencephalon

- Metencephalon—pons and cerebellum
  - ○ Pons—cranial nerves V, VI, VII, VIII, and respiratory centers
  - ○ Cerebellum—proprioceptors connect here
- Myelencephalon
  - ○ Medulla oblongata
  - ○ Cranial nerves—VIII, IX, X, XI, and XII
  - ○ Vital centers involved in regulation of breathing and cardiovascular responses

> **Quick fact** The rhombencephalon is also known as the *hindbrain*.

Thalamus

- Part of diencephalon
- Gray matter
- Sorts impulses and directs to appropriate areas in cerebral cortex

Hypothalamus

- Part of diencephalon
- Maintains homeostasis
- Controls body temperature
- Maintains water balance
- Controls sleep
- Controls appetite
- Controls emotions of fear and pleasure
- Controls pituitary gland
- Controls both portions of ANS
- Influences many major body functions

SENSES

Sensory Receptors

- Chemoreceptors—chemicals (e.g., taste, smell)
- Mechanoreceptors—movement
- Photoreceptors—light
- Thermoreceptors—temperature

General Senses

- Touch
- Pain
- Position
- Temperature
- Pressure

Special Senses

- Vision
- Hearing
- Taste
- Equilibrium
- Smell

Eyes

Eyeball Tunics (Three)

- Sclera (see Fig. 1.17)
  - ○ Outermost layer
  - ○ White of the eye (due to collagen)
  - ○ No blood vessels
- Choroid
  - ○ Middle layer
  - ○ Lots of blood vessels
  - ○ Delicate connective tissue
- Retina
  - ○ Innermost layer
  - ○ Receptor layer
  - ○ Contains rods and cones

> **Quick fact** The dark brown pigment of the choroid prevents the reflection of light.

Light and the Eye

- Cornea
  - ○ "Window" of the eye
  - ○ Main refracting structure
  - ○ No blood vessels
  - ○ Anterior continuation with sclera
- Aqueous humor
  - ○ Constantly produced and drained
  - ○ Fluid filling eyeball anterior to lens
  - ○ Gives eye forward curve
- Lens
  - ○ Elastic and firm
  - ○ Biconvex
  - ○ Thickness can be adjusted for far and near vision
- Vitreous body
  - ○ "Jelly-like" substance
  - ○ Fills posterior space
  - ○ Maintains eye shape

Retina

- Pigmented layer next to choroids
- Rods and cones (photoreceptors)
- Optic disc ("blind spot")—no rods and cones here
- Connecting neurons—carry impulses to optic nerve
- Optic nerve fibers

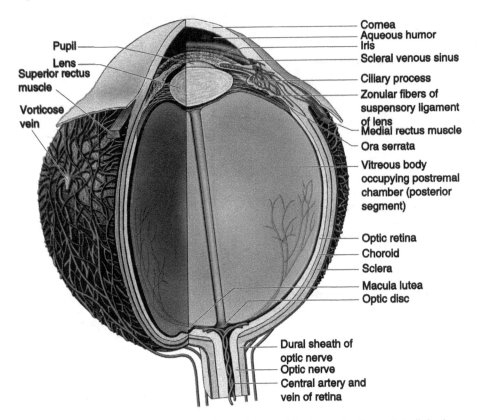

Pupil
Lens
Superior rectus muscle
Vorticose vein

Cornea
Aqueous humor
Iris
Scleral venous sinus
Ciliary process
Zonular fibers of suspensory ligament of lens
Medial rectus muscle
Ora serrata
Vitreous body occupying postremal chamber (posterior segment)
Optic retina
Choroid
Sclera
Macula lutea
Optic disc
Dural sheath of optic nerve
Optic nerve
Central artery and vein of retina

Figure 1.17 Structures of the Eye. (From Moore KL, Agur A. *Essential clinical anatomy*, 2nd ed. Philadelphia: Lippincott Williams & Wilkins; 2002.)

Rods
- Distributed around periphery of retina
- Active in dim light
- Visual acuity is low
- Cannot perceive color, only shades
- Vitamin A needed to manufacture a pigment to trigger rods

> **Quick fact** The deficiency of vitamin A can cause night blindness.

Cones
- Concentrated near the center of retina
- Active in bright light
- Visual acuity is high
- Perceive red, green, or blue
- Color blindness caused by malfunctioning cones

> **Quick fact** Color blindness occurs more frequently in males versus females.

Extrinsic Eye Muscles
- Originate on orbit and insert on the sclera
- Voluntary
- Contribute to convergence

- Extrinsic eye muscles (six)
  - Superior and inferior oblique
  - Superior and inferior rectus
  - Lateral and medial rectus

Intrinsic Eye Muscles
- Two circular structures within the eye
- Involuntary
- Iris
  - Colored part of the eye
  - Circular muscles—contract to constrict pupil in bright light
  - Radial muscles—contract in dim light to dilate pupil
- Ciliary muscle
  - Holds lens in place through suspensory ligaments
  - Controls the shape of the lens allowing for far/near vision
    - Contraction of ciliary muscle relaxes suspensory ligament and elastic lens thickens (see close)
    - Relaxation of ciliary muscle causes suspensory ligament tension; flattens lens (see far)

Accommodation for Near Vision
- Lens more rounded
- Light more focused on retina
- Controlled by ciliary muscle

Nerves of the Eye
- Sensory nerves
  - Optic nerve (CN II)
  - Trigeminal nerve (CN V)
- Motor nerves
  - Oculomotor nerve (CN III)—supplies all but two muscles
  - Trochlear nerve (CN IV)—supplies superior oblique muscle
  - Abducens nerve (CN VI)—supplies lateral rectus muscle

Steps in the Visual Process
- Light refracts
- Iris adjusts pupil
- Ciliary muscle adjusts lens
- Extrinsic muscles produce convergence
- Photoreceptors stimulated by light
- Optic nerve sends impulse to brain
- Occipital lobe cortex interprets optic nerve information

Ears

Sections of the Ear (Three)
- Outer ear (see Fig. 1.18)
  - Pinna (auricle)
    - External auditory (meatus) canal
    - Tympanic membrane (eardrum)
- Middle ear
  - Three (ossicles) bones—incus, malleus, and stapes
- Inner ear
  - Sensory receptors—semicircular canals, cochlea, and vestibule

Ceruminous Glands
- Wax-producing glands that secrete cerumen
- Found in external auditory canal

Middle Ear Ossicles (Three)
- Incus ("anvil"), malleus ("mallet"), and stapes ("stirrup")
- Amplifying sound waves on tympanic membrane
- Handle of malleus attaches to tympanic membrane
- Base of stapes connected to inner ear
- Incus between malleus and stapes (attached to both)

Eustachian Tube
- Connects middle ear with pharynx
- Opens and closes to equalize pressure on either side of tympanic membrane

Inner Ear (Labyrinth)
- Most important and complex portion of the ear
- Contains three areas
  - Vestibule
    - Equilibrium receptors
    - Two bony chambers

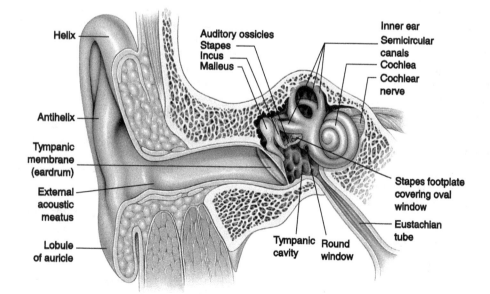

Figure 1.18 Structures of the Ear. (Asset provided by Anatomical Chart Co.)

- ○ Semicircular canals
  - Equilibrium receptors
  - Three bony tubes
- ○ Cochlea
  - Hearing receptors
  - Appearance of a "snail shell"

Organ of Corti
- "Hearing organ"
- Ciliated receptors
- Located within the cochlea

Process of Hearing (Cochlea)
- Sound waves captured in external auditory canal
- Tympanic membrane vibrates
- Tympanum → malleus → incus → stapes
- Stapes triggers inner ear
- Vibrations move cilia in cochlear duct
- Nerve impulse generated by movement of cilia against tectorial membrane
- Cranial nerve VIII takes AP to the brain
- Temporal lobe cortex interprets information

Equilibrium (Vestibule and Semicircular Canals)
- Static equilibrium—moving in straight line
- Dynamic equilibrium—body spinning or moving in multiple directions

Use the DVD or visit the website at http://thePoint.lww.com/Long for additional materials about *equilibrium*.

Taste (Gustation)
- Fluid must be present to taste (chemicals in solution to taste)
- Nerves involved with taste
  - ○ Facial nerve (CN VII)
  - ○ Glossopharyngeal nerve (CN IX)

Tongue Taste Map
- Sweet—tip of the tongue
- Salty—anterior sides of tongue
- Sour—laterally on tongue
- Bitter—posterior part of tongue

Olfaction (Smell)
- Chemicals in solution to smell
- Olfactory nerve (CN I) takes information to the olfactory center (temporal lobe cortex)

CARDIOVASCULAR SYSTEM

Layers of the Heart (Three)
- Endocardium
  - ○ Smooth epithelial cells
  - ○ Lines the chambers
  - ○ Covers the valves

- Myocardium
  - ○ Cardiac muscle
  - ○ Thickest layer
  - ○ Pumps blood
  - ○ Lightly striated
  - ○ Involuntary
  - ○ Single nuclei in cardiac cells
  - ○ Branching cellular networks
  - ○ Intercalated disc—modified plasma membranes transfer electrical impulses
- Epicardium
  - ○ Serous membrane
  - ○ Visceral layer of the pericardium

Pericardium
- Sac enclosing the heart
- Pericardial portions
  - ○ Fibrous pericardium
    - Outer layer
    - Heaviest layer
    - Anchor heart to diaphragm, sternum, and so on
  - ○ Serous pericardium
    - Parietal pericardium—outer layer of serous pericardium
    - Parietal cavity—contains thin layer of fluid to decrease friction
    - Visceral pericardium is same as epicardium

Structures of the Heart
- Atria (two)—receive venous blood (see Fig. 1.19)
  - ○ Right atrium—deoxygenated blood from body through superior/inferior vena cava and coronary sinus (pumps blood to right ventricle)
  - ○ Left atrium—oxygen from lungs through pulmonary vein (pumps blood to left ventricle)
- Ventricles (two)—eject blood into arteries
  - ○ Right ventricle—pumps blood to lungs for O$_2$ through pulmonary artery
  - ○ Left ventricle—pumps blood to entire body for O$_2$ delivery
- One-way valves (four)
  - ○ Tricuspid—between right atrium and ventricle; right atrioventricular (AV) valve
  - ○ Bicuspid (mitral valve)—between left atrium and ventricle; left AV valve
  - ○ Semilunar valves—open during ventricular contraction and close during ventricular relaxation (pulmonary valve—right ventricle and pulmonary artery and aortic valve—left ventricle and aorta)
- Chamber divisions
  - ○ Interatrial septum—separates atria
  - ○ Interventricular septum—separates ventricles

Quick fact The left ventricle is the thickest of the heart walls and forms the apex of the heart.

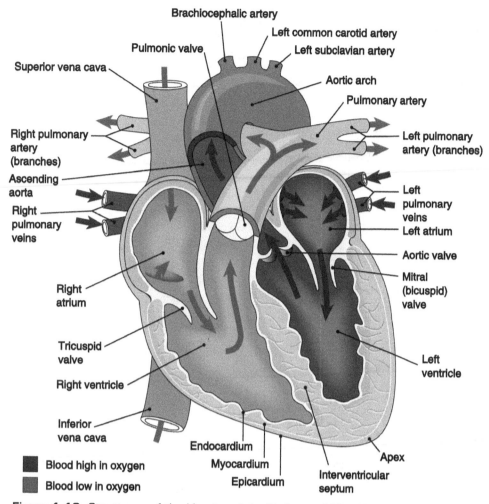

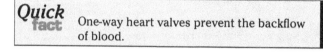

Figure 1.19 Structures of the Heart and the Pathway of Blood Flow. (Reprinted with permission from Cohen BJ, Wood DL. *Memmler's the human body in health and disease*, 9th ed. Philadelphia: Lippincott Williams & Wilkins; 2000.)

Quick fact One-way heart valves prevent the backflow of blood.

Quick fact The heart is slightly bigger than a person's fist.

Quick fact The left lung is slightly smaller than right lung due to the area of the cardiac notch, where the heart rests.

Quick fact The left ventricle is stronger and larger and is more detrimental to a person's health if damaged by a myocardial infarction (heart attack).

Coronary Arteries
- Right and left coronary arteries supply oxygenated blood to myocardium
- First branch from aorta
- Fill when heart is relaxed

Quick fact Cornary artery disease (CAD) is the most common type of heart disease and is the leading cause of death in the United States.

Systemic Circulation
- Greater resistance to blood flow than pulmonary circulation
- Flow must be consistent so force in left ventricle must be greater

Sinoatrial Node
- Pacemaker in right atrium near opening of superior vena cava

- Slow spontaneous depolarization
- Membrane potential –60 mV and depolarizes to –40 mV (threshold for AP of these cells)

Atrioventricular Node

- Between the atria and the ventricles
- Part of heart conduction system
- Slower process than sinoatrial (SA) node
- AV bundle (bundle of His)
  - Branches to all portions of the ventricles
  - Purkinje fibers—myofibers that conduct impulse to the myocardium of the ventricles

Conduction Pathway of the Heart

- SA node sends AP
- Atria contract with AV node triggered
- AV node sends AP
  - Slower to allow atria to contract completely filling ventricles
- Bundle of His triggers Purkinje fibers to cause ventricles to contract
- All the ventricles contract at once

Autonomic Nervous System Heart Control

- Sympathetic nervous system
  - Increases heart rate
  - Increases contraction force of myocardium
  - Acts on SA/AV nodes
  - Cardiac output can increase two to three times normal
- Parasympathetic nervous system
  - Decreases heart rate to restore homeostasis through CN X (vagus)
  - Acts on SA/AV nodes

Cardiac Cycle

- Repeating pattern of contraction and relaxation (systole + diastole = single heart beat)
- Systole (phase of contraction)—AV valves close → blood from ventricle through aortic/pulmonary valves
- Diastole (phase of relaxation)—AV valves open → blood to ventricle/pulmonary and aortic valves close

Heart Sounds

- "Lub"
  - First sound
  - AV valve closes and blood vibration makes sound
  - Longer, lower-pitched sound
  - Start of ventricular systole
- "Dub"
  - Second sound
  - Semilunar valves closing
  - Shorter, sharper sound
  - Ventricular relaxation

Pulmonary Circuit

- Right ventricle → Pulmonary artery → Lungs → Pulmonary veins → Left atrium

Systemic Circuit

- Left ventricle → Aorta → Tissues → System veins → Superior or inferior vena cava → Right atrium

Total Blood Volume

- 5.5 L
- At rest, the average ventricle pumps equivalent of total blood volume
  - 5,500 mL (5.5 L) = 70 – 80 mL per beat × 70 beats per minute

Factors that Affect Blood Pressure

- Vessel diameter
- Vessel elasticity—arteries expand
- Blood viscosity—thickness
  - Increased viscosity = increased BP (e.g., dehydration, increased red blood cells [RBCs])
- Blood volume
  - Decreased volume = decreased BP
  - Increased volume = increased BP

Regulation of Stroke Volume

- End-diastolic volume (EDV)—volume of blood in the ventricles at the end of diastole
- Total peripheral resistance—frictional resistance, or impedance, to blood flow in the arteries
- Contractility—strength of ventricular contraction

RESPIRATORY SYSTEM

Phases of Respiration

- Pulmonary ventilation
  - Inhalation and exhalation
  - Exchange of atmospheric and alveoli air
- External gas exchange
  - Occurs in lungs
  - Oxygen diffusion from alveoli into blood
  - Carbon dioxide diffusion from blood for elimination
- Internal gas exchange
  - Occurs in tissues
  - Oxygen diffuses from blood to tissues
  - Carbon dioxide diffuses from tissues to blood

Air Pathway

- Nose → Pharynx → Larynx → Trachea → Right and left primary bronchi → Right and left secondary bronchi (each lobe) → Right and left tertiary bronchi (segmental) → Right and left bronchioles → Right and left alveoli

Structures of the Respiratory System

Nasal Cavities
- Nares (nostrils) (see Figs. 1.20 and 1.21)
  - Opening to nose
- Nasal septum
  - Divides nasal cavities
  - Plate of ethmoid—superior portion
  - Vomer—inferior portion
- Conchae
  - Three projections
  - Lateral wall of each nasal cavity
  - Increases surface area
- Mucous membrane
  - Lines nasal cavity
  - Increases warmth and moisture of air
  - Decreased foreign body penetration

> *Quick* fact The mucous membranes of the nose contain a large number of blood vessels.

Pharynx
- Muscular
- Three portions
  - Nasopharynx—behind nose
  - Oropharynx—posterior to mouth
  - Laryngopharynx—opens into larynx and esophagus

Larynx
- Between trachea and pharynx
- Thyroid cartilage including Adam apple
- Vocal cords
  - Mucous membrane folds
  - Vibrate with air
- Glottis
  - Space between vocal cords
  - Epiglottis covers larynx
  - Glottis and epiglottis keep fluid and food out of trachea
- Cricoid cartilage—ring of cartilage forming inferior wall of larynx

> *Quick* fact The larynx is more commonly referred to as the *voice box*.

Trachea
- C-shaped cartilage with posterior opening
- Allows increased room for esophagus when swallowing
- Anterior to esophagus
  - Travels from larynx to T5
- Divides into right and left primary bronchi

Bronchi
- Two right and left primary bronchi
- Branch from trachea
- Right bigger than left
- Bronchi enter lungs through hilum
- Lined by epithelial cells with cilia
- Small bits of cartilage help keep bronchi open
- Right bronchus shorter, wider, and more vertical than left

> *Quick* fact Most foreign particles that enter the lungs travel through the right bronchus.

Lungs
- Located in thoracic cavity
- Mediastinum—space between lungs for other vessels (e.g., heart, trachea, esophagus)
- Left lung
  - Two lobes (superior and inferior)
  - Cardiac notch—indentation where the heart rests
  - Bronchus subdivides into two secondary bronchi
- Right lung
  - Three lobes (superior, middle, and inferior)
  - Bronchus subdivides into three secondary bronchi

Lung Pleura
- Covering of lungs
- Two layers
  - Parietal pleura—attached to chest wall
  - Visceral pleura—attached to lung surface
- Pleural space
  - Between two pleural layers
  - Fluid for lubrication
    - Resists separation of tissues
    - Allows frictionless movement

Bronchioles
- Smallest tubes
- No cartilage
- Smooth muscle
- ANS control

Alveoli
- Tiny air sacs
- Walls are single cell thickness
- Increased ability for gas exchange
- Capillaries cover alveoli
- Three times more lung tissue than needed for life

> *Quick* fact Surfactant is a substance produced in the alveoli to decrease surface tension of fluids.

Inhalation (Inspiration)
- Takes 1 to 2 seconds
- Active phase—requires energy
- Requires muscle activity
- Diaphragm flattens (contracts)—stimulated by I neurons
- Gas pressure within thoracic cavity decreases as size increases
- Lungs are expanded
- Oxygen concentrations in inhaled air is 21%
- Carbon dioxide concentrations in inhaled air is 0.04%

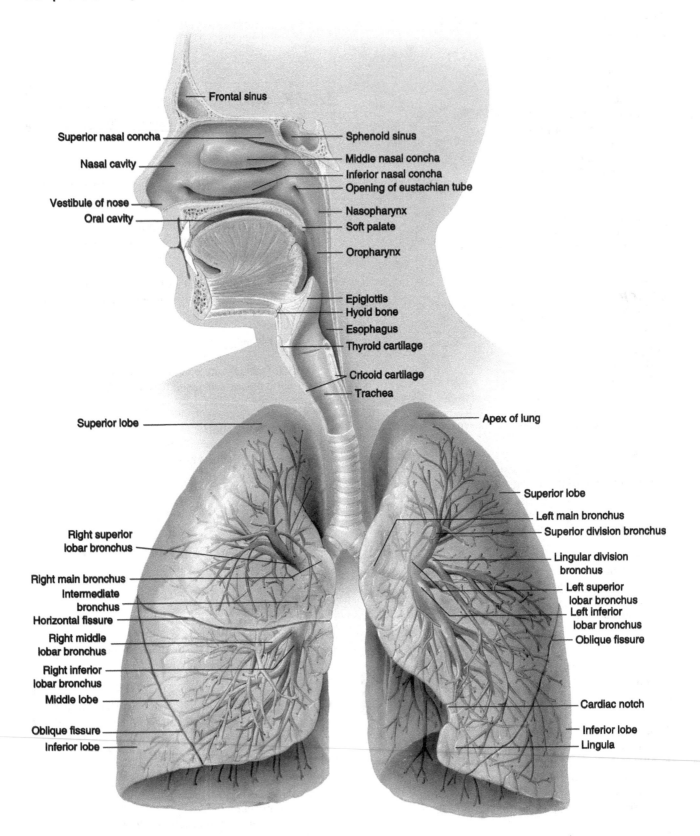

Figure 1.20 Structures of the Respiratory System. (Asset provided by Anatomical Chart Co.)

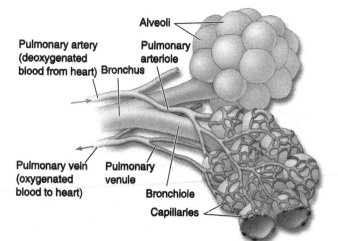

Figure 1.21 Terminal Structures of the Respiratory System. (From McArdle WD, Katch FI, Katch VL. *Essentials of exercise physiology*, 2nd ed. Baltimore: Lippincott Williams & Wilkins; 2000.)

- Lung pressure is less than air pressure
- Motor impulses from medulla increase
- Inhalation prolonged by pons (apneustic center)
- Intrapleural pressure becomes even greater negative gradient because of suction between pleural membranes
- Normal inspiration stops when pressure gradient equalizes

Exhalation (Expiration)

- Takes 2 to 3 seconds (longer than inspiration)
- Passive phase—no energy requirement
- Respiratory muscles relax
- Lung and air pressure equalizes to stop expiration
- Lungs are compressed as diaphragm relaxes (fills thorax)
- Motor impulses decrease with expiration
- Forced exhalation requires energy—active process
- E neurons inhibit I neurons (medulla)
- Pneumotaxic center interrupts impulses from apneustic center (pons)
- Air pressure is less than lung pressure
- Oxygen concentration in exhaled air is 16%
- Carbon dioxide concentration in exhaled air is 4.5%

Quick fact The cerebral cortex can allow for voluntary changes in respiration, such as when singing.

Hyperventilation

- Increased air in the alveoli
- Increased oxygen and decreased carbon dioxide
- Increased pH of blood (alkalosis)
- Dizziness and fainting may occur

Hypoventilation

- Decreased air in alveoli
- Decreased oxygen and increased carbon dioxide
- Decreased blood pH (acidosis)

Oxygen Transport

- Plasma (1.5% volume of oxygen)
- Hemoglobin (98.5% volume of oxygen)
- Oxygenated blood is saturated with 97% oxygen
- Deoxygenated blood is saturated with 70% oxygen
- Blood is never totally depleted of oxygen
- Carbon monoxide binds to hemoglobin with a stronger bond than oxygen (displaces oxygen)

Quick fact Blood oxygen saturation (SpO_2) levels can be indirectly measured using a device known as a *pulse oximeter*.

Carbon Dioxide Transport

- Carbon dioxide is a by-product of cellular metabolism
- Three ways to transport
  ○ Dissolved in plasma (10%)
  ○ Hemoglobin and plasma proteins (15%)
  ○ Bicarbonate ion HCO_3^- (75%)

Bicarbonate Ion

- Occurs when carbon dioxide dissolves in blood
- Carbonic anhydrase—enzyme-increasing rate of bicarbonate formation
- Reactions are reversible as bicarbonate reforms carbon dioxide in the lungs for expiration
- $CO_2 + H_2O \longleftrightarrow H_2CO_3 \longleftrightarrow H^+ + HCO_3^-$
- Each bicarbonate ion formed equals release of H^+ and causes blood to become acidic
- Bicarbonate ion is blood buffer keeping pH around 7.35 to 7.45

Respiratory Regulation

- Nervous system control
- Chemical control

 Use the DVD or visit the website at http://thePoint.lww.com/Long for additional materials about *respiratory regulation*.

DIGESTIVE SYSTEM

Functions of the Digestive System

- Digestion—breakdown
- Absorption—transfer of nutrients into blood
- Elimination—elimination of unused by-products in body

Walls of the Digestive Tract

- Mucosa
  - Mucous membrane
  - Contains digestive juices
  - Secretion cells
- Submucosa
  - Blood vessels
  - Nerves
  - Helps regulate digestion
  - Small intestine submucosa has glands to protect from acidic atmosphere
- Smooth muscle (two layers)
  - Circular (inner layer)—contraction narrows lumen
  - Longitudinal (outer layer)—contraction shortens and widens lumen
- Serosa
  - Serous membrane
  - Found in abdominopelvic cavity organs
  - Thin, moist tissue
  - Forms part of peritoneum

 Quick fact Peristalsis is the wave-like propulsion of food through the digestive tract.

Peritoneum

- Lines abdominopelvic cavity
- Thin, shiny serous membrane
- Separates and/or binds organs to one another
- Carries blood, lymphatic vessels, and nerves

Peritoneum Portions

- Parietal peritoneum
  - Outer portion
  - Lines cavity
- Visceral peritoneum
  - Inner portion
  - Covers organs

 Quick fact The visceral peritoneum allows organs to move over one another.

Divisions of Peritoneum

- Mesentery
- Mesocolon
- Greater omentum
- Lesser omentum

Mesentery

- Double-layered, fan-shaped portion
- Attaches posterior abdominal wall to small intestines
- Between layers are nerves and vessels supplying small intestine

Mesocolon

- Colon to posterior abdominal wall

Omentums

- Greater omentum
  - Double layer
  - Contains significant fat
  - Hangs like an apron over intestines
  - Attaches lower border of stomach to pelvic part of abdomen to transverse colon
- Lesser omentum
  - Located between stomach and liver

Alimentary (Gastrointestinal or Digestive) Tract

- Mouth → Pharynx → Esophagus → Stomach → Small intestine (Duodenum → Jejunum → Ileum) → Large intestine (Cecum → Ascending colon → Transverse colon → Descending colon → Sigmoid colon → Rectum → Anal canal) → Anus

Mouth

- Oral cavity
- Ingestion—receives food
- Mastication—breaks down food
- Mixes food with saliva
  - Salivary amylase—enzyme breaks down starches
- Deglutition—swallowing
- Tongue (taste and speech)
- Permanent teeth (32 total)
  - Incisors (eight)—cutting
  - Cuspids/canine/eye (four)—pointed with deep roots
  - Molars (20)—grinding

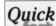 **Quick fact** From the ages of 2 to 6 years a child has 20 deciduous ("baby") teeth.

Esophagus

- Muscular tube
- Food mixes with mucus
- Esophageal hiatus
  - Esophagus transverses diaphragm
  - Weakness leads to a hiatal hernia

Quick fact The esophagus is approximately 10 in. long.

Stomach

- Upper left cavity
- J shaped
- Muscular layers
  - Oblique—grinds/mixes food
  - Circular—narrows lumen
  - Longitudinal—shorten/widens lumen

Portions of Stomach

- Fundus
  - Superior
  - Rounded
  - Under diaphragm
  - Left side

- Greater curvature
- Lesser curvature
- Pylorus
  - Slows food entering small intestine

Stomach Functions

- Storage—0.5 gal liquid/food
- Digestion
  - Hydrochloric acid—destroys pathologic microorganisms and denatures proteins
  - Pepsin—protein-digesting enzyme

Small Intestine

- Up to 20 ft (and 1 in in diameter)
- Duodenum → Jejunum → Ileum
- Pancreatic juices and mucus prevalent
- Mucus increases pH
- Secretes enzymes that digest carbohydrates and proteins
- Absorbs water, food, and minerals
- Villi and microvilli increase surface area

 Quick fact A lacteal is a lymphatic that absorbs fats into lymph.

Large Intestine

- 5-ft long (2.5 in. in diameter)
- Cecum attaches to small intestine
- Ileocecal valve—sphincter prevents backward travel of food
- Vermiform (appendix)—attaches to cecum
- Cecum → Ascending colon → Transverse colon → Descending colon → Sigmoid → Rectum → Anal canal
- Mucus—no enzyme secretions
- Water reabsorption
- No food digestion
- Storage of undigested food
  - Feces—solid waste
  - Defecation—waste elimination
  - Anal sphincter—voluntary defecation

Quick fact Bacteria in the large intestine produce vitamin K and some B complex vitamins.

Digestive Accessory Organs

- Salivary glands
- Liver
- Gallbladder
- Pancreas

Salivary Glands

- Parotid glands
  - Largest
  - Inferior and anterior to ear
- Submaxillary (submandibular) glands
  - Near lower jaw

- Sublingual glands
  - Under tongue

Liver

- Found in upper right quadrant of abdomen (see Fig. 1.22)
- Right and left lobes
  - Right lobe is the largest and has two inferior lobe divisions
- Blood supplied by two structures
  - Portal vein—deoxygenated and digestive end products
  - Hepatic artery—oxygenated

Quick fact The liver is the largest glandular organ.

Liver Functions

- Manufactures bile
- Stores vitamins and iron
- Modifies fats
- Destroys old RBCs
- Synthesizes urea
- Detoxifies body

Gallbladder

- Stores bile (Fig. 1.22)
- Inferior surface of the liver
- Dumps into duodenum

Pancreas

- Extends from duodenum to spleen
- Produces enzymes to digest carbohydrates, proteins, fats, and nucleic acids
- Produces alkaline fluid to decrease acidic chyme

URINARY SYSTEM

Parts of Urinary System

- Kidneys (two)
  - Form urine
  - Remove waste from blood
  - Balance body fluid
- Ureters (two)
  - Tubes
  - Transport urine from kidneys to urinary bladder
- Urinary bladder
  - Reservoir of urine
- Urethra
  - Transports urine from bladder to outside

Kidneys

- Retroperitoneal space T12-L3 (see Fig. 1.23)
- Hilum—medial notch where renal vein/artery and ureter attach
- Renal cortex—outer kidney
- Renal medulla—inner kidney
  - Renal pyramids
  - Renal pelvis—connects with ureter
  - Calyces—tips of pyramids that collect urine

Anterior view

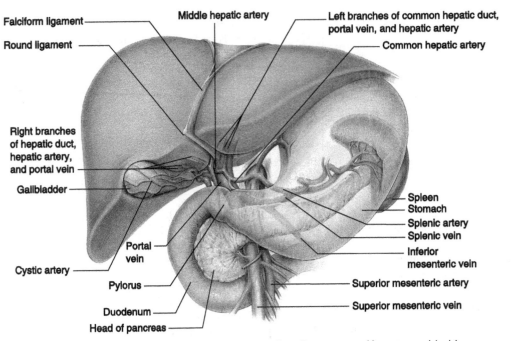

Figure 1.22 Liver, Gall Bladder, and Surrounding Structures. (Asset provided by Anatomical Chart Co.)

- Renal capsule—membrane surrounding kidney
- Adipose kidney—protective fat layer
- Renal artery—oxygenated blood from abdominal aorta
- Renal vein—transports blood from kidney to inferior vena cava
- Nephron—functional unit of kidney

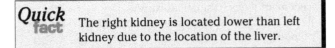

Quick fact The right kidney is located lower than left kidney due to the location of the liver.

Nephron
- Coiled tube with end bulb (glomerular or Bowman capsule)
- Glomerulus—cluster of capillaries
- Afferent arteriole—oxygenated blood to glomerulus
- Efferent arteriole—deoxygenated blood from glomerulus

Tubular portions of nephron
- Proximal convoluted tubule
  - Reabsorbs most water and NaCl into blood
  - Reabsorbs all of glucose, small proteins, and amino acids into blood
- Loop of Henle
  - Reabsorbs approximately 25% water and NaCl
  - Descending limb—reabsorbs water (osmosis) and salt impermeable
  - Ascending limb—reabsorbs salt, urea, and water impermeable
- Distal convoluted tubule
  - Urine transport

Juxtaglomerular apparatus
- Formed by afferent arteriole and distal convoluted tubule
- Specialized cells
- Regulates kidney function
- Low BP triggers renin secretion

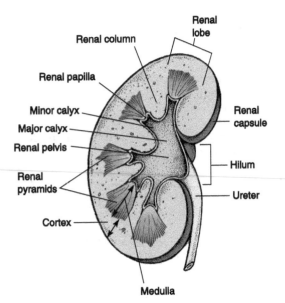

Figure 1.23 Structures of the Kidney. (From *Stedman's Medical Dictionary*, 27th ed. Baltimore: Lippincott Williams & Wilkins; 2000.)

Kidney Function
- Excretes metabolic wastes
- Maintains water balance
- Regulates pH of body fluids (7.35 to 7.45)
- Regulates RBC production through erythropoietin
- Regulates BP through renin-angiotensin pathway

Urine Formation
- Glomerular filtration
  - BP dependent (three to four times BP of capillaries)
  - Soluble items out of blood
  - Blood cells and proteins too large—stay in blood
- Tubular reabsorption
  - Filtrate leaves nephron by osmosis, diffusion, and active transport
  - Renal threshold—if body cannot reabsorb quickly enough—materials excreted in urine
- Tubular secretions
  - Final filtrate adjustments
  - Regulation of pH
- Urine concentration

Urethra
- Female—opening to vagina
- Male—carry semen and urine
  - Passes through prostate gland

Urination (Micturition) and Urine
- Voluntary and involuntary sphincter muscles
- 95% water and 5% solids and gases
- Specific gravity (Usg) between 1.002 and 1.040
- Pathway of urine flow in kidneys
  - Renal pyramids → Calyces → Renal pelvis → Ureter

Quick fact A Usg of 1.030 classifies a person as being severely dehydrated.

Antidiuretic Hormone
- Regulates permeability to water
- Released by posterior pituitary gland
- Produced by hypothalamus and released by posterior pituitary gland
- ↑ Antidiuretic hormone (ADH) = ↑ Permeability = ↑ Water reabsorption

Parathyroid Hormone
- Acts on kidneys to promote calcium ion reabsorption
- Promotes reabsorption of sodium ions
- Promotes excretion of phosphate ions
- Produced in the parathyroid gland

Aldosterone
- Promotes excretion of potassium ions
- Promotes reabsorption of sodium ions
- Produced by adrenal cortex

Renin-Angiotensin Pathway
- Decreased BP simulates renin secretion
- Renin splits plasma protein angiotensinogen to angiotensin I
- Angiotensin I is converted to angiotensin II
- Angiotensin II causes vasoconstriction and stimulates adrenal cortex to secrete aldosterone
- BP increases

Erythropoietin
- Hormone secreted by kidneys
- Secreted because of hypoxia
- Stimulates red bone marrow to increase RBC production
- Increases oxygen-carrying capacity of blood

ENDOCRINE SYSTEM

Endocrine Gland Function
- Secretes hormones directly into the blood
- Has no ducts—why they must secrete directly into the blood
- Blood carries the hormones to the target organ(s)

Quick fact Hormones are delivered by the blood to every cell in the body, but only the target cells are able to respond to those hormones.

Endocrine Glands
- Pineal gland (see Fig. 1.24)
- Pituitary gland (hypophysis)
- Thyroid gland
- Parathyroid gland
- Thymus
- Adrenal gland
- Pancreas
- Ovaries or testes

General Categories of Hormones (Three)
- Catecholamines
  - Epinephrine and norepinephrine
- Polypeptides and glycoproteins
  - All hormones except hormones of sex glands and adrenal cortex, for example, anti-diuretic hormone, insulin, and thyroid-stimulating hormone (TSH)
  - Amino acid components
- Steroids
  - Types of lipids
  - Adrenal cortex and sex glands (e.g., corticosteroids, testosterone)

Quick fact When two or more hormones work together to produce a particular result, their effects are said to be synergistic.

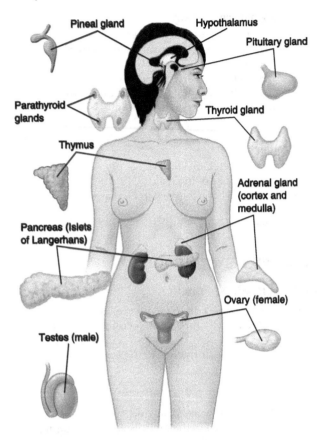

Figure 1.24 Major Endocrine Glands of the Body. (From Anderson MK, Parr GP, Hall SJ, et al. *Foundations of athletic training: prevention, assessment, and management*, 4th ed. Baltimore: Lippincott Williams & Wilkins; 2009.)

Synergistic Hormones

- Synergistic hormones can be (a) additive or (b) complementary
  - Additive—all do the same thing like epinephrine and norepinephrine, both increase heart rate
  - Complementary—all stimulate separate processes of the same action (e.g., follicle-stimulating hormone [FSH] and testosterone are involved in spermogenesis)

> **Quick fact** The hypothalamus has releasing and inhibiting hormones that trigger the pituitary gland to release or inhibit hormones (e.g., growth hormone–releasing hormone triggers GH release and growth hormone–inhibiting hormone inhibits GH release).

Pituitary Gland (Hypophysis)

- Located in sphenoid bone
- Called the *master gland*

- Controlled by hypothalamus through the infundibulum
- Anterior pituitary—produces and secretes hormones
- Posterior pituitary—secretes hormones produced by the hypothalamus

Anterior Pituitary Hormones (Six)

- Growth hormone (GH or somatatrophin)
  - Stimulates movement of amino acids to tissue cells
  - Incorporates amino acids into tissue protein
  - Stimulates growth of all tissues
  - Stimulates protein synthesis
  - Needed for maintenance and repair of cells
  - Stimulates liver to release fatty acids for energy during stress
- TSH or thytrophin
  - Thyroid gland produces and excretes thyroxine (T_4)
- Adrenocorticotropic hormone (ACTH or corticotropin)
  - Stimulates adrenal cortex to secrete glucocorticoids (hydrocortisone or cortisol)
  - Aids in protecting body in stress situations (e.g., pain/injury)
- FSH or folliculotrophin
  - Stimulates the growth of ovarian follicles in females and production of sperm in males
- Luteinizing hormone (LH or luteotrophin)
  - Stimulates ovulation in females
  - Stimulates secretion of testosterone in males
  - Causes corpus luteum development
- Prolactin
  - Stimulates milk production from mammary glands in females after birth
  - In males, supports the regulation of reproduction system gonadotrophins
  - Acts on the kidneys to help regulate water and electrolyte balance

Posterior Pituitary Hormones (Two)

- Antidiuretic hormone (ADH or arginine vasopression [AVP])
  - Stimulates the kidneys to retain water by reabsorption in kidney tubules (decreases excretions)
  - Increased ADH causes smooth muscle contractions that increase blood pressure
- Oxytocin
  - In females, stimulates the contraction of the uterus during labor
  - Stimulates the mammary gland to eject milk (ejection reflex)

> **Quick fact** A decrease in ADH increases water loss, and too much can cause diabetes insipidus.

Adrenal Glands

- Paired organs that rest on top of the kidneys
- Adrenal cortex—secretes steroid hormones that participate in the regulation of mineral and energy balance

- Adrenal medulla—secretes catecholamine hormones that complement the sympathetic nervous system

Adrenal Medulla Hormones
- Epinephrine (adrenaline) and norepinephrine (noradrenaline)
- Fight or flight hormones
- These hormones can be released as neurotransmitters from nerve endings

Effects of Epinephrine and Norepinephrine
- Increase BP because of arteriole contraction
- Dilate of bronchioles
- Increase cell metabolism
- Increase heart rate
- Convert glycogen to glucose for energy

Adrenal Cortex Hormones
- Glucocorticoids
  - Maintain carbohydrate reserve
  - Stimulate liver to convert amino acids into glucose instead of protein
  - Suppress inflammatory response cortisol (hydrocortisone)
  - Increase free-floating amino acids and fatty acids from tissues (e.g., muscle and adipose)
- Mineralocorticoids
  - Example—aldosterone
  - Regulate electrolyte balance
  - Increase potassium secretions and control sodium reabsorption in the kidneys
- Sex hormones

Thyroid Gland
- Found around the pharynx
- Produces and secretes thyroxine (T_4), triiodothronine (T_3), and calcitonin
- T_3 and T_4 are used for proper growth and development
- T_3 and T_4 determine BMR
- Calcitonin used for calcium metabolism by decreasing circulating blood calcium and increasing bone deposits of Ca^{2+}

Parathyroid Gland
- Embedded in the posterior thyroid gland
- Secretes parathyroid hormone
- Helps raise the blood Ca^{2+} concentration by releasing it from bone

Pancreas
- Within the abdomen
- Functions as both an endocrine and exocrine gland
- Endocrine portion is called the *islets of Langerhans* (*pancreatic islets*)

Islets of Langerhans
- Two types of cells
  - α Cells—secrete the hormone glucagon
  - β Cells—secrete the hormone insulin

> **Quick fact** Glucagon and insulin actions are antagonistic.

α Cells
- Secrete glucagon when blood glucose concentration falls
- Glucagon stimulates the liver to hydrolyze glucagons to glucose (glycogenolysis)—this causes the blood glucose levels to rise
- Glucagon also stimulates the hydrolysis of stored fat (lipolysis) and the release of free fatty acids into the blood
- Glucagon plus other hormones stimulate the conversion of fatty acids to ketone bodies, which can be secreted by the liver into the blood and used by other organs as an emergency energy source

> **Quick fact** Glucagon is a hormone that helps maintain homeostasis during times of fasting, when the bodies energy reserves must be used.

β Cells
- Secrete insulin in response to a rise in blood glucose concentrations
- Insulin promotes glucose entry into tissue cells
- Conversion of glucose into energy storage molecules of glycogen and fat

> **Quick fact** After a meal, insulin secretion increases and glucagon secretion decreases.

Pineal Gland
- Found in the brain
- Produces and secretes melatonin during dark periods
- Melatonin secretions are highest at night secondary to their triggers decreasing with visual light (e.g., sunlight)
- Melatonin delays onset of puberty

Circadian Rhythms
- Daily rhythms within the body secondary to cycles of light and dark
- Jet lag and seasonal affective disorder (SAD) may be worse secondary to an increased production and secretion of melatonin

Thymus
- In front of the aorta
- Production site for T cells (thymus-dependent cells)
- T cells are lymphocytes involved in cell-mediated immunity
- Hormone thymosin—maturation of some white blood cells

Sex Glands

- Ovaries (female)—estrogen and progesterone
- Testes (male)—testosterone
- Secondary sex characteristics
  - Male—deep voice and facial hair
  - Female—increase ratio fat/muscle, wider hips, and breast development

Female Reproductive System

Female Reproductive System Organs

- Uterus (see Fig. 1.25)
  - Location of embryo development
- Fallopian tubes (two)
  - Transport ova (egg)
- Ovaries (two)
  - Produce ova

Layers of the Uterus (Three)

- Perimetrium—outer cover
- Myometrium—middle layer of smooth muscle
- Endometrium—inner layer

Endometrium

- Stratified, squamous, nonkeratinized epithelium
- Cyclically grows thicker as a result of estrogen and progesterone levels
- Sheds with bleeding at menstruation

> **Quick fact** Endometriosis is a condition involving an ectopic endometrium found in various sites within the pelvic cavity.

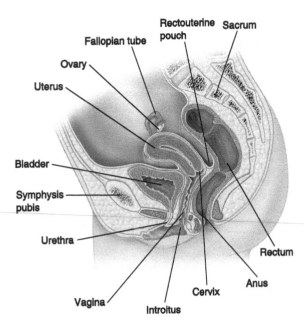

Figure 1.25 Female Reproductive System. (From Anderson MK, Parr GP, Hall SJ, et al. *Foundations of athletic training: prevention, assessment, and management*, 4th ed. Baltimore: Lippincott Williams & Wilkins; 2009.)

Menstrual Cycle

- Average 28-day cycle (see Fig. 1.26)
- First day of menstruation is day one of the cycle
- Phases of menstruation
  - Follicular phase
  - Ovulation
  - Luteal phase

> **Quick fact** The prefix menstru- means month.

Follicular Phase

- Day 1 of menstruation until the day of ovulation (usually days 1 to 13)
- Menstruation occurs days 1 to 4 or 5
- Estrogen highest at day 12
- FSH stimulates secretion of estradoil
- Positive feedback system
- FSH and estradoil stimulate the production of LH receptors
- LH surges approximately 24 hours before ovulation
- LH peaks at approximately 16 hours before ovulation

Ovulation

- Approximately day 14
- Rupture of a membrane

Luteal Phase

- Corpus luteum secretes estradiol and progesterone
- Progesterone peaks approximately 1 week after ovulation
- Negative feedback inhibition of FSH and LH secretion (prevents multiple pregnancies)
- Estrogen and progesterone levels fall late in luteal phase (approximately 22 days)

Male Reproductive System

Male Reproductive System Organs

- Gonads (testes)—primary (see Fig. 1.27)
- Epididymis—accessory
  - Stores sperm
- Ductus deferens—accessory
  - Previously called *vas deferens*
  - Allows sperm to travel through spermatic cord
- Ejaculatory duct—accessory
  - Empties into urethra

Testes

- Two, suspended in scrotum
- Spermatic cord
  - Contains blood/lymphatic vessels, nerves, and ductus deferens
- Seminiferous tubules
  - Sperm production
- Interstitial cells
  - Hormone secretion

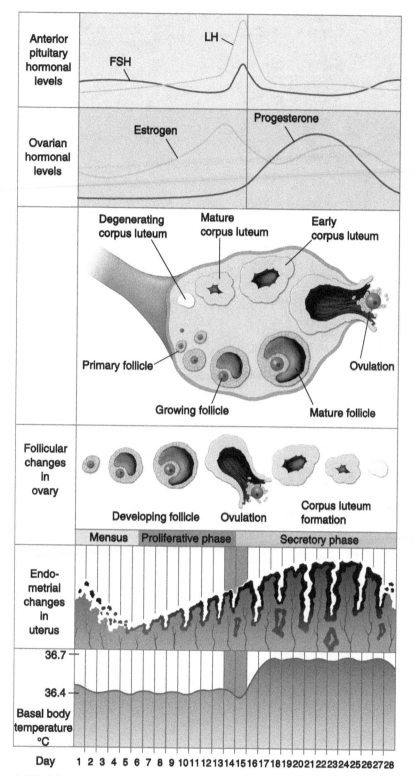

Figure 1.26 Menstrual Cycle. FSH, follicle-stimulating hormone; LH, luteinizing hormone (From Premkumar K. *The massage connection anatomy and physiology*. Baltimore: Lippincott Williams & Wilkins; 2004.)

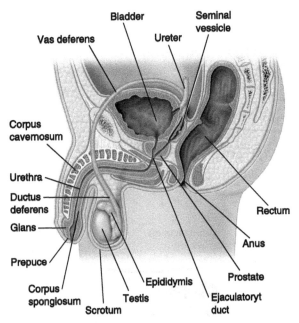

Figure 1.27 Male Reproductive System. (From Anderson MK, Parr GP, Hall SJ, et al. *Foundations of athletic training: prevention, assessment, and management*, 4th ed. Baltimore: Lippincott Williams & Wilkins; 2009.)

Hormones

- Testosterone
  - Secondary sex characteristics
  - Maintains reproductive components
- FSH
  - Promotes sperm formation
  - Stimulates cells used to develop sperm
- LH
  - Triggers interstitial cells to produce testosterone

Semen

- Helps transport sperm
- Nourishes sperm
- Neutralizes acidity level of urethra
- Lubricates during intercourse
- Prevents infection

P A R T **2** Anatomy of the Head, Neck, Spine, and Thorax

KEY TERMS

- Abducent nerve
- Accessory nerve
- Bifid
- Bifurcation
- Cauda equine
- Cerebrospinal fluid (CSF)
- Gray matter
- Insertion
- Interneurons
- Origin
- Pars interarticularis
- Sacral plexus

BONES OF THE HEAD, NECK, SPINE, AND THORAX

See Table 1.2.
See Figures 1.28 to 1.33.

MAJOR LIGAMENTS OF THE HEAD, NECK, SPINE, AND THORAX

See Table 1.3.
See Figure 1.34.

Table 1.2 Bones of the Head, Neck, Spine, and Thorax

Head and Neck	Spine	Thorax
Frontal	Cervical vertebra C1	Manubrium of sternum
Parietal	(atlas)	Body of sternum
Temporal	Cervical vertebra C2	Xiphoid process of
Occipital	(axis)	sternum
Sphenoid	Cervical vertebrae C3-7	Ribs 1–7 (true ribs)
Ethmoid	Thoracic vertebrae	Ribs 8–12 (false ribs) and
Lacrimal	T1-12	(10–11 are floating ribs)
Nasal	Lumbar vertebra L1-5	
Vomer	Sacral vertebrae S1-5	
Inferior nasal	Coccygeal vertebrae	
concha	Co1-4	
Zygomatic		
Maxilla		
Palatine		
Mandible		
Hyoid		

Quick **fact** The transverse ligament of the atlas is also known as the *hangman's ligment* because it supports the odontoid process of the axis.

MUSCLES OF THE HEAD, NECK, SPINE, AND THORAX

Sternocleidomastoid

- Origin: Sternal head—manubrium of sternum; clavicular head—medial clavicle (see Fig. 1.35)
- Insertion: Mastoid process of temporal bone, superior nuchal line of occipital bone
- Action: One side—neck flexion, neck lateral flexion, neck contralateral rotation
- Innervation: Spinal accessory (CN XI), C2-3
- Arterial Supply: Occipital, superior thyroid

Anterior Scalene

- Origin: Transverse processes of C3-6 vertebrae
- Insertion: First rib
- Action: Neck flexion, neck lateral flexion, neck contralateral rotation, and first rib elevation
- Innervation: Ventral rami of C4-6
- Arterial Supply: Transverse cervical, inferior thyroid

Splenius Capitis

- Origin: Ligamentum nuchae, spinous processes of C7 vertebra, and spinous processes of T1-4 vertebrae
- Insertion: Mastoid process of temporal bone, superior nuchal line of occiput
- Action: Neck extension, neck lateral flexion, and neck rotation

- Innervation: C2-4
- Arterial Supply: Occipital, transverse cervical

Splenius Cervicis

- Origin: Spinous processes of T3-6 vertebrae
- Insertion: Transverse processes of C1-3 vertebrae
- Action: Neck extension, neck lateral flexion, and neck rotation
- Innervation: C4-8
- Arterial Supply: Occipital, transverse cervical

Trapezius

- Origin: Upper portion—superior nuchal line, external occipital protuberance, ligamentum nuchae, C7 spinous process of vertebra; middle portion—T1-5 spinous processes of vertebrae; lower portion—T6-12 spinous processes of vertebrae
- Insertion: Upper portion—lateral clavicle; middle portion—acromion process of scapula, spine of scapula; lower portion—root of spine of scapula
- Action: Upper portion—neck extension, neck lateral flexion, neck contralateral rotation, scapular elevation, scapular upward rotation; middle portion—scapular retraction, scapular upward rotation; lower portion—scapular depression, scapular upward rotation
- Innervation: Spinal accessory (CN XI), C2-4
- Arterial Supply: Transverse cervical, dorsal scapular

Quadratus Lumborum

- Origin: Posterior iliac crest, iliolumbar ligament
- Insertion: 12th rib, transverse processes of L1-4 vertebrae
- Action: Trunk lateral flexion, trunk extension, pelvic elevation, pelvic anterior tilt, and 12th rib depression
- Innervation: T12, L1-4
- Arterial Supply: Lumbar, iliolumbar

Rectus Abdominis

- Origin: Pubic crest, pubic symphysis
- Insertion: Fifth to seventh costal cartilage, xiphoid process of sternum
- Action: Trunk flexion, pelvic posterior tilt, and trunk lateral flexion
- Innervation: Intercostals (T7-12)
- Arterial Supply: Lower intercostals, inferior epigastric

Transverse Abdominis

- Origin: Inguinal ligament, iliac crest, 7th to 12th costal cartilage, and thoracolumbar fascia
- Insertion: Pubic crest, abdominal aponeurosis, and linea alba
- Action: Compresses abdominal contents

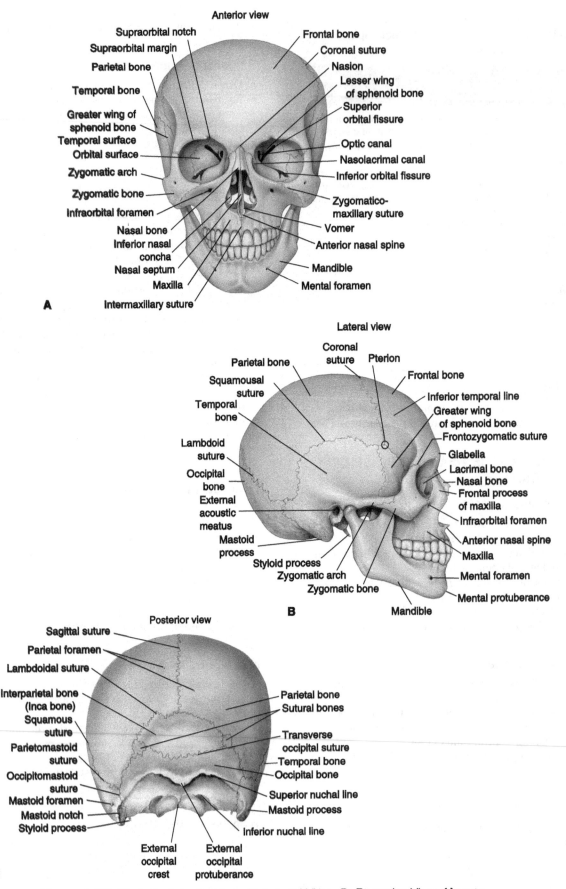

Anterior view

- Supraorbital notch
- Supraorbital margin
- Parietal bone
- Temporal bone
- Greater wing of sphenoid bone
- Temporal surface
- Orbital surface
- Zygomatic arch
- Zygomatic bone
- Infraorbital foramen
- Nasal bone
- Inferior nasal concha
- Nasal septum
- Maxilla
- Intermaxillary suture

- Frontal bone
- Coronal suture
- Nasion
- Lesser wing of sphenoid bone
- Superior orbital fissure
- Optic canal
- Nasolacrimal canal
- Inferior orbital fissure
- Zygomatico-maxillary suture
- Vomer
- Anterior nasal spine
- Mandible
- Mental foramen

A

Lateral view

- Parietal bone
- Squamousal suture
- Temporal bone
- Lambdoid suture
- Occipital bone
- External acoustic meatus
- Mastoid process
- Styloid process
- Zygomatic arch
- Zygomatic bone

- Coronal suture
- Pterion
- Frontal bone
- Inferior temporal line
- Greater wing of sphenoid bone
- Frontozygomatic suture
- Glabella
- Lacrimal bone
- Nasal bone
- Frontal process of maxilla
- Infraorbital foramen
- Anterior nasal spine
- Maxilla
- Mental foramen
- Mental protuberance
- Mandible

B

Posterior view

- Sagittal suture
- Parietal foramen
- Lambdoidal suture
- Interparietal bone (Inca bone)
- Squamous suture
- Parietomastoid suture
- Occipitomastoid suture
- Mastoid foramen
- Mastoid notch
- Styloid process
- External occipital crest
- External occipital protuberance

- Parietal bone
- Sutural bones
- Transverse occipital suture
- Temporal bone
- Occipital bone
- Superior nuchal line
- Mastoid process
- Inferior nuchal line

C

Figure 1.28 Skull. **A:** Anterior View. **B:** Lateral View. **C:** Posterior View. (Assets provided by Anatomical Chart Co.)

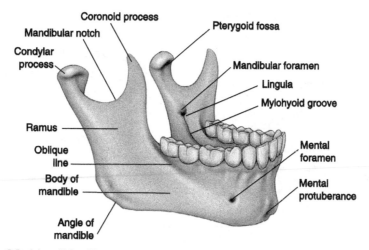

Figure 1.29 Mandible. (Assets provided by Anatomical Chart Co.)

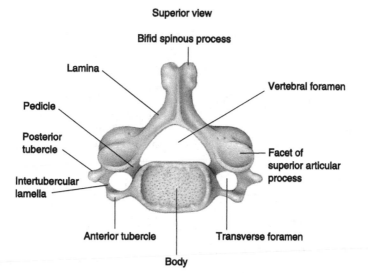

Figure 1.30 Fifth Cervical Vertebra (Superior View). (Assets provided by Anatomical Chart Co.)

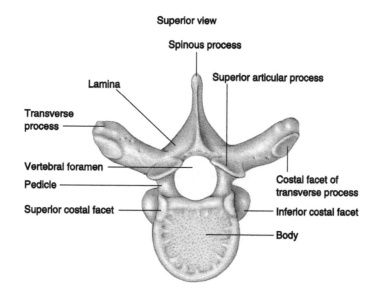

Figure 1.31 Seventh Thoracic Vertebra (Superior View). (Assets provided by Anatomical Chart Co.)

Superior view

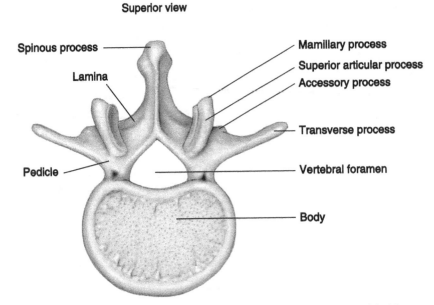

Spinous process

Lamina

Pedicle

Mamillary process

Superior articular process

Accessory process

Transverse process

Vertebral foramen

Body

Figure 1.32 Second Lumbar Vertebra (Superior View). (Assets provided by Anatomical Chart Co.)

- Innervation: Intercostals (T7-12), iliohypogastric (T12, L1), and ilioinguinal (L1)
- Arterial Supply: Inferior epigastric

External Abdominal Oblique

- Origin: 5th to 12th ribs
- Insertion: Iliac crest, pubic crest, inguinal ligament, abdominal aponeurosis, and linea alba
- Action: Trunk flexion, trunk lateral flexion, trunk contralateral rotation, pelvic posterior tilt, and compresses abdominal contents
- Innervation: Intercostals (T8-12), iliohypogastric (T12, L1), and ilioinguinal (L1)
- Arterial Supply: Lower intercostals, inferior epigastric

Internal Abdominal Oblique

- Origin: Inguinal ligament, iliac crest, and thoracolumbar fascia

- Insertion: Pubic crest, 10th to 12th costal cartilage, abdominal aponeurosis, and linea alba
- Action: Trunk flexion, trunk lateral flexion, trunk ipsilateral rotation, pelvic posterior tilt, and compresses abdominal contents
- Innervation: Intercostals (T8 – T12), iliohypogastric (T12, L1), and ilioinguinal (L1)
- Arterial Supply: Subcostal and posterior intercostal, inferior epigastric

 Use the DVD or visit the website at http://thePoint.lww.com/Long for additional material about muscles of the head, neck, spine, and thorax.

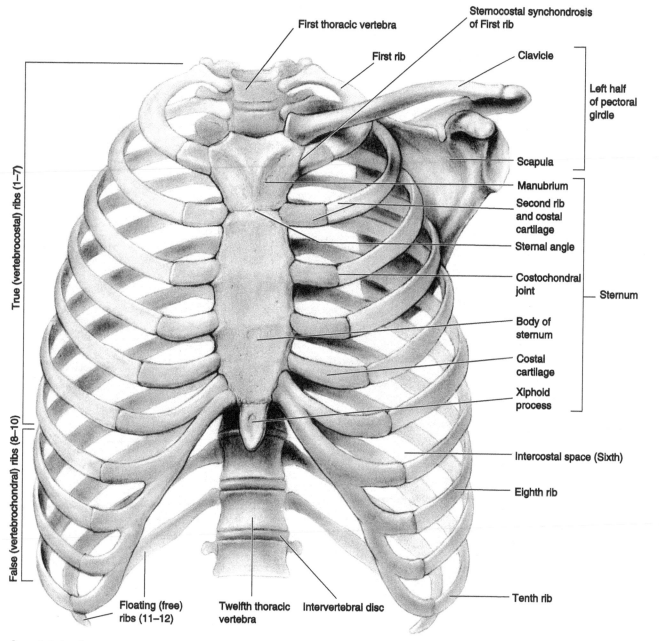

A Anterior view

Figure 1.33 Thoracic Skeleton. **A:** Anterior View. **B:** Posterior View. (From Moore KL, Dalley AF. *Clinical oriented anatomy*, 4th ed. Baltimore: Lippincott Williams & Wilkins; 1999.)

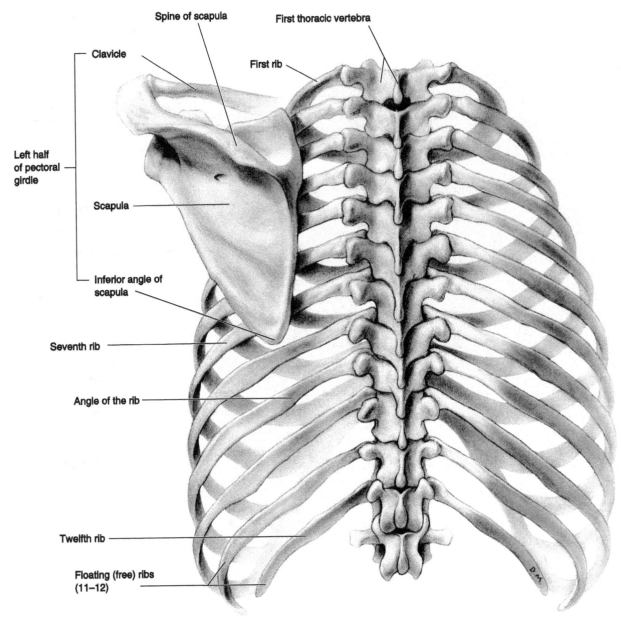

B Posterior view

Figure 1.33 *Continued*

Table 1.3 Major Ligaments of the Head, Neck, Spine, and Thorax

Head and Neck	Spine	Thorax
Atlantooccipital	Anterior longitudinal	Costoclavicular
Atlantoaxial	Posterior longitudinal	Interclavicular
Occipitoaxial	Ligamentum flavum	Sternoclavicular (SC)
Ligamentum nuchae	Intertransverse	
	Capsular	
	Interspinous	
	Supraspinous	
	Iliolumbar	
	Lumbosacral	
	Sacrospinous	
	Sacrotuberous	

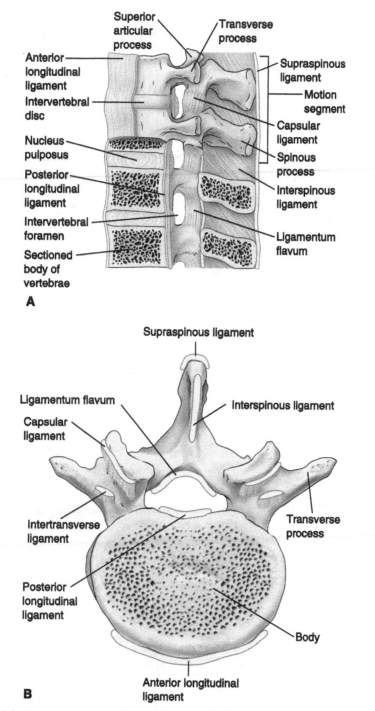

Figure 1.34 Ligaments of the Spine. **A:** Sagittal View. **B:** Transverse View. (From Anderson MK, Parr GP, Hall SJ, et al. *Foundations of athletic training: prevention, assessment, and management*, 4th ed. Baltimore: Lippincott Williams & Wilkins; 2009.)

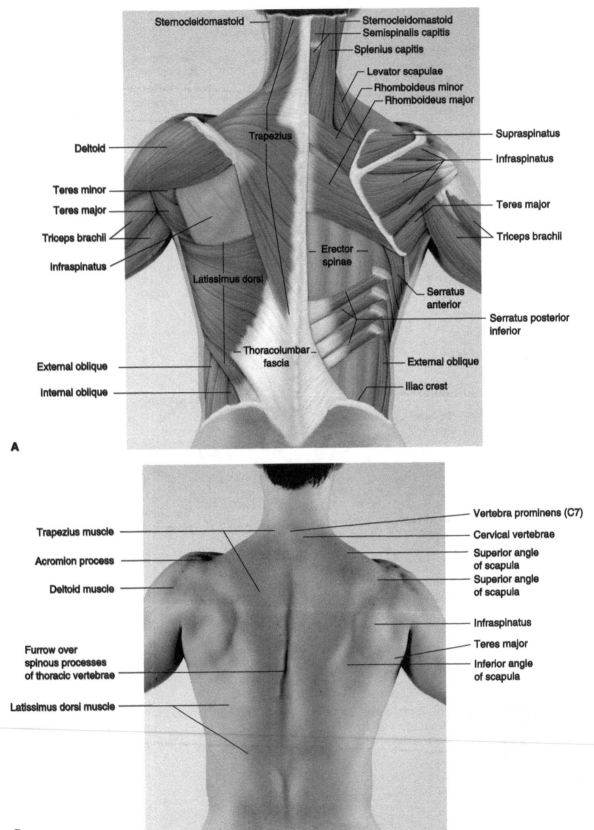

Figure 1.35 Muscles of the Head, Neck, Spine, and Thorax. **A:** Posterior View. **B:** Posterior View-Surface. **C:** Anterior View. **D:** Anterior View-Surface. (From Premkumar K. *The massage connection anatomy and physiology*. Baltimore: Lippincott Williams & Wilkins; 2004.)

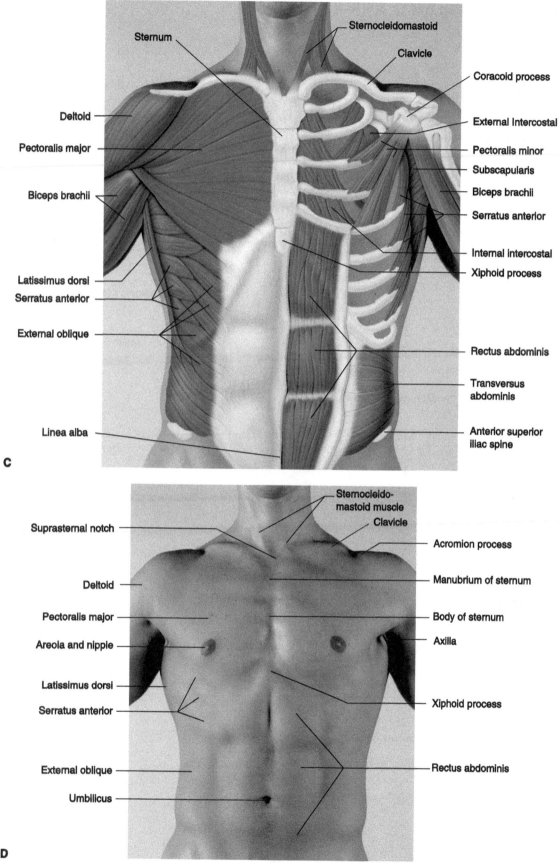

C

- Sternum
- Sternocleidomastoid
- Clavicle
- Coracoid process
- Deltoid
- External Intercostal
- Pectoralis major
- Pectoralis minor
- Subscapularis
- Biceps brachii
- Biceps brachii
- Serratus anterior
- Internal intercostal
- Xiphoid process
- Latissimus dorsi
- Serratus anterior
- External oblique
- Rectus abdominis
- Transversus abdominis
- Linea alba
- Anterior superior iliac spine

D

- Suprasternal notch
- Sternocleido-mastoid muscle
- Clavicle
- Acromion process
- Deltoid
- Manubrium of sternum
- Pectoralis major
- Body of sternum
- Areola and nipple
- Axilla
- Latissimus dorsi
- Serratus anterior
- Xiphoid process
- External oblique
- Rectus abdominis
- Umbilicus

Figure 1.35 *Continued*

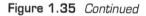

ARTERIES OF THE HEAD, NECK, SPINE, AND THORAX

See Figure 1.36.

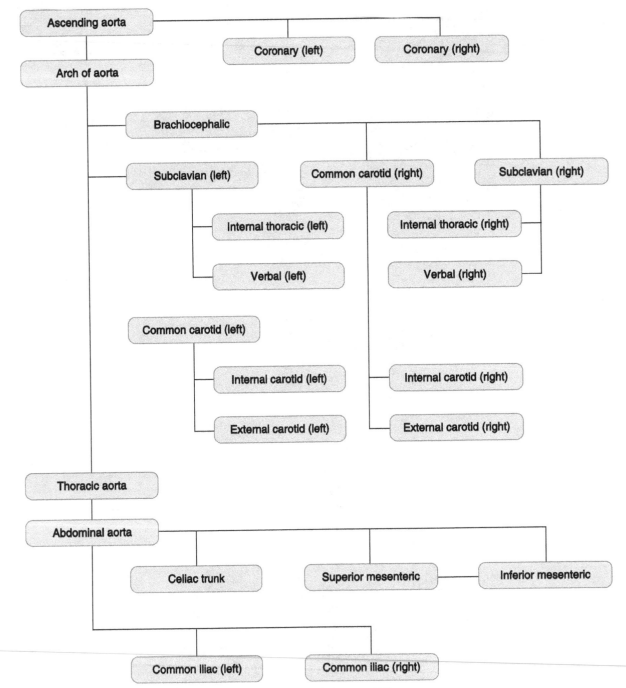

Figure 1.36 Arteries of the Head, Neck, Spine, and Thorax.

NERVES OF THE HEAD, NECK, SPINE, AND THORAX

Nerves of the Cervical Plexus

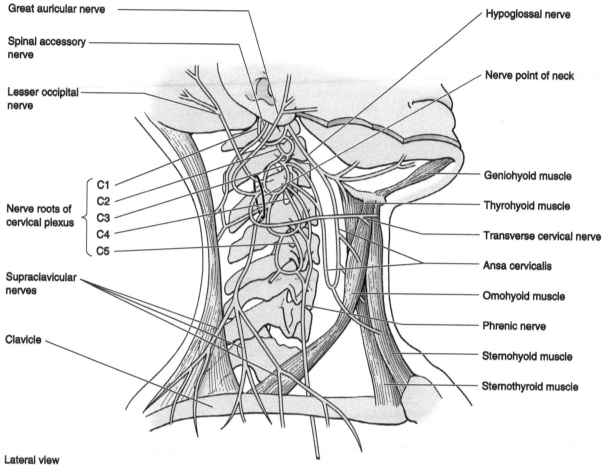

Great auricular nerve

Spinal accessory nerve

Lesser occipital nerve

Nerve roots of cervical plexus
- C1
- C2
- C3
- C4
- C5

Supraclavicular nerves

Clavicle

Hypoglossal nerve

Nerve point of neck

Geniohyoid muscle

Thyrohyoid muscle

Transverse cervical nerve

Ansa cervicalis

Omohyoid muscle

Phrenic nerve

Sternohyoid muscle

Sternothyroid muscle

Lateral view

Figure 1.37 Nerves of the Cervical Plexus. (From Moore KL, Dalley AF. *Clinical oriented anatomy*, 4th ed. Baltimore: Lippincott Williams & Wilkins; 1999.)

Nerves of the Lumbar Plexus

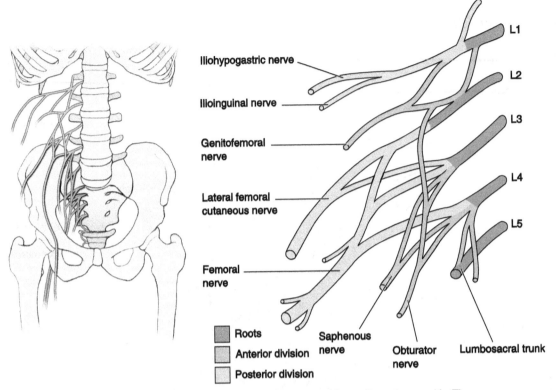

Figure 1.38 Nerves of the Lumbar Plexus. (Adapted from Premkumar K. *The massage connection anatomy and physiology*. Baltimore: Lippincott Williams & Wilkins; 2004.)

Nerves of the Sacral Plexus

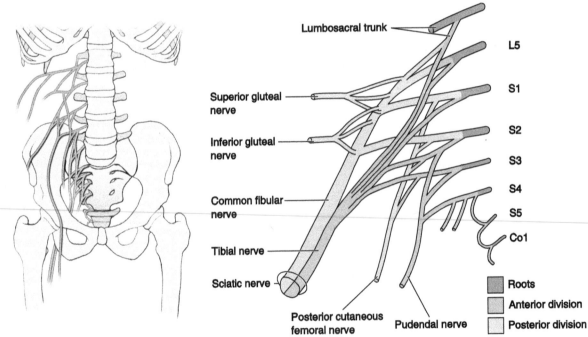

Figure 1.39 Nerves of the Sacral Plexus. (Adapted from Premkumar K. *The massage connection anatomy and physiology*. Baltimore: Lippincott Williams & Wilkins; 2004.)

Anatomy of the Upper Extremity

KEY TERMS

- Circumflex
- Labrum
- Prehension

BONES OF THE UPPER EXTREMITY

See Table 1.4.
See Figures 1.40 to 1.44.

> **Quick fact**
> Most of the force transmitted through the forearm goes through the radius.

MAJOR LIGAMENTS OF THE UPPER EXTREMITY

See Table 1.5.
See Figures 1.45 to 1.48.

> **Quick fact**
> The coracoacromial, or "arch" ligament, forms part of the roof of the subacromial space.

MAJOR ARTERIES OF THE UPPER EXTREMITY

See Figure 1.49.

Table 1.4 Bones of the Upper Extremity

Shoulder Girdle	Upper Arm and Forearm	Wrist and Hand
Scapula	Humerus	Scaphoid
Clavicle	Radius	Lunate
	Ulna	Triquetrum
		Pisiform
		Trapezium
		Trapezoid
		Capitate
		Hamate
		First to fifth metacarpals
		First to fifth proximal, middle, and distal phalanges

MAJOR NERVES OF THE UPPER EXTREMITY

Nerves of the Brachial Plexus

See Figure 1.50.

Major Nerves of the Arm

See Figure 1.51.

MUSCLES OF THE SHOULDER COMPLEX, UPPER ARM, ELBOW, FOREARM, WRIST, AND HAND

See Figure 1.52.

Pectoralis Major

- Origin: Clavicular portion—medial clavicle; sternocostal portion—sternum, first to sixth costal cartilage
- Insertion: Lateral lip of intertubercular (bicipital) groove of humerus
- Action: Shoulder flexion, shoulder adduction, shoulder internal rotation, shoulder extension, shoulder abduction, scapular depression, and scapular protraction
- Innervation: Lateral pectoral (C5-7), medial pectoral (C8, T1)
- Arterial Supply: Pectoral branches of thoracoacromial trunk, posterior intercostals, and lateral thoracic

Deltoid

- Origin: Anterior portion—lateral clavicle; middle portion—acromion process of scapula; posterior portion—spine of scapula
- Insertion: Deltoid tuberosity of humerus
- Action: Anterior portion—shoulder abduction, shoulder flexion, shoulder internal rotation; middle portion—shoulder abduction; posterior portion—shoulder abduction, shoulder extension, shoulder external rotation
- Innervation: Axillary (C5-6)
- Arterial Supply: Anterior humeral circumflex, posterior humeral circumflex, and thoracoacromial

Lattisimus Dorsi

- Origin: T7-12 spinous process of vertebrae, L1-5 spinous processes of vertebrae, sacrum, iliac crest, 10th to 12th ribs, and inferior angle of scapula
- Insertion: Medial lip of intertubercular (bicipital) groove of humerus

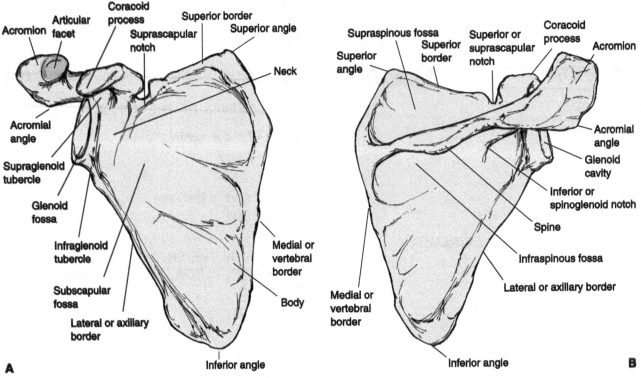

Figure 1.40 Scapula. **A:** Anterior View. **B:** Posterior View. (From Oatis CA. *Kinesiology: the mechanics and pathomechanics of human movement.* Baltimore: Lippincott Williams & Wilkins; 2003.)

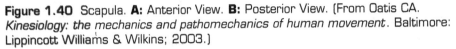

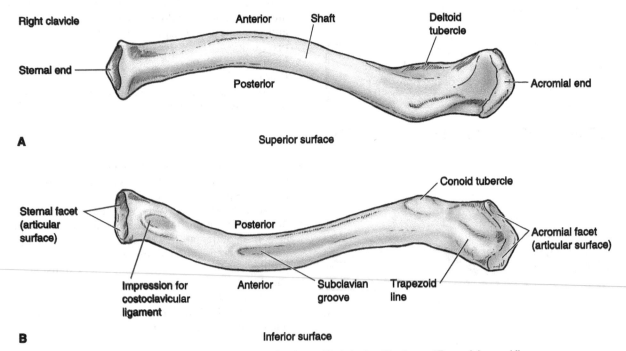

Figure 1.41 Clavicle. **A:** Superior Surface. **B:** Inferior Surface. (From Moore KL, Dalley AF. *Clinical oriented anatomy*, 4th ed. Baltimore: Lippincott Williams & Wilkins; 1999.)

Anterior view

Posterior view

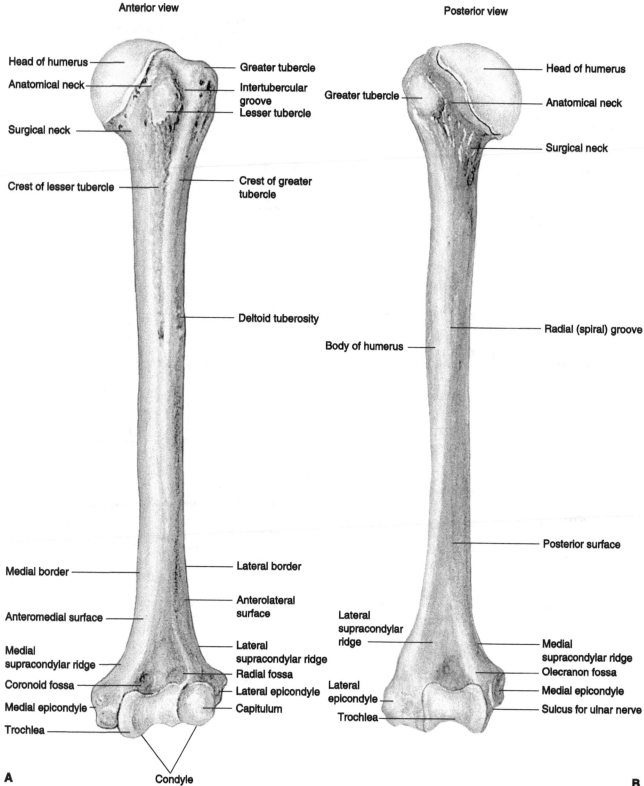

Head of humerus

Greater tubercle

Anatomical neck

Intertubercular groove

Lesser tubercle

Surgical neck

Crest of lesser tubercle

Crest of greater tubercle

Deltoid tuberosity

Greater tubercle

Head of humerus

Anatomical neck

Surgical neck

Body of humerus

Radial (spiral) groove

Posterior surface

Medial border

Lateral border

Anterolateral surface

Anteromedial surface

Lateral supracondylar ridge

Medial supracondylar ridge

Radial fossa

Coronoid fossa

Lateral epicondyle

Medial epicondyle

Capitulum

Trochlea

Condyle

Lateral supracondylar ridge

Lateral epicondyle

Trochlea

Medial supracondylar ridge

Olecranon fossa

Medial epicondyle

Sulcus for ulnar nerve

A

B

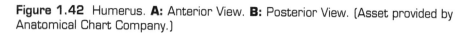

Figure 1.42 Humerus. **A:** Anterior View. **B:** Posterior View. (Asset provided by Anatomical Chart Company.)

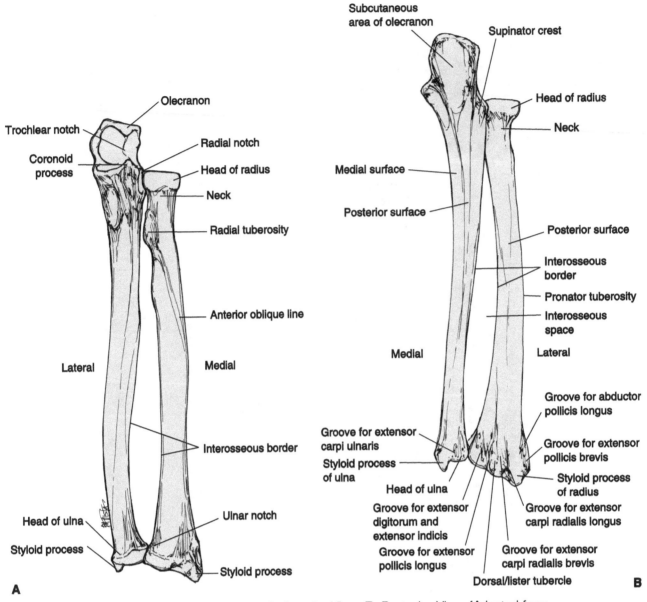

Figure 1.43 Radius and Ulna. **A:** Anterior View. **B:** Posterior View. (Adapted from Premkumar K. *The massage connection anatomy and physiology*. Baltimore: Lippincott Williams & Wilkins; 2004.)

Palmar view

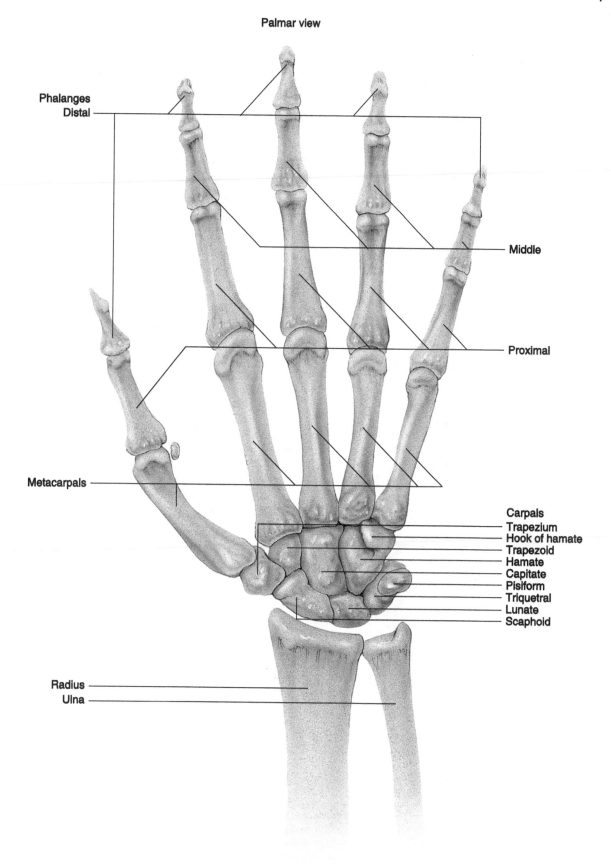

Phalanges
Distal

Middle

Proximal

Metacarpals

Carpals
Trapezium
Hook of hamate
Trapezoid
Hamate
Capitate
Pisiform
Triquetral
Lunate
Scaphoid

Radius
Ulna

Figure 1.44 Bones of the Wrist and Hand (Palmar View). (Asset provided by Anatomical Chart Company.)

Table 1.5 Major Ligaments of the Upper Extremity

Shoulder Complex	Elbow	Wrist and Hand
Coracoclavicular (CC)—Trapezoid and Conoid	Radial collateral (RCL)	Ulnar collateral of wrist
Acromioclavicular (AC)	Lateral ulnar collateral	Radial collateral of wrist
Coracoacromial (Arch)	Accessory lateral collateral	Capitotriquetral
Coracohumeral	Ulnar collateral (UCL)	Lunotriquetral
Superior glenohumeral	Annular	Ulnolunate
Middle glenohumeral		(Ulnolunate–triquetral)
Inferior glenohumeral		Capitoscaphoid
Transverse humeral		Radioscaphocapitate
		Scapulolunate
		Radiolunate (radiolunotriquetral)
		Radioscapholunate
		Palmar
		Dorsal
		Interossei
		Radial collateral of finger
		Ulnar collateral of finger

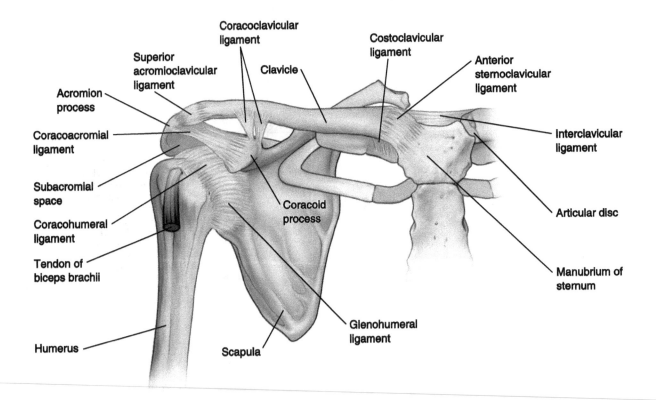

Figure 1.45 Ligaments of the Shoulder Complex (Anterior View). (From Anderson MK, Parr GP, Hall SJ, et al. *Foundations of athletic training: prevention, assessment, and management*, 4th ed. Baltimore: Lippincott Williams & Wilkins; 2009.)

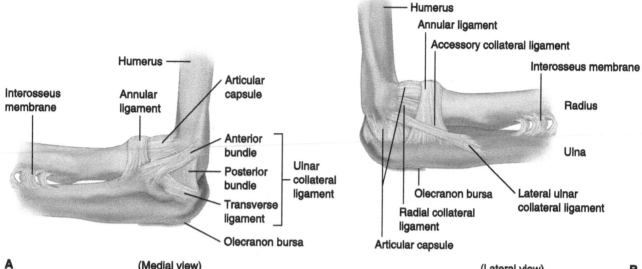

A (Medial view) (Lateral view) **B**

Figure 1.46 Ligaments of the Elbow. **A:** Medial View. **B:** Lateral View. (From Anderson MK, Parr GP, Hall SJ, et al. *Foundations of athletic training: prevention, assessment, and management*, 4th ed. Baltimore: Lippincott Williams & Wilkins; 2009.)

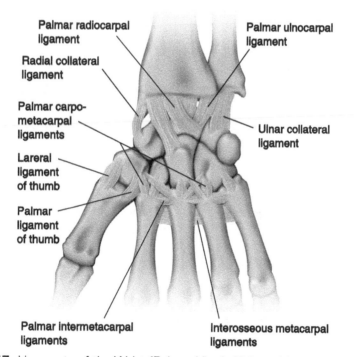

Figure 1.47 Ligaments of the Wrist (Palmar View). (Adapted from Premkumar K. *The massage connection anatomy and physiology*. Baltimore: Lippincott Williams & Wilkins; 2004.)

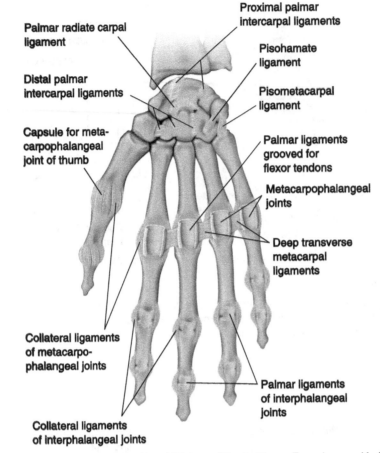

Palmar radiate carpal ligament

Distal palmar intercarpal ligaments

Capsule for meta- carpophalangeal joint of thumb

Proximal palmar intercarpal ligaments

Pisohamate ligament

Pisometacarpal ligament

Palmar ligaments grooved for flexor tendons

Metacarpophalangeal joints

Deep transverse metacarpal ligaments

Collateral ligaments of metacarpo- phalangeal joints

Collateral ligaments of interphalangeal joints

Palmar ligaments of interphalangeal joints

Figure 1.48 Ligaments of the Hand (Palmar View). (From Premkumar K. *The massage connection anatomy and physiology.* Baltimore: Lippincott Williams & Wilkins; 2004.)

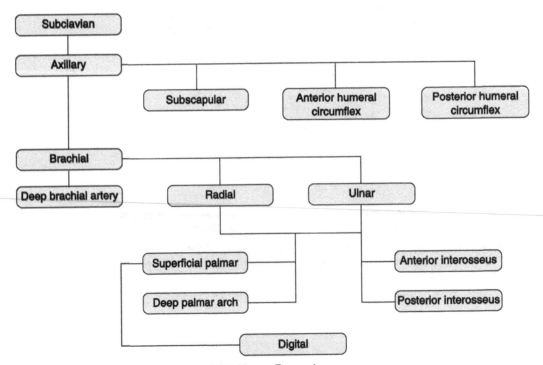

Figure 1.49 Major Arteries of the Upper Extremity.

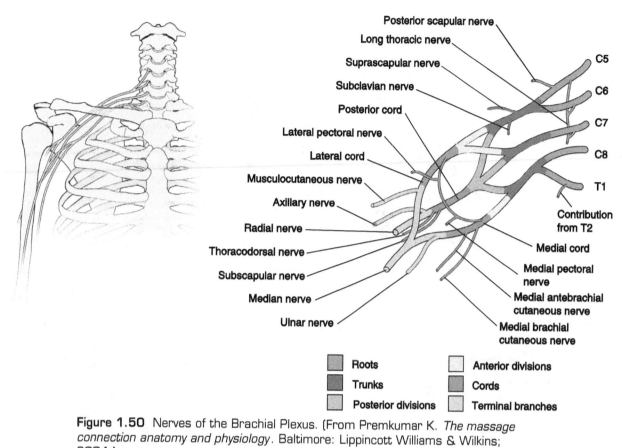

Figure 1.50 Nerves of the Brachial Plexus. (From Premkumar K. *The massage connection anatomy and physiology*. Baltimore: Lippincott Williams & Wilkins; 2004.)

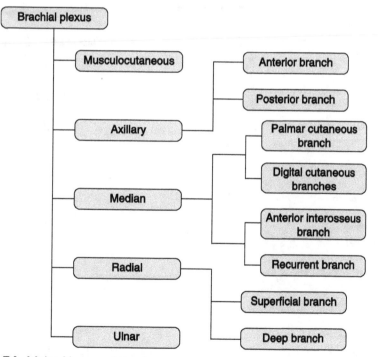

Figure 1.51 Major Nerves of the Arm.

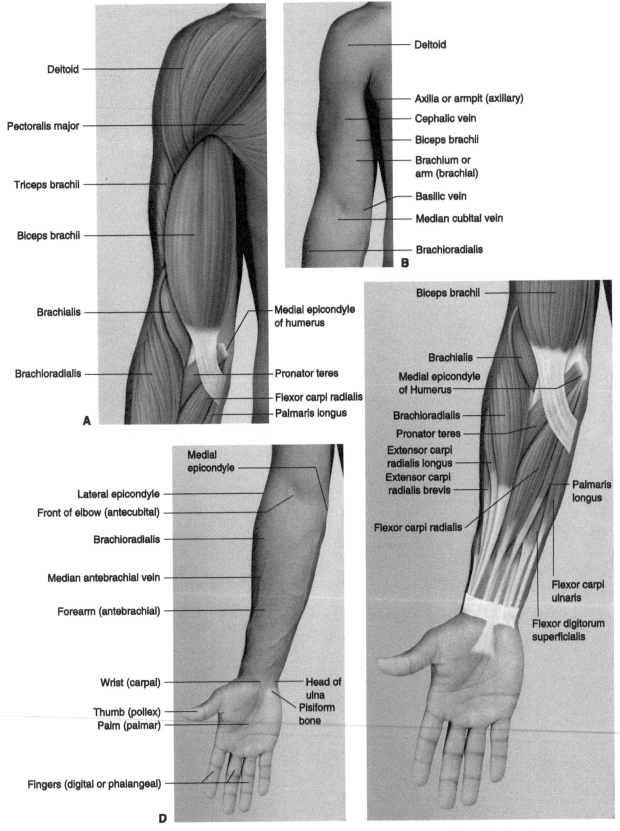

Figure 1.52 Muscles of the Upper Limb. **A:** Anterior View-Upper Arm. **B:** Anterior View-Upper Arm Surface. **C:** Anterior View-Lower Arm. **D:** Anterior View-Lower Arm Surface. **E:** Posterior View-Upper Arm. **F:** Posterior View-Upper Arm Surface. **G:** Posterior View-Lower Arm. **H:** Posterior View-Lower Arm Surface. (From Premkumar K. *The massage connection anatomy and physiology*. Baltimore: Lippincott Williams & Wilkins; 2004.)

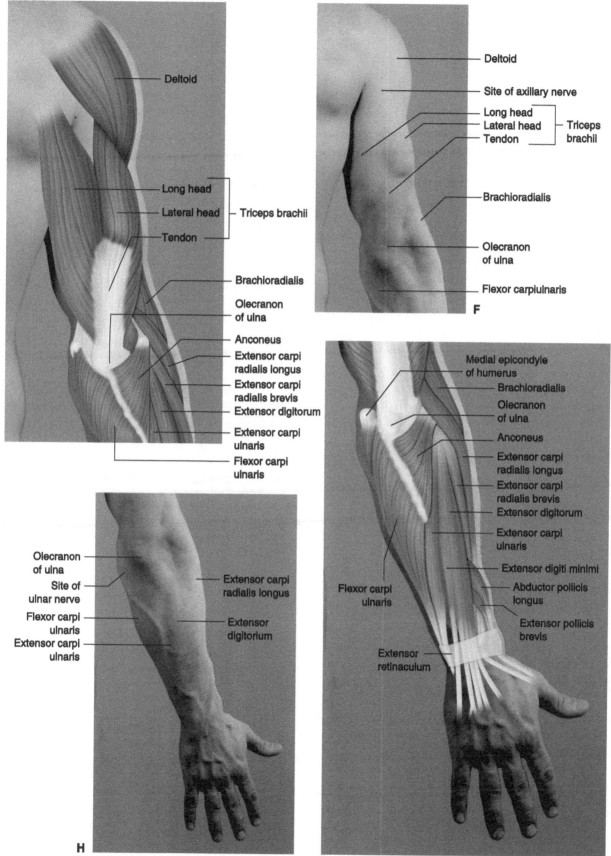

Figure 1.52 *Continued*

- Action: Shoulder extension, shoulder adduction, shoulder internal rotation, and pelvic anterior tilt
- Innervation: Thoracodorsal (C6-8)
- Arterial Supply: Subscapular, transverse cervical, and thoracodorsal

Supraspinatus

- Origin: Supraspinous fossa of scapula
- Insertion: Greater tuberosity of humerus
- Action: Shoulder abduction
- Innervation: Suprascapular (C5-6)
- Arterial Supply: Suprascapular

Infraspinatus

- Origin: Infraspinous fossa of scapula
- Insertion: Greater tuberosity of humerus
- Action: Shoulder external rotation
- Innervation: Suprascapular (C5-6)
- Arterial Supply: Suprascapular, circumflex scapular

Teres Minor

- Origin: Axillary border of scapula
- Insertion: Greater tuberosity of humerus
- Action: Shoulder external rotation
- Innervation: Axillary (C5-6)
- Arterial Supply: Circumflex scapular, posterior circumflex humeral

Subscapularis

- Origin: Subscapular fossa of scapula
- Insertion: Lesser tuberosity of humerus
- Action: Shoulder internal rotation
- Innervation: Upper and lower subscapular (C5-6)
- Arterial Supply: Subscapular, transverse cervical

> **Quick fact** The supraspinatus, infraspinatus, teres minor, and subscapularis (S.I.T.S. muscles) comprise the rotator cuff.

Teres Major

- Origin: Axillary border of scapula
- Insertion: Medial lip of intertubercular (bicipital) groove of humerus
- Action: Shoulder internal rotation, shoulder adduction, shoulder extension, and scapular upward rotation
- Innervation: Lower subscapular (C5-6)
- Arterial Supply: Subscapular

Rhomboid Major

- Origin: T2-5 spinous processes of vertebrae
- Insertion: Vertebral border of scapula
- Action: Scapular retraction, scapular elevation, and scapular downward rotation
- Innervation: Dorsal scapular (C4-5)
- Arterial Supply: Dorsal scapular

Rhomboid Minor

- Origin: C7 spinous process of vertebra, spinous process of T1 vertebra
- Insertion: Vertebral border of scapula
- Action: Scapular retraction, scapular elevation, and scapular downward rotation
- Innervation: Dorsal scapular (C4-5)
- Arterial Supply: Dorsal scapular

Serratus Anterior

- Origin: First to ninth ribs
- Insertion: Vertebral border of scapula
- Action: Scapular protraction, scapular upward rotation
- Innervation: Long thoracic (C5-7)
- Arterial Supply: Lateral thoracic, thoracodorsal

> **Quick fact** The muscles of the "shoulder girdle" do not attach to the humerus.

Coracobrachialis

- Origin: Coracoid process of scapula
- Insertion: Middle one third of humerus
- Action: Shoulder flexion, shoulder adduction
- Innervation: Musculocutaneous (C5-7)
- Arterial Supply: Brachial

Biceps Brachii

- Origin: Long head—supraglenoid tubercle of scapula; short head—coracoid process of scapula
- Insertion: Radial tuberosity
- Action: Long head—elbow flexion, forearm supination, shoulder flexion, shoulder abduction; short head—elbow flexion, forearm supination, shoulder flexion, shoulder adduction
- Innervation: Musculocutaneous (C5, C6)
- Arterial Supply: Brachial

> **Quick fact** The long head of the biceps tendon attaches to the glenoid labrum.

Brachialis

- Origin: Distal one half of humerus
- Insertion: Coronoid process of ulna, ulnar tuberosity
- Action: Elbow flexion
- Innervation: Musculocutaneous (C5-6)
- Arterial Supply: Brachial

Triceps Brachii

- Origin: Long head—infraglenoid tubercle of scapula; lateral head—proximal one half of humerus; medial head—distal one half of humerus

- Insertion: Olecranon process of ulna
- Action: Long head—elbow extension, shoulder extension, shoulder adduction; lateral head—elbow extension; medial head—elbow extension
- Innervation: Radial (C7-8)
- Arterial Supply: Deep brachial, posterior humeral circumflex

Brachioradialis
- Origin: Lateral supracondylar ridge of humerus
- Insertion: Radial styloid process
- Action: Elbow flexion, forearm supination, forearm pronation
- Innervation: Radial (C5, C6)
- Arterial Supply: Radial

Pronator Teres
- Origin: Medial supracondylar ridge of humerus, coronoid process of ulna
- Insertion: Middle one third of lateral radius
- Action: Forearm pronation, elbow flexion
- Innervation: Median (C6-7)
- Arterial Supply: Radial, ulnar

Supinator
- Origin: Lateral epicondyle of humerus, supinator crest of ulna
- Insertion: Proximal one third of lateral radius
- Action: Forearm supination
- Innervation: Radial (C6)
- Arterial Supply: Radial, posterior interosseus

Flexor Carpi Ulnaris
- Origin: Medial epicondyle of humerus, proximal two thirds of posterior ulna
- Insertion: Pisiform, hook of hamate, base of fifth metacarpal
- Action: Wrist flexion, wrist ulnar deviation, and elbow flexion
- Innervation: Ulnar (C7-8)
- Arterial Supply: Ulnar

Flexor Carpi Radialis
- Origin: Medial epicondyle of humerus
- Insertion: Base of second metacarpal, base of third metacarpal
- Action: Wrist flexion, wrist radial deviation, elbow flexion, and forearm pronation
- Innervation: Median (C6-7)
- Arterial Supply: Ulnar

Palmaris Longus
- Origin: Medial epicondyle of humerus
- Insertion: Palmar aponeurosis
- Action: Wrist flexion, forearm pronation, and elbow flexion

- Innervation: Median nerve (C6-7)
- Arterial Supply: Ulnar

 Quick fact The palmaris longus muscle is absent in some people.

Flexor Digitorum Superficialis
- Origin: Ulnar head—medial epicondyle of humerus, coronoid process of ulna; radial head—proximal two thirds of anterior radius
- Insertion: Palmar aspect of second to fifth middle phalanges
- Action: Finger flexion at second to fifth metacarpophalangeal joints, finger flexion at second to fifth proximal interphalangeal joints, wrist flexion, elbow flexion
- Innervation: Median (C7-8, T1)
- Arterial Supply: Ulnar

Flexor Digitorum Profundus
- Origin: Proximal three fourths of anteromedial ulna
- Insertion: Base of second to fifth distal phalanges
- Action: Finger flexion at second to fifth metacarpophalangeal joints, finger flexion at second to fifth proximal interphalangeal joints, finger flexion at second to fifth distal interphalangeal joints, wrist flexion
- Innervation: Median (C8, T1), ulnar (C8, T1)
- Arterial Supply: Anterior interosseus

Quick fact A rupture of the flexor digitorum profundus tendon is known as *jersey finger*.

Flexor Pollicis Longus
- Origin: Middle anterior aspect of radius, medial epicondyle of humerus, and coronoid process of ulna
- Insertion: Base of distal phalanx of thumb
- Action: Thumb flexion at the carpometacarpal joint, thumb flexion at metacarpophalangeal joint, thumb flexion at interphalangeal joint, wrist flexion, wrist radial deviation, and elbow flexion
- Innervation: Median, anterior interosseous branch (C8, T1)
- Arterial Supply: Radial, anterior interosseus

Extensor Digitorum
- Origin: Lateral epicondyle of humerus
- Insertion: Dorsal aspect of base of second to fifth middle phalanges, dorsal aspect of base of second to fifth distal phalanges
- Action: Finger extension at second to fifth metacarpophalangeal joints, finger extension at second to fifth proximal interphalangeal joints, finger extension at second to fifth distal PIP joints, wrist extension, and elbow extension

- Innervation: Radial (C6-8), posterior interosseus
- Arterial Supply: Ulnar

Extensor Carpi Ulnaris
- Origin: Lateral epicondyle of humerus, middle one third of posterior ulnar
- Insertion: Dorsal aspect of base of the fifth metacarpal
- Action: Wrist extension, wrist ulnar deviation, and elbow extension
- Innervation: Radial (C6-8), posterior interosseus
- Arterial Supply: Ulnar

Extensor Carpi Radialis Longus
- Origin: Distal one third of lateral supracondylar ridge of humerus, lateral epicondyle of humerus
- Insertion: Dorsal aspect of base of the second metacarpal
- Action: Wrist extension, wrist radial deviation, forearm pronation, and elbow extension
- Innervation: Radial (C6-7)
- Arterial Supply: Radial

Extensor Pollicis Longus
- Origin: Posterolateral aspect of middle one third of ulna
- Insertion: Dorsal aspect of base of first distal phalanx
- Action: Thumb extension at carpometacarpal joint, thumb extension at metacarpophalangeal joint, thumb extension at proximal interphalangeal joint, wrist extension, wrist radial deviation, and forearm supination

- Innervation: Radial (C6-8), posterior interosseus
- Arterial Supply: Posterior interosseus

Extensor Pollicis Brevis
- Origin: Posterior radius
- Insertion: Dorsal aspect of base of first proximal phalanx
- Action: Thumb extension at carpometacarpal joint, thumb extension at metacarpophalangeal joint, thumb abduction, wrist radial deviation, and wrist extension
- Innervation: Radial (C6-7), posterior interosseus
- Arterial Supply: Posterior interosseus

Abductor Pollicis Longus
- Origin: Middle one third of posterior radius, middle posterior ulna
- Insertion: Dorsal aspect of base of first metacarpal
- Action: Thumb abduction, thumb extension at carpometacarpal joint, wrist radial deviation, and forearm supination
- Innervation: Radial (C6-7), posterior interosseus
- Arterial Supply: Posterior interosseus

 Use the DVD or visit the website at http://thePoint.lww.com/Long for additional material about the *muscles of the shoulder, upper arm, elbow, forearm, wrist, and hand.*

PART 4 Anatomy of the Lower Extremity

BONES OF THE LOWER EXTREMITY

See Table 1.6.
See Figures 1.53 to 1.57.

> **Quick fact** The sesamoid bones of the great toe are embedded in the flexor hallucis longus tendon, which provides the muscle with a mechanical advantage.

MAJOR LIGAMENTS OF THE LOWER EXTREMITY

See Table 1.7.
See Figures 1.58 to 1.61.

> **Quick fact** The calcaneonavicular, or "spring," ligament helps support the medial longitudinal arch.

MAJOR ARTERIES OF THE LOWER EXTREMITY

See Figure 1.62.

MAJOR NERVES OF THE LOWER EXTREMITY

See Figure 1.63.

Table 1.6 Bones of the Lower Extremity

Pelvic Girdle	Upper and Lower Leg	Ankle and Foot
Ilium	Femur	Talus
Ischium	Tibia	Calcaneus
Pubis	Fibula	Navicular
	Patella	First to third (medial, intermediate, lateral) cuneiforms
		Cuboid
		First to fifth metatarsals
		First to fifth proximal, middle, and distal phalanges
		Sesamoids bones of the great toe

MUSCLES OF THE HIP, THIGH, KNEE, LOWER LEG, ANKLE, AND FOOT

Iliacus

- Origin: Iliac fossa, anterior inferior iliac spine, and sacral ala
- Insertion: Lesser trochanter of femur
- Action: Hip flexion, hip external rotation, and pelvic anterior tilt
- Innervation: Femoral (L2-4)
- Arterial Supply: External iliac, hypogastric, iliolumbar, and medial femoral circumflex

Psoas Major

- Origin: T12 body of vertebra, L1-5 transverse processes of vertebra, L1-5 bodies of vertebrae
- Insertion: Lesser trochanter of femur
- Action: Hip flexion, hip external rotation, trunk flexion, trunk lateral flexion, trunk contralateral rotation, and pelvic anterior tilt
- Innervation: Lumbar plexus, anterior branches (L2-4)
- Arterial Supply: External iliac, internal iliac, lumbar, and iliolumbar

> *Quick* **fact** The iliacus, psoas major, and psoas minor comprise the iliopsoas muscle group.

Gluteus Medius

- Origin: Lateral aspect of ilium
- Insertion: Greater trochanter of femur
- Action: Anterior portion—hip abduction, hip flexion, hip internal rotation, pelvic anterior tilt; posterior portion—hip abduction, hip extension, hip external rotation, pelvic posterior tilt
- Innervation: Superior gluteal (L4-5, S1)
- Arterial Supply: Superior gluteal

Gluteus Minimus

- Origin: Lateral aspect of ilium
- Insertion: Greater trochanter of femur
- Action: Anterior portion—hip abduction, hip flexion, hip internal rotation, pelvic anterior tilt; posterior portion—hip abduction, hip extension, hip external rotation, pelvic posterior tilt
- Innervation: Superior gluteal (L4-5, S1)
- Arterial Supply: Superior gluteal

Gluteus Maximus

- Origin: Sacrum, coccyx, posterior iliac crest, and thoracolumbar fascia
- Insertion: Gluteal tuberosity of femur, iliotibial band, and Gerdy tubercle of tibia
- Action: Upper portion—hip extension, hip external rotation, hip abduction, pelvic posterior tilt; lower portion—hip extension, hip internal rotation, hip adduction, pelvic posterior tilt
- Innervation: Inferior gluteal (L5, S1-2)
- Arterial Supply: Superior gluteal, inferior gluteal, and medial femoral circumflex

Piriformis

- Origin: Anterior sacrum, posterior ischium, greater sciatic notch, and obturator foramen (see Fig. 1.64)
- Insertion: Greater trochanter of femur
- Action: Hip external rotation, hip abduction, and hip extension
- Innervation: First sacral (S1), second sacral (S2)
- Arterial Supply: Superior gluteal, inferior gluteal

> *Quick* **fact** A tight piriformis muscle can place pressure on the sciatic nerve, resulting in neurologic symptoms that radiate down the posterior thigh.

Rectus Femoris

- Origin: Anterior inferior iliac spine, superior to acetabulum
- Insertion: Patella, patellar tendon, and tibial tuberosity
- Action: Hip flexion, pelvic anterior tilt, and knee extension
- Innervation: Femoral (L2-4)
- Arterial Supply: Femoral

Vastus Medialis

- Origin: Intertrochanteric line of the femur, linea aspera of the femur, and medial supracondylar ridge
- Insertion: Patella, patella tendon, and tibial tuberosity

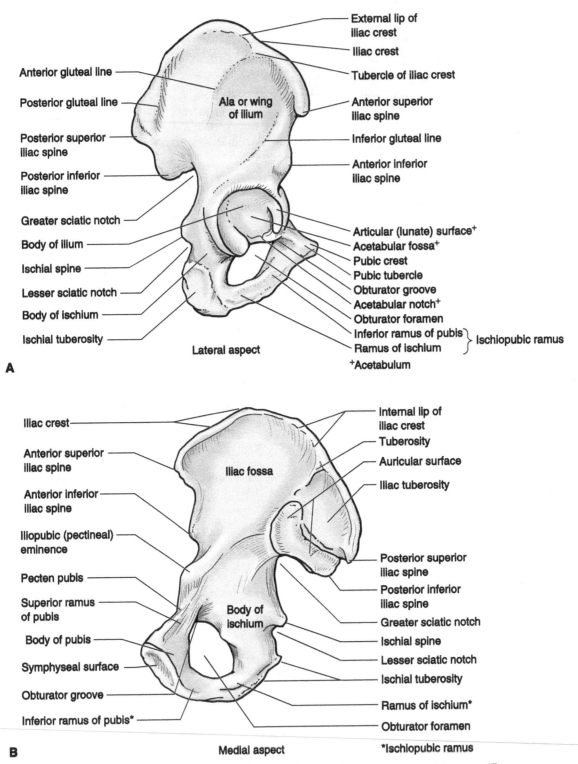

External lip of
iliac crest

Iliac crest

Tubercle of iliac crest

Anterior superior
iliac spine

Inferior gluteal line

Anterior inferior
iliac spine

Anterior gluteal line

Posterior gluteal line

Posterior superior
iliac spine

Posterior inferior
iliac spine

Greater sciatic notch

Body of ilium

Ischial spine

Lesser sciatic notch

Body of ischium

Ischial tuberosity

Ala or wing
of ilium

Articular (lunate) surface+

Acetabular fossa+

Pubic crest

Pubic tubercle

Obturator groove

Acetabular notch+

Obturator foramen

Inferior ramus of pubis
Ramus of ischium } Ischiopubic ramus

+Acetabulum

Lateral aspect

A

Iliac crest

Anterior superior
iliac spine

Anterior inferior
iliac spine

Iliopubic (pectineal)
eminence

Pecten pubis

Superior ramus
of pubis

Body of pubis

Symphyseal surface

Obturator groove

Inferior ramus of pubis*

Iliac fossa

Body of
ischium

Internal lip of
iliac crest

Tuberosity

Auricular surface

Iliac tuberosity

Posterior superior
iliac spine

Posterior inferior
iliac spine

Greater sciatic notch

Ischial spine

Lesser sciatic notch

Ischial tuberosity

Ramus of ischium*

Obturator foramen

B

Medial aspect

*Ischiopubic ramus

Figure 1.53 Bones of the Pelvic Girdle. **A:** Lateral Aspect. **B:** Medial Aspect. (From Moore KL, Dalley AF. *Clinical oriented anatomy*, 4th ed. Baltimore: Lippincott Williams & Wilkins; 1999.)

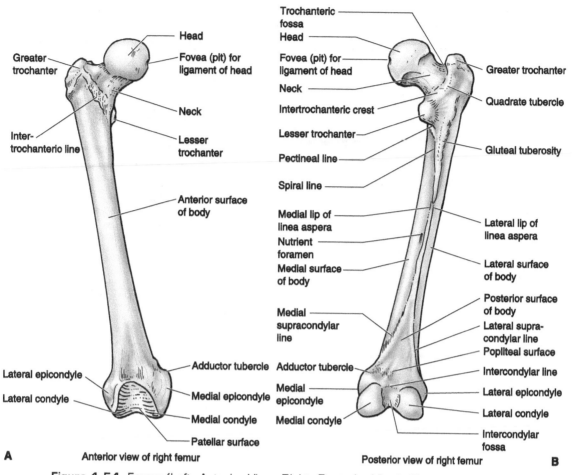

Greater trochanter

Head

Fovea (pit) for ligament of head

Neck

Lesser trochanter

Inter-trochanteric line

Anterior surface of body

Lateral epicondyle

Lateral condyle

Adductor tubercle

Medial epicondyle

Medial condyle

Patellar surface

A   Anterior view of right femur

Trochanteric fossa

Head

Fovea (pit) for ligament of head

Neck

Intertrochanteric crest

Lesser trochanter

Pectineal line

Spiral line

Medial lip of linea aspera

Nutrient foramen

Medial surface of body

Medial supracondylar line

Adductor tubercle

Medial epicondyle

Medial condyle

Greater trochanter

Quadrate tubercle

Gluteal tuberosity

Lateral lip of linea aspera

Lateral surface of body

Posterior surface of body

Lateral supra-condylar line

Popliteal surface

Intercondylar line

Lateral epicondyle

Lateral condyle

Intercondylar fossa

Posterior view of right femur   **B**

Figure 1.54 Femur (Left, Anterior View; Right, Posterior View). (From Moore KL, Dalley AF. *Clinical oriented anatomy*, 4th ed. Baltimore: Lippincott Williams & Wilkins; 1999.)

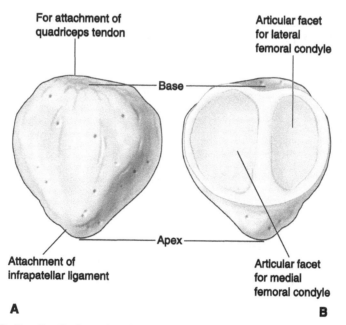

For attachment of quadriceps tendon

Articular facet for lateral femoral condyle

Base

Apex

Attachment of infrapatellar ligament

Articular facet for medial femoral condyle

A

B

Figure 1.55 Patella. **A:** Anterior View. **B:** Posterior View. (From Anderson MK, Parr GP, Hall SJ, et al. *Foundations of athletic training: prevention, assessment, and management*, 4th ed. Baltimore: Lippincott Williams & Wilkins; 2009.)

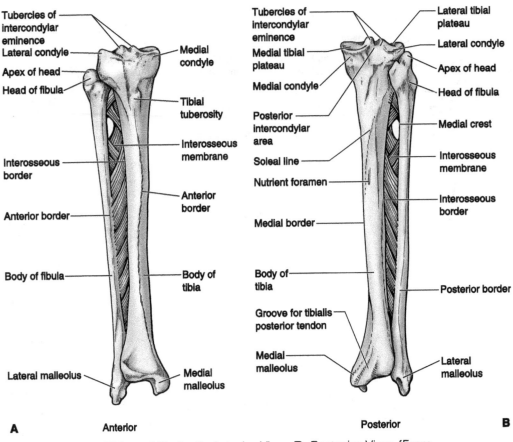

Figure 1.56 Tibia and Fibula. **A:** Anterior View. **B:** Posterior View. (From Moore KL, Dalley AF. *Clinical oriented anatomy*, 4th ed. Baltimore: Lippincott Williams & Wilkins; 1999.)

Table 1.7 Major Ligaments of the Lower Extremity

Pelvis and Hip	Knee	Lower Leg, Ankle, and Foot
Inguinal	Anterior cruciate (ACL)	Anterior tibiofibular
Ligamentum teres	Posterior cruciate (PCL)	Posterior tibiofibular
Ischiofemoral	Medial (tibial) collateral (MCL)	Crural interosseus
Iliofemoral (Y ligament of Bigalow)	Lateral (fibular) collateral (LCL)	Anterior talofibular (ATF)
Pubofemoral	Transverse	Calcaneofibular (CF)
	Coronary	Posterior talofibular (PTF)
	Patellomeniscal	Deltoid
	Ligament of Wrisberg	Calcaneonavicular ("spring")
	Ligament of Humphrey	Long plantar
	Oblique popliteal	Bifurcate
	Arcuate popliteal	Dorsal tarsal
	Posterior meniscofemoral	Plantar tarsal
	Posterior ligament of the fibular head	Interosseous tarsal
		Plantar calcaneocuboid
		Dorsal calcaneocuboid
		Dorsal
		Plantar
		Interosseous
		Deep transverse
		Collateral of toes

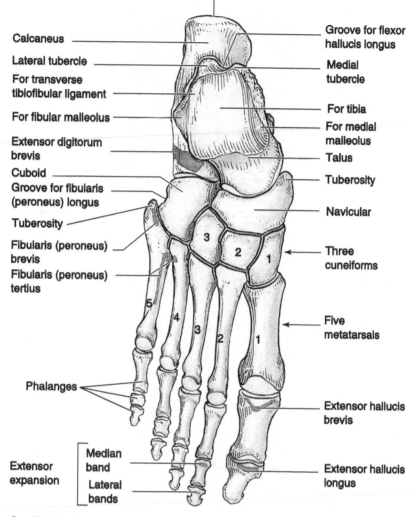

Calcaneal tuberosity (posterior surface)

Calcaneus

Lateral tubercle

For transverse tibiofibular ligament

For fibular malleolus

Extensor digitorum brevis

Cuboid

Groove for fibularis (peroneus) longus

Tuberosity

Fibularis (peroneus) brevis

Fibularis (peroneus) tertius

Phalanges

Extensor expansion

Median band

Lateral bands

Groove for flexor hallucis longus

Medial tubercle

For tibia

For medial malleolus

Talus

Tuberosity

Navicular

Three cuneiforms

Five metatarsals

Extensor hallucis brevis

Extensor hallucis longus

A Dorsal view

Figure 1.57 Bones of the Foot. **A:** Dorsal View. **B:** Plantar View. (From Moore KL, Dalley AF. *Clinical oriented anatomy*, 4th ed. Baltimore: Lippincott Williams & Wilkins; 1999.)

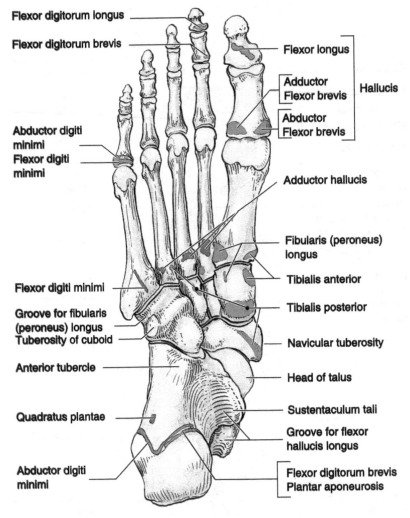

Flexor digitorum longus

Flexor digitorum brevis

Flexor longus

Adductor
Flexor brevis

Abductor
Flexor brevis

Hallucis

Abductor digiti minimi
Flexor digiti minimi

Adductor hallucis

Fibularis (peroneus) longus

Tibialis anterior

Flexor digiti minimi

Tibialis posterior

Groove for fibularis (peroneus) longus
Tuberosity of cuboid

Navicular tuberosity

Anterior tubercle

Head of talus

Quadratus plantae

Sustentaculum tali

Groove for flexor hallucis longus

Abductor digiti minimi

Flexor digitorum brevis
Plantar aponeurosis

B   Plantar view

Figure 1.57 *Continued*

Anterior view

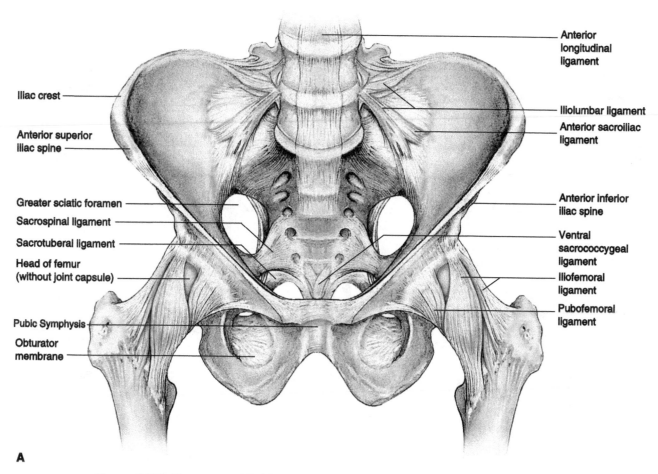

Iliac crest

Anterior superior
iliac spine

Greater sciatic foramen

Sacrospinal ligament

Sacrotuberal ligament

Head of femur
(without joint capsule)

Pubic Symphysis

Obturator
membrane

Anterior
longitudinal
ligament

Iliolumbar ligament

Anterior sacroiliac
ligament

Anterior inferior
iliac spine

Ventral
sacrococcygeal
ligament

Iliofemoral
ligament

Pubofemoral
ligament

A

Figure 1.58 Ligaments of Pelvis and Hip. **A:** Anterior View. **B:** Posterior View.
(Asset provided by Anatomical Chart Company.)

Posterior view

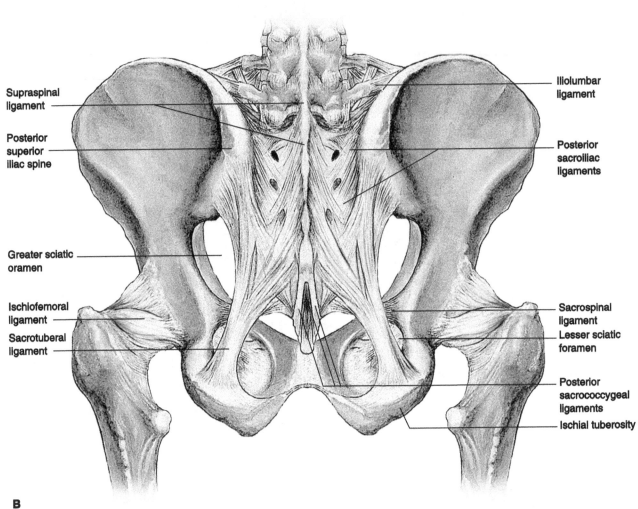

Supraspinal
ligament

Posterior
superior
iliac spine

Greater sciatic
foramen

Ischiofemoral
ligament

Sacrotuberal
ligament

Iliolumbar
ligament

Posterior
sacroiliac
ligaments

Sacrospinal
ligament

Lesser sciatic
foramen

Posterior
sacrococcygeal
ligaments

Ischial tuberosity

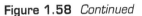

Figure 1.58 *Continued*

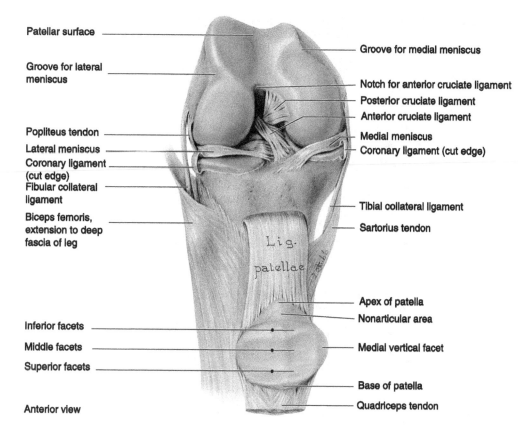

Patellar surface

Groove for lateral meniscus

Popliteus tendon

Lateral meniscus

Coronary ligament (cut edge)

Fibular collateral ligament

Biceps femoris, extension to deep fascia of leg

Inferior facets

Middle facets

Superior facets

Anterior view

Groove for medial meniscus

Notch for anterior cruciate ligament

Posterior cruciate ligament

Anterior cruciate ligament

Medial meniscus

Coronary ligament (cut edge)

Tibial collateral ligament

Sartorius tendon

Lig. patellae

Apex of patella

Nonarticular area

Medial vertical facet

Base of patella

Quadriceps tendon

Figure 1.59 Ligaments of the Knee (Anterior View). (From Moore KL, Dalley AF. *Clinical oriented anatomy*, 4th ed. Baltimore: Lippincott Williams & Wilkins; 1999.)

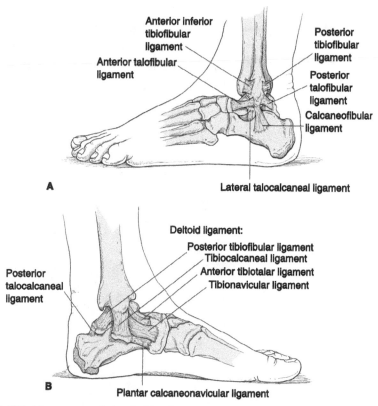

Anterior inferior tibiofibular ligament

Anterior talofibular ligament

Posterior tibiofibular ligament

Posterior talofibular ligament

Calcaneofibular ligament

Lateral talocalcaneal ligament

A

Deltoid ligament:
Posterior tibiofibular ligament
Tibiocalcaneal ligament
Anterior tibiotalar ligament
Tibionavicular ligament

Posterior talocalcaneal ligament

Plantar calcaneonavicular ligament

B

Figure 1.60 Ligaments of the Ankle. **A:** Lateral View. **B:** Medial View. (Cipriano J. *Photographic manual of regional orthopaedic and neurological tests*, 2nd ed. Baltimore: Lippincott Williams & Wilkins; 1991.)

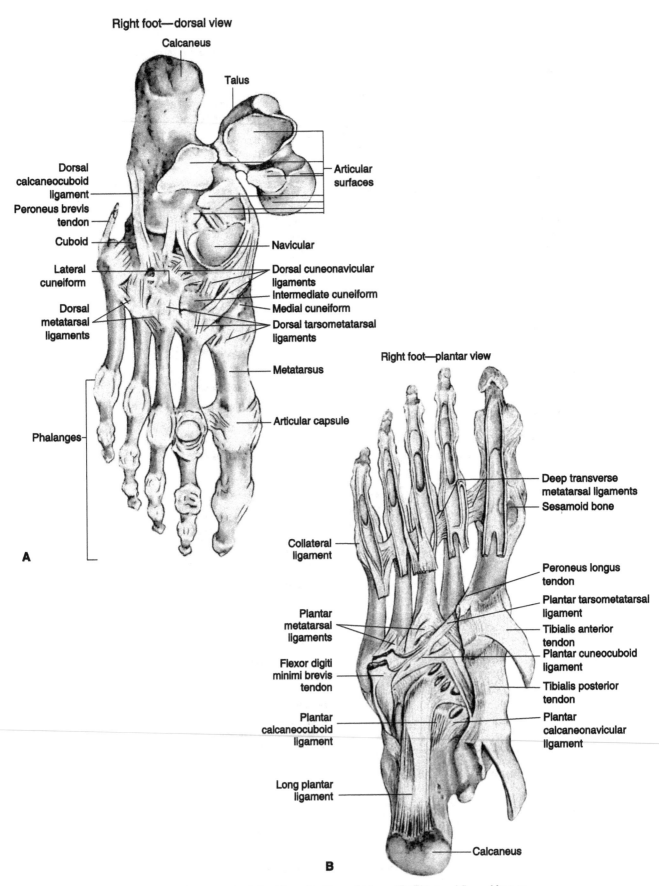

Figure 1.61 Ligaments of the Foot. **A:** Dorsal View. **B:** Plantar View. (Asset provided by Anatomical Chart Company.)

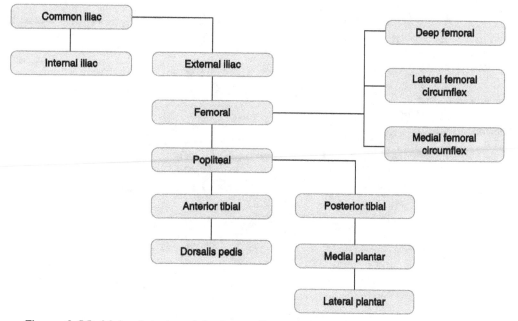

Figure 1.62 Major Arteries of the Lower Extremity.

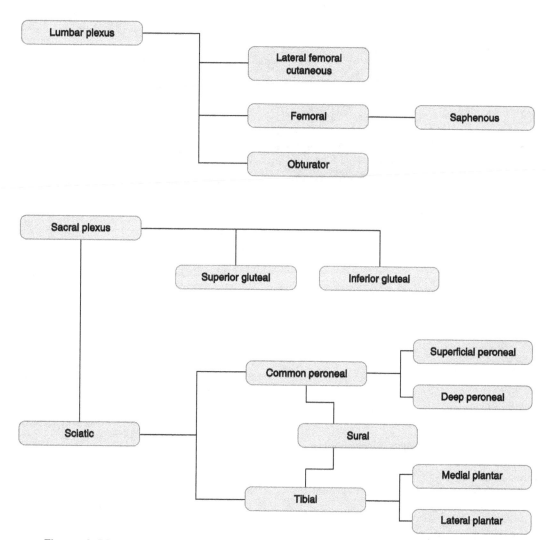

Figure 1.63 Major Nerves of the Lower Extremity.

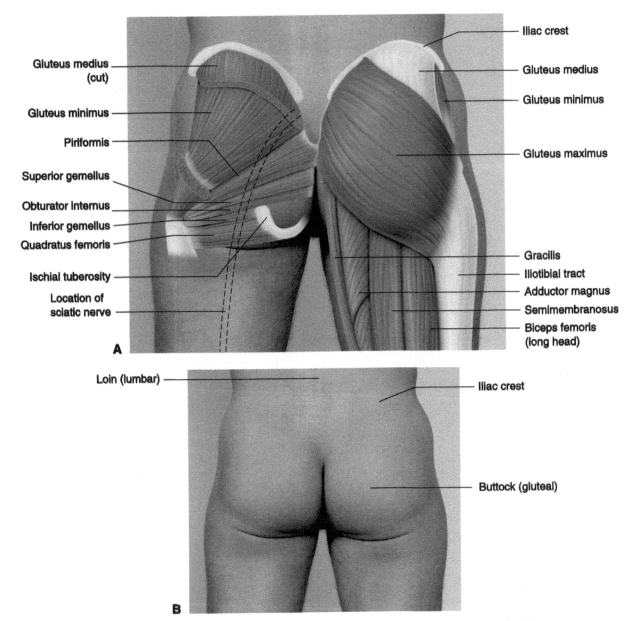

Gluteus medius (cut)

Gluteus minimus

Piriformis

Superior gemellus

Obturator internus

Inferior gemellus

Quadratus femoris

Ischial tuberosity

Location of sciatic nerve

A

Iliac crest

Gluteus medius

Gluteus minimus

Gluteus maximus

Gracilis

Iliotibial tract

Adductor magnus

Semimembranosus

Biceps femoris (long head)

Loin (lumbar)

Iliac crest

Buttock (gluteal)

B

Figure 1.64 Muscles of the Posterior Hip and Buttock. (From Premkumar K. *The massage connection anatomy and physiology*. Baltimore: Lippincott Williams & Wilkins; 2004.)

- Action: Knee extension
- Innervation: Femoral (L2-4)
- Arterial Supply: Femoral

Vastus Lateralis

- Origin: Greater trochanter of femur, intertrochanteric line of femur, gluteal tuberosity of femur, and linea aspera of the femur
- Insertion: Lateral patella, patellar tendon, and tibial tuberosity
- Action: Knee extension
- Innervation: Femoral (L2-L4)
- Arterial Supply: Femoral

Vastus Intermedius

- Origin: Proximal two thirds of anterior femur, linea aspera of femur (see Fig. 1.65)
- Insertion: Patella, patellar tendon, and tibial tuberosity
- Action: Knee extension
- Innervation: Femoral (L2-4)
- Arterial Supply: Femoral

Biceps Femoris

- Origin: Long head—ischial tuberosity; short head—linea aspera of femur, lateral supracondylar ridge
- Insertion: Head of fibula, lateral tibial condyle

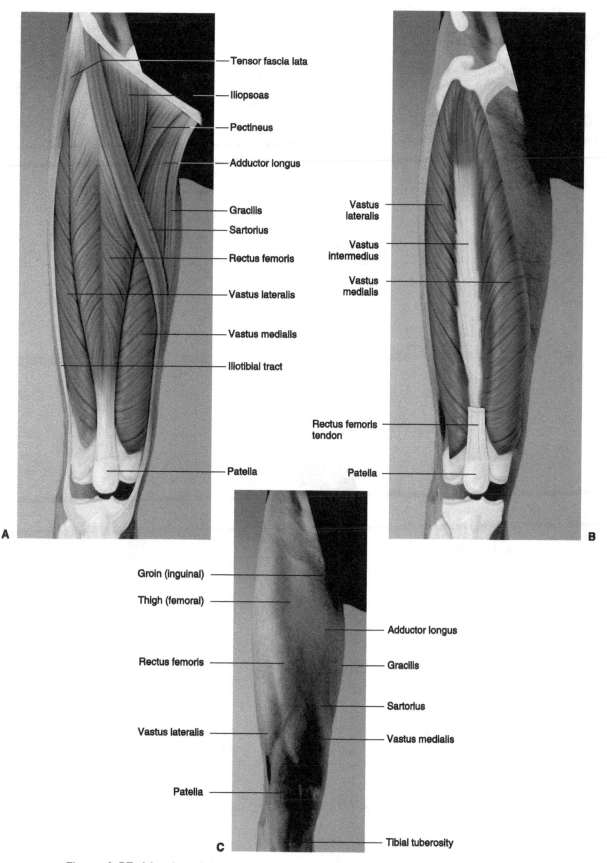

Figure 1.65 Muscles of the Hip and Thigh. **A:** Anterior View-Superficial. **B:** Anterior View-Deep. **C:** Anterior View-Surface. **D:** Posterior View-Superficial. **E:** Posterior View-Deep. **F:** Posterior View-Surface. **G:** Lateral View-Superficial. **H:** Lateral View-Surface. (From Premkumar K. *The massage connection anatomy and physiology*. Baltimore: Lippincott Williams & Wilkins; 2004.)

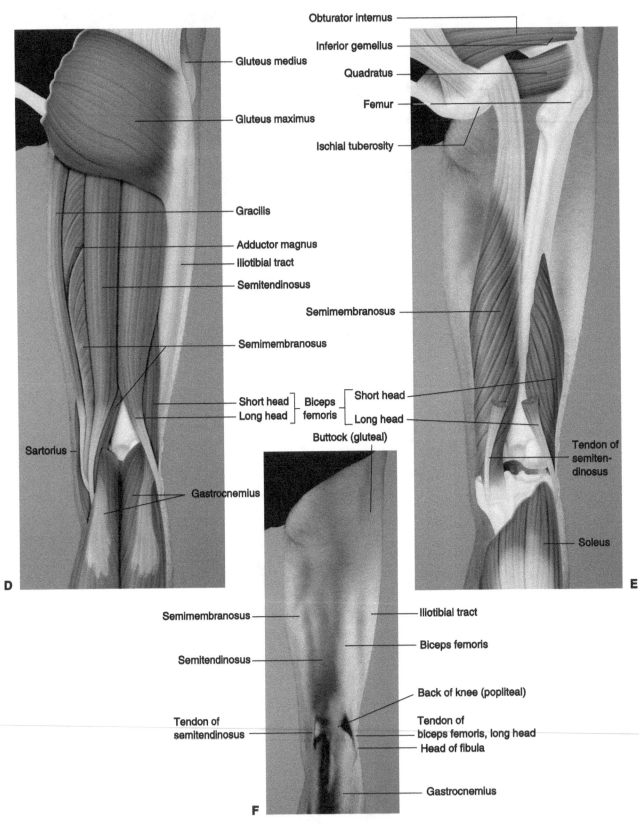

Figure 1.65 *Continued*

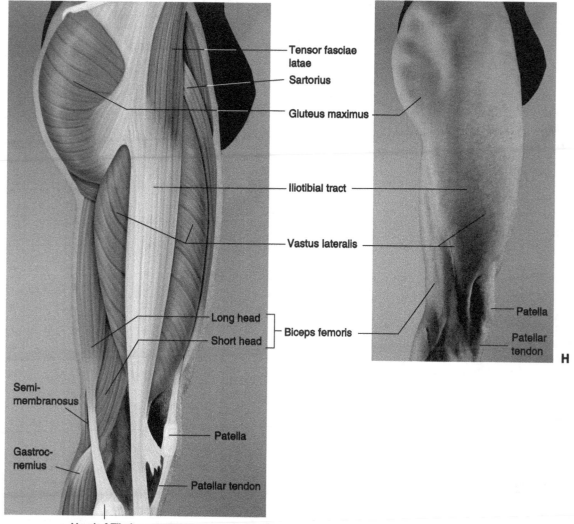

Tensor fasciae latae

Sartorius

Gluteus maximus

Iliotibial tract

Vastus lateralis

Long head

Short head

Biceps femoris

Semi-membranosus

Gastroc-nemius

Patella

Patellar tendon

Head of Fibula

Patella

Patellar tendon

G

H

Figure 1.65 *Continued*

- Action: Long head—hip extension, hip adduction, hip external rotation, knee flexion, knee external rotation, pelvic posterior tilt; short head—knee flexion, knee external rotation
- Innervation: Long head—sciatic, tibial (S1-3); short head—sciatic, peroneal (L5, S1-2)
- Arterial Supply: Long head—deep femoral, inferior gluteal, popliteal

Semimembranosus

- Origin: Ischial tuberosity
- Insertion: Posterior aspect of medial tibial condyle
- Action: Hip extension, hip internal rotation, knee flexion, knee internal rotation, and pelvic posterior tilt
- Innervation: Sciatic, tibial (L5, S1-2)
- Arterial Supply: Deep femoral, inferior gluteal, popliteal

Semitendinosus

- Origin: Ischial tuberosity
- Insertion: Pes anserine of tibia
- Action: Hip extension, hip internal rotation, knee flexion, knee internal rotation, pelvic posterior tilt
- Innervation: Sciatic, tibial (L5, S1-2)
- Arterial Supply: Deep femoral, inferior gluteal, popliteal

Quick **fact** The biceps femoris, semimembranosus, and semitendinosus comprise the muscle group known as the *hamstrings*.

All of the hamstring muscles share a common origin at the ischial tuberosity.

Adductor Magnus

- Origin: Anterior portion—inferior pubic ramus, ischial ramus; posterior portion—ischial tuberosity
- Insertion: Linea aspera of femur, adductor tubercle of femur, gluteal tuberosity, and medial supracondylar ridge
- Action: Hip adduction, hip extension, hip external rotation, hip internal rotation, pelvic posterior tilt, and pelvic elevation
- Innervation: Anterior portion—obturator (L2-4), posterior portion—sciatic (L4-5, S1-3)
- Arterial Supply: Femoral, obturator

Gracilis

- Origin: Pubic symphysis, inferior pubic ramus
- Insertion: Pes anserine of tibia
- Action: Hip adduction, hip flexion, hip internal rotation, knee flexion, knee internal rotation, pelvis anterior tilt, and pelvic elevation
- Innervation: Obturator (L2-4)
- Arterial Supply: Femoral, obturator

Sartorius

- Origin: Anterior superior iliac spine (see Fig. 1.66)
- Insertion: Pes anserine of tibia
- Action: Hip flexion, hip abduction, hip external rotation, pelvic anterior tilt, and knee flexion knee internal rotation
- Innervation: Femoral (L2-3)
- Arterial Supply: Femoral

Quick fact The sartorius is the longest muscle in the body.

Quick fact The semitendinosus, gracilis, and sartorius all insert at the pes anserine of the tibia.

Gastrocnemius

- Origin: Lateral head—posterior aspect of lateral femoral condyle; medial head—posterior aspect of medial femoral condyle
- Insertion: Achilles tendon, calcaneus
- Action: Ankle plantar flexion, knee flexion
- Innervation: Tibial (S1-2)
- Arterial Supply: Posterior tibial, peroneal, and sural branches of popliteal

Soleus

- Origin: Fibular head, proximal one third of fibula, middle one third of tibia

- Insertion: Achilles tendon, calcaneus
- Action: Ankle plantar flexion
- Innervation: Tibial (S1-2)
- Arterial Supply: Posterior tibial, peroneal, and sural branches of popliteal

Quick fact The gastrocnemius and soleus muscles are located within the superficial posterior compartment.

Quick fact The gastrocnemius and the soleus muscles comprise the triceps surae muscle group.

Tibialis Posterior

- Origin: Proximal two thirds of posterior tibia, proximal two thirds of posterior fibula, interosseus membrane
- Insertion: Navicular, cuboid, first cuneiform, second cuneiform, third cuneiform, and base of second to fourth metatarsals
- Action: Ankle plantar flexion, foot inversion
- Innervation: Tibial (L4-5, S1)
- Arterial Supply: Posterior tibial

Flexor Digitorum Longus

- Origin: Middle one third of posterior tibia
- Insertion: Plantar aspect of base of second to fifth distal phalanges
- Action: Ankle plantar flexion, foot inversion, toe flexion at second to fifth metatarsophalangeal joints, toe flexion at second to fifth proximal interphalangeal joints, and toe flexion at second to fifth distal interphalangeal joints
- Innervation: Tibial (L5, S1-2)
- Arterial Supply: Posterior tibial

Flexor Hallucis Longus

- Origin: Distal two thirds of posterior fibula, interosseus membrane
- Insertion: Base of first distal phalanx
- Action: Ankle plantar flexion, foot inversion, great toe flexion at first metatarsophalangeal joint, and great toe flexion at first interphalangeal joint
- Innervation: Tibial (L5, S1-2)
- Arterial Supply: Posterior tibial

Quick fact The tibialis posterior, flexor digitorum longus, and flexor hallucis longus are located within the deep posterior compartment of the lower leg.

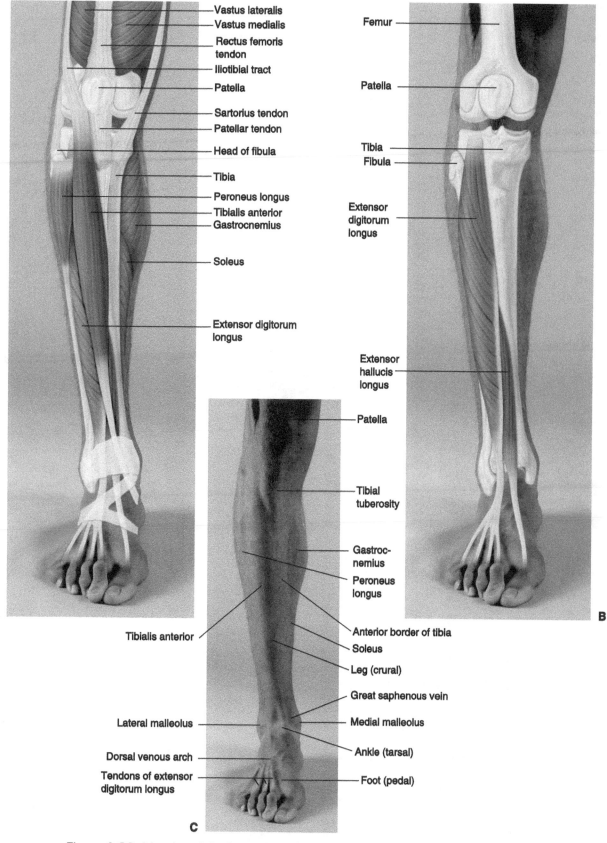

Figure 1.66 Muscles of the Lower Leg. **A:** Anterior View-Superficial. **B:** Anterior View-Deep. **C:** Anterior View-Surface. **D:** Posterior View-Superficial. **E:** Posterior View-Deep. **F:** Posterior View-Surface. **G:** Lateral View-Superficial. **H:** Lateral View-Surface. (From Premkumar K. *The massage connection anatomy and physiology*. Baltimore: Lippincott Williams & Wilkins; 2004.)

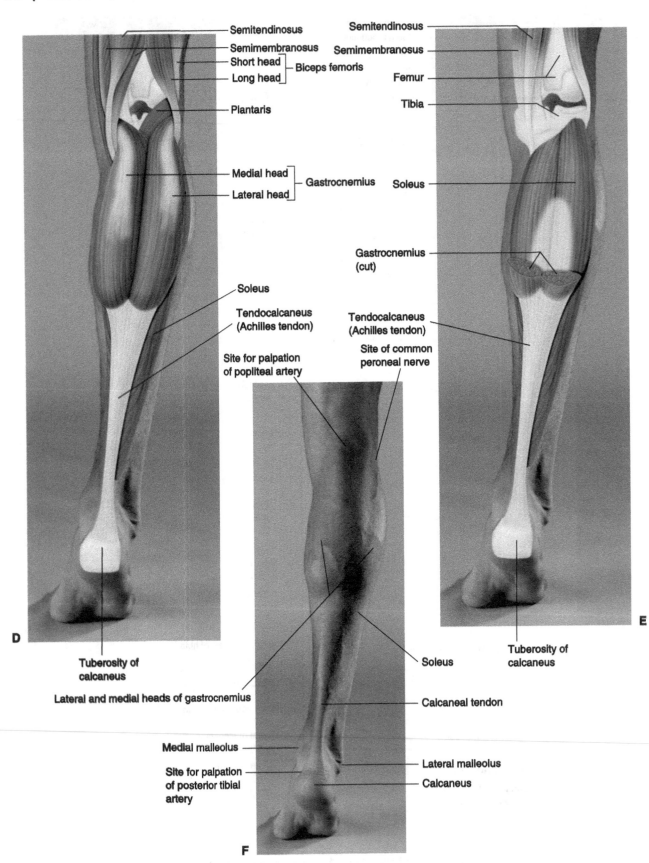

Semitendinosus
Semimembranosus
Short head
Long head ⎤ Biceps femoris
Plantaris
Medial head
Lateral head ⎤ Gastrocnemius
Soleus
Tendocalcaneus (Achilles tendon)
Site for palpation of popliteal artery

Semitendinosus
Semimembranosus
Femur
Tibia
Soleus
Gastrocnemius (cut)
Tendocalcaneus (Achilles tendon)
Site of common peroneal nerve

D

Tuberosity of calcaneus

Lateral and medial heads of gastrocnemius

Medial malleolus

Site for palpation of posterior tibial artery

F

Soleus

Calcaneal tendon

Lateral malleolus

Calcaneus

E

Tuberosity of calcaneus

Figure 1.66 *Continued*

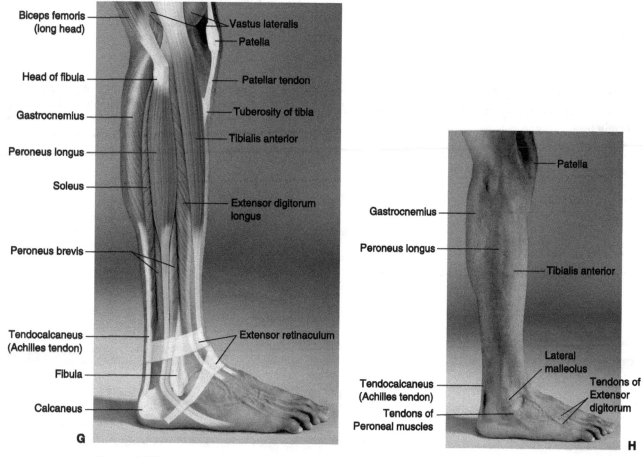

Figure 1.66 *Continued*

Peroneus Longus

- Origin: Fibular head, proximal two thirds of lateral fibula
- Insertion: First cuneiform, base of first metatarsal
- Action: Ankle plantar flexion, foot eversion
- Innervation: Superficial peroneal (L4-5, S1)
- Arterial Supply: Peroneal

Peroneus Brevis

- Origin: Distal two thirds of lateral fibula
- Insertion: Base of fifth metatarsal
- Action: Ankle plantar flexion, foot eversion
- Innervation: Superficial peroneal (L4-5, S1)
- Arterial Supply: Peroneal

Tibialis Anterior

- Origin: Lateral tibial condyle, proximal two thirds of lateral tibia
- Insertion: First cuneiform, base of first metatarsal
- Actions: Ankle dorsiflexion, foot inversion
- Innervation: Deep peroneal (L4-5, S1)
- Arterial Supply: Anterior tibial

Extensor Digitorum Longus

- Origin: Lateral tibial condyle, fibular head, proximal two thirds of anterior fibula, and interosseus membrane
- Insertion: Dorsal aspect of second to fifth middle phalanges, dorsal aspect of second to fifth distal phalanges
- Action: Ankle dorsiflexion, foot eversion, toe extension at second to fifth metatarsophalangeal joints, toe extension at second to fifth proximal interphalangeal

joints, and toe extension at second to fifth distal
interphalangeal joints
- Innervation: Deep peroneal (L4 – L5, S1)
- Arterial Supply: Anterior tibial

Extensor Hallucis Longus

- Origin: Middle one third of anterior fibula, interosseous
  membrane
- Insertion: Base of first distal phalanx
- Action: Ankle dorsiflexion, foot inversion, great toe
  extension at first metatarsophalangeal joint, and great
  toe extension at first interphalangeal joint
- Innervation: Deep peroneal (L4-5, S1)
- Arterial Supply: Anterior tibial

Peroneus Tertius

- Origin: Distal one third of anterior fibula, interosseus
  membrane
- Insertion: Base of fifth metatarsal

- Action: Ankle dorsiflexion, foot eversion
- Innervation: Deep peroneal (L4-5, S1)
- Arterial Supply: Anterior tibial

> **Quick fact** The anterior tibialis, extensor digitorum
> longus, extensor hallucis longus, and
> peroneus tertius are located within the
> anterior compartment of the
> lower leg.

 Use the DVD or visit the website at
http://thePoint.lww.com/Long for additional
material about the *muscles of the hip, thigh, knee,
lower leg, ankle, and foot.*

PART 5   Kinesiology

KEY TERMS

- Ginglymoid joint
- Gomphosis

KINESIOLOGY REFERENCE TERMS

Anatomic Position

- Standing erect (see Fig. 1.67 and
  Table 1.8)
- Facing forward
- Feet parallel and close to each other
- Arms by side
- Palms facing forward
- Fingers and thumbs extended

> **Quick fact** The only difference between the anatomic
> and fundamental positions is that the palms
> of the hands face the side of the body in the
> fundamental position.

 Use the DVD or visit the website at
http://thePoint.lww.com/Long for additional
material about *directional terminology.*

JOINTS

Roles of Joints

- Allow joint movement
- Limit movement
- Provide stability
- Bear body weight
- Absorb shock

Classification of Joints by Structure

See Table 1.9.

Classification of Joints by Function

See Table 1.10.

Anatomy of Synovial Joints

- Joint (synovial) cavity (see Fig. 1.68)
  - Space between articulating surfaces of joint
  - Filled with synovial fluid
- Synovial fluid
  - Fluid within the joint cavity
  - Secreted by synovial membrane
- Joint (articular) capsule
  - Connects bones of synovial joint
  - Encloses joint cavity
  - Composed of two layers—(a) fibrous capsule and
    (b) synovial membrane

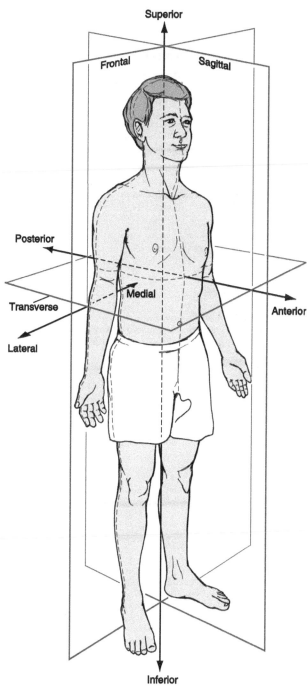

Figure 1.67 Planes of Motion and Axes of Rotation from the Anatomical Position. (From Oatis CA. *Kinesiology: the mechanics and pathomechanics of human movement.* Baltimore: Lippincott Williams & Wilkins; 2003.)

Table 1.8 Planes of Motions and Axes of Rotation

Plane of Motion	Axis of Rotation	Examples of Movements
Sagittal or anteroposterior	Frontal, coronal, or mediolateral	Shoulder flexion, hip extension, Ankle dorsiflexion
Frontal, coronal, or lateral	Sagittal or anteroposterior	Shoulder abduction, wrist adduction, hip adduction
Transverse or horizontal	Vertical, longitudinal, or superoinferior	Neck rotation, trunk rotation, Forearm pronation

- ○ Connect bone to bone
- ○ Primarily collagen fibers
- ○ Act to limit ROM and provide static joint stability
- ○ May blend into fibrous portion of the joint capsule
- ○ Classified as either extra-articular (outside capsule) or intra-articular (located inside capsule)
- Muscles
  - ○ Soft tissue structures
  - ○ Possess ability to contract
  - ○ Connect to bones through their tendons
  - ○ Provide dynamic joint stability

Quick fact The degeneration of articular cartilage is known as *osteoarthritis*.

Classification of Synovial Joints

- Uniaxial (see Fig. 1.69)
  - ○ One axis of rotation, one plane
  - ○ Includes ginglymus and trochoidal joints
- Biaxial
  - ○ Two axes of rotation, two planes
  - ○ Includes condyloidal and sellar joints
- Triaxial (polyaxial or multiaxial)
  - ○ Three axes of rotation, three planes
  - ○ Includes enarthrodial joints
- Nonaxial
  - ○ Does not occur about an axis, instead involves gliding movement
  - ○ Arthrodial (gliding or plane) joints

Joint Motion

- Joint structure dictates motion
- ROM—range through which a joint moves
  - ○ Active range of motion (AROM)—achieved by muscle contraction
  - ○ Active assistive range of motion (AAROM)—achieved by combination of muscle contractions and assistance by external force
  - ○ Passive range of motion (PROM)—achieved by an external force without muscle contraction

- ○ Fibrous capsule—outer layer of joint capsule
- ○ Synovial membrane—secretes synovial fluid within joint
- Articular (hyaline) cartilage
  - ○ Lines articulating joint surfaces
- Ligaments
  - ○ Fibrous structures

Table 1.9 Joint Structure Classification

Classification	Subclassification	Movement	Example
Fibrous	Gomphosis	Minimal	Tooth socket
	Suture	Immovable	Cranial sutures
	Syndesmosis	Slight	Inferior tibiofibular joint
Cartilaginous	Synchondrosis	Slight	Costochondral joints
	Symphysis	Slight	Pubis symphysis
Synovial	Arthrodial (gliding)	Gliding	Carpal joints
	Trochoidal (pivot)	Rotational	Proximal radioulnar joint
	Ginglymus (hinge)	Uniplaner	Humeroulnar joint
	Condyloidal (biaxial ball and socket)	Biplaner	Radiocarpal joint
	Sellar (saddle)	Biaxial	Carpometacarpal joint of thumb
	Enarthrodial (multiaxial ball and socket)	Triplaner	Coxafemoral joint

- Resistive range of motion (RROM)—performed against a resistance applied by an external force
- Goniometry
  - Method of measuring joint motion
  - Performed using a goniometer
  - Measured in degrees
- Axial (circular, angular, or rotary) motion
  - Occurs about an axis of rotation
  - Example—flexion of forearm at elbow joint
  - Axial motion can be classified as being—(a) uniaxial, (b) biaxial, or (c) triaxial
- Nonaxial (gliding, sliding, or linear) motion
  - Does not occur about or around an axis of rotation
  - Gliding motion
  - Example—movement of one carpal bone on another carpal bone
- Physiological movement
  - Bones move through planes of motion about an axis of rotation at joint
  - Example—flexion and extension

- Osteokinematic motion
  - Bones of a joint move relative to the three cardinal planes of motion
- Joint arthrokinematics
  - Occurs between articular surfaces of joint
  - Necessary for osteokinematic motion to occur
  - Includes three types of accessory motions

 Use the DVD or visit the website at http://thePoint.lww.com/Long about *joint motion terminology.*

> **Quick fact** Accessory joint motions are known as *spin, roll, and glide.*

Table 1.10 Joint Function Classification

Classification	Subclassification	Movement	Example
Synarthrosis	Gomphosis	Minimal	Tooth socket
	Suture	Immovable	Cranial sutures
Amphiarthrosis	Syndesmosis	Slight	Inferior tibiofibular joint
	Synchondrosis	Slight	Costochondral joints
	Symphysis	Slight	Pubis symphysis
Diarthrosis	Arthrodial (gliding)	Gliding	Carpal joints
	Trochoidal (pivot)	Rotational	Proximal radioulnar joint
	Ginglymus (hinge)	Uniplaner	Humeroulnar joint
	Condyloidal (biaxial ball and socket)	Biaxial	Radiocarpal joint
	Sellar (saddle)	Biaxial	Carpometacarpal joint of thumb
	Enarthrodial (multiaxial ball and socket)	Triplaner	Coxafemoral joint

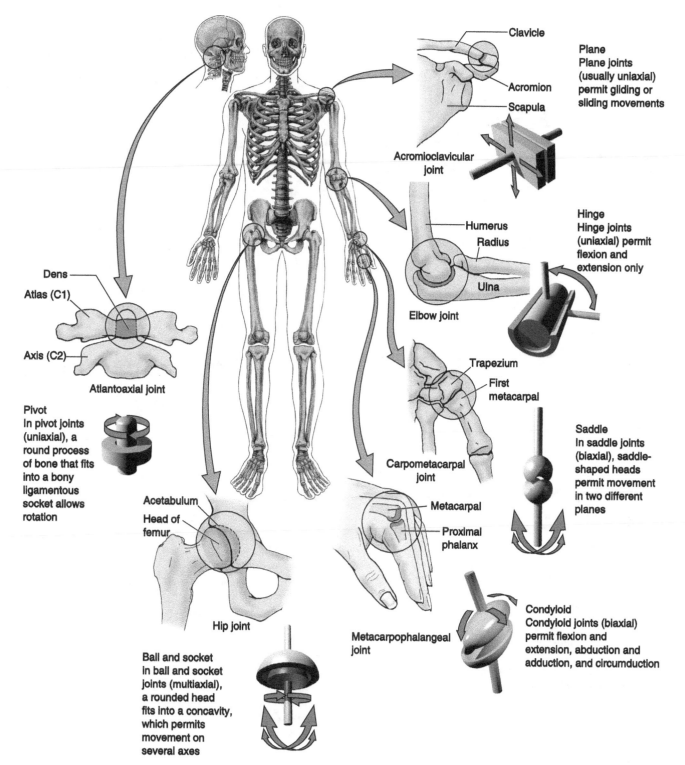

Figure 1.68 Types of Synovial Joints. (From Moore KL, Dalley AF. *Clinical oriented anatomy*, 4th ed. Baltimore: Lippincott Williams & Wilkins; 1999.)

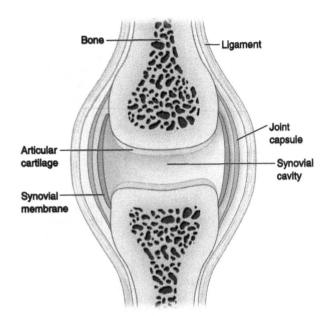

Figure 1.69 Synovial Joint Anatomy. (From Anderson MK, Parr GP, Hall SJ, et al. *Foundations of athletic training: prevention, assessment, and management*, 4th ed. Baltimore: Lippincott Williams & Wilkins; 2009.)

Quick fact
Normal ROM for a particular joint may vary from person to person.

MAJOR JOINTS OF THE BODY

See Table 1.11.

BASIC BIOMECHANICAL PRINCIPLES

Lever Systems in the Body

- First-class lever (see Fig. 1.70)
  - Fulcrum is between the resistance and applied force
  - Example within the body—neck extension
  - Example outside the body—see saw
- Second-class lever
  - Resistance is between the fulcrum and applied force
  - Very efficient lever system
  - Example within the body—standing heel raise
  - Example outside the body—wheelbarrow
- Third-class lever
  - Applied force is between the fulcrum and resistance
  - Very inefficient system
  - Example within the body—elbow flexion
  - Example outside the body—swinging door

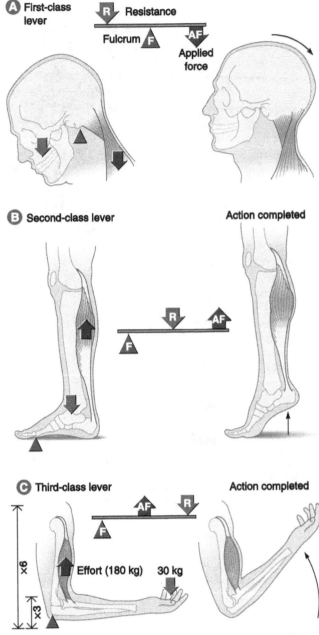

Figure 1.70 Lever Systems in the Body. **A:** First-Class Lever. **B:** Second-Class Lever. **C:** Third-Class Lever. (From Premkumar K. *The massage connection anatomy and physiology*. Baltimore: Lippincott Williams & Wilkins; 2004.)

Newton's Laws

- Newton's first law (law of inertia)
  - An object will remain at rest or continue at a constant velocity unless an external force acts upon it
- Newton's second law (law of acceleration and momentum)
  - Net force = mass × acceleration

Table 1.11 Major Joints of the Body by Region

Head, Neck, and Spine	Thorax and Pelvis	Upper Extremity	Lower Extremity
Temperomandibular	Sternoclavicular	Coracoclavicular	Coxafemoral
Atlantooccipital	Chondrosternal	Acromioclavicular	Tibiofemoral
Atlantoaxial	Costochondral	Scapulothoracic	Patellofemoral
Vertebral facet	Sacroiliac	Glenohumeral	Proximal tibiofibular
		Humeroulnar	Distal tibiofibular
		Humeroradial	Talocrural
		Proximal radioulnar	Subtalar
		Distal radioulnar	Tarsometatarsal
		Radiocarpal	Intermetatarsal
		Carpometacarpal	Metatarsophalangeal
		Intermetacarpal	Interphalangeal
		Metacarpophalangeal	Proximal interphalangeal
		Interphalangeal	Distal interphalangeal
		Proximal interphalangeal	
		Distal interphalangeal	

- Newton's third law (law of action–reaction)
  - Every action has an equal and opposite reaction

Gravity

- Center of gravity
  - Point of an object where weight is balanced
  - Lower center of gravity = increased stability
  - Center of gravity changes with motion
- Base of support
  - Point of contact with supporting surface
  - Large base of support = increased stability
- Line of gravity
  - Vertical line through center of gravity
  - Stability increases when line of gravity falls within base of support

1. The all or none response law states which of the following?
   a. When a muscle contracts, all the fibers will contract maximally at the same time or not at all
   b. All the muscle fibers that make up a muscle will always fire regardless of the resistance applied
   c. When an individual muscle fiber fires, the fiber will contract maximally or not at all
   d. When a muscle is contracting against a maximal resistance, the muscle fibers will fire only as much as they need to
   e. A muscle fiber will fire with more force eccentrically than it will concentrically

2. Which of the following is *not* a function of the muscular system?
   a. Production of heat
   b. Movement of the body
   c. Ligament attachment
   d. Support to joints
   e. Maintenance of posture

3. In the anatomic position, the wrist is considered to be in what anatomic position to the hip?
   a. Superficial
   b. Lateral
   c. Dorsal
   d. Proximal
   e. Medial

4. What is the most efficient energy system for a marathon runner?
   a. ATP-PC system
   b. Phosphagen system
   c. Aerobic respiration system
   d. Glycolytic system
   e. Lactic acid system

5. The act of performing the lower body exercise known as a squat occurs in what plane of motion?
   a. Sagittal
   b. Coronal
   c. Transverse
   d. Frontal
   e. Horizontal

6. Which of the following best describes the concept of reciprocal inhibition?
   a. The physiological process of how a muscle contracts at the cellular level
   b. The amount of force a muscle can produce is dependent on the length of the muscle during contraction
   c. Some fibers of a muscle will remain in a noncontractile state if they are not needed to move a resistance during a concentric muscle contraction
   d. A muscle will recruit other muscle fibers within itself if it cannot move a resistance with a given number of muscle fibers
   e. When the agonist muscle group concentrically contracts, the antagonist muscle group relaxes

7. What is the appropriate term for a hole that is found within a bone?
   a. Process
   b. Fossa
   c. Facet
   d. Epicondyle
   e. Foramen

8. Which of the following is considered to be a diarthrotic joint?
   a. Ginglymus
   b. Trochoidal
   c. Arthrodial
   d. Sellar
   e. All of the above

9. Which of the following is *false* regarding an antagonistic muscle?
   a. It has the opposite action of the agonist muscle
   b. It lengthens as the agonist muscle shortens
   c. It is positioned opposite of the agonist muscle
   d. It relaxes as the agonist muscle contracts
   e. None of the above

10. Performing a full range of motion resistive band strengthening exercise for the shoulder is an example of what type of muscle contraction?
    a. Isometric
    b. Isokinetic
    c. Static

d. Isotonic
e. All of the above

11. Which of the following is an example of a sesamoid bone?
    a. Vertebra
    b. Metatarsal
    c. Patella
    d. Scapula
    e. Humerus

12. What is the term for a bundle of muscle fibers within a muscle?
    a. Sarcolemma
    b. Fasiculus
    c. Tendon sheath
    d. Fascia
    e. Myofibril

13. Which of the following statements is *true* regarding the insertion of a muscle?
    a. A muscle's line of pull is directed toward from the muscle insertion
    b. It is usually the part that attaches closest to the midline of the body
    c. It is usually the most distal attachment point
    d. A muscle can only have one insertion point
    e. All of the above

14. A ginglymus joint produces what type of joint motion?
    a. Nonaxial
    b. Uniaxial
    c. Biaxial
    d. Triaxial
    e. All of the above

15. Moving the scapula toward the midline of the body is known as what type of shoulder girdle movement?
    a. Retraction
    b. Abduction
    c. Extension
    d. Protraction
    e. Flexion

16. Which of the following forms of muscle are spindle shaped with a central muscular belly?
    a. Multipennate
    b. Triangular
    c. Fusiform
    d. Quadrate
    e. None of the above

17. Which of the following is *true* regarding slow-twitch muscle fibers?
    a. They have a high level of aerobic endurance
    b. They have low motor unit strength
    c. They appear smaller than fast-twitch muscle fibers

d. They have a slow contractile speed
e. All of the above

18. The carpometacarpal joint of the thumb is an example of what type of joint?
    a. Ginglymus
    b. Sellar
    c. Trochoidal
    d. Condyloidal
    e. Enarthrodial

19. The amount of electrical impulse needed in order for a muscle fiber to fire is termed as which of the following?
    a. Myoneural junction
    b. Motor unit conductivity
    c. Threshold
    d. Lactic acid level
    e. Myoneural level

20. A bone acts as which of the following in regard to lever systems in the body?
    a. Resistance
    b. Axis
    c. Force
    d. Lever
    e. Effort

21. From the anatomic position, what movement of the wrist involves moving the hand in the direction of the fifth digit?
    a. Radial deviation
    b. Flexion
    c. Extension
    d. Supination
    e. Ulnar deviation

22. A decrease in muscle fiber size is best termed by which of the following?
    a. Synergy
    b. Atrophy
    c. Hypertrophy
    d. Hyperplasia
    e. None of the above

23. Shoulder flexion is an example of which of the following joint motions?
    a. Rotation motion
    b. Curvilinear motion
    c. Rolling motion
    d. Linear motion
    e. Spinning motion

24. Which of the following statements is *true* regarding ligaments?
    a. They are made up primarily of an elastic type of tissue
    b. They can only be found outside of the joint capsule

c. They secrete synovial fluid to help lubricate the joint
d. They may blend with the fibrous portion of the joint capsule
e. They provide dynamic support to the joint

25. Which of the following statements is *false* regarding lever systems in the body?
a. A lever is a rigid bar that turns about an axis of rotation
b. The effort is representative of the resistance that has to be overcome
c. The arrangement of the lever, axis, and force determine the type of lever
d. The axis and fulcrum are synonymous with each other
e. Leverage is the mechanical advantage a force can have when moving an object

26. The ability of a muscle to return to its original length after it has been stretched is termed which of the following?
a. Contractility
b. Extensibility
c. Sensitivity
d. Conductivity
e. None of the above

27. Which of the following joints are *not* considered to be a "true" joint?
a. Scapulothoracic joint
b. Acromioclavicular joint
c. Sternoclavicular joint
d. Glenohumeral joint
e. All of the above

28. What motions occur at the proximal radioulnar joint?
a. Elbow flexion and extension
b. Shoulder internal and external rotation
c. Wrist radial and ulnar deviation
d. Wrist flexion and extension
e. None of the above

29. Which joint of the shoulder complex has the largest range of motion?
a. Scapulothoracic joint
b. Acromioclavicular joint
c. Glenohumeral joint
d. Sternoclavicular joint
e. None of the above

30. Shoulder flexion occurs on what axis of rotation?
a. Sagittal
b. Multiaxial
c. Frontal
d. Vertical
e. None of the above

31. What structure plays a primary role in preventing hyperextension of the proximal interphalangeal (PIP) joint of the ring finger?
a. Flexor pollicis longus tendon
b. Intercarpal ligament
c. Ulnar collateral ligament
d. Volar plate
e. Extensor indices tendon

32. Which of the following factors plays a primary role in glenohumeral injuries?
a. The weakness of the triceps brachii
b. The tightness of the upper trapezius muscle
c. The shape of the clavicle
d. The shape of the scapula
e. The shallowness of the glenoid fossa

33. Which of the following is *false* regarding the first carpometacarpal joint?
a. It is classified as a sellar joint
b. Part of its articulation includes a bone from the distal carpal row
c. Flexion and extension motion occur at this joint
d. This joint is part of the thumb
e. It provides very little movement for the thumb

34. What would be the most effective exercise to strengthen the subscapularis muscle?
a. Using a dumbbell, flexing the shoulder with the elbow bent at 90 degrees
b. Using theraband, adducting the shoulder
c. Using a dumbbell, externally rotating the shoulder
d. Using theraband, internally rotating the shoulder
e. Using the resistance of another person, isometrically elevating the shoulder

35. The medial (ulnar) collateral ligament complex of the elbow is primarily responsible for restraining what type of force at the elbow?
a. Anterior
b. Varus
c. Valgus
d. Posterior
e. Axial

36. Which of the following is *false* regarding the supraspinatus muscle?
a. It assists in the stabilization of the humeral head within the glenoid fossa
b. It travels through the subacromial space
c. It is part of the rotator cuff muscle complex
d. It is located posteriorly in relationship to the subscapularis muscle
e. It is classified as one of the "power" muscles of the shoulder complex

37. The humeroulnar joint is classified as what type of joint?
a. Sellar
b. Condyloidal

c. Arthrodial
d. Enarthrodial
e. Ginglymus

38. Which of the following statements is *true* regarding the muscles of the shoulder girdle?
    a. They are only found on the anterior side of the body
    b. They help provide static stability to the shoulder complex
    c. None of them attach to the humerus
    d. There are only three shoulder girdle muscles
    e. They are all responsible for glenohumeral joint motion

39. Which of the following bones of the wrist are included in the proximal carpal row?
    a. Capitate
    b. Hamate
    c. Trapezoid
    d. Trapezium
    e. None of the above

40. Which of the following is an articulation of the sternoclavicular joint?
    a. Humerus
    b. Manubrium
    c. Scapular spine
    d. Coracoid process
    e. Glenoid fossa

41. What muscle is the only pure flexor of the elbow?
    a. Brachialis
    b. Biceps brachii
    c. Supinator
    d. Brachioradialis
    e. Coracobrachialis

42. Elbow extension occurs on which of the following planes of movement?
    a. Frontal
    b. Horizontal
    c. Sagittal
    d. Transverse
    e. Coronal

43. Which of the following is *false* regarding the carrying angle of the elbow?
    a. Cubitus valgus is an increase in the carrying angle of the elbow
    b. Baseball pitchers may typically exhibit cubitus valgus of their throwing arm
    c. A normal carrying angle for a female is between 10 and 15 degrees
    d. Males have a greater carrying angle than females
    e. None of the above

44. When evaluating a patient's shoulder and back, you notice a "winging" of the right scapula. This sign most likely indicates weakness of what muscle?
    a. Subscapularis
    b. Serratus anterior
    c. Rhomboid minor
    d. Teres minor
    e. Supraspinatus

45. Which of the following positions would work the brachioradialis muscle most effectively when performing biceps curl exercises?
    a. With the forearm in full pronation
    b. With the forearm in a neutral position
    c. With the wrist in radial deviation
    d. With the forearm in full supination
    e. With the shoulder in full extension

46. The radiocarpal joint is classified as what type of joint?
    a. Sellar
    b. Condyloidal
    c. Arthrodial
    d. Enarthrodial
    e. Ginglymus

47. Which of the following would best describe the term *cubitus recurvatum*?
    a. Hyperextension of the elbow joint
    b. Hyperflexion of the elbow joint
    c. Hyperextension of the wrist joint
    d. Hyperflexion of the wrist joint
    e. Hyperflexion of the glenohumeral joint

48. Which of the following is *true* regarding the characteristics of a tendon sheath in the hand?
    a. It is sealed at both ends
    b. It is a hollow tube
    c. It is double walled
    d. It is filled with synovial fluid
    e. All of the above

49. What ligament is classified as being part of the coracoclavicular joint?
    a. Coracoacromial ligament
    b. Conoid ligament
    c. Glenohumeral ligament
    d. Costoclavicular ligament
    e. Interclavicular ligament

50. What is the name of the first cervical vertebra?
    a. Cervicis
    b. Axis
    c. Splenius
    d. Inion
    e. Atlas

51. Which of the following statements is *false* regarding the vertebrae of the spine?
    a. The individual movements between each vertebra are relatively large
    b. There are seven vertebrae in the cervical spine
    c. The vertebral foramen is the passageway for the spinal cord
    d. The vertebrae of the sacrum are fused
    e. There are 12 thoracic vertebrae

52. Which of the following movements occur at the atlantoocipital joint?
    a. Thoracic flexion
    b. Lumbar rotation
    c. Lumbar lateral flexion
    d. Cervical extension
    e. Cervical rotation

53. The vertebral facet joints of the lumbar vertebrae are considered to be what type of joint?
    a. Sellar
    b. Condyloidal
    c. Arthrodial
    d. Enarthrodial
    e. Ginglymus

54. How many pairs of ribs are classified as being the "true" ribs?
    a. 2
    b. 5
    c. 7
    d. 10
    e. 12

55. Which of the following best describes the annulus fibrosis of the intervertebral discs?
    a. Soft, pulpy substance
    b. Hard, immobile
    c. Dense, fibrocartilaginous
    d. Soft, liquid-like
    e. None of the above

56. What is the term for an increased anterior curvature of the lumbar spine?
    a. Scoliosis
    b. Lordosis
    c. Kyphosis
    d. Humpback
    e. Gibbus

57. Right cervical rotation movement occurs on which of the following axes of rotation?
    a. Sagittal
    b. Frontal
    c. Transverse
    d. Vertical
    e. Coronal

58. How many vertebrae are considered to be part of the lumbar spine?
    a. 4
    b. 7
    c. 9
    d. 12
    e. None of the above

59. Which of the following muscles of the shoulder girdle *do not* play a role in cervical motion?
    a. Rhomboid major
    b. Levator scapulae
    c. Infraspinatus
    d. Trapezius
    e. Rhomboid minor

60. The longissimus dorsi muscle is responsible for movements in which of the following vertebral segments?
    a. Lumbar
    b. Coccyx
    c. Thoracic
    d. Cervical
    e. Sacral

61. What is the sacrospinalis muscle group also known as?
    a. Multifidus
    b. Scalenes
    c. Sternocleidomastoid
    d. Quadratus lumborum
    e. Erector spinae

62. Which of the following muscles acts as an extensor of the vertebral column?
    a. Scalenus anterior
    b. Rectus abdominis
    c. Rectus capitis anterior
    d. Iliocostalis lumborum
    e. Longus colli

63. The costal facets of which vertebrae articulate with the ribs?
    a. Sacral
    b. Lumbar
    c. Thoracic
    d. Cervical
    e. None of the above

64. Which of the following muscles are considered to be part of the prevertebral muscle group?
    a. Scalenus medius
    b. Obliquus capitus inferior
    c. Rectus capitis anterior
    d. Spinalis cervicis
    e. All of the above

65. The innominate bones are connected posteriorly by which of the following structures?
    a. Sacrum
    b. Coccyx
    c. Acetabulum
    d. Posterior superior iliac spine
    e. Pubis symphysis

66. Which of the following is the longest muscle in the body?
    a. Adductor magnus
    b. Semitendinosus
    c. Semimembranosus
    d. Gracilis
    e. Sartorius

67. What gluteal muscle is responsible for extending the hip?
    a. Gluteus medius
    b. Gluteus minimus
    c. Gluteus maximus
    d. All of the above
    e. None of the above

68. Which of the following best describes the angle of inclination of the femur?
    a. Relationship between the greater trochanter and the femoral neck
    b. Relationship between the anterior superior iliac spine and the femoral neck
    c. Relationship between the femoral head and the femoral shaft
    d. Relationship between the greater trochanter and the lesser trochanter
    e. Relationship between the femoral head and the acetabulum

69. Which muscle is *not* a part of the deep external rotators of the hip?
    a. Gemellus superior
    b. Piriformis
    c. Obturator internus
    d. Quadratus femoris
    e. Pectineus

70. What structure makes up the medial border of the femoral triangle?
    a. Iliotibial band
    b. Adductor magnus muscle
    c. Inguinal ligament
    d. Adductor longus muscle
    e. Sartorius muscle

71. What type of movement occurs at the acetabular femoral joint?
    a. Flexion and extension
    b. Multidirectional
    c. Internal rotation and external rotation
    d. Adduction and abduction
    e. None of the above

72. Which of the following muscles are considered to be biarticulate?
    a. Adductor brevis
    b. Gracilis
    c. Pectineus
    d. Adductor longus
    e. Gluteus medius

73. On what plane of movement does hip abduction occur?
    a. Frontal
    b. Horizontal
    c. Sagittal
    d. Transverse
    e. None of the above

74. What type of movement occurs at the tibiofemoral joint?
    a. Knee flexion
    b. Knee extension
    c. Knee internal rotation
    d. Knee external rotation
    e. All of the above

75. Which of the following bones is least responsible for transmitting ground forces through the leg?
    a. Fibula
    b. Talus
    c. Tibia
    d. Calcaneus
    e. None of the above

76. Which of the following occurs in the swing phase of the walking gait cycle?
    a. Toe off
    b. Heel strike
    c. Heel off
    d. Midstance
    e. None of the above

77. The patella provides a mechanical advantage to what muscle?
    a. Semimembranosus
    b. Biceps femoris
    c. Gastrocnemius
    d. Rectus femoris
    e. All of the above

78. What axis of rotation does ankle plantar flexion occur on?
    a. Frontal
    b. Sagittal
    c. Transverse
    d. All of the above
    e. None of the above

79. A person who has excessive hyperextension of the knees is termed as having which of the following?
    a. Genu varum
    b. Genu valgum
    c. Genu recurvatum
    d. Patella alta
    e. Patella baja

80. Which of the following is *false* regarding the talus bone?
    a. It articulates with the calcaneus
    b. Several muscles attach there to provide stability for ankle and foot
    c. It is considered to be part of the region known as the *hindfoot*
    d. It fits inside the ankle mortise
    e. It makes up part of the talocrural joint

81. Which of the following is *true* regarding the screw home mechanism of the knee?
    a. As the knee extends during the last few degrees of extension the tibia externally rotates
    b. As the knee extends during the last few degrees of extension the tibia internally rotates
    c. This mechanism places the knee in the open packed position
    d. This mechanism places the knee in full flexion
    e. This mechanism places the tibiofemoral joint in its least congruent position

82. Which of the following is *true* regarding the motion of supination?
    a. It occurs at the metatarsophalangeal joints
    b. It is another name for the motion of eversion
    c. It is a triplaner movement
    d. It only occurs in the transverse plane
    e. None of the above

83. Which of the following best describes the range of motion for knee external rotation?
    a. 30 degrees
    b. 145 degrees
    c. 90 degrees
    d. 60 degrees
    e. 45 degrees

84. Which of the following joints is located proximal to the knee?
    a. The first metatarsophalangeal joint
    b. The subtalar joint
    c. The distal interphalangeal joint
    d. The inferior tibiofibular joint
    e. The proximal interphalangeal joint

85. What tendon helps reinforce the medial longitudinal arch of the foot?
    a. Extensor hallucis longus
    b. Plantaris
    c. Posterior tibialis
    d. Peroneus brevis
    e. Extensor digitorum longus

86. Which of the following muscles is considered to be part of the triceps surae muscle group?
    a. Posterior tibialis
    b. Soleus
    c. Biceps femoris
    d. Flexor hallucis longus
    e. Anterior tibialis

87. What tendon passes directly behind the lateral malleolus of the ankle?
    a. Anterior tibialis tendon
    b. Extensor hallucis longus tendon
    c. Achilles tendon
    d. Posterior tibialis tendon
    e. Peroneus longus tendon

88. Which muscle is *not* located within the anterior compartment of the lower leg?
    a. Peroneus brevis
    b. Peroneus tertius
    c. Anterior tibialis
    d. Extensor hallucis longus
    e. Extensor digitorum longus

89. Which of the following structures insert at the Gerdy tubercle?
    a. Adductor brevis
    b. Sartorius
    c. Lateral collateral ligament
    d. Iliotibial band
    e. None of the above

90. What structure surrounds the muscular compartments of the lower leg?
    a. Fascia
    b. Retinaculum
    c. Ligament
    d. Tendon
    e. Periosteum

91. All three of the muscles that insert at the pes anserine are responsible for what movements?
    a. Knee extension and external rotation
    b. Knee flexion and external rotation
    c. Knee internal and external rotation
    d. Knee extension and internal rotation
    e. Knee flexion and internal rotation

92. What plane of motion does knee internal rotation occur on?
    a. Sagittal
    b. Lateral
    c. Frontal
    d. Coronal
    e. None of the above

93. Eversion of the ankle occurs at which of the following joints?
    a. Ankle joint
    b. Subtalar joint
    c. Tarsometatarsal joint
    d. Metatarsophalangeal joint
    e. Talocrural joint

94. The medial collateral ligament serves as a primary restraint for which of the following types of forces placed on the knee?
    a. Varus force
    b. Valgus force
    c. Rotary force
    d. Anterior translation force
    e. Posterior translation force

95. What muscles make up the hamstring muscle group?
    a. Rectus femoris, semitendinosus, and semimembranosus
    b. Sartorius, biceps femoris, and semitendinosus
    c. Semimembranosus, semitendinosus, and gracilis
    d. Sartorius, gracilis, and semitendinosus
    e. None of the above

96. What is the only intrinsic muscle that is located on the dorsum of the foot?
    a. Quadratus plantae
    b. Plantar interossei
    c. Peroneus tertius
    d. Extensor digitorum brevis
    e. Lumbricales

97. Which is not a *glial* cell?
    a. Astrocytes
    b. Macroglia
    c. Oligodendroglia
    d. Microglia
    e. Perikaryon

98. Which of the following muscles plays the most important role in moving the knee through the last 15 degrees of extension?
    a. Biceps femoris
    b. Rectus femoris
    c. Vastus medialis oblique
    d. Vastus lateralis
    e. Rectus intermedius

99. What term identifies a reflex that involves skeletal muscle?
    a. Spinal reflex
    b. Peripheral reflex
    c. Somatic reflex
    d. Autonomic reflex
    e. Visceral reflex

100. Which spinal nerve root contains motor fibers?
    a. The ventral nerve root
    b. The dorsal nerve root
    c. The posterior nerve root
    d. The lateral gray horn
    e. The ascending tract

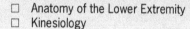

STUDY CHECKLIST

☐ Systemic Anatomy and Physiology
☐ Anatomy of the Head, Neck, Spine, and Thorax
☐ Anatomy of the Upper Extremity
☐ Anatomy of the Lower Extremity
☐ Kinesiology

Use the DVD or visit the website at http://thePoint.lww.com/Long to take the *online examination*.

2

Risk Management and Injury Prevention

Part 1   Risk Factors for Activity

Part 2   Preparticipation Examinations

Part 3   Protective Devices and Procedures

Part 4   Environmental Factors

Section 2 Examination

OVERVIEW

Risk management and injury prevention is arguably the most important area of knowledge and skills within the competencies. While at work, the athletic trainer should be constantly thinking about what the next step should be to maintain the safety of the athletes. Prophylactic taping, assisting in fluid replacement, and instructing on flexibility exercises are just a few of the tasks that athletic trainers perform on a daily basis to help decrease injury risk. Athletic trainers should have sound skills in protective equipment fitting, be able to identify common diseases and disabilities, and educate athletes on the importance of health maintenance and wellness. Whether the athletic trainer is monitoring environmental hazards during practice, fitting football helmets, or educating an athlete on the warning signs of cancer, he or she should take positive steps to keep the athletes healthy. Proactive and sound risk management and injury prevention practices can make a significant impact on the health of the athletes and the success of their teams.

CLINICAL PROFICIENCIES

- Plan, implement, evaluate, and modify a fitness program specific to the physical status of the patient. This will include instructing the patient in proper performance of the activities and the warning signs and symptoms of potential injury that may be sustained. Effective lines of communication shall be established to elicit and convey information about the patient's status and the prescribed program. While maintaining patient confidentiality, all aspects of the fitness program shall be documented using standardized record-keeping methods.

- Select, apply, evaluate, and modify appropriate standard protective equipment and other customer devices for the patient in order to prevent and/or minimize the risk of injury to the head, torso, spine, and extremities for safe participation in sport and/or physical activity. Effective lines of communication shall be established to elicit and convey information about the patient's situation and the importance of protective devices to prevent and/or minimize injury.

- Demonstrate the ability to develop, implement, and communicate effective policies and procedures to allow safe and efficient physical activity in a variety of environmental conditions. This will include obtaining, interpreting, and recognizing potentially hazardous environmental conditions and making the appropriate recommendations for the patient and/or activity. Effective lines of communication shall be established with the patient, coaches, and/or appropriate officials to elicit and convey information about the potential hazard of the environmental condition and the importance of implementing appropriate strategies to prevent injury. (Reproduced with permission of the National Athletic Trainers' Association.)

Risk Factors for Activity

CARDIAC RISK FACTORS

Cardiac Risk Factors Associated with Physical Activity (American College of Sports Medicine)

- Risks of exercise in adults are higher than in younger persons
  - Increased prevalence of atherosclerotic cardiovascular disease
- Risks of physical activity
  - Exertion-related sudden cardiac death
  - Acute myocardial infarction
- Common causes of sudden cardiac death in high school/college athletes
  - Aortic stenosis
  - Cardiomyopathy
  - Coronary artery anomalies
  - Hypertrophic cardiomyopathy
  - Myocarditis
- Risks during exercise testing
  - Exertion-related sudden cardiac death
  - Acute myocardial infarction

> **Quick fact** According to the ACSM, there is a higher incidence of exertion-related sudden death in individuals with sickle cell trait.

Prevention of Exercise-Related Cardiac Deaths (American College of Sports Medicine)

- Preparticipation examination (PPE) physical examination
- Medical clearance for persons with cardiovascular disease or other conditions with cardiac death risk
- Educate adults in symptoms of coronary artery disease (CAD)
- Slow progression when starting new exercise programs
- Physician evaluation if younger or older participants experience angina, dyspnea, or syncope from exercising
- Staff should be trained in cardiopulmonary resuscitation (CPR) and automated external defibrillator (AED) use
- Routine exercise stress testing—not recommended by all experts
- PPE echocardiography—not recommended by all experts

Risks and Precautions Associated with Physical Activity in Special Populations

- Refer to Section 3: Pathology of Injuries and Illnesses

Preparticipation Examinations

KEY TERMS
• Lean body mass
• Skinfold measurement
• Sun protection factor (SPF)

PURPOSE OF THE PREPARTICIPATION EXAMINATION

- General medical health
- Medical and orthopaedic conditions
- Health risks
- Immunization status

- Level of participation
- Fitness level
- Injury prevention
- Legal necessities
- Establish sports medicine team–athlete relationship

 Ideally, the preparticipation examination should be conducted by the athlete's primary care physician (PCP) because he or she will have the most knowledge in regard to the athlete's medical history.

ASSOCIATIONS AND ORGANIZATIONS ASSOCIATED WITH THE PREPARTICIPATION EXAMINATION

- American Academy of Family Physicians (AAFP)
- American Academy of Orthopaedic Surgeons (AAOS)
- American Academy of Pediatrics (AAP)
- American College of Sports Medicine (ACSM)
- American Medical Society of Sports Medicine (AMSSM)
- American Orthopaedic Society for Sports Medicine (AOSSM)
- American Osteopathic Academy of Sports Medicine (AOASM)
- National Athletic Trainers' Association (NATA)
- National Collegiate Athletic Association (NCAA)

PERSONNEL

- Essential personnel
  - PCP
  - Certified athletic trainer (ATC)
- Ancillary personnel
  - Orthopaedists, dentists, dermatologists

PREPARTICIPATION EXAMINATION DOCUMENTATION

- Medical record
  - Physical
  - Participation clearance
  - Immunization record
  - Medical history questionnaire
  - Emergency contact information
  - Authorization for emergency medical treatment
  - Health insurance information
  - Prior consultations, surgeries, treatments, and/or rehabilitation
- Ancillary questionnaires
  - Asthma
  - Abnormal menses
  - Disordered eating
  - Heat illness

 The PPE physical examination should be conducted by a doctor of medicine (MD), a doctor of osteopathic medicine (DO), physician assistants (PAs), or nurse practitioner (NP).

PRIMARY CARE PHYSICIAN EXAMINATION FORMAT

- Advantages
  - More comprehensive from a general medical standpoint
  - Greater understanding of medical/family history
  - Greater privacy
  - More cost effective for schools/organizations
- Disadvantages
  - May not be as comprehensive from an orthopaedic standpoint
  - Greater time commitment for PCP
  - Higher athlete cost
- Efficient site use
  - Area where athlete can complete PPE forms
  - Private area for PCP examination

STATION EXAMINATION FORMAT

- Advantages
  - Allows for assessment of large number of athletes at one time
  - More comprehensive from an orthopaedic standpoint
  - Lower athlete cost
  - Establishes sports medicine team–athlete relationship
  - Involvement of entire sports medicine team
- Disadvantages
  - Brief time allowed for each athlete
  - May be less comprehensive from a general medical standpoint
  - Decreased privacy
  - Following up on medical health issues
  - Has to be well coordinated
- Efficient site use
  - Area where athlete can complete PPE forms
  - Quiet area for assessing vital signs
  - Private area for assessing anthropometric measurements
  - Private area for physician examinations
  - Weight room and gymnasium for fitness testing

EXAMINATION FREQUENCY

- Annual medical examination
  - May be dictated by individual state policies for high school athletes
  - Ideally performed at least 6 weeks before sports activity

- AAFP, AAP, AMSSM, and AOASM recommendations
  - Entry-level complete physical examination
  - Limited annual reevaluation
- NCAA recommendations
  - Entrance into collegiate athletics program: medical examination
  - Subsequent years: updated medical history annually
  - Event of significant injury or illness: follow-up examination
- American Heart Association (AHA) recommendations
  - Entrance into collegiate athletics program: cardiovascular examination
  - Subsequent years: interim cardiovascular history and blood pressure assessment
  - Significant changes in medical status or abnormalities: may require more formal cardiovascular examination

PREPARTICIPATION EXAMINATION COMPONENTS

- Comprehensive medical history questionnaire
- Physical examination
- Fitness assessment

Use the DVD or visit the website at http://thePoint.lww.com/Long for additional materials about *components of the preparticipation examination*.

P A R T 3 Protective Devices and Procedures

KEY TERMS
- Health record
- Health risk appraisal

SPORTS EQUIPMENT

Associations and Organizations Associated with Sports Safety Equipment Standards
- American Society for Testing Materials (ASTM)
- NATA
- NCAA
- National Federation of State High School Athletic Associations (NFHS)
- National Operating Committee on Standards for Athletic Equipment (NOCSAE)

Mouth Guards
- Types of mouth guards
  - Stock—ready to use, but cannot customize
  - Commercial mouth-formed—thermoplastic material that can be customized through "boil and bite" method
  - Custom fabricated—teeth impression obtained and constructed by dentist or mouth guard manufacturer
- Worn to help prevent:
  - Mouth soft tissue trauma
  - Dental trauma
  - Mandible fractures
  - Temperomandibular joint trauma

Quick fact There are custom-fabricated mouth guards on the market now that allow the athlete to fit himself or herself for the guard and mail it off to be fabricated.

Use the DVD or visit the website at http://thePoint.lww.com/Long for additional materials about *how to fit a mouth guard*.

FOOTBALL HELMET FITTING
- Follow manufacturer's instructions
- Measure head circumference
- Wet hair—stimulates playing conditions
- Tighten chin strap appropriately—equal in distance and tension on each side
- Appropriate-sized cheek pads—no space between pad and cheek
- Inflator needle—lubricated with glycerine
- Insert inflator needle with twisting motion
- Ear openings centered with external auditory meatus
- Back of helmet—cover base of skull
- Eyebrows—1 to 2 finger widths below front edge of helmet

- Face mask—2 to 3 finger widths from nose/forehead
- Helmet does not slip/rotate when head is moved
- Appropriate face mask for position
- Face mask clips—secured and in good condition

> **Quick fact** All football helmets must be NOCSAE certified and have a visible warning label on the helmet.

FOOTBALL SHOULDER PAD FITTING

- Follow manufacturer's instructions
- Appropriate type pads for position
- Measure athlete
- Axillary straps and breastplate laces—appropriately tightened for a snug fit
- Adequate space on each side of neck collar—be able to abduct arms overhead without impinging neck
- Internal foam padding—channel over acromioclavicular joint
- Pads completely cover clavicle, acromioclavicular joint, and glenohumeral joint
- Shoulder cups—cover the deltoid
- Breast plate—completely covers sternum
- Back plate—completely covers scapula

PROTECTIVE BRACES

- Manufactured
  - Off-the-shelf—ready to use (less expensive)
  - Custom made—measured, fabricated, and fitted (more expensive)
- Function/purpose
  - Prophylactic—prevent injury
  - Rehabilitative—used following surgery during rehabilitation process
  - Functional—protection after injury and/or surgery
- Body area
  - Foot—orthotics, plantar fascia night splint
  - Ankle—lace-up ankle brace, semirigid ankle brace
  - Lower leg—neoprene sleeve
  - Knee—hinged knee brace, rotary instability knee brace
  - Thigh—neoprene sleeve
  - Shoulder—shoulder glenohumeral instability brace
  - Elbow—hinged elbow brace
  - Wrist—semirigid wrist brace
  - Fingers—neoprene buddy strap

CUSTOM PROTECTIVE DEVICES

- Types of materials
  - Low density (soft)—moleskin, foam, felt, sponge rubber
  - High density (nonyielding)—fiberglass, thermomoldable plastic, plaster

- Types of foam
  - Open cell—deforms quickly and provides minimal shock absorption
  - Closed cell—rebounds and returns to original shape quickly
- Pads
  - Friction pad—doughnut pad
  - Soft pad—bony prominence pad
  - Hard-shell pad—muscular contusion pad
- Splints
  - Static splint
  - Dynamic splint
- Casts
  - Soft cast
  - Hard cast

> **Quick fact** Dynamic splints are frequently used in the management of hand and finger injuries.

ATHLETIC FOOTWEAR

- Toe box
  - ½ in. to ¾ in. between longest toe and end of toe box
  - Width of toe box depends on sport
- Sole
  - Layers: (a) thick and spongy, (b) midsole, (c) hard rubber layer
  - Shock absorption
  - Durable
  - Provides good traction
- Heal counter
  - Controls foot inversion and eversion
  - Firm
  - Well fitted
- Shoe uppers
  - Typically combination of nylon and leather
  - Lightweight
  - Well ventilated
  - Padded above heel counter
- Arch support
  - Durable, yet soft supportive material
  - Smooth seams
- Shoe lasts
  - Framework from which shoes are built
  - Three general categories
    - Straight (motion control, hyperpronated, flexible foot)
    - Semicurved (normal foot)
    - Curved (cushioning, hypersupinated, rigid foot)

ATHLETIC WRAPPING AND TAPING

Principles of Athletic Wrapping

- Quick-drying tape adherent to skin—prevents slipping of wrap
- Contracting muscle during wrapping—prevents wrap from becoming too tight
- Wrap from distal to proximal—promotes venous return

Table 2.1 Athletic Wrapping Techniques

Upper Extremity	Lower Extremity
Shoulder spica	Foot and ankle spica
Elbow figure-eight	Cloth ankle wrap
Lower arm spiral	Lower leg spiral
Hand/wrist spiral	Upper leg spiral
Hand/wrist figure-eight	Quadriceps support/spica
Cloth wrist wrap	Hip flexor support/spica
	Hamstring support/spica
	Groin/adductor support/spica
	Gluteal support/spica

Table 2.2 Athletic Taping Techniques

Upper Extremity	Lower Extremity
Acromioclavicular joint sprain	Toe spica
Elbow collateral ligament sprain	Turf toe
Elbow hyperextension	Medial longitudinal arch
Circular wrist	LowDye arch
Wrist "X" tape	Transverse arch
Thumb spica	Achilles' tendon
Finger buddy tape	Closed basket weave
Finger collateral ligament sprain	Open basket weave
	Shin splints
	Patellofemoral (McConnell) taping
	Knee collateral ligament sprain
	Knee rotary instability
	Knee hyperextension

- Apply wrap from bottom of roll—prevents wrap from being too restrictive
- Alternate wrap from hand to hand
- Overlap wrap ½ of the width of wrap below
- Large number of turns with moderate, uniform tension—decreases chance of compromising circulation
- Do not cover tips of fingers/toes—need to be visible for circulation check
- Assess for adequate circulation and sensation

Athletic Wrapping Techniques

See Table 2.1

Principles of Taping

See Table 2.2
- Clean and dry skin
- Cover open wounds
- If possible, shave body hair and apply tape directly to skin—increases support
- For joint areas—place body part in desired position of stabilization

- For muscular areas—contract muscle to prevent tape from becoming too tight
- Use quick-drying tape adherent on skin—decreases slipping of tape
- Lubricate and pad areas of high friction
- To avoid skin irritation, use thin layer of underwrap (prewrap)
- Use uniform tension and smooth out tape when applying
- Avoid continuous taping—may impede circulation
- Overlap tape strips ½ of the width of tape strip below
- Avoid making gaps or wrinkles—can cause blisters
- Assess for adequate circulation and sensation
- Techniques for tape removal include (a) manual, (b) tape cutter, and (c) tape scissors
- When removing tape, pull skin from tape—not tape from skin
- When needed, use tape removal product

PART 4 Environmental Factors

MONITORING HEAT AND HUMIDITY

- Wet Bulb Globe Temperature (WBGT) index
  - WBGT risk chart—objective means for determining risk and necessary precautions
  - Measuring instruments—WBGT meter
  - Instrument readings: (a) dry bulb (ambient temperature), (b) wet bulb (humidity), and (c) globe (sun's radiation)
  - $WBGT = (0.1 \times DBT) + (0.7 \times WBT) + (GT \times 0.2)$
- Temperature-Humidity Activity Index
  - Provides risk level and activity recommendations
  - Measuring instruments: sling or digital psychrometer
  - Temperature and relative humidity

HEAT ILLNESS PREVENTION

- Availability of appropriate medical care
- Emergency action plan
- Protocol for treating heat illnesses
- Protocol for modification of activity level based on heat and humidity readings
- Include history of heat illnesses as part of PPE
- Educate staff on prevention, recognition, and treatment
- Educate athletes on hydration and appropriate fluid intake
- Appropriate amount of sleep (6 to 8 hours) in cool environment and well-balanced diet

- Schedule practices to avoid the hottest times of the day (10 AM to 5 PM)
- Allow for appropriate acclimatization to heat
- Assess athlete weight before and after practice
- Check athlete hydration level (urine specific gravity [Usg])
- Monitor heat and humidity before and during practices/events
- Clothing should allow for adequate cooling of body
- Maintain appropriate hydration during practices/events
- Easy access to water and electrolyte drinks
- Frequent rest and water breaks during practices
- Cooling methods available on-site

HYDRATION STATUS ASSESSMENT

- Weight charts
- Urine color
- Usg

 Quick fact Athletes should be gradually acclimated to exercising in the heat over a 10- to 14-day period.

TYPES OF HEAT ILLNESSES

- Dehydration
- Heat syncope
- Heat cramps
- Heat exhaustion
- Exertional heat stroke
- Exertional hyponatremia

Use the DVD or visit the website at http://thePoint.lww.com/Long for additional materials about *signs and symptoms of heat illnesses.*

Treatment of Heat Illnesses

- Refer to Section 6: Acute Care of Injuries and Illnesses (see Fig. 2.1)

HYPOTHERMIA

- Hypothermia—a decrease in core body temperature
- Factors that increase occurrence
  - Low temperature
  - Wind
  - Wet/damp

Quick fact The absence of shivering in a hypothermic patient is a sign of severe hypothermia.

Prevention of Hypothermia

- Appropriate clothing
  - Water proof
  - Wind proof
  - "Breathes" well
- Dress in layers
- Engage in good warm-up
- Assure athlete is well hydrated
- Avoid exercise outside when the ambient temperature and/or wind-chill factor is at a potentially dangerous level

Quick fact When exercising outdoors, keep in consideration the wind-chill factor, not just the ambient temperature.

TYPES OF COLD INJURIES AND ILLNESSES

- Hypothermia
- Frost nip
- Chilblains (pernio)
- Superficial (early) frostbite
- Deep (late) frostbite

 Use the DVD or visit the website at http://thePoint.lww.com/Long for additional materials about *signs and symptoms of cold injuries and illnesses.*

TREATMENT OF COLD INJURIES AND ILLNESSES

- Refer to Section 6: Acute Care of Injuries and Illnesses

LIGHTNING HAZARDS

Lightning Hazard Prevention (National Athletic Trainers' Association and National Collegiate Athletic Association)

- A proactive lightning safety policy
- An emergency action plan
- Educate staff, coaches, and athletes
- Monitor weather
  - Daily before practice/events
  - Thunder "watch" versus "warning"
  - Resources—National Weather Service (NWS), news, Internet, radio, etc.
- Preestablished safe shelter
  - The closest "safe" structure or location
  - A building with plumbing and/or electricity
  - In the absence of a building, a vehicle is the next best option

 Quick fact Athletic dugouts are not a safe shelter from lightning strikes, and should be avoided during a thunder/lightning storm.

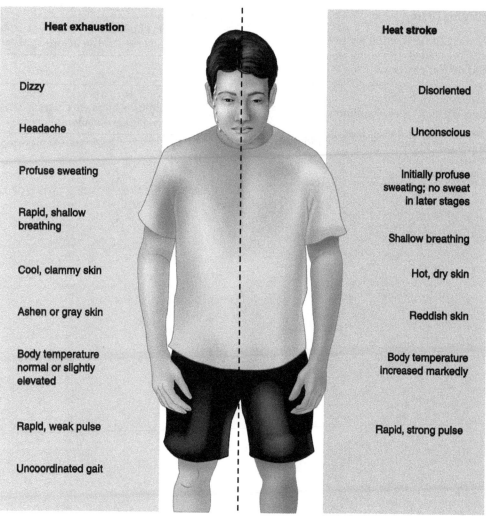

Heat exhaustion

Dizzy

Headache

Profuse sweating

Rapid, shallow breathing

Cool, clammy skin

Ashen or gray skin

Body temperature normal or slightly elevated

Rapid, weak pulse

Uncoordinated gait

Heat stroke

Disoriented

Unconscious

Initially profuse sweating; no sweat in later stages

Shallow breathing

Hot, dry skin

Reddish skin

Body temperature increased markedly

Rapid, strong pulse

Figure 2.1 Signs and Symptoms of Heat Illnesses.

LIGHTNING MONITORING AND DETECTION

- Flash-to-bang method
  - Strike of lightning—count in seconds until you hear the clap of thunder, then divide number of seconds by 5 = estimated number of miles away
  - A building with plumbing and/or electricity
- Weather radios and Internet
- Handheld lightning detectors

 Quick **fact** Thunder may be not be heard due to atmospheric and environmental disturbances.

LIGHTNING SAFETY RECOMMENDATIONS

- NATA position statement
  - Postpone or suspend activities, if thunderstorm appears imminent, until hazard has passed
  - Highly recommend seeking safe structure or location at first sign of lightning or thunder
  - 30–30 rule

- 30–30 rule
  - By the time flash-to-bang count approaches 30 seconds or less, everyone should be in safe location
  - Before resuming activities, 30 minutes should pass after last sound of thunder heard or last flash of lightning seen
- NCAA Sports Medicine Handbook
  - Lightning awareness should increase with the first flash of lightning, sound of thunder, and/or other signs of storms
  - As a minimum, by the time there is a flash-to-bang count of 30 seconds, everyone should be in safe location
  - Before resuming athletic activities, wait 30 minutes after last sound of thunder and last flash of lightning

Quick **fact** Lightning strikes can occur as far as 10 miles away from the location of the rain shaft.

SUNBURN PREVENTION

- Sunscreen—at least sun protection factor (SPF) 15 (higher SPF may be needed depending on skin complexion and time of sun exposure)
- Apply sunscreen 30 minutes before sun exposure
- Reapply sunscreen every 2 hours
- Avoid times that are high risk for sunburns (10 AM to 4 PM)
- Appropriately cover skin and head when outdoors
- Avoid tanning beds
- Frequent skin examinations

 Quick fact It is important to check the expiration on the sunscreen bottle before application.

Quick fact Sunburns increase a person's risk of developing melanoma.

SECTION 2 Examination

1. Which of the following is the best method for testing the upper body muscular strength of an athlete?
   a. A 30-second pull-up test
   b. A 1-RM bench press
   c. A 1-minute push-up test
   d. A 10-RM bench press
   e. A 1-minute sit-up test

2. What is the correct formula for calculating the WBGT index?
   a. WBGT = (0.4 × DBT) + (0.5 × WBT) + (0.6 × GT)
   b. WBGT = (0.3 × DBT) + (0.9 × WBT) + (0.2 × GT)
   c. WBGT = (0.8 × DBT) + (0.4 × WBT) + (0.7 × GT)
   d. WBGT = (0.2 × DBT) + (0.1 × WBT) + (0.6 × GT)
   e. WBGT = (0.1 × DBT) + (0.7 × WBT) + (0.2 × GT)

3. The Donjoy Playmaker is an example of what type of brace?
   a. Semirigid wrist brace
   b. Lace-up ankle brace
   c. Hinged knee brace
   d. Shoulder instability
   e. Rigid night splint

4. What body structure is involved with the general medical condition known as *meningitis*?
   a. Myelin sheath of peripheral nerves
   b. Covering of the brain and spinal cord
   c. Outer layer of the heart
   d. Pleural lining of the lungs
   e. Inner lining of the ureters and urinary bladder

5. Which test would be most appropriate for assessing cardiorespiratory fitness?
   a. Zigzag test
   b. Illinois test
   c. Harvard step test
   d. Shuttle run test
   e. 40-yard dash

6. What is the term for the thickening of the heart muscle?
   a. Myocarditis
   b. Aortic stenosis
   c. Hypertrophic cardiomyopathy
   d. Angina pectoris
   e. Endocarditis

7. Keratitis is the inflammation of which of the following eye structures?
   a. Pupil
   b. Cornea
   c. Retina
   d. Choroid
   e. Conjunctiva

8. Which of the following materials used in the construction of custom protective devices is *not* classified as a low-density material?
   a. Moleskin
   b. Gauze
   c. Polycarbonate
   d. Closed-cell foam
   e. Adhesive sponge rubber

9. A stadiometer is used to assess which of the following?
   a. Speed
   b. Agility
   c. Weight
   d. Rhythm
   e. Height

10. Which statement best describes the AHA recommendations regarding preparticipation evaluations for athletes?
    a. An athlete must have a physical examination before each athletic season
    b. An athlete must have an echocardiography before entrance into a college athletics program
    c. An athlete must have a cardiovascular examination before entrance into a college athletics program
    d. An athlete must have an echocardiography before each athletic season
    e. An athlete must have a yearly follow-up examination with the PCP

11. What is the normal carrying angle of the elbow for females?
    a. 0 to 5 degrees
    b. 5 to 10 degrees
    c. 10 to 15 degrees
    d. 15 to 20 degrees
    e. 20 to 25 degrees

12. Which of the following is *false* regarding the skin disorder tinea versicolor?
    a. It is caused by a fungal infection
    b. Lesions will not tan when exposed to the sun
    c. Presents itself as red scaling papules
    d. It is usually asymptomatic
    e. Usually found on the abdomen, neck, or chest

13. The globe thermometer temperature reading of a WBGT meter represents which of the following?
    a. Ambient temperature
    b. Sun's radiation
    c. Relative humidity
    d. Water vapor
    e. Absolute humidity

14. A written guarantee from the manufacturer that a product is safe for use is termed which of the following?
    a. Expressed warranty
    b. Product liability
    c. Strict liability
    d. Implied warranty
    e. Foreseeability of harm

15. What type of mouth guard offers the athlete the least amount of protection?
    a. Mouth formed
    b. Thermoplastic
    c. Commercial
    d. Custom fabricated
    e. Stock

16. Which of the following types of stretching techniques is not considered a safe way to improve flexibility?
    a. Yoga
    b. Ballistic stretching
    c. Static stretching
    d. Passive range of motion
    e. PNF stretching

17. Which of the following guidelines would be *false* when fitting football shoulder pads on an athlete?
    a. Allow an approximately 1 to 1½ in. space on each side of the neck collar
    b. Lateral shoulder flap should cover the deltoid region
    c. Sternum should be completely covered by the breast plate
    d. Anterior shoulder flap should completely cover the anterior glenohumeral joint
    e. Athlete should be able to abduct the arms overhead without impinging the neck

18. Measuring limb girth can assess which of the following?
    a. Muscular hypertrophy
    b. Muscular endurance
    c. Muscular strength

    d. Muscular power
    e. Muscular hyperplasia

19. A "doughnut" pad is typically constructed to prevent further irritation of what types of injury?
    a. Ligament sprain
    b. Blister
    c. Muscle strain
    d. Tendinitis
    e. Stress fracture

20. Which of the following is *false* regarding the application of an elastic wrap?
    a. Each turn of the wrap should be overlapped by at least half of the underlying wrap
    b. Wraps should be applied from a distal to proximal direction
    c. The body part should be wrapped with the involved muscles in a relaxed position
    d. Application of an adherent tape spray is appropriate when attempting to prevent slipping of the wrap
    e. It is best to use a large number of turns with moderate tension when applying the wrap

21. What test best assesses for the flexibility of the hip flexors?
    a. Thomas test
    b. Thompson test
    c. V-sit test
    d. Sit-and-reach test
    e. Ober test

22. Which of the following is *true* regarding the fitting of an athlete with crutches?
    a. The underarm crutch brace should be 3 in. below the anterior fold of the axilla
    b. The elbow should be flexed at a 60-degree angle
    c. Crutch tips should be 4 in. in front of the shoe
    d. Crutch tips should be 6 in. from the outer margin of the shoe
    e. The athlete should have both the shoes off

23. The internal foam padding of the shoulder pads should create a channel over what structure in order to protect it?
    a. Deltoid muscle
    b. Sternum
    c. AC joint
    d. Scapula
    e. GH joint

24. Which of the following is a sign of heat exhaustion?
    a. Swelling of the extremities
    b. Slow and bounding pulse
    c. Pale, moist, cool skin
    d. Increase in body temperature above 104°F
    e. Tachycardia

25. What percentage of thunder cannot be heard due to atmospheric disturbances?
    a. 10% to 25%
    b. 20% to 40%
    c. 50% to 60%
    d. 60% to 85%
    e. 70% to 95%

26. Which of the following types of mouth guards are typically the most expensive?
    a. Custom fabricated
    b. Stock
    c. Mouth formed
    d. Commercial
    e. Thermoplastic

27. Which of the following statements is *true* regarding hypothermia?
    a. Can be prevented by assuring proper hydration
    b. Is defined as an increase in core body temperature
    c. Is increased by factors including high temperature and humidity
    d. Will cause death when core body temperature reaches 90°
    e. Is not influenced by the wind chill factor

28. Protective ear guards are worn in wrestling to help prevent which of the following types of conditions?
    a. Otitis externa
    b. Vertigo
    c. Concussions
    d. Auricular hematoma
    e. Tinnitus

29. Which of the following is a sign of chilblains?
    a. Pale skin
    b. Red skin
    c. Excessive shivering
    d. Gangrene
    e. Cyanotic skin

30. An athlete approaches you at football practice with dry, red skin; severe fatigue; and an altered level of consciousness. As you evaluate him you find that he has a strong, rapid pulse, and shallow respirations. Which of the following heat illnesses is the athlete most likely suffering from?
    a. Hypothermia
    b. Exertional hyponatremia
    c. Heat syncope
    d. Heat exhaustion
    e. Exertional heat stroke

31. What should be signed by an athlete who has been advised not to participate in sports due to a preexisting medical condition, but has made the personal decision to participate despite the advisement of medical personal?
    a. A deemed consent form
    b. A consent to treat form

    c. An assumption of risk form
    d. An exculpatory waiver form
    e. An implied consent form

32. The clean and jerk test would be most appropriate in assessing which of the following components of fitness?
    a. Upper body muscular endurance
    b. Upper and lower body muscular power
    c. Upper and lower body muscular strength
    d. Lower body muscular strength
    e. Lower body muscular endurance

33. Which of the following conditions would most likely disqualify an athlete from participation in a contact sport?
    a. Asthma
    b. Mononucleosis
    c. History of heat illness
    d. Diabetes mellitus
    e. Convulsive disorder

34. What is the term for 20/20 vision?
    a. Farsightedness
    b. Hypermetropia
    c. Myopia
    d. Nearsightedness
    e. Emmetropia

35. Concentration is assessed, during the standardized assessment of concussion (SAC) tool, by doing which of the following?
    a. Repeating five words at the end of test that were given at beginning of the test by the examiner
    b. Performing the Romberg test for the examiner
    c. Repeating multiple strings of digits to the examiner in reverse order
    d. Providing the month, date, day of the weak, year, and time to the examiner
    e. Repeating five words provided by the examiner in three successive trials

36. Which of the following best indicates a heart rate that is considered to be bradycardia?
    a. 50 bpm
    b. 70 bpm
    c. 80 bpm
    d. 95 bpm
    e. 105 bpm

37. Pectus excavatum could be an indication of what general medical condition?
    a. Marfan syndrome
    b. Systemic lupus erythematosus
    c. Cushing syndrome
    d. Juvenile rheumatoid arthritis
    e. Osteomyelitis

38. A non–cantilevered-type shoulder pad is most likely to be equipped on which of the following types of position players in football?
    a. Offensive lineman
    b. Defensive end
    c. Wide receiver
    d. Linebacker
    e. Running back

39. A history of pneumothorax would be questioned during what part of the preparticipation examination?
    a. Neurologic examination
    b. Cardiovascular examination
    c. Orthopaedic examination
    d. Pulmonary examination
    e. Gastrointestinal examination

40. What orthopaedic special test can be used to screen for shoulder impingement syndrome?
    a. Apley scratch test
    b. Fagin test
    c. Hawkins-Kennedy test
    d. Roo test
    e. Drop arm test

41. What ligamentous stress test can be used to screen for calcaneofibular ligament laxity?
    a. Lachman test
    b. Anterior drawer test
    c. Kleiger test
    d. Thompson test
    e. Inversion talar-tilt test

42. A hyporeflexive patellar tendon reflex would indicate pathology at what spinal nerve root level?
    a. C6
    b. C8
    c. L2
    d. L4
    e. S2

43. Which of the following is *not* an advantage of using a station format for preparticipation examinations?
    a. Lower cost for the athlete
    b. May be more comprehensive from an orthopaedic standpoint
    c. Allows for greater athlete privacy
    d. Can involve the entire sports medicine team
    e. Allows for assessment of a large number of athletes at one time

44. Which of the following would *not* be part of a lipid profile blood test?
    a. Total cholesterol level
    b. HDL level
    c. LDL level
    d. Hemoglobin level
    e. Tryglyceride level

45. Before taking part in the first practice of the season, what simple device could you use to obtain baseline data on an asthmatic athlete's peak expiratory volume?
    a. A metabolic cart
    b. A stadiometer
    c. A sphygmamometer
    d. A pulse oximeter
    e. A peak flow meter

46. Which would be the most appropriate number of sets and reps for an athlete who wanted to engage in a resistant training program to improve the muscular endurance of the quadriceps muscle group?
    a. 1 set of 15 reps
    b. 4 sets of 5 reps
    c. 2 sets of 10 reps
    d. 5 sets of 3 reps
    e. 3 sets of 20 reps

47. During the preparticipation examination, an orthopaedist or athletic trainer may assess the ACL for laxity. Which best describes what laxity is?
    a. Amount of accessory motion within a joint
    b. Amount of "give" within a joint
    c. Amount of passive range of motion available at a joint
    d. Amount of resistance within a joint
    e. Amount of active range of motion available at a joint

48. An athlete with genu valgum is more commonly referred to as having what?
    a. Knee hyperextension
    b. Frog-eyed patella
    c. Knock-knees
    d. Bowlegs
    e. "Squinting" patella

49. What is the correct rule for covering a hard cast worn on the forearm in football?
    a. No less than ½ in. thick, low-density, open-cell material on all exterior surfaces of the hard cast
    b. No less than 1 in. thick, low-density, open-cell material on all exterior surfaces of the hard cast
    c. No less than ½ in. thick, high-density, closed-cell material on all exterior surfaces of the hard cast
    d. No less than 1 in. thick, high-density, closed-cell material on all exterior surfaces of the hard cast
    e. No less than 2 in. thick, high-density, open-cell material on all exterior surfaces of the hard cast

50. Ideally, who should perform an athlete's preparticipation examination?
    a. An athletic trainer
    b. A primary care physician
    c. A school nurse
    d. A team physician
    e. An orthopaedic physician

51. At what point of dehydration do you start to see a decrease in athletic performance and thermoregulatory function?
    a. 2% BWL
    b. 4% BWL
    c. 5% BWL
    d. 6% BWL
    e. 9% BWL

52. Which of the following immunizations prevent the disease commonly known as *lock jaw*?
    a. MMR
    b. Hepatitis-B
    c. Tetanus
    d. Meningococcus
    e. Varicella

53. What structure does the Feiss line assess?
    a. Deltoid ligament complex
    b. Metatarsals
    c. Great toe
    d. Medial longitudinal arch
    e. Achilles' tendon

54. Which of the following is the medical field that specializes in the treatment of eye injuries and disorders?
    a. Endodontics
    b. Ophthalmology
    c. Optometry
    d. Osteopathy
    e. Orthopaedics

55. What type of taping procedure would you use to prevent a sprain of the anterior talofibular ligament?
    a. Open basket weave
    b. Closed basket weave
    c. Medial longitudinal arch
    d. LowDye arch
    e. Transverse arch

56. How would you do assess for cranial nerve XII function?
    a. Identify familiar taste on anterior tongue
    b. Pupillary reaction to light
    c. Resisted shoulder shrug
    d. Clenching of the teeth
    e. Lateral gaze

57. Which of the following would best describe a hammer-toe deformity?
    a. Hyperextension of the MTP joint, flexion of the PIP joint, and flexion of the DIP joint
    b. Hyperextension of the MTP joint, flexion of the PIP joint, and hyperextension of the DIP joint
    c. Flexion of the MTP joint, flexion of the PIP joint, and flexion of the DIP joint
    d. Flexion of the MTP joint, hyperextension of the PIP joint, and flexion of the DIP joint
    e. Flexion of the MTP joint, hyperextension of the PIP joint, and hyperextension of the DIP joint

58. Which organization sets the standards for football helmet certification?
    a. NCAA
    b. NATA
    c. NFHS
    d. NOCSAE
    e. OSHA

59. When performing a myotome assessment on an athlete, what component of the segmental nerve are you testing?
    a. Visceral component
    b. Sensory component
    c. Motor component
    d. Proprioceptive component
    e. Mechanoreceptor component

60. What part of the athletic shoe is responsible for controlling excessive amounts of foot inversion and eversion?
    a. Sole
    b. Toe box
    c. Heal counter
    d. Shoe uppers
    e. Arch support

61. What virus is responsible for causing shingles?
    a. Rhinovirus
    b. HBV
    c. HPV
    d. Herpes simplex virus
    e. Varicella zoster virus

62. Which of the following represents a normal Q-angle in a female?
    a. 13 degrees
    b. 18 degrees
    c. 20 degrees
    d. 25 degrees
    e. 28 degrees

63. Hepatomegaly is the enlargement of what organ?
    a. Liver
    b. Spleen
    c. Kidney
    d. Pancreas
    e. Gall bladder

64. A mesomorph body build is best described as which of the following?
    a. Thin build with a low body mass
    b. Stocky build with a high body mass
    c. Stocky build and short in height
    d. Athletic build with an average body mass
    e. Athletic build with a low body mass

65. Which of the following types of examinations would be used to test the integrity of noncontractile tissues in an injured body part?
    a. Passive range of motion
    b. Active range of motion
    c. Resistive range of motion
    d. Manual muscle tests
    e. None of the above

66. During the preparticipation examination, a physician informed a high school diver that the diver had "swimmer's ear." What structure of the ear is involved in this condition?
    a. Tympanic membrane
    b. Ear ossicles
    c. External auditory meatus
    d. Internal auditory meatus
    e. Semicircular canals

67. Which of the following is *true* regarding an increased angle of inclination?
    a. It may be manifested through genu valgum
    b. An increased angle of inclination is termed *coxa vara*
    c. It is more commonly found in males
    d. It may be manifested through a laterally positioned patella
    e. It can increase the mechanical advantage of the gluteus medius muscle

68. Where are the check-reins placed when taping an athlete who has suffered a reverse turf toe injury?
    a. Spanning the dorsum of the great toe
    b. Spanning the plantar aspect of the great toe
    c. Along the medial border of the great toe
    d. Along the lateral border of the great toe
    e. Circumferentially, just proximal to the interphalangeal joint

69. Which of the following would be of the highest priority when establishing a policies and procedures manual?
    a. Treating athletes with asthma
    b. Emergency action plan
    c. Treating heat-related illnesses
    d. Immobilizing and splinting fractures
    e. Practice coverage for athletic teams

70. What term best describes a viral infection that causes a total body skin rash for 2 to 3 days?
    a. Rubella
    b. Varicella
    c. Eczema
    d. Rubeola
    e. Ringworm

71. Which of the following would be the most appropriate test to assess an athlete's agility?
    a. The 50-yard dash
    b. The Stork test

c. The 12-minute walk/run test
d. The T-drill test
e. The Harvard step test

72. Which is an early sign of hypothermia?
    a. Pain
    b. Numbness
    c. Shivering
    d. Disorientation
    e. Burning sensation

73. What is the term for the development of tension within a muscle as it shortens?
    a. Isokinetic
    b. Eccentric
    c. Static
    d. Isometric
    e. Concentric

74. Neck rolls are used primarily to prevent what type of athletic injury?
    a. Throat injuries
    b. Contusions
    c. Brachial plexus injuries
    d. Shoulder sprains
    e. Concussions

75. Prickly heat is usually due to what mechanism and/or environmental condition?
    a. Continuously wet skin and unevaporated sweat
    b. Skin reaction to atmospheric allergens
    c. Direct, prolonged sun exposure to the skin
    d. Extremely moist air with very little air movement
    e. Low relative humidity and low ambient temperature

76. Which would *not* be an appropriate reason for applying an elastic wrap to the ankle joint?
    a. To hold a custom protective pad in place
    b. To provide stability and protection after a ligament sprain
    c. To provide support to soft tissue structures
    d. To hold a wound dressing in place
    e. To provide compression to decrease swelling

77. Which of the following is *false* regarding athletic taping?
    a. Open wounds should always be covered before taping
    b. After cryotherapy, allow the athlete's skin to return to normal temperature before taping
    c. Prewrap should always be used
    d. Avoid continuous taping
    e. Use a heel and lace pad over the Achille's tendon area

78. Which of the following is *false* regarding the appropriate fitting of a football helmet?
    a. Ear openings should be centered with the external auditory meatus
    b. Eyebrows should be two finger widths below the front edge of the helmet
    c. Back of helmet should cover base of skull
    d. You should not be able to slide your finger between the cheek pads and skin
    e. Helmet should not move or slip when rotated

79. What is the term for a lateral curvature of the thoracic spine?
    a. Kyphosis
    b. Humpback
    c. Lordosis
    d. Scoliosis
    e. Swayback

80. What type of cardiorespiratory training involves participating in a type of exercise that varies from athlete's normal exercise routine in order to improve performance?
    a. Cross training
    b. Interval training
    c. Fartlek training
    d. Plyometric training
    e. Continuous training

81. Which of the following is *false* regarding the overload principle?
    a. The overload principle can be applied to cardiorespiratory training
    b. To improve a physiological performance, the body must work harder than it is accustomed to
    c. When the body is subjected to overload, it will only result in physiological damage
    d. The overload principle can be applied to progressive resistance training
    e. The overload principle is incorporated into conditioning exercises to improve performance

82. What type of stretching technique involves a combination of alternating periods of stretching with periods of muscular contraction?
    a. Yoga
    b. Ballistic
    c. Progressive
    d. PNF
    e. Static

83. Which of the following is best described as the ability to rapidly and accurately change body position?
    a. Flexibility
    b. Agility
    c. Balance
    d. Muscular endurance
    e. Proprioception

84. What piece of equipment is needed to perform the Harvard step test?
    a. Metronome
    b. Cones
    c. VO$_{2max}$ analyzer
    d. Medicine ball
    e. Wooden block

85. How much time should an athlete allow, after applying sunscreen, before exercising outdoors?
    a. 10 minutes
    b. 20 minutes
    c. 40 minutes
    d. 50 minutes
    e. 60 minutes

86. In a set of shoulder pads with a cantilever system, where is the actual cantilever located in relation to the athlete's body?
    a. Across the shoulder blade
    b. Along the upper arm
    c. Across the top of the shoulder
    d. Across the breast bone
    e. Along the spine

87. Nitrogen dioxide, stagnant air, and sunlight are responsible for producing which of the following?
    a. Sulfur dioxide
    b. Smog
    c. Photochemical haze
    d. Carbon monoxide
    e. Nitrous oxide

88. An abnormally high hemoglobin reading, when a dipstick urinalysis test is performed, is most likely due to which of the following?
    a. Diabetes
    b. Urinary tract infection
    c. Dehydration
    d. Excessive hydration
    e. Alcoholism

89. Which of the following pieces of protective equipment are *not* required for their respective sport in college athletics?
    a. Protective eyewear—women's lacrosse
    b. Protective ear guard—wrestling
    c. Mouth guard—field hockey
    d. Knee pads—volleyball
    e. Shin guards—soccer

90. What instrument is used to determine the Temperature-Humidity Activity Index?
    a. Spirometer
    b. Dry-bulb thermometer
    c. Peak flow meter
    d. Stadiometer
    e. Sling psychrometer

91. What does the abbreviation PMH stand for?
    a. Premenstrual history
    b. Previous mental health
    c. Postworkout muscular hypertrophy
    d. Past medical history
    e. Postural muscle hypertrophy

92. Which of the following is the most necessary piece of documentation needed before allowing a college student to compete in intercollegiate athletics?
    a. Immunization record
    b. Health insurance information
    c. Authorization for emergency medical treatment
    d. Medical history questionnaire
    e. Participation clearance

93. Protective eyewear worn in college women's lacrosse must meet the standards of what organization?
    a. AOASM
    b. ASTM
    c. NFHS
    d. NCAA
    e. NOCSAE

94. A recent change in the color and size of a mole could indicate which of the following medical conditions?
    a. Diabetes
    b. Cancer
    c. AIDS
    d. Cystic fibrosis
    e. RSD

95. How long should athletic play be suspended after the last occurrence of thunder or lightning?
    a. 10 minutes
    b. 15 minutes
    c. 20 minutes
    d. 30 minutes
    e. 45 minutes

96. The Snellen chart is used in during what portion of the preparticipation examination?
    a. Eye examination
    b. Neurologic examination
    c. Musculoskeletal examination
    d. Pulmonary examination
    e. Dermatologic examination

97. What is measured when performing the pull-up test for upper body endurance?
    a. The number of repetitions completed in a 15-second period
    b. The number of repetitions completed in a 30-second period
    c. The length of time the chin can be held at the level of the pull-up bar
    d. The length of time the chin can be held just beneath the pull-up bar
    e. The number of repetitions completed until complete fatigue

98. What body composition assessment technique involves submerging the subject under water on a large scale?
    a. Bod Pod
    b. Bioelectrical impedance
    c. Hydrostatic weighing
    d. Skinfold thickness
    e. DEXA

99. When assessing resistive range of motion for a body part, what is the name of the test that is performed at the end of the range of motion, in which you apply overload pressure to the body part in a static position?
    a. Manual muscle test
    b. Strength test
    c. Break test
    d. Pressure test
    e. Stability test

100. When should the physical fitness examination be performed for incoming athletes?
    a. Before arriving at school
    b. Before their orthopaedic examination
    c. After their orthopaedic examination
    d. Before their preparticipation examination
    e. After their preparticipation examination

 Use the DVD or visit the website at http://thePoint.lww.com/Long to take the *online examination.*

✓ STUDY CHECKLIST

I have studied:
☐ Risk factors for activity
☐ Preparticipation examination
☐ Mouth guards
☐ Football helmet fitting
☐ Football shoulder pad fitting

☐ Protective devices and braces
☐ Athletic footwear
☐ Athletic wrapping
☐ Taping principles
☐ Environmental concerns

SECTION 2

SUPPLEMENTAL READING

1. Anderson MK, Parr GP, Hall SJ. *Foundations of athletic training: prevention, assessment, and management*, 4th ed. Philadelphia: Lippincott Williams & Wilkins; 2009.

2. Beam JW. *Orthopedic taping, wrapping, bracing and padding*. Philadelphia: FA Davis Co; 2006.

3. Binkley HM, Beckett J, Casa DJ, et al. National Athletic Trainers' Association position statement: Exertional heat illnesses. *J Athl Train*. 2002;347(3):329–343.

4. Casa DJ, Almquist J, Anderson S, et al. Inter-association task force on exertional heat illnesses consensus statement. *NATA News*. 2003;6:24–29.

5. Hillman SK. *Introduction to athletic training*, 2nd ed. Champaign: Human Kinetics; 2005.

6. National Athletic Trainers' Association. *Athletic training educational competencies*, 4th ed. Dallas: National Athletic Trainers' Association; 2006.

7. NCAA. *2006-07 NCAA sports medicine handbook*, 18th ed. Indianapolis: NCAA; 2006.

8. Perrin DH. *Athletic taping and bracing*, 2nd ed. Champaign: Human Kinetics; 2005.

9. Prentice WE. *Arnheim's principles of athletic training: a competency-based approach*. New York: McGraw-Hill; 2006.

10. Street S, Runkle D. *Athletic protective equipment care, selection, and fitting*. Boston: McGraw-Hill; 2000.

11. Walsh KM, Bennett B, Cooper MA, et al. National Athletic Trainers' Association position statement: Lightning safety for athletics and recreation. *J Athl Train*. 2000;35(4):471–477.

SECTION

3

Pathology of Injuries and Illnesses

Part 1   Human Cell Function and Dysfunction

Part 2   Inflammation and Infection

Part 3   Circulation and Homeostasis

Part 4   Exercise and Illness, Injury, or Disease

Part 5   Common Injuries

Section 3 Examination

OVERVIEW

Having a good understanding of the body's physiological and pathological response to injury and illness plays an important role in both the diagnosing process and in the formulation of a treatment and rehabilitation plan. Therefore, the athletic trainer should be able to describe the etiology, signs, symptoms, and epidemiology of common injuries and illnesses of the human body. To accomplish this, the athletic trainer must have fundamental knowledge on topics such as the body's inflammatory response, healing process, and cellular function. This knowledge is the first step in effectively treating your athletes and patients.

CLINICAL PROFICIENCIES

There are no proficiencies assigned by the *Athletic Training Educational Competencies*, 4th edition for this section.

Human Cell Function and Dysfunction

KEY TERMS

- Neuroglia
- Osmosis
- Pathogenesis
- Phagocyte
- Phagocytosis
- Ribonucleic acid (RNA)

CELLS

- Simplest unit of life (see Fig. 3.1)
- Plasma membrane
  - Outer layer
  - Lipid/protein composition
  - Contains microvilli
- Cytoplasm
  - Cytosol
    - Fluid
  - Endoplasmic reticulum
    - Rough endoplasmic reticulum
      - Contains ribosomes
      - Forms complex compounds
    - Smooth endoplasmic reticulum
      - Does not contain ribosomes
      - Lipid synthesis
  - Ribosomes
    - Manufacture proteins
    - Comprise protein and ribonucleic acid (RNA)
  - Mitochondria
    - Cell "powerhouse"
    - Convert nutrients to ATP
  - Golgi apparatus
    - Forms complex compounds from proteins
  - Centrioles
    - Separate chromosomes during cell division
  - Lysosomes
    - Sacs with digestive enzymes
    - Digest cell substances
  - Vesicles
    - Store and move bulk material in/out of cells
  - Peroxisomes
    - Contain enzymes
    - Break down harmful substance
- Nucleus
  - Contains chromosomes
  - Comprises DNA and protein
  - Nucleolus
    - Small body in nucleus
    - Makes ribosomes
    - Comprises RNA, DNA, and proteins

- Cell extensions
  - Flagellum
    - A whip-like projection
    - Moves cell
  - Cilia
    - Hair-like projections
    - Move fluid around cell
    - Move cell

Use the DVD or visit the website at http://thePoint.lww.com/Long for additional materials about *cell division*.

ENERGY TRANSPORT

- Glycolysis (see Figs. 3.2 to 3.4)
  - Converts glucose to pyruvic acid
  - Net gain of 2 adenosine triphosphate (ATP)
- Lactic acid pathway
  - Anaerobic
  - Lactic acid converted to glucose in liver
- Aerobic respiration
  - Krebs cycle
  - 30 to 32 ATP formed
- Lipid metabolism
  - Glycerol converted to phosphoglyceraldehyde for energy
- Protein metabolism
  - Amino acids derived from hydrolysis

TRANSPORT MECHANISMS

- Diffusion
  - Lower concentration to higher concentration
  - Passive transport
  - No energy requirement
  - Diffusion stops when concentrations are equal
- Osmosis (see Fig. 3.5)
  - Water moves from solution more dilute to one with higher solute concentration
  - Passive transport
  - No energy required
- Facilitated diffusion
  - Membrane carriers
  - Passive transport
  - Properties of saturation, specificity, and competition
- Active transport
  - Requires energy—ATP
  - Sodium-potassium pump
- Bulk transport
  - Large molecules
  - Envelops molecule

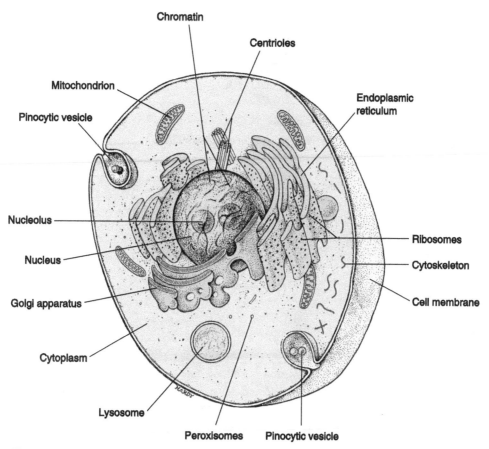

Figure 3.1 The structure of a typical cell. (From *Stedman's medical dictionary*, 27th ed. Baltimore: Lippincott Williams & Wilkins; 2000.)

- Exocytosis
- Endocytosis

SELECTED CELL ADAPTATIONS

- Atrophy—decreased muscle fiber size
- Hypertrophy—increased muscle fiber size
- Differentiation—change from one functional state to another
- Hyperplasia—increased muscle fiber numbers
- Metaplasia—converting one tissue into an abnormal other form
- Tumors—malignant or benign mass

SEGMENTS OF A NEURON

- Dendrite—an impulse toward cell body
- Axon—an impulse from cell body
- Presynaptic neuron—an impulse toward synapse
- Postsynaptic neuron—an impulse from synapse

SYNAPTIC JUNCTIONS

- Electrical
  - Gap junctions
  - Smooth muscle

- Chemical
  - Synaptic cleft
  - Most common
  - Chemical neurotransmitters

NERVE IMPULSES

- Resting potential
- Depolarization of nerve cell membrane
- Reverse membrane polarity
- Myelinated versus unmyelinated
- Large-diameter versus small-diameter nerves

Quick **fact** At rest, a nerve has a positive charge outside the cell membrane and a negative charge inside the cell membrane.

REFRACTORY PERIOD

- Repolarization following depolarization
- A change in sodium permeability
- Absolute refractory period—nothing triggers action potential
- Relative refractory period—increased stimulus will trigger action potential

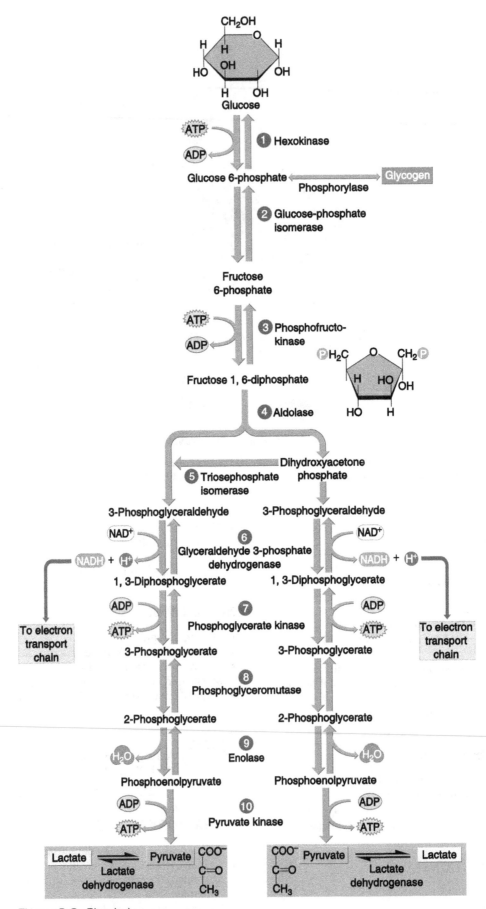

Figure 3.2 Glycolysis.

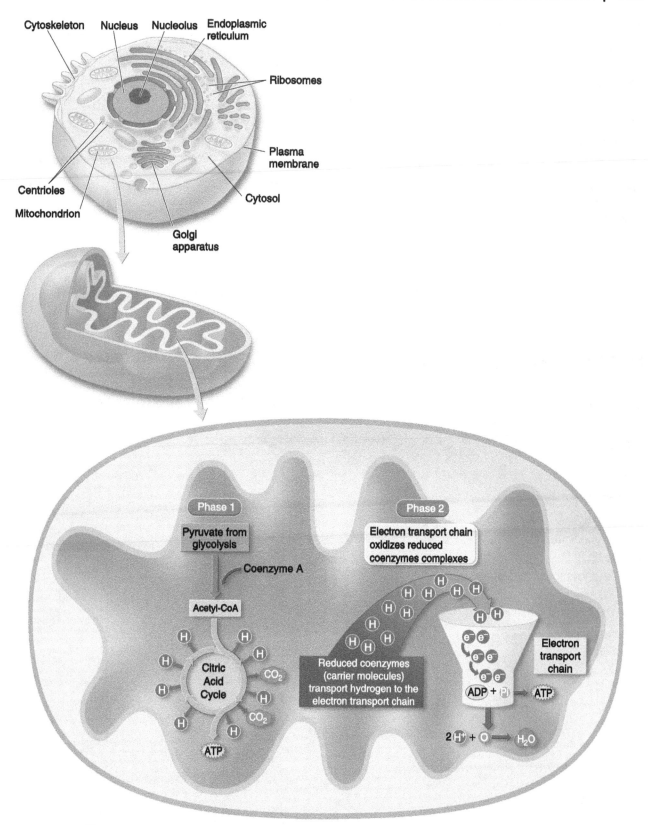

Figure 3.3 Electron Transport Chain.

ATP-PCr
Glycolysis
Oxidative
% Capacity of energy systems
100
80
60
40
20
40
80
120
160
Work time (s)

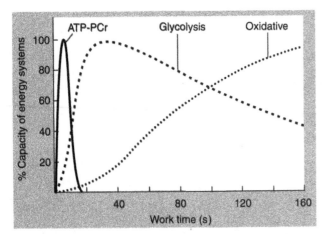

Figure 3.4 Metabolic Pathways Energy Production.

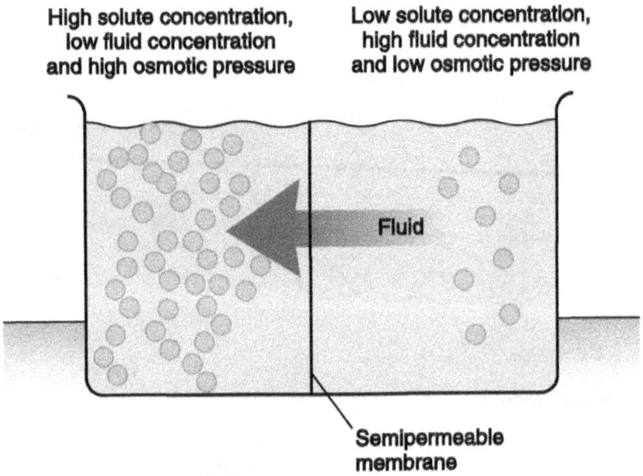

High solute concentration, low fluid concentration and high osmotic pressure
Low solute concentration, high fluid concentration and low osmotic pressure
Fluid
Semipermeable membrane

Figure 3.5 Osmosis. (Adapted from Metheny NM. *Fluid and electrolyte balance: nursing consideration*, 3rd ed. Philadelphia: Lippincott-Raven, 1996.)

PART 2 Inflammation and Infection

KEY TERMS

- Acute inflammation
- Angiogenesis
- Antibody (Ab)
- Antigen (Ag)
- Arteriovenous anastomosis (Ava)
- Bacterium, bacteria
- Chemotaxis
- Coagulation
- Debridement
- Endolymph
- Fibrin
- Fibrinogen
- Fibrinolysin
- Granulation tissue
- Immune response
- Kallikrein
- Keloid
- Kinin
- Leukotrienes (LT)
- Mast cell
- Memory B cells
- Memory T cells
- Neutrophil
- Plasmin
- Plasminogen
- Polymorphonuclear leukocyte, polynuclear leukocyte
- Prodromal stage
- Prodrome
- Proteoglycans
- Prothrombin
- Releasing factors
- Reticular formation
- Reticulin
- Thrombin
- Viscosity

INJURY PROCESS

- Stress overcomes body's ability to adapt
- Microtrauma versus macrotrauma
- Primary versus secondary damage

WOLFF LAW

- Changes in bone architecture related to weight bearing
- Increased weight bearing = increased bone strength
- Decreased weight bearing = decreased bone strength
- Osteoblasts versus osteoclast activity

TISSUE RECOVERY PROCESS

- Healing by primary and secondary intention
- Limits the pain→spasm→loss of motion→loss of function cycle
- Often lasts longer than outward signs/symptoms
- Three phases of healing
  ○ Inflammatory
  ○ Proliferation/repair/revascularization/rebuilding/fibroblastic
  ○ Maturation/remodeling

OUTSIDE FACTORS AFFECTING HEALING

- Age
- Chronic disease
- Dehydration
- Infection
- Malnutrition
- Smoking
- Substance use

INFLAMMATORY PHASE

- Maintain homeostasis (see Fig. 3.6)
- Stabilize and contain the injured areas
- Mobilize natural defenses
- Quick vasoconstriction
- Initial coagulation through platelets
- Vascular permeability changes
- Vasodilation

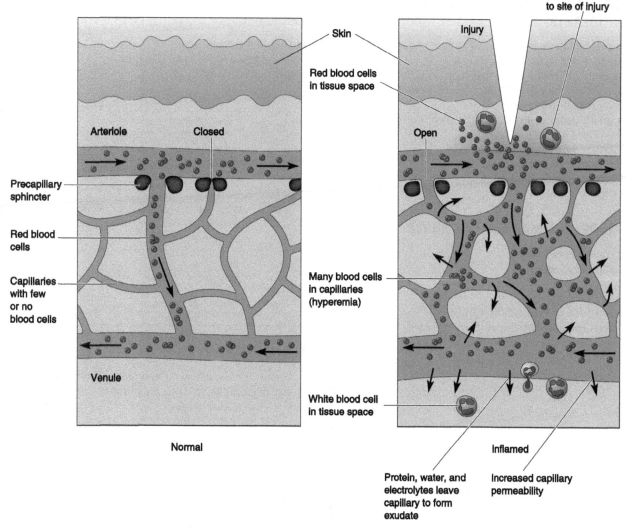

Figure 3.6 Acute Inflammatory Process. (From Premkumar K. *The massage connection anatomy and physiology*. Baltimore: Lippincott Williams & Wilkins; 2004.)

- Chemotactin
- Initial debridement
- Damaged lymphatic vessels precipitate extracellular fluid retention
- Lasts up to 5 days

Quick fact Avoid thinking of the inflammatory phase as the enemy to recovery. It is a necessary component of healing unless it is not limited.

SIGNS OF INFLAMMATION

- Heat
- Loss of function
- Pain
- Redness (hyperemia)
- Swelling (edema)

PROLIFERATION/REPAIR/ REVASCULARIZATION/REBUILDING/ FIBROBLASTIC PHASE

- Dispose of dead cells (see Fig. 3.7)
- Restore circulation
- Granulation tissue formation
- Transition from debridement to angiogenesis
- Increased fibroblasts
- Increased extracellular collagen (type III→type I) (see Fig. 3.8)
- Increased proteoglycans
- Increased epithelial cell mitosis
- Decreased polymorphonuclear leukocytes (PMN)
- Lasts up to 4 weeks

REMODELING/MATURATION PHASE

- Capillary recession
- Return to function
- Increased tensile strength
- Decreased glycoproteins
- Decreased glycosaminoglycan (GAG)
- Decreased fibroblasts and myofibroblasts
- May take a year or more for completion

Quick fact Inflammatory mediators include heparin, histamine, kinin, leukotrienes, neutrophils, prostaglandin, and serotonin.

Quick fact Many of the early cells of wound healing are considered chemotaxis or attract other cells toward the site.

Use the DVD or visit the website at http://thePoint.lww.com/Long for additional materials about *substances of wound healing.*

COLONIZATION VERSUS INFECTION

- Colonization implies that a microorganism is present without causing illness
- Infection occurs when a microorganism causes disease

Quick fact People are frequently colonized with various "bugs"—*Streptococcus, Staphylococcus,* but healthy immune systems are able to fight infection or an adequate portal of entry so that the infection does not occur.

CHAIN OF INFECTION

- Pathogen
- Reservoir
- Portal of exit
- Means of transmission
- Portal of entry
- New host

Quick fact The infectious disease cycle begins with a pathogenic microorganism.

Quick fact Many microorganisms cause disease because of the toxins they produce while living in the body.

Quick fact Pathogens have natural environments in which they prosper.

TRANSMISSION

- Must leave the reservoir and move through a portal of exit (e.g., saliva, mucous membranes, blood, feces, and nose/throat discharges)
- Direct (contact) or indirect (vector, e.g., mosquitoes or ticks)

PORTAL OF ENTRY

- Penetration of the skin or direct contact
- Inhalation through the mouth or nose
- Ingestion of contaminated food or water

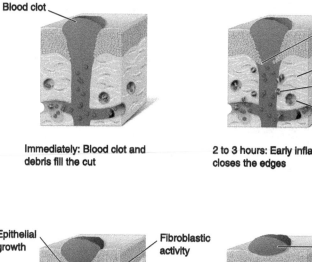

Immediately: Blood clot and
debris fill the cut

2 to 3 hours: Early inflammation
closes the edges

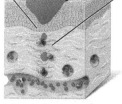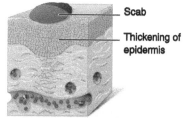

2 to 3 days: Macrophages remove
blood clot; Increased fibroblastic
activity and epithelial growth
close gap

10 to 14 days: Scab formation—
epithelial covering is complete
and edges of wound unite by
fibrous tissue; however, the
wound is still weak

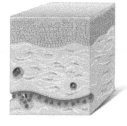

Weeks: The scar tissue is still
hyperemic; union of edges is
good but not full strength

Months to Years: Very little or
no scars; collagen tissue
remodeled by enzymes;
normal blood flow

Figure 3.7 Healing of Skin Wounds by First Intention. (From Premkumar K. *The massage connection anatomy and physiology*. Baltimore: Lippincott Williams & Wilkins; 2004.)

Quick fact The number of microorganisms present and/or a compromised immune system enhances chance of infection.

Quick fact If the environment is right—the new host may become a reservoir for the disease.

BODY'S DEFENSE SYSTEM

- Skin
- Mucous membranes
- Cilia
- Inflammatory and immune response

Use the DVD or visit the website at http://thePoint.lww.com/Long for additional materials about *inflammatory immune response*.

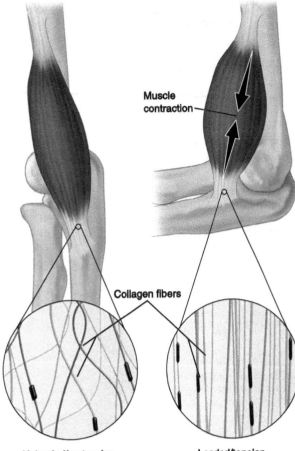

Figure 3.8 Collagen Fibers.

LYMPHATIC SYSTEM AND INFECTION

Lymphatic Functions
- Fluid balance
  - Retrieves excess fluid and protein left in the interstitial spaces
- Infection protection
  - Lymphocytes (white blood cells [WBCs]) attack pathogens
  - Filtration of foreign/harmful debris
- Fat absorption
  - Brings large products of digestion, for example, fats to the blood stream

Lymphatic Capillaries
- More permeable (larger pores) particularly to proteins
- Similar to blood capillaries
- One-way valves of overlapping cells

Right Lymphatic Duct
- Lymph from right superior quadrant (right head, neck, thorax, and extremity)
- Empties into right subclavian vein
- Smaller duct than thoracic duct

Thoracic Duct
- Lymph from the entire body except right superior quadrant
- Opens into the left subclavian vein

Main Lymph Node Location
- Inguinal
- Mesenteric (largest number)
- Tracheobronchial
- Axillary
- Cervical

Spleen Functions
- Cleanse blood
- Destroy red blood cells (RBCs)
- Prebirth RBC production
- Blood reservoir
- Huge blood supply

Thymus
- Key in immunity prebirth to early infancy
- T lymphocytes develop influences by thymosin (hormone)
- Shrinks after puberty

Tonsils
- Located near pharynx
- Grooves housing lymphocytes
- Tonsil location
  - Lingual tonsils—back of tongue
  - Pharyngeal tonsils (adenoids)—behind nose
  - Palatine—either side of soft palate; one thinks of as a tonsil

Appendix
- Lymphoid tissue
- Attached to large intestine
- May play a role in developmental immunity
- Appendicitis causes pain at the McBurney point

IMMUNITY DEFENSE MECHANISMS

- Nonspecific defenses
  - Attack pathological organisms regardless of type
- Specific defenses
  - Attack only certain pathological organisms but not others

Types of Nonspecific Defenses
- Chemical and mechanical barriers
  - Skin, mucous membranes, cilia, tears, perspiration, saliva, digestive juices, sneezing, coughing, vomiting, and diarrhea
- Phagocytes
  - Destroy WBC and remove foreign material

- Natural killer cells
  - Found in lymph nodes, spleen, blood, and bone marrow
  - Recognize dangerous cells, for example, tumor cells by membranes and destroy them
- Inflammation
  - Get rid of irritants
  - Triggered by histamine
- Fever
  - Results from and boosts immune system activity
  - Controlling fever, unless extremely high, is merely an act of decreasing uncomfortable symptoms
- Interferon
  - Substances released by some cells
  - Prevent viral multiplication and spreading

Types of Specific Defenses

- Inborn immunity
  - Inherited or genetic immunity
  - Species and individual immunity
- Acquired immunity (occurs after birth)
  - Natural immunity
    - Active—contact with the disease
    - Passive—antibodies in placenta or through nursing
  - Artificial immunity
    - Active—vaccine
    - Passive—immune serum

ATTENUATED VACCINE

- One that is from a live organism but weakened for use
- Heat or chemical alteration
- Takes several weeks for this immunity to occur
- Altered toxin is called *toxoid*

IMMUNE SERUM (ANTISERUM)

- Used in emergencies when there is no time to wait for active immunity
- Used when a person is exposed to toxic amounts of a virulent organism
- Contains counteracting antibodies
- Short-term protection

PART 3 # Circulation and Homeostasis

KEY TERMS

- Erythropoiesis
- Hemiparesis
- Hemodynamometer
- Hemopoiesis
- Hemopoietic

CIRCULATION

Functions of the Circulatory System

- Transportation—substances necessary for cellular metabolism
  - Respiratory—RBC for O_2 transport
  - Nutritive—absorbed products of digestion through liver and into cells of the body
  - Excretory—metabolic wastes, excessive water, and ions
- Regulation—carries hormones from site of origin to target tissue
- Protection—clotting to decrease blood loss, WBC for immunity

Major Components of the Circulatory System

- Cardiovascular system—heart and blood vessels
- Lymphatic system—lymph vessels, lymph nodes, lymphoid organs (spleen, tonsils, and thymus)

Components of Blood

- Erythrocytes (RBCs)—O_2 transport (see Fig. 3.9)
- Leukocytes (WBCs)—immune defense
- Thrombocytes (platelets)—blood clotting; cell fragments
- Plasma—contains proteins and many water-soluble molecules (glucose and electrolytes); 55% total blood volume; 91% water

> **Quick fact** Five liters of blood (8% of body weight) in adult.

Plasma Proteins

- Albumins—produced by liver and provide osmotic pressure needed to draw water from surrounding tissue fluid into the capillaries
- Globulins
  - α-Globulins—formed by the liver and function to transport lipids and fat-soluble vitamins in blood

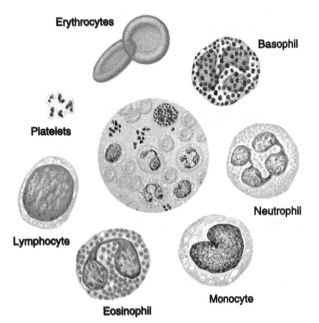

Erythrocytes

Basophil

Platelets

Neutrophil

Lymphocyte

Eosinophil

Monocyte

Figure 3.9 White Blood Cells and Platelets. (From Smeltzer SC, Bare BG. *Brunner and Suddarth's textbook of medical-surgical nursing,* 9th ed. Philadelphia: Lippincott Williams & Wilkins; 2002.)

- ○ β-Globulins—formed by the liver and function to transport lipids and fat-soluble vitamins in blood
- ○ γ-Globulins—antibodies produced by lymphocytes
- Fibrinogen—produced by the liver used in clotting by converting to fibrin

Plasma Volume
- Decreased water then remaining plasma becomes excessively concentrated (osmolality increases)
- Osmoreceptors in the hypothalamus detect decreases in water and stimulate thirst sensation and release of antidiuretic hormone (ADH) from posterior pituitary (improves water retention by kidneys)

Erythrocytes
- Flattened, biconcave discs
- Production of RBC requires vitamins B and C, folic acid, iron, and copper
- Most numerous of blood cells
- Live 120 days—destroyed by liver and spleen
- Shape allows increased surface area for oxygen transport and gas diffusion
- No nuclei or mitochondria (anuclear)—need more space for oxygen carrying
- Get energy through anaerobic respiration
- Hemoglobin molecules give blood red color—"heme" iron and "globin" protein
- Cannot move independently
- Erythropoietin—hormone stimulates RBC production; released by kidney when oxygen supply decreases

Hemoglobin
- Iron-containing protein
- Carries oxygen, carbon dioxide, and H^+

- Four amino acid chains—each with one heme group
- Four heme groups on each RBC bind to four oxygen molecules

Leukocytes
- Contain nuclei and mitochondria
- Round in shape
- Move like amoeba toward infection site and through pores in capillary walls
- Diapedesis—movement of leukocytes through capillary walls
- WBCs are invisible under microscope unless stained

 Use the DVD or visit the website at http://thePoint.lww.com/Long for additional information about *leukocytes.*

Thrombocytes (Platelets)
- Smallest are actually fragments of large cells found in bone marrow (megakaryocytes)
- Life span 10 days
- No nucleus or DNA
- Do have mitochondria
- Can move like amoeba
- Important role in blood clotting
  - ○ Phospholipids in platelet cell membrane activate clotting factors in plasma (plasma fibrin)
  - ○ Release serotonin which constricts blood vessels and decreases blood flow in injured areas
  - ○ Secrete growth factors

Anemia
- Condition characterized by abnormally low concentration of hemoglobin or RBC content
- Iron-deficiency anemia—decreased iron which is crucial component to hemoglobin
- Pernicious anemia—inadequate availability of vitamin B_{12}, which is needed for RBC production
- Aplastic anemia—destruction of bone marrow by chemicals (e.g., chemotherapy, x-rays)

Hemopoiesis
- A process by which blood cells are formed
- Erythropoiesis—RBC formation
- Leukopoiesis—WBC formation

Two Areas of Hemopoiesis After Birth
- Myeloid tissue—red bone marrow of long bones, ribs, sternum, bodies of vertebrae, and portions of skull (form all types of blood cells)
- Lymphoid tissue—lymph nodes, tonsils, spleen, and thymus (form lymphocytes)

 Quick fact Destruction of aging RBC in spleen and liver.

Quick fact The pH of blood plasma averages 7.40 and is regulated by *lungs* and *kidneys.*

Hemostasis
- Prevents blood loss when damage occurs to a blood vessel
- Process of hemostasis
  - Vasoconstriction of smooth muscles in blood vessels—decrease blood flow
  - Platelet plug formation—coagulation
  - Blood clot

Final Steps of Blood Clotting

- Prothrombinase with Ca^{2+} converts prothrombin to thrombin
- Thrombin converts fibrinogen to fibrin
- Fibrin plus blood cells and plasma forms blood clot

ABO Blood Type Groups

- Four blood types
  - A
  - B
  - AB
  - O
- A blood type has A antigen
- B blood type has B antigen
- AB blood type has AB antigen
- O blood type has no antigen
- People with O blood type are universal donors
- People with AB blood type are universal recipients

> **Quick fact** Agglutination (clumping)—occurs if giving a person blood from a different blood type group.

Rh Factor (D Antigen)

- Rh negative—no D antigen
- Rh positive—contains D antigen
- Named for Rhesus monkeys in which it was first identified
- Contributes to complications with transfusions and pregnancy

> **Quick fact** Blood can be stored for 35 days.

Types of Blood Vessels

- Arteries—from heart to tissues
- Arterioles—oxygenated blood into capillaries
- Capillaries—gas exchange
  - Connect arterioles and venules
  - Single cell thickness
- Venules—deoxygenated blood from capillaries back toward heart
- Veins—blood from tissues to heart

Three Tunics (Layers) of Artery

- Endothelium
  - Inner tunic
  - Smooth epithelial cells
  - Smooth cells prevent blood clotting
- Middle tunic
  - Smooth muscle
  - Thickest layer
  - Under autonomic nervous system (ANS) control
- Outer tunic
  - Connective tissue

Arteries

- Arteries have thick walls because blood is pumped under pressure
- Arteries are deep

Veins

- Same three layers as artery
- Much thinner than artery
- One-way valves
- Deep veins tend to parallel arteries
- Veins are both superficial and deep

Anastomoses

- Communication areas between vessels
- Blood can reach vital centers with more than a single pathway
- Arteriovenous anastomoses (Ava) have no capillary but rather connected through a thoroughfare called a *metarteriole*
  - Increase blood flow
  - Increase blood volume
  - Prevent tissue freezing, for example, feet, hands, earlobes

Portal Systems

- Blood leaving capillary bed does not go back to heart
- Blood moves toward another capillary bed in another tissue, for example, hepatic portal system
- Hepatic portal system
  - Blood from abdominal organs goes to the liver
  - Blood collected in sinus networks (sinusoids)
  - Nutrients in blood are processed in liver

Capillary Exchange

- Diffusion is main method
- Interstitial fluid—slightly salty
- Blood pressure—pushes fluids into interstitial spaces
- Osmotic pressure pulls fluids into capillaries

Blood Pressure

- Force of blood against vessel walls
- BP = Cardiac output × peripheral resistance

PART 4

Exercise and Illness, Injury, or Disease

KEY TERMS

- Atlantoaxial
- Obese
- Prosthesis, prostheses
- Quadraplegia

Exercise suggestions are given as ranges. At no time should a health care professional push someone beyond his or her physical capabilities. In many instances, for example, working with the elderly, the suggestions are more aggressive than the person's physical starting point. Meet the person at his or her physical capability and gradually yet progressively enhance the well-being. Specific special populations are listed in the following text with recommendations. Frequency, intensity, duration, and mode of exercise are not identified for some populations as limitations may only be dictated by the individual's ability and not the diagnosis.

AGING

Etiology: Increasing biological age, poor lifestyle choices, environment, malnutrition, and/or chronic disease states
Characteristics:
- Decreased number and size of muscle and nerve fibers
- Decreased flexibility and motor control
- Increased heart rate, blood pressure, and cardiac work
- Decreased functional capacity and stroke volume
- Decreased ATP, creatinine phosphate (CP), and glycogen stores
- Decreased VO_2max and fat-free body mass
- Increased osteoporosis

Exercise Precautions:
- Avoid high-intensity exercise
- Decreased adaptability and recovery from exercise
- Increase warm-up and cool-down
- Self-directed pace
- Avoid isometrics or Valsalva with resistance training

Frequency:
- Aerobics—3 to 5 days per week
- Resistance—2 to 3 days per week
- Flexibility—daily
- Motor Control—2 to 3 days per week

Intensity: 40% to 70% VO_2max; 60% to 80% HR_{max}
Duration: 30 to 60 minutes
Mode: Flexibility, motor control, resistance, and low-impact aerobic activities

> **Quick fact** Strength decreases 15% per decade between ages 50 and 70 and 30% per decade thereafter.

AMPUTATIONS

Etiology: Varied causes, for example, chronic disease, trauma, and birth abnormality
Characteristics:
- Surgically or traumatically removed body part, often an extremity or part of an extremity
- Often requires prosthetic device

Exercise Precautions:
- Stump breakdown
- Balance issues because of altered center of gravity
- Phantom pain syndrome

ARTHRITIS

Etiology: Inflammatory joint and rheumatologic disease
Characteristics:
- Pain
- Stiffness
- Muscle weakness
- Fatigue
- Inflamed joints, tendons, ligaments, and bones
- Joint degeneration

Exercise Precautions:
- Increased pain and stiffness may prevent early day exercise
- Nonsteroidal anti-inflammatory drug (NSAID) use may cause anemia and gastrointestinal bleeding
- Musculoskeletal pain may be decreased with NSAID usage
- No exercise during flare-ups

Frequency:
- Aerobics—3 to 5 days per week
- Resistance—2 to 3 days per week
- Flexibility—daily

Intensity: 40% to 70% VO_2max; 60% to 80% HR_{max}
Duration: 30 to 60 minutes
Mode: Low-intensity aerobic, resistance, and flexibility exercises

CANCER

Etiology: Uncontrolled proliferation of cells
Characteristics:
- Multitude of differing disease states
- May or may not be invasive
- Often requires surgery, radiation, and/or chemotherapy

Exercise Precautions:
- Precautions vary with stage of treatment or recovery
- Self-paced low-intensity programs initially
- Increase intensity of programs as strength and endurance develops

CEREBRAL PALSY

Etiology: Varied causes, for example, chronic disease, trauma, and birth abnormality
Characteristics:
- Chronic neurologic disorder
- Pathological reflexes
- Seizures
- Brain lesion

Exercise Precautions:
- Unpredictable hypertonic and hypotonic muscle contractions
- Balance issues require even ground and open eye training

CYSTIC FIBROSIS

Etiology: Genetic disability primarily in whites
Characteristics:
- Pulmonary symptoms (initially similar to asthma)
- High mucus production
- Lower airway infections
- Gastrointestinal and pancreatic duct obstructions
- Digestive enzyme secretion abnormalities

Exercise Precautions:
- Assure arterial O_2 concentrations do not decrease with activity
- Competitive sports may alter perception of safe participation
- Consider avoiding strenuous resistance training

Quick fact Exercising for the patient with cystic fibrosis results in increased productive discharge of mucus.

DIABETES MELLITUS

Etiology: Type 1—genetic and autoimmune link; type 2—changeable risk factors and sedentary lifestyle
Characteristics:
- Polyuria
- Polydipsia
- Polyphagia
- Hyperglycemia
- Varied glucose levels

Exercise Precautions:
- Decreased circulation
- Look for signs of skin breakdown and wounds frequently
- Vision changes may affect balance
- Increased nerve deterioration
- Avoid late-night exercise (hypoglycemia while sleeping)
- No exercise of insulin injection sites for 60 minutes following injection
- A light meal before exercise
- Dehydration
- 10 to 30 g carbohydrate snacks for every 45 to 60 minutes of exercise
- Check blood glucose levels frequently
- Exercise with a partner
- Caution intense resistance exercises

Frequency: 3 to 4 days per week
Intensity: 40% to 70% VO_2max; 60% to 80% HR_{max}
Duration: 30 to 60 minutes per day
Mode: Aerobic, flexibility, and resistance exercises

Quick fact Diabetic patients should consider exercising at the same time each day.

DOWN SYNDROME

Etiology: Genetic
Characteristics:
- Intellectual disability
- Decreased coordination, balance, and vision
- Commonly, cardiac defects are present
- Hypothyroidism
- Atlantoaxial instability
- Pain insensitivity

Exercise Precautions:
- Increased time for noticeable aerobic gains
- Heart rate lower than normal (30 to 35 beats per minute less)
- Require clear directions, task demonstration, and constant reinforcement
- Medical clearance for contact activities, for example, diving

HEARING IMPAIRMENT

Etiology: Varied causes, for example, chronic disease, trauma, and birth abnormality
Characteristics:
- Inability to hear normally

Exercise Precautions:
- Communications
- Decreased balance
- Patients with cochlear implants should not use plastic equipment (static)

HYPERTENSION

Etiology: Increased vascular resistance
Characteristics: Increased systolic and/or diastolic blood pressure
Exercise Precautions:
- In stage 3 hypertension, begin medication before exercise
- No exercise if systolic reading >200 mm Hg or diastolic >110 mm Hg
- Avoid isometric and Valsalva maneuvers with resistance training
- Know results of hypertension medications, for example, diuretics and β-blockers
- Medication may impair thermoregulation
Frequency: 3 to 7 days per week
Intensity: 40% to 70% VO_2max; 60% to 80% HR_{max}
Duration: 30 to 60 minutes
Mode: Aerobic exercise primary mode; circuit training resistance programs possible

> **Quick fact** Stage 1 and 2 hypertension responds to aerobic activity by decreasing blood pressure on average 10 mm Hg.

OBESITY

Etiology: Genetic and/or environmental
Characteristics:
- Body mass index of 30 or above
- Other associated chronic conditions
Exercise Precautions:
- Increased hyperthermia with exercise
- May begin non–weight bearing and progress as tolerated
- Increased risk for orthopaedic injuries
Frequency: 5 to 7 days per week
Intensity: 60% to 85% VO_2max; 50% to 70% HR_{max}
Duration: 45 to 60 minutes
Mode: Aerobic activities (large muscle groups)

OSTEOPOROSIS

Etiology: Low bone mass caused by systemic skeletal disease
Characteristics:
- Skeletal fragility
- Skeletal fractures
- Postural changes
Exercise Precautions:
- Explosive exercises
- Excessive trunk flexion
- Dynamic abdominal exercises
- Twisting motions
- Postural deviations change center of gravity
- Balance deterioration
Frequency:
- Aerobics—3 to 5 days per week
- Resistance—2 to 3 days per week
- Flexibility—daily

Intensity: 40% to 70% VO_2max; 40% to 70% HR_{max}
Duration: 30 to 60 minutes
Mode: Weight-bearing aerobic and resistance exercises; flexibility training

PARAPLEGIA

Etiology: Varied causes, for example, chronic disease, trauma, and birth abnormality
Characteristics: Inability to have sensory and/or motor function in two of four extremities and surrounding structures
Exercise Precautions:
- Skin breakdown
- Increased resting heart rate
- Decreased blood pressure
- Autonomic dysreflexia (hyperreflexia)
- Spasms
- Bladder/bowel dysfunction
- Sensation deficits prevent pain recognition

POLIOMYELITIS

Etiology: Viral infection
Characteristics:
- Nonfunctioning motor nerves
- Intact sensory nerves
- Partial paralysis where virus invades
Exercise Precautions:
- Avoid overfatigue
- Postpolio syndrome

PREGNANCY

Etiology: Gestational condition resulting from fertilized egg implant
Characteristics:
- Increased weight gain
- Changes in hormonal levels
- Altered center of gravity
Exercise Precautions:
- Avoid abdominal trauma risks
- Increase carbohydrate intake in last trimester
- Avoid static standing
- Dehydration risk
- Thermoregulatory risk
- Heart rate decreases to heavy submaximal conditioning
- Sedentary women may start exercise in second trimester with medical approval
- Altered metabolic and cardiopulmonary functions
- Hypermobility (related to hormones) may contribute to joint dysfunction
Frequency: 3 to 7 days per week
Intensity: Use rating of perceived exertion (RPE) scale and not heart rate
Duration: 30 to 60 minutes
Mode: Aerobic and resistance exercises

> **Quick fact** Regular exercise may be useful in decreasing preeclampsia and gestational diabetes.

PULMONARY DISEASE

Etiology: Lung obstruction or restriction
   conditions
Characteristics:
   ○ Dyspnea
   ○ Shortness of breath
Exercise Precautions:
   ○ Arterial oxygen saturation levels may
      decrease
   ○ Use pulse oximetry initially
   ○ Supplemental oxygen may be warranted
   ○ Upper extremity exercises especially critical to
      training
   ○ Inspiratory muscle training
   ○ Skeletal muscle deterioration because of oxygen
      decreases
Frequency: 3 to 5 days weekly
Intensity: No concluding recommendations; 50% VO$_2$max;
   50% HR$_{max}$
Duration: Intermittent, repetitive exercises with rest;
   exercise up to 30 minutes daily
Mode: Aerobic and resistance training

RHABDOMYOLYSIS

Etiology: Medications, supplements, trauma, toxins,
   and other disease state or genetic
   conditions
Characteristics:
   ○ Hyperkalemia
   ○ Dark urine
   ○ Cramping
   ○ Cardiac arrhythmias
   ○ Acute renal failure
   ○ Clotting cascade failure
Exercise Precautions:
   ○ Assure proper hydration
   ○ Avoid precipitating factors

SICKLE CELL TRAIT

Etiology: Genetic (see Fig. 3.10)
Characteristics:
   ○ Malformed RBCs
   ○ Decreased oxygen binding to RBCs
Exercise Precautions:
   ○ Thermoregulatory deficiency
   ○ Avoid high-intensity exercise
   ○ Hypotension
   ○ Tachycardia
   ○ Muscle cramping
   ○ Hyperventilation
   ○ Ischemia

SPINA BIFIDA

Etiology: Congenital neural tube defect
Characteristics:
   ○ Altered sensory and motor function
   ○ Open or skin-covered spinal neural tube
   ○ Cerebral shunts may be present

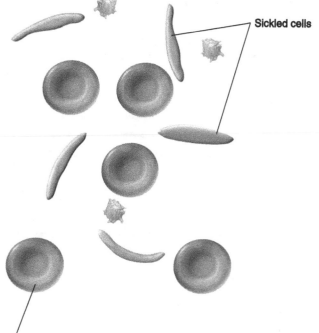

Sickled cells

Normal red
blood cell

Figure 3.10 Sickle Cell Anemia. (Asset provided by
Anatomical Chart Co.)

Exercise Precautions:
   ○ Increased latex sensitivity
   ○ Headgear required if cerebral shunts
      present
   ○ Increased gag reflex
   ○ Bladder/bowel dysfunctions
   ○ Spasms
   ○ Skin lesions may go unnoticed

TETRAPLEGIA (QUADRAPLEGIA)

Etiology: Varied causes, for example, chronic disease,
   trauma, and birth abnormality
Characteristics: Inability to have sensory and/or motor
   function in four extremities and surrounding
   structures
Exercise Precautions:
   ○ Skin breakdown
   ○ Increased resting heart rate
   ○ Decreased blood pressure
   ○ Autonomic dysreflexia (hyperreflexia)
   ○ Spasms
   ○ Bladder/bowel dysfunction
   ○ Sensation deficits prevent pain
      recognition

Quick fact Decreased venous return in nonfunctioning
extremities raises resting heart rate in
athletes with tetraplegia.

VISUAL IMPAIRMENT

Etiology: Varied causes, for example, chronic disease, trauma, and birth abnormality
Characteristics: Inability to see normally
Exercise Precautions:
- Communications
- Postural deviations
- Decreased balance in newly blind
- Nystagmus
- Glaucoma patients should avoid all underwater activities, swimming, and isometrics

---

PART 5 Common Injuries

KEY TERMS

- Abscess
- Ankylosing spondylitis
- Axonotmesis
- Bankart lesion
- Battle sign
- Bimalleolar fracture
- Bone scan
- Bucket-handle tear
- Calcific bursitis
- Calcific tendinitis
- Computed tomography (CT)
- Epistasis
- External fixation
- Fluorescein
- Gamekeeper's thumb
- Gunstock deformity
- Herniated disc
- Hill-Sachs lesion
- Internal fixation
- Laminectomy
- Lisfranc injury
- Loose bodies
- Lumbar puncture
- Magnetic resonance imaging (MRI)
- Mallet finger
- Mallet toe
- Malocclusion
- March fracture
- Meniscectomy
- Meniscus, menisci
- Neurapraxia
- Neuropathy
- Neurotmesis
- Plexopathy
- Plica
- Pneumothorax
- Pott fracture
- Scotty dog
- Sinding-Larsen-Johansson syndrome
- SLAP lesion
- Spina bifida occulta
- Spinal stenosis
- Spondylitis
- Spondylolisthesis
- Spondylolysis
- Spondylopathy
- Spondylosis
- Tetraplegia

COMMON PATHOLOGY TERMS

- Ape Hand Deformity: Extension of the thumb and alignment in the same plane as the fingers
- Athlete Foot: Tinea pedis—fungal infection
- Baker Cyst: Synovial membrane herniation into the popliteal fossa
- Bankart Lesion: Damage to the anterior lip of the glenoid
- Baseball Finger: Rupture of extensor tendon from distal interphalangeal (DIP) joint (mallet finger)
- Battle Sign: Discoloration behind the ear due to a basilar skull fracture
- Benediction Deformity: Wasting of the hypothenar, dorsal interossei and fourth and fifth lumbrical muscles resulting from ulnar nerve palsy (Bishop deformity)
- Bennett Fracture: Fracture-dislocation to the proximal end of the first metacarpal at the carpal-metacarpal joint

- Bishop Deformity: Wasting of the hypothenar, dorsal interossei and fourth and fifth lumbrical muscles resulting from ulnar nerve palsy (Benediction deformity)
- Blow-Out Fracture: Fracture of the orbital floor occurring as a result of a sudden increase in orbital pressure from a direct blow to the eye
- Blow-Out Injury: An injury occurring from a hard blow to the chest while the glottis is closed, which results in rupturing of the alveoli
- Bouchard Nodes: Nodules or bony enlargement of the proximal interphalangeal (PIP) joint of the hand
- Boutonniere Deformity: Rupture of the central slip of the extensor tendon at the PIP resulting in no active extensor mechanism at the PIP joint
- Bowler's Thumb: Compression of the digital nerve on the medial aspect of the thumb, leading to paresthesia in the thumb
- Boxer's Fracture: Fracture of the fifth metacarpal
- Bucket-Handle Tear: Longitudinal meniscal tear
- Cheyne-Stokes Respirations: Abnormal breathing pattern of hyperpnea and apnea
- Claw Hand Deformity: Injury to the median and ulnar nerves, hyperextension of metacarpophalangeal (MCP) joints, and flexion of PIP and DIP
- Claw Toe: Hyperextension of metatarsophalangeal (MTP) joint and hyperflexion of interphalangeal (IP) joints
- Coach Finger: Fixed flexion deformity resulting from dislocation at the PIP joint
- Colle Fracture: Fracture involving a displaced radius 1.5 in. from the wrist
- Cyclist's Nipples: Nipple irritation due to perspiration and wind-chill
- Cyclist's Palsy: Paresthesia in the ulnar nerve distribution
- de Quervain's Syndrome: Inflammatory stenosing tenosynovitis of the abductor pollicis longus and extensor pollicis brevis tendons
- Dead Arm Syndrome: Common sensation felt with recurrent anterior shoulder dislocation
- Dupuytren Contracture: Fibrosis of the palmar fascia with flexion deformity of the fourth and fifth digits
- Faun Beard: Hairy patch over lumbar spine indicating spina bifida occulta
- Forearm Splints: Chronic strain to the forearm muscles
- Freiberg Disease: Avascular necrosis to the second metatarsal head in some adolescents
- Frozen Shoulder: Adhesive capsulitis of the shoulder
- Gamekeeper's Thumb: Rupture of the ulnar collateral ligament (UCL) (volar ligament) of the thumb secondary to hyperextension and abduction
- Golfer's Elbow: Medial epicondylitis
- Gunstock Deformity: A carrying angle of less than the 5 to 15 degrees valgus angulation
- Hammer Toe: Flexion deformity of DIP
- Heberden Nodes: Nodules or bony enlargement of the DIP of the hand
- Hill-Sachs Lesion: Defect on the posterior aspect of the articular cartilage of the humeral head
- Hip Pointer: Contusions of the iliac crest
- Hump Back: Increased kyphotic curve

- Jersey Finger: Rupture of flexor digitorum profundus
- Jock Itch: Tinea cruris—fungal infection
- Joint Mice: Loose fragments within a joint
- Jones Fracture: A transverse stress fracture of the proximal fifth metatarsal
- Kehr Sign: Referred pain down the left shoulder indicative of a ruptured spleen
- Kienböck Disease: Avascular necrosis of the lunate
- Larsen-Johansson Disease: Inflammation or partial avulsion of the apex of the patella
- Legg-Calvé-Perthes Disease: Avascular necrosis of the proximal epiphysis
- Lisfrank Injury: Injury to the tarsometatarsal joint
- Little Leaguer's Shoulder: Fracture of the proximal humeral growth plate
- Little Leaguer's Elbow: Tension stress injury of the medial epicondyle
- Maisonneuve Fracture: An external rotation injury of the ankle with an associated fracture of the proximal third of the fibula
- Mallet Finger: Rupture of extensor tendon from DIP
- Mallet Toe: MTP and PIP neutral and flexed DIP of toe
- Marfan Syndrome: Connective tissue disorder
- McBurney Point: A point one third of the distance between the anterior superior iliac spine (ASIS) and umbilicus. Indicates appendicitis
- Nightstick Fracture: Fracture to the ulna due to a direct blow
- Osgood-Schlatter Disease: Inflammation or partial avulsion of the tibial apophysis
- Parrot-Break Tear: Horizontal meniscal tear
- Plantar Warts: Verrucae plantaris
- Pott Fracture: Fracture of the lower part of the fibula and of the malleolus of the tibia, with lateral displacement of the foot
- Prickly Heat: Miliaria
- Pronator Syndrome: Median nerve entrapped by the pronator teres
- Raccoon Eyes: Delayed discoloration around the eyes from skull fracture
- Raynaud Disease: Condition characterized by intermittent bilateral attacks of ischemia of the fingers or toes, marked by severe pallor, numbness and pain
- Reye Syndrome: Disorder in kids following acute illness that may result in coma and increased intracranial hypertension
- Runner's Nipples: Nipple irritation due to friction as the shirt rubs over the nipples
- Scheuermann Disease: Osteochondrosis of the spine allowing disc herniation
- Sever Disease: Osteochondrosis of the calcaneal apophysis
- Silver Fork Deformity: Colle fracture
- Skier's Thumb: Gamekeeper's thumb
- Superior Labral Anterior Posterior (SLAP) Lesion: An injury to the superior labrum that typically begins posterior and extends anterior
- Snapping Hip Syndrome: A snapping sensation either heard or felt during motion of the hip
- Snowball Crepitation: Sound of crunching with tenosynovitis

- Spear Tackler's Spine: Cervical spine is placed at risk for serious injury due to excessive axial loading with spear-tackling
- Sprengel Deformity: Undersized scapula that sits high on the posterior chest wall
- Spring Ligament: Plantar calcaneonavicular ligament
- Stener Lesion: A complication of UCL injury to the thumb in which the adductor aponeurosis gets caught between the ruptured ends of the ligament and prevents healing
- Swan Neck Deformity: Hyperextension of the PIP and hyperflexion of the DIP due to disruption of the volar plate and tensioning of the flexor tendons
- Sway Back: Increased lordotic curve
- Tackler's Exostosis: Bony outgrowth on anterolateral humerus (Blocker's exostosis)
- Tennis Elbow: Epicondylitis of extensor/supinator muscles lateral condyle
- Trigger Finger: Stenosing of tendon sheath in finger flexors
- Turf Toe: Sprain of the first MTP joint
- Unhappy Triad: Anterior cruciate ligament (ACL), medial collateral ligament (MCL), and medial meniscus knee injury
- Valsalva Effect: Holding one's breath against a closed glottis
- Volkmann Contractures: Ischemic necrosis of the forearm muscles
- Wedge Fracture: Vertebral compression fracture with anterior vertebral narrowing
- Wrist Drop: Radial nerve damage causing weakness and/or paralysis of the wrist and finger extensors

 Use the DVD or visit the website at http://thePoint.lww.com/Long for additional materials about *identification, etiology, signs/symptoms, and management.*

GENERAL INJURY CONDITIONS

Identification, Etiology, Signs/Symptoms, and Management

- Apophysitis: Inflammation of bony outgrowth
- Bursitis: Inflammation of bursa
- Capsulitis: Inflamed joint capsule
- Chondral Fracture: Articular cartilage fracture
- Chondromalacia: Articular cartilage softening
- Contusion: Bruise
- Dislocation: Joint displacement
- Enthesitis: Inflammation at tendon/muscle attachment
- Epicondylitis: Inflammation of epicondyle and associated tissues
- Epiphyseal Plate Injury: Injury to cartilaginous growth plate (classified as Salter Harris injuries)
- Epiphysitis: Inflammation of the epiphysis
- Exostosis: Bony outgrowth from surface
- Fasciitis: Inflamed fascia
- Fracture: Broken bone (see Fig. 3.11)
- Myositis: Inflammatory condition of muscle

- Myositis Ossificans: Ectopic calcification of muscle
- Neuritis: Inflammatory condition of nerve
- Osteochondral Fracture: Fracture to joint cartilage and underlying bone
- Osteochondritis: Inflamed bone and cartilage
- Osteochondritis Dissecans: Separation of articular cartilage from bone
- Osteomyelitis: Inflammation of bone and marrow
- Periostitis: Inflammation of bone covering
- Radiculitis: Inflammation of spinal nerve root
- Salter Harris Epiphyseal Plate Injuries: 1-5 Grade for growth plate injuries (see Fig. 3.12)
- Sprain: Ligamentous or capsular stretch or tear
- Strain: Muscle or tendon stretch or tear
- Subluxation: Incomplete or partial dislocation
- Synovitis: Inflammation of synovial membrane
- Tendinitis: Inflammation of tendon
- Tenosynovitis: Inflammation of tendon sheath

Head and Face

Facial Laceration: Jagged cut on face
Scalp Laceration: Jagged cut on scalp

Spine

Brachial Plexus Stretch: Stinger or burner
Cervical Strain: Cervical muscle/tendon stretch or tear
Intervertebral Disc Herniation: Varied levels of protrusion, extrusion, or sequestration
Intervertebral Disc Rupture: Tear of intervertebral disc
Intervertebral Sprain: Stretching or tearing of ligaments between vertebrae
Lumbosacral Sprain: Stretching or tearing of ligaments between L5-S1
Lumbosacral Strain: Stretching or tearing of muscles affecting lumbosacral region
Nerve Root Compression (Radiculopathy): Compression of peripheral nerve at intervertebral foramen
Sacroiliac Sprain: Stretching or tearing ligaments between sacrum and ilium
Spinal Cord Concussion: Transient disturbance of spinal cord functions
Spinal Cord Contusion: Bruise of spinal cord
Spondylolisthesis ("Step Defect"): Pars interarticularis defect with forward vertebral slippage
Spondylitis: Inflammation of vertebral synovial joints
Spondylosis: Ankylosis of vertebra
Spondylolysis: Vertebral degenerations; pars interarticularis defect
Torticollis (Wry Neck): Stiff neck
Vertebral Dislocation: Intervertebral joint discontinuation
Vertebral Fracture: Break in a vertebra
Vertebral Subluxation: Incomplete or partial dislocation of vertebrae

Shoulder

Acromioclavicular Joint Sprain (Shoulder Pointer): Stretching or tearing of acromioclavicular and/or coracoclavicular ligament

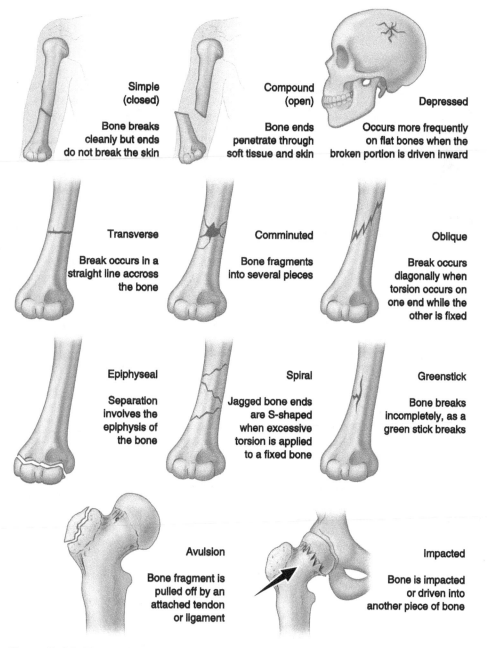

Simple (closed)

Bone breaks cleanly but ends do not break the skin

Compound (open)

Bone ends penetrate through soft tissue and skin

Depressed

Occurs more frequently on flat bones when the broken portion is driven inward

Transverse

Break occurs in a straight line accross the bone

Comminuted

Bone fragments into several pieces

Oblique

Break occurs diagonally when torsion occurs on one end while the other is fixed

Epiphyseal

Separation involves the epiphysis of the bone

Spiral

Jagged bone ends are S-shaped when excessive torsion is applied to a fixed bone

Greenstick

Bone breaks incompletely, as a green stick breaks

Avulsion

Bone fragment is pulled off by an attached tendon or ligament

Impacted

Bone is impacted or driven into another piece of bone

Figure 3.11 Types of Fractures.

Adhesive Capsulitis: Capsular adhesions, most commonly in shoulder

Axillary Nerve Contusion: Axillary nerve bruise

Bankart Lesion: Avulsion of inferior glenohumeral ligament from anterior labrum

Biceps Tendon Rupture: Tearing of biceps tendon

Bicipital Tendinitis: Inflammation of the biceps tendon

Bicipital Tenosynovitis: Inflammation of the biceps tendon synovial sheath

Blocker's Exostosis: Bony outgrowth of humerus

Glenohumeral Dislocation: Shoulder joint displacement

Glenohumeral Joint Sprain: Stretching or tearing of glenohumeral ligaments

Glenoid Labrum Tear: Tearing of shoulder labrum

Hill-Sachs Lesion: Defect in articular cartilage of humeral head

Humeral Fracture: Broken upper arm

Impingement Syndrome: Chronic shoulder pain within subacromial space and bursa

Long Thoracic Nerve Contusion: Bruising of long thoracic nerve

Rotator Cuff Tear: Tearing of muscle or tendon within rotator cuff (subscapularis, supraspinatus, infraspinatus, teres minor)

Rotator Cuff Tendinitis: Inflammation of the rotator cuff tendons

Scapular Fracture: Broken scapula

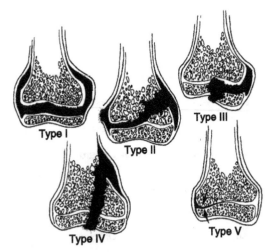

Figure 3.12 Salter Harris Classification of Epiphyseal Plate injuries. (From Blackbourne LH. *Advanced surgical recall*, 2nd ed. Baltimore: Lippincott Williams & Wilkins; 2004.)

SLAP Lesion: Superior labral tear from posterior to anterior and long head of biceps tendon pathology

Sternoclavicular Joint Sprain: Tearing or stretching capsule or ligaments of sternoclavicular joint

Subacromial Bursitis: Inflammation of subacromial bursa

Subdeltoid Bursitis: Inflammation of subdeltoid bursa

Thoracic Outlet Compression Syndrome: Compression of neurovascular bundle in neck and shoulder

Elbow

Anterior Capsulitis: Inflammation of anterior elbow capsule

Compartment Syndrome: Inflammation of forearm with increased neurovascular pressure

Cubital Tunnel Syndrome (Ulnar Neuropathy): Ulnar nerve entrapment

Elbow Dislocation: Elbow joint displacement

Elbow Subluxation: Incomplete or partial dislocation of the elbow

Lateral Collateral Ligament Sprain: Tearing or stretching of lateral collateral ligament of elbow

Lateral Epicondylitis (Extensor Tendonitis): Inflammation of lateral epicondyle of elbow

MCL Sprain: Tearing or stretching of MCL of elbow

Medial Epicondylitis (Flexor Tendonitis): Inflammation of medial epicondyle of elbow

Olecranon Bursitis: Inflammation of olecranon bursa of the elbow

Radial Nerve Contusion: Bruise of radial nerve

Ulnar Nerve Contusion: Bruise of radial nerve

Ulnar Stress Fracture: Partial fracture of the ulna

Forearm, Wrist, and Hand

Barton Fracture: Fracture of distal radius

Bennett Fracture: Avulsion fracture of the first metacarpal

Boutonniere Deformity: Ruptured extensor tendon

Bowler's Thumb: Ulnar nerve compression

Boxer's Fracture: Fracture of fifth metacarpal

Colle Fracture: Fracture to distal radius with dorsal displacement

de Quervain Syndrome: Tenosynovitis of abductor pollicus longus and extensor pollicus brevis tendons

Dupuytren Contracture: Nodules in palmar aponeurosis

Felon: Cellulitis of the finger

Finger Dislocations: Finger joint displacement at DIP, PIP, or MCP

Finger Fracture: Broken phalanx

Finger Subluxations: Incomplete or partial dislocation of finger

Galeazzi Fracture: Fracture of distal radius with subluxation or dislocation of distal radioulnar joint

Gamekeeper's Thumb: Sprain to UCL of the thumb

Hamate Fracture: Fracture of the hamate (carpal bone)

Jersey Finger: Avulsion flexor digitorum profundus tendon

Kienböck Disease: Avascular necrosis of the lunate

Mallet Finger: Avulsion of extensor tendon

Median Nerve Palsy: Damage to median nerve usually in carpal tunnel

Monteggia Fracture: Distal ulnar fracture with dislocation of radial head

Radial Nerve Palsy (Wrist Drop): Damage to radial nerve usually from midhumerus fracture

Scaphoid Fracture: Most common carpal bone fracture

Smith Fracture: Fracture to distal radius with volar displacement

Subungual Hematoma: Blood under fingernail or toenail

Swan Neck Deformity: MCP flexion, PIP extension, DIP flexion

Triangular Fibrocartilage Complex Tear: Tear of wrist cartilage between ulna and fifth metacarpal

Trigger Finger: Tenosynovitis of flexor tendons (usually third and fourth digits)

Ulnar Nerve Palsy: Sensory changes along ulnar nerve distribution in hand

Volkmann Ischemic Contracture: Ischemic necrosis of forearm muscles

Wrist Ganglion: Synovial cyst

Thigh, Hip, and Pelvis

Adductor Strain: Muscle or tendon stretch/tear of adductor longus, brevis, magnus, gracilis, pectineus

Adductor Tendinitis: Inflammation of tendons of adductor longus, brevis, magnus, gracilis, pectineus

Femoral Stress Fracture: Incomplete break of the femur, particularly the neck

Femur Fracture: Broken femur

Hamstring Strain: Muscle or tendon stretching/tearing to biceps femoris, semimembranosus, semitendinosus

Hamstring Tendinitis: Inflammation of tendons of biceps femoris, semimembranosus, and semitendinosus

Hip Dislocation: Femoral acetabular joint displacement

Hip Sprain: Stretching or tearing of hip ligament

Iliac Crest Contusion (Hip Pointer): Bruise to iliac crest and attaching musculature

Iliopectineal Bursitis: Inflammation of the iliopectineal bursa

Iliotibial (IT) "Band" Syndrome: Friction of IT band over lateral femoral epicondyle

Legg-Calvés-Perthes Disease: Avascular necrosis of femoral head

Osteitis Pubis: Inflamed pubic bone

Pelvic Fracture: Break among any of all bones of the pelvis

Pelvic Stress Fracture: Incomplete break of a bone within pelvis

Piriformis Syndrome: Inflammation of the piriformis muscle with radiating pain

Quadriceps Contusion: Bruise of the quadriceps muscles

Quadriceps Strain: Stretching or tearing to the muscle/tendon of quadriceps muscles

Quadriceps Tendinitis: Inflammation of tendon of quadriceps muscles

Slipped Capital Femoral Epiphysis: Injured growth plate of proximal femur; femoral neck moved up and forward

Trochanteric Bursitis: Inflamed bursa around greater trochanter

Knee

Anterior Cruciate Ligament (ACL) Sprain: Stretching or tearing of ACL

Chondromalacia Patella: Softening of articular cartilage behind the patella

Distal Femur Epiphyseal Plate Injury: Injury to distal femur cartilaginous growth plate

Fat Pad Contusion: Bruise of infrapatellar fat pad

Fibula Fracture: Break to fibula

Fibular Collateral Ligament (Lateral Collateral Ligament [LCL]) Sprain: Stretch or tear to LCL

IT Band Friction Syndrome: Inflammatory condition affecting entire length of IT band

Infrapatellar Bursitis: Inflammation of infrapatellar bursa

Meniscal Tear: Torn knee cartilage

Osgood-Schlatter Disease: Tibial tubercle apophysitis

Patella Fracture: Fracture of the kneecap

Patella Subluxation: Incomplete or partial dislocation to kneecap

Patella Tendinitis (Jumper's Knee): Inflammation of patella tendon

Patellar Dislocation: Patellofemoral joint displacement

Patellar Tendon Rupture: Tear of the patella tendon

Peroneal Nerve Contusion: Bruise to peroneal nerve behind fibula

Pes Anserine Bursitis: Inflammation of the pes anserine bursa

Plica Syndrome: Synovial fold inflammation of the knee

Popliteal Cyst (Baker's Cyst): Accumulation of fluid in popliteal space of knee

Popliteus Tendinitis: Inflammation of popliteus tendon

Posterior Cruciate Ligament (PCL) Sprain: Stretching or tearing of PCL

Sinding-Larsen-Johansson Disease: Traction injury to inferior pole of patella at tendon origin

Suprapatellar Bursitis: Inflammation of bursa above patella

Tibial Collateral Ligament (MCL) Sprain: Stretch or tear of MCL

Tibial Fracture: Broken tibia

Tibiofemoral Dislocation (Knee): Tibiofemoral joint disarticulation

Ankle, Foot, and Leg

Achilles Bursitis: Inflammation of Achilles bursa

Achilles Tendinitis: Inflammation of Achilles tendon

Achilles Tendon Rupture: Complete or incomplete tear of Achilles tendon

Achilles Tenosynovitis: Inflammation of Achilles tendon sheath

Ankle Dislocation: Displacement of one or more bones in the ankle

Anterior Compartment Syndrome: Increased pressure in lower leg compresses neurovascular vessels

Anterior Talofibular Sprain: Stretch or tear of anterior talofibular ligament

Bifurcated Ligament Sprain: Midtarsal joint stretch or tear of calcaneocuboid/calcaneonavicular ligament

Bunion (Hallus Valgus): Hallux valgus of first MTP joint causing bony outgrowth

Bunionette (Tailor's Bunion): Angulation of fifth metatarsophalangeal joint

Calcaneofibular Ligament Sprain: Tearing or stretching of calcaneofibular ligament of ankle

Chondral Ankle Fracture: Articular cartilage fracture in ankle

Corn—Hard (Callus Durum): Thickening of the soft tissue on dorsum of toes

Corn—Soft (Callus Molle): Thickening of soft tissue between toes (usually fourth and fifth)

Deltoid Ligament Sprain: Tearing or stretching of deltoid ligament of ankle

Fibular Fracture: Broken fibula

Fibular Stress Fracture: Incomplete break of fibula

Great Toe Sprain (Turf Toe): Stretching or tearing of extensor or flexor tendon of first toe

Hallux Rigidus: Stiffness or fusion of first MTP joint

Hammer Toe: Hyperflexion of PIP with hyperextension of DIP

Heel Spur: Bony outgrowth on plantar surface of calcaneus

Ingrown Toenail: Toenail edges embed in soft tissue

Jones Fracture: Fracture of base of fifth metatarsal

Longitudinal Arch Sprain: Stretching or tearing of the longitudinal arch

Medial Tibial Stress Syndrome: Anterior shin pain often termed *shin splints*

Metatarsal Arch Sprain: Stretching or tearing of the transverse arch

Metatarsal Fracture: Broken metatarsal bone

Metatarsal Stress Fracture: Overload-induced discontinuation of metatarsal bone

Osteochondral Ankle Fracture: Fracture extending from cartilaginous surface into bony matrix

Osteochondritis Dissecans (Joint Mice): Fragments of cartilage/bone in the joint

Peroneal Tendinitis: Inflammation of one of the peroneal tendons (usually longus)

Peroneal Tendon Dislocation: Displacement of peroneal tendon (usually longus)

Peroneal Tendon Subluxation: Partial displacement of peroneal tendon (usually longus)

Pes Cavus: High longitudinal arch; rigid foot

Pes Planus: Flat longitudinal arch; pliable foot

Plantar Fasciitis: Inflammation of the plantar fascia

Plantar Neuroma: Morton neuroma; interdigital neuroma

Plantar Wart: Inward growing wart common to sole of foot

Plantaris Muscle Rupture: Complete or incomplete tear of plantaris tendon; tennis leg

Retrocalcaneal Bursitis: Inflammation of bursa between Achilles tendon and calcaneus

Shin Splints: Anterior shin pain often termed *medial tibial stress syndrome*

Subungual Hematoma: Blood under fingernail or toenail

Syndesmosis Sprain: Stretching or tearing of anterior and/or posterior tibiofibular ligaments

Talar Dome Fracture: Broken dome of the talus resulting from significant inversion or eversion sprains

Talotibial Exostosis: Bony outgrowth from surface or talus

Tarsal Fracture: Broken tarsal bone

Tarsal Tunnel Syndrome: Entrapped posterior tibial nerve along medial malleolus

Tibial Fracture: Broken tibia bone

Tibial Stress Fracture: Overload-induced discontinuation of tibial bone

Transverse Arch Sprain: Stretching or tearing of the metatarsal arch

1. During a preparticipation physical, the team physician comes across a basketball player with the following profile: The athlete is tall with an arm span greater than his height, pectus carinatum or excavatum, high-arched palate and myopia. What is the probable diagnosis?
   a. Paget disease
   b. Milch disease
   c. Marfan syndrome
   d. Gigantism
   e. Lisfranc syndrome

2. An athlete's pulmonary function is tested through a spirometer. Several measurements are taken during this test. The maximum amount of air that can be expired after a maximum inspiration is known as:
   a. Maximum expiratory flow rate
   b. Forced expiratory volume
   c. Vital capacity
   d. Tidal volume
   e. Stroke volume

3. When should MMR immunization first be administered?
   a. At birth
   b. 3 to 4 months
   c. 12 to 15 months
   d. 6 to 9 months
   e. 18 to 24 months

4. How is pediculosis spread between individuals?
   a. Coughing and sneezing
   b. Poor hand washing/hygiene
   c. Airborne droplets
   d. Close sexual contact
   e. Contact with open sores

5. All of the following conditions would disqualify an athlete from competition except:
   a. Renal disease
   b. Uncontrolled hypertension
   c. Marfan syndrome
   d. Acute mononucleosis
   e. The absence of one testicle

6. You have a lacrosse player who has been experiencing bouts of coughing following sprinting activities on the field. You have noticed that these bouts are less likely to occur when the player has a lengthy warm-up. What might be this player's problem?
   a. Influenza
   b. Exercise-induced bronchiospasm
   c. Pleurisy
   d. Umbilication
   e. Malingering

7. A member of the equestrian team visits the athletic training room with the following symptoms—fever, malaise, myalgia, and a rash. The athlete notes that she was riding some cross-country trails recently. What might be this athlete's medical problem?
   a. General trail fatigue
   b. Lyme disease
   c. Rocky Mountain spotted fever
   d. A and B
   e. B and C

8. Charles is a member of the football team who has postprandial symptoms of nausea. A mild fever, aches, and chills accompany the symptoms. Charles is suffering from:
   a. Mononucleosis
   b. Influenza
   c. Molluscum contagiosum
   d. Herpes simplex I
   e. Chlamydia

9. One of your athletes steps on a nail but neglects telling you. The athlete is rushed to the hospital with symptoms of lockjaw. The organism that causes this disorder is called?
   a. Staphylococcus
   b. *Streptococcus*
   c. *Bacillus*
   d. HPV
   e. Cytokine

10. Kevin is a wrestler and presents with a large infection on the back of his neck. There is evidence of purulent formation, increased white blood count, and fever. What is the medical diagnosis for Kevin? What is the most common organism cause?
    a. Scabies and dermatophyte
    b. Carbuncle and *Staphylococci*
    c. Tinea neckius and fungaris

    d. Pediculosis capitus and pediculosis humanus capitis

    e. MRSA and *Staphylococcus*

11. Jane is a rugby player who recently ended a long-term relationship with her boyfriend. She presents with localized, painful blisters along one side of her body from the upper half of the spine to the breastbone. She mentions that she is experiencing burning and tingling with some flu-like symptoms. What might her symptoms imply?

    a. Pediculosis pubis

    b. Herpes zoster

    c. West Nile virus

    d. Group A *Streptococcus*

    e. HIV

12. Which characteristic defines moderate hypertension?

    a. Diastolic pressure 90 to 104 mm Hg and systolic pressure 140 to 159 mm Hg

    b. Diastolic pressure 125 to 130 mm Hg and systolic pressure 185 to 200 mm Hg

    c. Diastolic pressure 100 to 109 mm Hg and systolic pressure 160 to 179 mm Hg

    d. Diastolic pressure 85 to 90 mm Hg and systolic pressure 125 to 135 mm Hg

    e. None are true of moderate hypertension

13. Which condition increases the risk of exertional rhabdomyolysis?

    a. Sickle cell anemia

    b. Hypertension

    c. Anemia

    d. Hematuria

    e. Down syndrome

14. A young athlete has lost a lot of weight in a short time, and she is tired and irritable. Which of the following is the most likely cause of her symptoms?

    a. Graves disease

    b. Gullain-Barré syndrome

    c. Myasthenia gravis

    d. Paget disease

    e. Charcot-Marie-Tooth

15. Jeff and Mike were recently roughhousing and Mike tackled Jeff to the ground by placing his head in his abdomen. Jeff began experiencing discomfort in his abdomen. Which is not a sign and symptom of acute trauma to the abdomen?

    a. Rigidity

    b. Tenderness

    c. Guarding

    d. Rebound tenderness

    e. Bowel sounds

16. A football player whose position on the team is tight end comes into the athletic training room after the game, walking with his torso bent to the right. He reports sustaining a blow to his right lower back during a play. He is experiencing pain throughout the right side of the back and the groin. You notice muscle spasms in the athlete's back after removal of his shirt. You suspect a kidney contusion. What should you instruct the athlete to watch for and report?

    a. Increased hunger

    b. Hematuria

    c. Dyspnea

    d. Vertigo

    e. Hemarthrosis

17. What common name is given to irritable bowel syndrome?

    a. Graves disease

    b. Crohn disease

    c. Hamman disease

    d. Celiac disease

    e. Guterack disease

18. A male athlete comes to the athletic trainer complaining of painful urination and pus discharge from the genitals and confides that he had unprotected sex approximately 1 week earlier. On the basis of his symptoms, what should the athletic trainer suspect is the athlete's immediate problem?

    a. Tinea capitis

    b. Gonorrhea

    c. Acquired immunodeficiency syndrome

    d. Impetigo contagiosa

    e. Hepatitis

19. Jill enters the athletic training room with a low-grade fever, tender lymph nodes, tender left side, low-grade fever, and sore throat. You might suspect:

    a. Strep throat

    b. Appendicitis

    c. Influenza

    d. Mononucleosis

    e. Pneumonia

20. What term identifies trapped feces within an intestinal herniation?

    a. Gastroenteritis

    b. Diverticulosis

    c. Diverticulitis

    d. Clindamycin

    e. Hernia

21. Which structure accepts blood once it leaves the mitral valve?

    a. Pulmonary vein

    b. Right ventricle

    c. Aorta

    d. Left ventricle

    e. Left atrium

    f. Right atrium

22. The right coronary artery is divided into?
    a. Right anterior descending and circumflex arteries
    b. Right posterior descending and ascending arteries
    c. Right surreal and popliteus arteries
    d. Right glossopharyngeal and renal arteries
    e. None of the above

23. On an ECG what does the P wave represent?
    a. Systole
    b. Diastole
    c. Atrial repolarization
    d. Ventricular depolarization
    e. None of the above

24. What portion of the two heart sounds is represented by the closure of the pulmonary and aortic valves?
    a. Lub
    b. Dub
    c. 1st sound
    d. 2nd sound
    e. a and d
    f. b and c
    g. b and d

25. What occurs with the T wave of an ECG?
    a. Ventricular depolarization
    b. Atrial depolarization
    c. Ventricular repolarization
    d. Atrial repolarization
    e. Systole

26. What generally causes a skipped heartbeat secondary to stress, too much caffeine or nicotine?
    a. Atrial fibrillation
    b. Premature atrial contraction
    c. AV nodal reentrant tachycardia
    d. Premature ventricular contraction
    e. Ventricular fibrillation

27. Which cardiomyopathy is least common?
    a. Hypertrophic cardiomyopathy
    b. Dilated cardiomyopathy
    c. Restrictive cardiomyopathy
    d. Atrial cardiomyopathy
    e. Compensatory cardiomyopathy

28. Which neuroglia attach neurons to their blood vessels?
    a. Microglia
    b. Oligodendrocytes
    c. Astrocytes
    d. Ependymocytes
    e. Schwann cells

29. Which portion of the brain is involved in language comprehension?
    a. Primary motor cortex
    b. Brocca area
    c. Wernicke area

    d. Somatosensory area
    e. Prefrontal cortex

30. Which portion of the brain is associated with the perception of touch, pressure, temperature, and pain?
    a. Parietal lobe
    b. Frontal lobe
    c. Temporal lobe
    d. Occipital lobe
    e. Motor association cortex

31. What structure connects Brocca and Wernicke areas?
    a. Primary motor cortex
    b. Arcuate fasciculus
    c. Amyotrophic articularis
    d. Visual cortex
    e. Temporal dopaminius

32. Which disorder is characterized by paroxysmal contractions?
    a. Parkinson disease
    b. Cerebral vascular accident
    c. Grade 3 concussions
    d. Epilepsy
    e. Neurocardiogenic syncope

33. What name is given to the previously characterized petit mal seizures?
    a. Complex partial seizure
    b. Partial seizure
    c. Focal seizure
    d. Absence seizure
    e. Tonic-clonic seizure

34. What are the two types of cerebral vascular accidents?
    a. Mild and hypertensive
    b. Ischemic and hemorrhagic
    c. Prodromal and atherosclerotic
    d. Apoplexic and syncopatic
    e. None of the above

35. All of the following are lymphoid organs except:
    a. Thalamus
    b. Adenoids
    c. Spleen
    d. Tonsils
    e. All are lymphoid organs

36. What terminology identifies cancer arising from connective tissue?
    a. Carcinoma
    b. Melanoma
    c. Sarcoma
    d. Cirrhosis
    e. Epiderma

37. Which type of leukemia best describes one with slow and progressively declining RBC/WBC count in an adult?
    a. Acute myeloid leukemia
    b. Hairy cell leukemia
    c. Acute lymphocytic leukemia
    d. Non-Hodgkin lymphoma
    e. Hodgkin disease

38. Which type of traumatic brain injury accounts for most athletic-related deaths?
    a. Epidural hematoma
    b. Mild traumatic brain injury
    c. Subdural hematoma
    d. Concussion
    e. Supradural hematoma

39. All of the following except one are important in judging potential melanomas:
    a. Diameter
    b. Color
    c. Symmetry
    d. Elevation
    e. Location

40. An athlete arrives with subcutaneous edema around her lips, which disappears within 24 hours of onset. She complains that these episodes are recurring and not related to any trauma. What might be the diagnosis?
    a. Leukoplakia
    b. Labial carcinoma
    c. Angioedema
    d. Kaposi sarcoma
    e. Fistularis

41. Which organism associated with genital warts may be implicated in cervical cancer?
    a. Neisseria gonorrhoeae
    b. Human papillomavirus
    c. Acyclovir
    d. Treponema pallidum
    e. Trichomonas vaginalis

42. During the immune response, which cells are probably responsible for the accompanying fever?
    a. Helper T cells
    b. Memory B cells
    c. Cytokines
    d. Suppressor T cells
    e. Killer T cells

43. Pertussis is commonly called:
    a. Laryngitis
    b. Pharangitis
    c. Tonsilitis
    d. Whooping cough
    e. Measles

44. On which days of the menstrual cycle does menstruation normally occur?
    a. 23 to 28
    b. 14 to 19
    c. 1 to 5
    d. 5 to 10
    e. 16 to 21

45. What is the source of follicle-stimulating hormone?
    a. Adenohypophysis
    b. Hypothalamus
    c. Ovary
    d. Posterior pituitary
    e. Pineal gland

46. In which phase of menstruation does progesterone levels peak?
    a. Ovulation
    b. Follicular phase
    c. Luteal phase
    d. Progesterone levels are steady throughout
    e. Estrogen

47. What name is given to the superior portion of the sternum?
    a. Xiphoid process
    b. Sternal presis
    c. Manubrium
    d. Anomaly
    e. Rib 3-4 interface

48. McBurney point refers to:
    a. Gallbladder pain referral
    b. Spleen injury referral
    c. Appendix pain referral
    d. Heart pain referral
    e. Epigastric referral

49. Bladder infections or injuries often refer to:
    a. Right shoulder
    b. Groin/adductor area
    c. Inguinal area
    d. Left upper quadrant
    e. Right upper quadrant

50. Which sounds are not considered to be adventitious sounds during lung auscultation?
    a. Mediastinal crunch
    b. Rhonci
    c. Rales
    d. Bronchiovesicular
    e. All are adventitious sounds

51. During lung auscultation, which breath sound is considered quieter in normal humans?
    a. Inspiration
    b. Expiration
    c. Both are equal in sound

52. Which normal breath sounds are heard over the majority of the lung?
    a. Tracheal sounds
    b. Vesicular sounds
    c. Bronchiovesicular sounds
    d. Bronchial sounds
    e. All sounds are divided equally

53. What is the exit order for food making way through the large intestines?
    a. Ileum, cecum, transverse colon, sigmoid, and rectum
    b. Cecum, jejunum, transverse colon, sigmoid, and rectum
    c. Duodenum, jejunum, ileum, sigmoid, and rectum
    d. Cecum, ascending colon, transverse colon, descending colon, sigmoid, and rectum
    e. Pylorus, ascending colon, transverse colon, descending colon, cecum, and rectum

54. Which pancreatic cells are most plentiful?
    a. δ Cells
    b. α Cells
    c. β Cells
    d. Cells producing glucagon
    e. Exocrine cells

55. Normal before meal blood sugar values are within which range according to the ADA?
    a. 50 to 120 mg/dL
    b. 70 to 180 mg/dL
    c. 90 to 130 mg/dL
    d. 105 to 155 mg/dL
    e. 40 to 180 mg/dL

56. Which disorder has a rapid onset?
    a. Hairy cell leukemia
    b. Hypoglycemia
    c. Hyperglycemia
    d. Amyotrophic lateral sclerosis
    e. Parkinson disease

57. Which disorder is characterized by polyuria?
    a. Apoplexy
    b. Epilepsy
    c. Hyperglycemia
    d. Cholecystitis
    e. Giganticism

58. Which of the following is not a category of hormones?
    a. Steroids
    b. Neurotransmitters
    c. Catecholamines
    d. Glycoproteins
    e. Polypeptides

59. What are the most common examples of catecholamines?
    a. Testosterone and progesterone
    b. Epinephrine and norepinephrine

c. Insulin and glucagon
    d. Antidiuretic hormone and thyroid-stimulating hormone
    e. Dopamine and seratonin

60. Which synergistic hormones are additive in nature?
    a. Gynecomastia and antidiuretic hormone
    b. Progesterone and follicle-stimulating hormone
    c. Testosterone and follicle-stimulating hormone
    d. Epinephrine and norepinephrine
    e. Insulin and glucagons

61. Which portion of the ECG represents ventricular depolarization?
    a. P wave
    b. T wave
    c. ST segment
    d. QRS segment
    e. PQ segment

62. What portion of the adrenal gland is crucial for sustained life?
    a. Adenohypophysis
    b. Cortex
    c. Medulla
    d. Apophysis
    e. Pulposus

63. Which organ does not have endocrine functions?
    a. Thymus
    b. Cecum
    c. Stomach
    d. Placenta
    e. Heart

64. Which organ produces bicarbonate to reduce acidity during digestion?
    a. Pancreas
    b. Gall bladder
    c. Liver
    d. Stomach
    e. Small intestine

65. Where is the thymus?
    a. Either side of the larynx
    b. In front of the aorta
    c. Above the kidney
    d. Below the bladder
    e. Under the right axilla

66. What does cortisol do?
    a. Triggers insulin release
    b. Triggers antidiuretic hormone release
    c. Triggers epinephrine release
    d. Increases blood glucose levels
    e. Conserves sodium and potassium ions in the body

67. Snacks for diabetic athletes should range in which of the following categories?
    a. 50 to 60 g CHO every 45 minutes
    b. 30 to 40 g CHO every 30 minutes
    c. 90 to 100 g CHO every 30 minutes
    d. 60 to 70 g CHO every 60 minutes
    e. 15 to 20 g CHO every 45 minutes

68. During auscultations, should the lung surfaces brush against each other, which adventitious sound should be heard?
    a. Stridor
    b. Rhonchi
    c. Mediastinal crunch
    d. Pleural rub
    e. Crackles

69. Which ribs have conjoined costal cartilage?
    a. 1-5
    b. 6-9
    c. 1-7
    d. 8-10
    e. 12-15

70. Where does the first rib interface with the spine?
    a. C5
    b. C6
    c. C7
    d. T1
    e. T2

71. Which sign may indicate a potential spleen injury?
    a. McBurney point
    b. Kehr sign
    c. Homan sign
    d. Frederick sign
    e. Thomas point

72. What organism is often responsible for mononucleosis?
    a. Trichinosis
    b. Human papillomavirus
    c. Rhinovirus
    d. Epstein-Barr virus
    e. Spirochete

73. Which sexually transmitted disease can have dementia, blindness, and death associated with it?
    a. Gonorrhea
    b. Chlamydia
    c. Syphilis
    d. Trichomoniasis
    e. Bacterial vaginosis

74. What hormone peaks triggering ovulation?
    a. FSH
    b. LH
    c. ADH
    d. Progesterone
    e. Estrogen

75. Which glial cells are star-shaped and digest parts of dead neurons?
    a. Astroglia
    b. Microglia
    c. Satellite cells
    d. Oligodendroglia
    e. Ependymal cells

76. Which glial cells are continuous with the ventricles of the brain and assist with cerebrospinal fluid circulation?
    a. Schwann cells
    b. Astrocytes
    c. Ependymal cells
    d. Oligodendroglia
    e. Microglia

77. What does heart failure mean?
    a. The heart has stopped working
    b. Heart effort is insufficient
    c. Heart's pumping power is too strong for the peripheral vessels
    d. Fluid is found in the pericardium
    e. Myocardial flatulence

78. Which disease is caused by the human papillomavirus?
    a. Syphilis
    b. Genital warts
    c. Rubella
    d. Whooping cough
    e. Amyotrophic lateral sclerosis

79. What name is given to a gland surrounding a hair follicle which secretes oily substances around the follicle protecting it from cold?
    a. Lipotic gland
    b. Sebaceous gland
    c. Paronychia gland
    d. Hyperhidrosis gland
    e. Subcutis gland

80. James comes into the athletic training room with a finger that is hot, swollen, and painful around the nail itself. There was no evidence of trauma. James most likely has:
    a. Hordeolum
    b. Paronychia
    c. Moniliasis
    d. Verruca planus
    e. Contagion

81. In order to disinfect surfaces, current thought is to use what ratio of water to bleach?
    a. 9:1
    b. 1:10
    c. 1:6
    d. 1:1
    e. 8:1

82. Which of the following is not a palpable pulse location?
    a. Dorsalis pedis
    b. Posterior tibialis
    c. Carotid
    d. Axillary
    e. Popliteal

83. Bradycardia is identified as:
    a. Respirations >15
    b. Heart rate >80 beats per minute
    c. Heart rate >60 beats per minute
    d. Respirations <12
    e. Heart rate <60 beats per minute

84. Which term identifies the fifth Korotkoff sound?
    a. Systolic pressure
    b. Auscultatory sound
    c. Arterial constriction
    d. Diastolic pressure
    e. Atrial repolarization

85. When measuring body temperature, in a suspected heat injured patient, which thermometer is considered most reliable and accurate?
    a. Tympanic
    b. Rectal
    c. Electronic
    d. Oral
    e. Intravenous

86. Tympanic thermometer readings are usually_____ compared to oral thermometers?
    a. 0.4° C lower
    b. 0.8° C higher
    c. 0.4° C higher
    d. 0.8° C lower
    e. 0.5° C higher

87. What are the mechanism measures and values given to normal vision?
    a. Waxler chart; 20/15
    b. Opthalmoscope; 20/200
    c. Otoscope; 20/20
    d. Snellen chart; 20/20
    e. Phlebogram; 20/15

88. Which value is given to slightly hyperactive deep tendon reflexes?
    a. 0
    b. 1
    c. 2
    d. 3
    e. 4

89. Which sound is produced when performing percussion over a normal liver?
    a. Tympany
    b. Dullness
    c. Flatness
    d. Hyperresonance
    e. Resonance

90. Which name best describes pectus carinatum?
    a. Barrel chest
    b. Funnel chest
    c. Pigeon chest
    d. Normal chest
    e. Wheelbarrow chest

91. Which disordered breathing pattern is considered hyperpnea?
    a. Biot
    b. Kussmaul
    c. Ataxia
    d. Cheyne-Stokes
    e. Tachypnea

92. What location is most ideal to auscultate the aortic valve?
    a. 2nd left intercostal space
    b. 3rd left intercostal space
    c. 5th right intercostal space
    d. 2nd right intercostal space
    e. 4th left intercostal space

93. What is the normal first course of treatment for an athlete with long QT syndrome?
    a. Surgically implant a defibrillator into the patient
    b. β-Blocker medications
    c. Daily use of Holter monitoring device
    d. Heart transplantation
    e. Cardiac bypass surgery

94. Which disorder has claudication as a primary symptom?
    a. Wolff-Parkinson-White syndrome
    b. Mitral valve prolapse
    c. Congenital aortic valve stenosis
    d. Kawasaki disease
    e. Peripheral arterial disease

95. Which of the following conditions is not associated with right upper quadrant pain?
    a. Hepatitis
    b. Cholecystitis
    c. Diverticulitis
    d. Pneumonia
    e. Duodenal ulcer

96. Which of the following is not a sign or symptom of gastroesophageal reflux disease (GERD)?
    a. Severe chest pain
    b. Chronic cough
    c. Adenomegaly
    d. Food regurgitation
    e. Belching

97. Which organism is most responsible for peptic ulcers?
    a. *Bacillus cereus*
    b. *Escherichia coli*
    c. *Salmonella*
    d. *Helicobacter pylori*
    e. *Staphylococcus aureus*

98. Which dysfunction is noted for the term bell clapper deformity?
    a. Dysuria
    b. Hematuria
    c. Testicular torsion
    d. Urethritis
    e. Hydrocele

99. Which is larger, a furuncle or carbuncle?
    a. Furuncle
    b. Carbuncle
    c. There is no difference

100. Which skin condition presents with small vesicles accompanied by itching and crust formation?
    a. Eczema
    b. Wheal
    c. Hordeolum
    d. Folliculitis
    e. Hidradenitis

 Use the DVD or visit the website at http://thePoint.lww.com/Long to take the *online examination.*

✔ STUDY CHECKLIST

I have studied:
- ☐ Percussion
- ☐ Auscultations
- ☐ Hearing tests
- ☐ Visual acuity
- ☐ Vital signs
- ☐ Blood analysis

- ☐ Inoculations and health screenings
- ☐ Birth control
- ☐ Skin conditions
- ☐ Thorax and abdomen conditions
- ☐ Eyes, ears, nose, head, face, and throat
- ☐ Common illnesses and disease

SECTION 3

SUPPLEMENTAL READING

1. American College of Sports Medicine. *ACSM's guidelines for exercise testing and prescription*, 7th ed. Baltimore: Lippincott Williams & Wilkins; 2006.

2. Anderson MK, Parr GP, Hall SJ. *Foundations of athletic training: prevention, assessment, and management*, 4th ed. Philadelphia: Lippincott Williams & Wilkins; 2009.

3. Bahr R, Machlum S. *Clinical guide to sports injuries: an illustrated guide to the management of injuries in physical activity.* Champaign: Human Kinetics; 2004.

4. Bernier J. *Quick reference dictionary for athletic training.* Thorofare: Slack Inc; 2005.

5. Binkley HM, Beckett J, Casa DJ, et al. National athletic trainers' association position statement: exertional heat illnesses. *J Athl Train.* 2002;347(3):329–343.

6. Clover J. *Sports medicine essentials core concepts in athletic training and fitness instruction*, 2nd ed. Clifton Park: Thomson-Delmar Learning; 2007.

7. Hillman SK. *Introduction to athletic training*, 2nd ed. Champaign: Human Kinetics; 2005.

8. Howard TM, Butcher JD. *The little black book of sports medicine*, 2nd ed. Sudbury: Jones and Bartlett Publishers; 2006.

9. National Athletic Trainers' Association. *Athletic training educational competencies*, 4th ed. Dallas: National Athletic Trainers' Association; 2006.

10. Prentice WE. *Arnheim's principles of athletic training: a competency-based approach.* New York: McGraw-Hill; 2006.

11. *Professional guide to signs and symptoms*, 5th ed. Baltimore: Lippincott Williams & Wilkins; 2007.

12. Skinner JS. *Exercise testing and exercise prescription for special cases theoretical basis and clinical applicator*, 3rd ed. Baltimore: Lippincott Williams & Wilkins; 2005.

13. *Steadman's medical dictionary for the health professions and nursing*, 5th ed. Philadelphia: Lippincott Williams & Wilkins; 2005.

14. Thomas CL, ed. *Taber's cyclopedic medical dictionary.* Philadelphia: FA Davis Co; 1993.

4

Orthopaedic Clinical Examination and Diagnosis

Part 1   Principles of Clinical Examination

Part 2   Examination of the Head, Neck, Spine, and Thorax

Part 3   Examination of the Upper Extremity

Part 4   Examination of the Lower Extremity

Section 4 Examination

OVERVIEW

This section is intended to focus the student's skills at orthopaedic examination and diagnosis. Information required of the student to make good decisions when evaluating an athlete is included. This information is separated in small, manageable sections focusing on each body region.

CLINICAL PROFICIENCY

Demonstrate a musculoskeletal assessment of upper extremity, lower extremity, head/face, and spine (including the ribs) for the purpose of identifying (a) common acquired or congenital risk factors that would predispose the patient to injury and (b) a musculoskeletal injury. This will include identification and recommendations for the correction of acquired or congenital risk factors for injury. At the conclusion of the assessment, the student will diagnose the patient's condition and determine and apply immediate treatment and/or referral in the management of the condition. Effective lines of communication should be established to elicit and convey information about the patient's status. While maintaining patient confidentiality, all aspects of the assessment should be documented using standardized record-keeping methods. (Reproduced with permission of the National Athletic Trainers' Association.)

Principles of Clinical Examination

KEY TERMS

- Babinski sign
- Brudzinski sign
- Chvostek sign
- Dermatome
- Differential diagnosis
- End feel
- Goniometer
- Hyperreflexia
- Jendrassik maneuver
- Laxity
- Myotome
- Oppenheim reflex
- Palpation
- Synergist
- Tendon reflex
- Tonic
- Valgus
- Varus

CLINICAL EXAMINATION PROCESS

Clinical Examination Components

- History
- Observation
- Palpation
- Range of motion (ROM) tests
- Ligamentous tests
- Special tests
- Neurologic tests
- Functional tests

> **Quick fact** A solid understanding of human anatomy is crucial in being able to perform an effective and thorough examination.

History

- Primary complaint
  - "What hurts?"
  - Location of symptoms—"Point with one finger where it hurts the most"
  - Description of symptoms—pain, tingling, numbness, grinding, popping
  - Onset of symptoms—acute, chronic, or insidious
  - "What makes it feel worse and better?"
- Type and level of pain
  - Example—sharp, shooting, throbbing, burning
  - Referred pain—for example, Kehr sign (see Fig. 4.1)
  - Pain scale from "0 to 10" ("0" being no pain and "10" being severe pain)
- Etiology/Mechanism
  - "How did the injury occur?"
  - Changes in training regimen, training surface, shoes, and equipment
- Past medical history
  - Injuries, illnesses, medical conditions, surgeries
  - Question patient
  - Review medical record

> **Quick fact** If a patient is having trouble identifying the pain level on a scale of 1 to 10, you can use a visual analog scale.

> **Quick fact** Burning and/or radiating pain can be an indication of neurologic pathology.

Observation

- Gait and functional movement
  - Gait movement—foot hyperpronation, leg limp, or hip hike
  - Functional movement—take off shirt, tie shoes
- General posture
  - Examples—slumping, self-splinting of body part
- Facial expressions
  - Example—grimacing
- Body fluids
  - Blood, cerebrospinal fluid (CSF), mucus, or purulent discharge
- Gross deformity
  - Indicates—fracture, dislocation, or muscle/tendon rupture
- Symmetry
  - Muscles, bones, and joints
  - Indicates—muscle atrophy, muscle/tendon rupture, fracture, or dislocation
- Swelling/Edema
  - Local versus diffuse
  - Intracapsular versus extracapsular

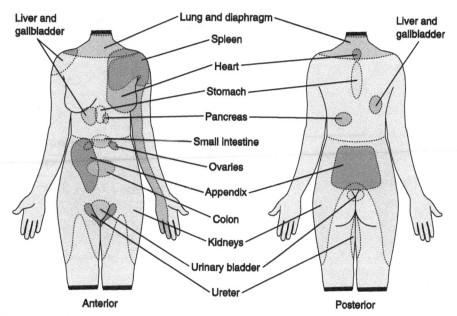

Figure 4.1 Patterns of Referred Organ Pain. Anderson MK, Parr GP, Hall SJ. *Foundations of athletic training: prevention, assessment, and management*, 4th ed. Baltimore: Lippincott Williams & Wilkins; 2009.

- Skin
  - Color—red, pale, cyanotic, jaundice, ecchymosis
  - Blisters, scars, skin infections
- Equipment and footwear
  - Equipment alterations, appropriate fit
  - Shoe-wear patterns

> **Quick fact** Swelling of the foot and hand can be objectively measured using an instrument known as a *volumeter*.

> **Quick fact** Assessing the wear pattern of a patient's shoe can provide clues in determining functional deviations of the foot.

Palpation

- Start away from injury site
  - Work toward primary site of injury
- Start with light pressure
  - Progress to deeper pressure as tolerated
- Bone and soft tissue structures
  - Muscles, tendons, ligaments, pulses
- Assess for:
  - Point tenderness
  - Pain
  - Muscle guarding
  - Swelling
  - Pitting edema
  - Deformity
  - Crepitus

- False motion
- Skin temperature/moisture level
- Vascular integrity

> **Quick fact** False motion describes movement at a point within a bone where there is no joint, thereby indicating a fracture.

> **Quick fact** When assessing skin temperature and moisture level, make sure you use the back of your hand.

Table 4.1 Vascular Integrity Assessment

Artery	Assessment Location
Carotid	Anterior to sternocleidomastoid
Brachial	Medial aspect of arm midway between shoulder and elbow
Radial	At wrist, lateral to flexor carpi radialis tendon
Ulnar	At wrist, between flexor digitorum and flexor carpi ulnaris tendon
Femoral	Within femoral triangle
Posterior tibialis	Posterior aspect of medial malleolus
Dorsalis pedis	Between first and second metatarsals on dorsal aspect of foot

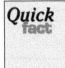

Quick fact The femoral artery can be palpated within the femoral triangle, which is bordered by the inguinal ligament, sartorius muscle, and adductor longus muscle.

Range of Motion Tests

- Active range of motion (AROM)
  - Assesses integrity/strength of muscles/ tendons
- Passive range of motion (PROM)
  - Assesses ligamentous/capsular integrity
  - Overpressure at end range
  - Pathological end feels—soft, firm, hard, and empty
- Resistive range of motion (RROM)
  - Assesses muscular strength
  - Large groups of muscles
  - Examples—wrist flexors and back extensors
  - Perform "break test" for 5 seconds
- Manual muscle tests (MMTs)
  - Assess muscular strength
  - Individual or smaller groups of muscles
  - Examples—palmaris longus, peroneus longus and brevis
  - Perform "break test" for 5 seconds
  - Grading scale—"0 to 5" (see Table 4.2)
- Goniometry
  - Measurement of joint angles
  - Measured in degrees with a goniometer
  - Intratester versus intertester reliability
  - Parts of goniometer: (a) body, (b) fulcrum, (c) stationary arm, and (d) movement arm (see Fig. 4.2)

Quick fact A plus/minus system may be incorporated into the manual muscle grading scale for a more detailed representation of motor function.

Table 4.2 Manual Muscle Test Grading Scale

Grade	Description
5 (Normal)	FROM vs. maximum R w/ (−) BT
4 (Good)	FROM vs. moderate R w/ (−) BT
3 (Fair)	FROM vs. G
2 (Poor)	FROM w/ G eliminated
1 (Trace)	No M but palpable MC
0 (Zero)	No M nor palpable MC

FROM, full range of motion; R, resistance; BT, break test; G, gravity; M, movement; MC, muscle contraction.

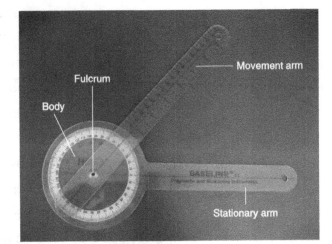

Figure 4.2 Parts of a Goniometer.

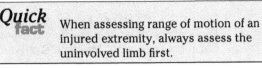

Quick fact When assessing range of motion of an injured extremity, always assess the uninvolved limb first.

Ligamentous Tests

- Assess for:
  - Ligament and/or joint capsule pathology
- Laxity
  - Usually described in millimeters of translation
- Examples
  - Anterior drawer test, valgus stress test
- Grading scale
  - First, second, or third degree
  - Mild, moderate, or severe

Special Tests

- Structures assessed
  - Muscles, cartilage, nerves, arteries
- Examples
  - McMurray test, vertebral artery test

Neurologic Tests

- Cranial nerves (CNs) (see Table 4.3)
  - CNs I to XII
  - Motor and/or sensory test
  - Assess for CN damage or head injury
- Dermatomes
  - Sensory function (see Table 4.4)
  - Eyes closed
  - Sharp, dull, and no sensation
  - Two-point discrimination
  - Hot versus cold discrimination
  - Bilateral comparison
  - Assess for nerve root, peripheral nerve, or spinal cord injury
- Myotomes
  - Motor function (Table 4.4)
  - RROM and/or MMTs

Table 4.3 Cranial Nerve Assessment

Name	Type	Function	Test
I. Olfactory	Sensory	Smell	Identify familiar odor
II. Optic	Sensory	Visual acuity and peripheral vision	Identify number of fingers held up Assess peripheral vision
III. Oculomotor	Motor	Pupillary reaction Upward and downward eye motion	Shine penlight in eye Perform upward and downward eye movement
IV. Trochlear	Motor	Upward eye motion	Perform upward eye movement
V. Trigeminal	Mixed	Sensory: sensation of forehead and lower jaw Motor: biting/chewing motion	Sensory: stroke forehead and lower jaw with finger Motor: bite down on tongue depressor and hold in place
VI. Abducens	Motor	Lateral eye motion	Perform lateral eye movement
VII. Facial	Mixed	Sensory: taste Motor: facial motions	Sensory: identify familiar taste on anterior tongue Motor: smile and whistle
VIII. Vestibulocochlear	Sensory	Hearing and balance	Sensory: lightly snap fingers behind ear Sensory: Romberg test
IX. Glossopharyngeal	Mixed	Sensory: taste Motor: muscles of pharynx	Sensory: identify familiar taste on posterior tongue Motor: instruct patient to swallow
X. Vagus	Mixed	Sensory: gag reflex Motor: muscles of pharynx and larynx	Sensory: place tongue depressor on back of tongue to produce gag reflex Motor: say "Ahh"
XI. Accessory	Motor	Shoulder elevation	Motor: shrug each shoulder against manual resistance
XII. Hypoglossal	Motor	Tongue motions	Motor: stick out the tongue

Cranial nerve tests should be performed bilaterally to assess the nerves on both sides of the brain.

Table 4.4 Spinal Nerve Root Assessment

Spinal Nerve Root	Myotome	Dermatome	Deep Tendon Reflex
C1	Neck flexion	Top of skull	N/A
C2	Neck flexion	External occipital protuberance	N/A
C3	Neck lateral flexion	Lateral aspect of neck	N/A
C4	Shoulder elevation	Clavicle	N/A
C5	Shoulder abduction	Lateral aspect of deltoid	Biceps brachii tendon
C6	Elbow flexion Wrist extension	Dorsal aspect of thumb	Brachioradialis tendon
C7	Elbow extension Wrist flexion	Dorsal aspect of third finger	Triceps brachii tendon
C8	Ulnar deviation Thumb extension	Palmar aspect of fifth digit	N/A
T1	Finger abduction Finger adduction	Medial epicondyle	N/A
L1	Hip flexion	Anterior aspect of hip	N/A
L2	Hip flexion	Anteromedial aspect of thigh	N/A
L3	Knee extension	Medial aspect of knee	Patellar tendon
L4	Ankle dorsiflexion	Dorsum of great toe	Patellar tendon
L5	Great toe extension	Dorsum of second to fifth toes	Medial hamstring tendon
S1	Ankle plantar flexion	Lateral aspect of fifth metatarsal	Achilles' tendon
S2	Knee flexion	Heel of foot	Lateral hamstring tendon

Only one dermatome area and one to two muscle actions have been provided in an attempt to prevent overlapping functions with other spinal nerve roots.

- ○ Perform "break test" for 5 seconds
- ○ Bilateral comparison
- ○ Assess for nerve root, peripheral nerve, or spinal cord injury
- Deep tendon reflexes (DTRs) (Table 4.4)
  - ○ Use neurologic or reflex hammer
  - ○ Hyperreflexia versus hyporeflexia (see Table 4.5)
  - ○ Examples—brachioradialis reflex and patellar reflex
  - ○ Assess for nerve root or spinal cord injury
- Pathologic reflexes (see Table 4.6)
  - ○ Examples—Babinski reflex and Oppenheim reflex
  - ○ Assess for head injury or spinal cord injury

Table 4.5 Deep Tendon Reflex (DTR) Grading Scale

Grade	Description
0	Absent
1	Diminished
2	Average (normal)
3	Exaggerated
4	Clonus—very brisk

 Quick fact A neurologic hammer has a sharp metal instrument and a dull brush built into it that can be removed and used for dermatome assessments.

Quick fact Ligamentous, special, and neurologic tests should always be performed bilaterally.

 Quick fact The vestibulocochlear nerve is also known as the *acoustic* or *auditory nerve*.

Quick fact Inventing your own "motor dance" is a helpful way to remember the myotomes of the spinal nerve root levels.

Quick fact A positive Babinski reflex test is a normal response in newborns.

Functional Tests

- Progress from low to high intensity
  - ○ Example—walk → jog → sprint → cutting
- Assess for:
  - ○ Flexibility, proprioception, endurance, strength, power
- Sports specific
  - ○ Return-to-running protocol
  - ○ Return-to-throwing protocol

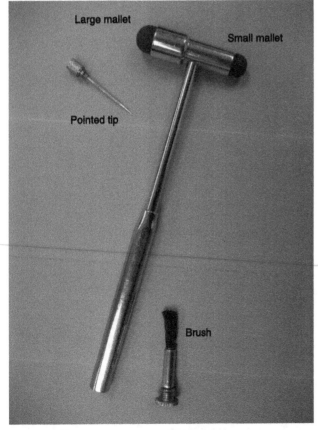

Figure 4.3 Parts of a Neurologic Hammer.

Table 4.6 Pathological Reflexes

Pathological Reflex	Maneuver	Positive Response	Indication
Babinski	Stroke lateral aspect of foot sole	Extension of big toe and fanning of four lesser toes	Pyramidal tract lesion
Oppenheim	Stroke anteromedial tibial surface	Extension of big toe and fanning of four lesser toes	Pyramidal tract lesion
Brudzinski	Passively flex lower limb	Similar movement occurs in contralateral limb	Meningitis

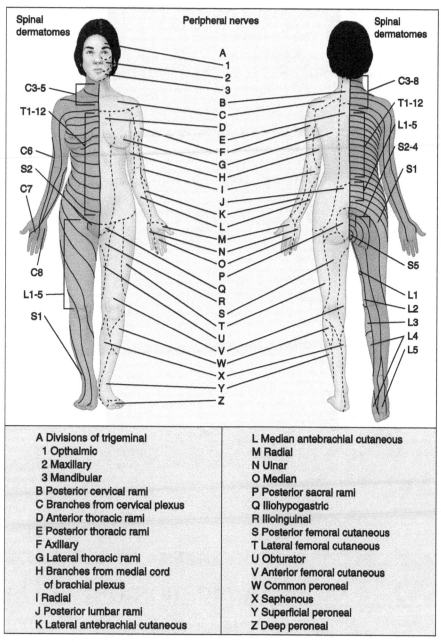

Spinal dermatomes

Peripheral nerves

Spinal dermatomes

C3-5
T1-12
C6
S2
C7
C8
L1-5
S1

A
1
2
3
B
C
D
E
F
G
H
I
J
K
L
M
N
O
P
Q
R
S
T
U
V
W
X
Y
Z

C3-8
T1-12
L1-5
S2-4
S1
S5
L1
L2
L3
L4
L5

A Divisions of trigeminal	L Median antebrachial cutaneous
1 Opthalmic	M Radial
2 Maxillary	N Ulnar
3 Mandibular	O Median
B Posterior cervical rami	P Posterior sacral rami
C Branches from cervical plexus	Q Iliohypogastric
D Anterior thoracic rami	R Ilioinguinal
E Posterior thoracic rami	S Posterior femoral cutaneous
F Axillary	T Lateral femoral cutaneous
G Lateral thoracic rami	U Obturator
H Branches from medial cord	V Anterior femoral cutaneous
of brachial plexus	W Common peroneal
I Radial	X Saphenous
J Posterior lumbar rami	Y Superficial peroneal
K Lateral antebrachial cutaneous	Z Deep peroneal

Figure 4.4 Dermatome Distribution for the Spinal and Peripheral Nerve Roots. Anderson MK, Parr GP, Hall SJ. *Foundations of athletic training: prevention, assessment, and management*, 4th ed. Baltimore: Lippincott Williams & Wilkins; 2009.

Quick fact Functional tests, which are sports specific in nature, should be performed before an athlete returns to play.

DOCUMENTATION PROCEDURE

SOAP Note Format

- Subjective
- Objective
- Assessment
- Plan

Subjective

- What the patient tells you
- Examples—primary complaint, mechanism of injury, past medical history

Objective

- What your findings are
- Examples—girth measurements, goniometry readings, MMT results

Table 4.7 Peripheral Nerve Assessment

Peripheral Nerve	Sensory Distribution	Motor Function
Suprascapular	Acromial end of clavicle	Shoulder external rotation
Axillary	Central aspect of deltoid	Shoulder abduction
Musculocutaneous	Anterolateral aspect of forearm	Elbow flexion
Radial	Dorsal aspect of second metacarpal	Wrist extension
Median	Palmar aspect of third finger	Thumb opposition
Ulnar	Palmar aspect of fifth finger	Fifth finger flexion
Femoral	Anteromedial aspect of thigh	Knee extension
Obturator	Anteromedial aspect of thigh	Hip adduction
Common peroneal	Fibular head	Ankle dorsiflexion
Deep peroneal	Webspace between great toe and second toe	Great toe extension
Superficial peroneal	Dorsum of third metatarsal	Ankle eversion
Tibial	Medial aspect of heel	Ankle plantar flexion

Only one dermatome area and one muscle action have been provided in an attempt to prevent overlapping functions with other peripheral nerves.

> *Quick* **fact** The information documented in the objective portion of the SOAP note should be measurable findings.

Assessment
- What you think is wrong

- Examples—structures injured, severity, short-/long-term goals

Plan
- What you are going to do?
- Examples—therapeutic exercises, therapeutic modalities, criteria for return to play

---

PART 2

Examination of the Head, Neck, Spine, and Thorax

KEY TERMS
- Kyphosis
- Lordosis
- Lumbar triangle
- Scoliosis
- Valsalva maneuver

PALPATIONS

Bony Palpations
See Table 4.8.

 Use the DVD or visit the website at http://thePoint .lww.com/Long for more information about *bony palpations of the head, neck, spine, and thorax.*

Table 4.8 Bony Palpations of the Head, Neck, Spine, and Thorax

Head and Neck	Spine	Thorax
Frontal bone	C1 transverse process	Sternal end of clavicle
Parietal bone	C2 transverse process	Sternoclavicular joint
Temporal bone	C3-7 spinous processes	Suprasternal (jugular) notch
Occipital bone	C3-7 transverse processes	Manubrium
Occiput	T1-12 spinous processes	Sternal body
Superior nuchal line	T1-12 transverse processes	Xiphoid process
External occipital protuberance	L1-5 spinous processes	Ribs
Mastoid process	L1-5 transverse processes	Costochondral joint
Temperomandibular joint	Sacrum	Sternocostal joint
Mandible	Coccyx	
Angle of the mandible		
Superior orbital margin		
Inferior orbital margin		
Nasal bone		
Zygoma		
Zygomatic arch		
Maxilla		
Teeth		
Hyoid bone		

Table 4.9 Soft Tissue Palpations of the Head, Neck, Spine, and Thorax

Head and Neck	Spine	Thorax
Scalp	Paraspinalsh	Sternoclavicular ligament
Ear auricle	Erector spinae	Costal cartilage
Ear helix	Ligamentum nuchae	Serratus anterior
Ear lobule	Supraspinous ligaments	Latissimus dorsi
Nose		Thoracolumbar fascia
Masseter		Pectoralis major
Parotid gland		External oblique
Lips		Internal oblique
Tongue		Rectus abdominis
Sternocleidomastoid		Abdominal quadrants
Anterior scalene		Liver
Upper trapezius		Spleen
Levator scapulae		McBurney point
Splenius cervicis		
Splenius capitis		
Lymph node chain		
Thyroid cartilage		
Thyroid gland		
Cricoid cartilage		
Trachea		
Carotid artery		

 Quick fact The external occipital protuberance is also known as the *inion*.

Soft Tissue Palpation

See Table 4.9.
See Table 4.10.

Use the DVD or visit the website at http://thePoint .lww.com/Long for additional information about *soft tissue palpations of the head, neck, spine, and thorax.*

 Quick fact When an individual has mononucleosis, the spleen may be palpable just inferior to the ribcage within the upper left abdominal quadrant.

Quick fact The McBurney point is located a third of the distance between the anterior superior iliac spine (ASIS) and the umbilicus.

GONIOMETRY

Cervical Flexion

- Patient Position: Sitting
- Fulcrum: External auditory meatus
- Movement Arm: Base of nares
- Stationary Arm: Perpendicular to floor
- Normal ROM: 45 to 50 degrees

Cervical Extension

- Patient Position: Sitting
- Fulcrum: External auditory meatus
- Movement Arm: Base of nares
- Stationary Arm: Perpendicular to floor
- Normal ROM: 45 to 60 degrees

Cervical Lateral Flexion

- Patient Position: Sitting
- Fulcrum: Spinous process of C7 vertebra

Table 4.10 Organ Location within the Abdominal Quadrants

Upper right quadrant	Upper left quadrant
Liver	Stomach
Gall bladder	Spleen
Kidney	Kidney
Pancreas	Pancreas
Lower right quadrant	Lower left quadrant
Intestines	Intestines
Ureter	Ureter
Urinary bladder	Urinary bladder
Gonads	Gonads
Appendix	

- Movement Arm: External occipital protuberance
- Stationary Arm: Perpendicular to floor
- Normal ROM: 45 degrees

Cervical Rotation

- Patient Position: Sitting
- Fulcrum: Center of skull
- Movement Arm: End of nose
- Stationary Arm: Between acromial processes
- Normal ROM: 60 to 80 degrees

 Use the DVD or visit the website at http://thePoint.lww.com/Long for additional materials about *goniometry of the head, neck, spine, and thorax.*

MANUAL MUSCLE TESTS

Sternocleidomastoid and Anterior Scalene

- Patient Position: Supine, head rotated, shoulder flexed 90 degrees, elbow flexed 90 degrees
- Stabilization: None
- Patient Cue: "Lift head up diagonally"
- Force Direction: Head—posterolaterally

> *Quick fact* Anterior scalene muscle tightness could be a potential cause of thoracic outlet syndrome.

Splenius Capitis and Cervicis

- Patient Position: Prone, head rotated, shoulder flexed 90 degrees, elbow flexed 90 degrees
- Stabilization: None
- Patient Cue: "Lift head up diagonally"
- Force Direction: Head—anterolaterally

Upper Trapezius

- Patient Position: Sitting, arms at side, face turned opposite direction
- Stabilization: None
- Patient Cue: "Bring ear and shoulder together"
- Force Direction: Shoulder—depression; head—anterolaterally flexion

Levator Scapulae

- Patient Position: Prone, elbow flexed, humerus adducted in slight extension, humerus slightly externally rotated
- Stabilization: None
- Patient Cue: "Maintain position as pressure is applied"
- Force Direction: Inner elbow—scapular abduction and downward rotation; shoulder—depression

> *Quick fact* In addition to cervical spine movement, the upper trapezius also plays a role in moving the scapula.

Lattisimus Dorsi

- Patient Position: Prone, arm at side, elbow extended, humerus internally rotated, palm facing the ceiling
- Stabilization: Pelvis
- Patient Cue: "Move arm backward and away from side of body"
- Force Direction: Distal forearm—abduction and flexion

Serratus Anterior

- Patient Position: Supine, elbow fully extended, shoulder flexed 90 degrees
- Stabilization: None
- Patient Cue: "Push entire arm off table"
- Force Direction: Fist—downward

> *Quick fact* Weakness of the serratus anterior muscle could be caused by long thoracic nerve pathology.

Erector Spinae

- Patient Position: Prone, hands behind head
- Stabilization: Above knee and ankle
- Patient Cue: "Lift trunk toward ceiling and hold"
- Force Direction: None

Quadratus Lumborum

- Patient Position: Prone, leg extended and abducted
- Stabilization: None
- Patient Cue: "Lift hip toward head"
- Force Direction: Leg—traction

Rectus Abdominis

- Patient Position: Supine, hands behind head
- Stabilization: None
- Patient Cue: "Do a sit-up and hold"
- Force Direction: None

Internal and External Oblique

- Patient Position: Supine, hands behind head
- Stabilization: Above knee and ankle
- Patient Cue: "Do a sit-up with rotation and hold"
- Force Direction: None

Upper Pectoralis Major

- Patient Position: Supine, elbow extended, shoulder flexed 90 degrees, slight shoulder internal rotation

- Stabilization: Contralateral shoulder
- Patient Cue: "Pull arm straight across body toward opposite shoulder"
- Force Direction: Proximal forearm—horizontal flexion

Lower Pectoralis Major

- Patient Position: Supine, elbow extended, shoulder flexed 90 degrees, slight shoulder internal rotation
- Stabilization: Opposite iliac crest
- Patient Cue: "Pull arm diagonally across body toward opposite hip"
- Force Direction: Forearm—obliquely in a flexion and horizontal extension

 Use the DVD or visit the website at http://thePoint.lww.com/Long for more information about *manual muscle tests of the head, neck, spine, and thorax.*

LIGAMENTOUS AND SPECIAL TESTS

Vertebral Artery Test

- Patient Position: Supine, head off table
- Hand Position: Both hands supporting occiput
- Maneuver: Passively extend, laterally flex, and rotate head to one side; hold for 30 seconds
- Positive Test: Vertigo, loss of consciousness, nausea, nystagmus, difficulty speaking, visual disturbances
- Indication: Vertebral artery occlusion

 Quick fact The vertebral artery test should be performed before conducting any other cervical spine tests.

Foraminal Compression (Spurling) Test

- Patient Position: Sitting
- Hand Position: Both hands interlocked on top of head
- Maneuver: Actively extend and laterally flex neck, apply downward pressure on head
- Positive Test: Neck pain radiating down arm ipsilateral to lateral neck flexion
- Indication: Nerve root impingement

Quick fact The cervical compression test is similar to the Spurling test, except the head is maintained in a neutral position while applying downward pressure on top of the head.

Foraminal Distraction Test

- Patient Position: Sitting
- Hand Position: One hand under chin, other hand supports occiput

- Maneuver: Slowly lift head upward
- Positive Test: Relief or decrease in pain
- Indication: Nerve root impingement

Quick fact The foraminal distraction test can be performed after a positive foraminal compression test to confirm the presence of nerve root impingement.

Brachial Plexus Stretch (Traction) Test

- Patient Position: Sitting or standing
- Hand Position: One hand on side of head, other hand on top of shoulder
- Maneuver: Passively laterally flex neck and depress shoulder
- Positive Test: Neck pain radiating down arm contralateral to lateral neck flexion, neck pain ipsilateral to lateral neck flexion
- Indication: Neck pain radiating down arm contralateral to lateral neck flexion indicates brachial plexus pathology, neck pain radiating down arm ipsilateral to lateral neck flexion indicates nerve root impingement

 Quick fact A stretching of the brachial plexus is commonly known as a *stinger* or *burner*.

Valsalva (Maneuver) Test

- Patient Position: Sitting
- Hand Position: None, but stand near patient
- Maneuver: Take and hold a deep breath, initiate pressure as if having a bowel movement
- Positive Test: Increased pain
- Indication: Herniated disc, osteophyte, tumor

Quick fact Valsalva test increases intrathecal pressure around the spinal cord.

Spring Test

- Patient Position: Prone
- Hand Position: Both thumbs over spinous process of vertebra
- Maneuver: Apply an anterior force to spinous process
- Positive Test: Decrease in vertebral movement, increase in vertebral movement
- Indication: Decrease in vertebral movement indicates hypomobility; increase in vertebral movement indicates hypermobility

Kernig-Brudzinski (Brudzinksi-Kernig) Test

- Patient Position: Supine, hands behind head
- Hand Position: None

- Maneuver: Actively flex neck; actively flex hip until pain is experienced; actively flex knee
- Positive Test: Radiating pain into leg with neck and hip flexion, followed by relief with knee flexion
- Indication: Nerve root impingement, dural or meningeal irritation

Slump Test

- Patient Position: Sitting, leaning forward, shoulders rounded forward, maintaining neck in neutral position
- Hand Position: One hand under chin, other hand behind head
- Maneuver: Passively flex neck, passively extend knee, passively dorsiflex ankle
- Positive Test: Buttock, posterior thigh, or calf pain/neurologic symptoms
- Indication: Nerve root impingement, spinal cord impingement, sciatic nerve pathology

> **Quick fact** The maneuver for the slump test can also be performed actively by the patient versus passively by the examiner.

Sitting Root Test

- Patient Position: Sitting, neck flexed
- Hand Position: None
- Maneuver: Actively extend knee
- Positive test: Buttock, posterior thigh, or calf pain; arching of back
- Indication: Sciatic nerve pathology

Stork Standing (One-Leg Standing Lumbar Extension) Test

- Patient Position: Standing on one leg, plantar aspect of opposite foot rests on medial knee of standing leg
- Hand Position: None, but stand behind patient
- Maneuver: Actively extend trunk
- Positive Test: Lumbar spine pain
- Indication: Pars interarticularis pathology

> **Quick fact** The stork standing test is also referred to the *single leg stance test.*

Unilateral Straight Leg Raise (Lasegue) Test

- Patient Position: Supine
- Hand Position: One hand on distal anterior thigh, other hand around heel
- Maneuver: Passively flex hip until pain or tightness occurs, lower leg until symptoms resolve, passively dorsiflex ankle, actively flex neck
- Positive Test: Low back or leg pain before 70-degree hip flexion, low back and/or radiating leg pain that reoccurs with ankle dorsiflexion and/or neck flexion, lack of

symptom reoccurrence with ankle dorsiflexion and/or neck flexion, symptoms occurring past 70-degree hip flexion
- Indication: Low back or leg pain before 70-degree hip flexion indicates intervetebral disc pathology, low back and/or radiating leg pain that reoccurs with ankle dorsiflexion and/or neck flexion indicates sciatic nerve or dural pathology, lack of symptom reoccurrence with ankle dorsiflexion and/or neck flexion indicates tight hamstrings, symptoms occurring past 70-degree hip flexion indicates lumbar spine or sacroiliac joint pathology

Bilateral Straight Leg Raise Test

- Patient Position: Supine
- Hand Position: One forearm under both heels, other forearm on both distal anterior thighs
- Maneuver: Passively flex both hips with knees extended
- Positive Test: Low back pain before 70-degree hip flexion, low back pain past 70-degree hip flexion
- Indication: Low back pain before 70-degree hip flexion indicates sacroiliac joint pathology, low back pain past 70-degree hip flexion indicates lumbar spine pathology

Hoover Test

- Patient Position: Supine
- Hand Position: Palms of hands under each heel
- Maneuver: Actively perform a straight leg raise
- Positive Test: Inability to perform straight leg raise, lack of pressure in palm under contralateral heel
- Indication: Inability to lift leg indicates muscular weakness, lack of increased pressure in palm under resting heel indicates malingering

Sacroiliac Joint Compression Test

- Patient Position: Supine
- Hand Position: Arms crossed, each palm of hand over each ASIS
- Maneuver: Apply outward and downward pressure
- Positive Test: Sacroiliac joint pain
- Indication: Sacroiliac joint pathology

> **Quick fact** The sacroiliac joint compression test is also known as the *gapping test.*

Sacroiliac Joint Distraction Test

- Patient Position: Sidelying
- Hand Position: Both hands over iliac crest
- Maneuver: Apply downward pressure
- Positive Test: Sacroiliac joint pain
- Indication: Sacroiliac joint pathology

Patrick (FABER) Test

- Patient Position: Supine; leg flexed, abducted, and externally rotated so that the foot rests on thigh just above knee
- Hand Position: One hand on iliac crest, other hand on opposite hip
- Maneuver: Passively abduct leg
- Positive Test: Sacroiliac joint pain, hip and/or inguinal pain, inability to abduct leg below level of contralateral leg
- Indication: Sacroiliac joint pain indicates sacroiliac joint pathology, hip and/or inguinal pain indicates hip pathology, inability to abduct leg below level of contralateral leg indicates iliopsoas muscle tightness

Quick fact FABER stands for flexion, abduction, and external rotation.

Lateral Rib Compression Test

- Patient Position: Supine or standing
- Hand Position: One hand on side of ribcage, other hand on side of opposite ribcage
- Maneuver: Compress both sides of ribcage simultaneously and quickly release
- Positive Test: Rib pain
- Indication: Rib contusion, rib fracture, and costochondral separation

Anterior/Posterior Rib Compression Test

- Patient Position: Supine or standing
- Hand Position: One hand on anterior ribcage, other hand on posterior rib cage
- Maneuver: Compress both sides of ribcage simultaneously and quickly release
- Positive Test: Rib pain
- Indication: Rib contusion, rib fracture, and costochondral separation

Use the DVD or visit the website at http://thePoint.lww.com/Long for additional materials about *ligamentous and special tests of the head, neck, spine, and thorax.*

PART 3

Examination of the Upper Extremity

KEY TERMS

- Triangular fibrocartilage complex
- Winged scapula

Quick fact The tunnel of Guyon is located between the pisiform and the hook of the hamate.

Use the DVD or visit the website at http://thePoint.lww.com/Long for additional materials about *bony palpations of the upper extremity.*

PALPATIONS

Bony Palpations

See Table 4.11.

Quick fact The bicipital groove is also known as the *intertubercular groove.*

Quick fact The carpal bones of the hand can be remembered by the pneumonic "Some Lions Take Prey That They Can't Handle."

Soft Tissue Palpations

See Table 4.12.

Quick fact The Erb point is located just superior to the clavicle within the supraclavicular fossa and is the location where the trunk of the brachial plexus is most superficial.

Table 4.11 Bony Palpations of the Upper Extremity

Shoulder Complex and Upper Arm	Elbow and Forearm	Wrist and Hand
Shaft of clavicle	Humeral shaft	Scaphoid
Acromial end of clavicle	Medial supracondylar ridge	Scaphoid tubercle
Acromioclavicular joint	Medial epicondyle	Lunate
Acromion process	Olecranon process	Triquetrum
Coracoid process	Lateral supracondylar ridge	Pisiform
Spine of scapula	Lateral epicondyle	Trapezium
Superior angle of scapula	Ulnar groove	Trapezoid
Vertebral border of scapula	Ulnar shaft	Capitate
Inferior angle of scapula	Radial head	Hamate
Axillary border of scapula	Proximal radioulnar joint	Hook of hamate
Humeral head	Radial shaft	Tunnel of Guyon
Greater tuberosity	Radial styloid process	First to fifth CMC joints
Bicipital groove	Lister tubercle	First to fifth metacarpal bases
Lesser tuberosity	Distal radioulnar joint	First to fifth metacarpal shafts
Deltoid tuberosity	Radiocarpal joint	First to fifth metacarpal heads
Humeral shaft		First to fifth MCP joints
		Proximal phalanx of thumb
		IP joint of thumb
		Distal phalanx of thumb
		Second to fifth proximal phalanges
		Second to fifth PIP joints
		Second to fifth middle phalanges
		Second to fifth DIP joints
		Second to fifth distal phalanges

CMC, carpometacarpal; MCP, metacarpophalangeal; PIP, proximal interphalangeal; DIP, distal interphalangeal.

Table 4.12 Soft Tissue Palpations of the Upper Extremity

Shoulder Complex and Upper Arm	Elbow and Forearm	Wrist and Hand
Acromioclavicular ligament	Cubital fossa	Radial artery
Subacromial bursa	Distal biceps brachii tendon	Ulnar artery
Coracoacromial ligament	Brachial artery	Anatomical snuffbox
Anterior deltoid	Ulnar collateral ligament complex	Abductor pollicis longus tendon
Middle deltoid	Radial collateral ligament complex	Extensor pollicis brevis tendon
Posterior deltoid	Annular ligament	Extensor pollicis longus tendon
Supraclavicular fossa	Ulnar nerve	Adductor pollicis muscle
Erb point	Distal triceps brachii tendon	Extensor carpi radialis longus tendon
Coracobrachialis	Anconeus	Extensor digitorum tendons
Long head of biceps brachii tendon	Brachioradialis	Flexor carpi radialis tendon
Biceps brachii (short head)	Pronator teres	Palmaris longus tendon
Biceps brachii (long head)	Flexor carpi radialis	Flexor carpi ulnaris tendon
Brachialis	Flexor carpi ulnaris	Thenar eminence
Triceps brachii	Pronator quadratus	Palmer aponeurosis
Teres minor	Palmaris longus	Hypothenar eminence
Teres major	Extensor carpi radialis longus	Flexor pollicis longus tendon
Rhomboid minor	Extensor carpi ulnaris	Volar plates of the IP joints
Rhomboid major	Extensor digitorum	UCL of MCP joint of thumb
Middle trapezius		RCL of the PIP joints
Lower trapezius		UCL of the PIP joint
Axilla		
Axillary lymph nodes		

IP, interphalangeal; UCL, ulnar collateral ligament; MCP, metacarpophalangeal joint; RCL, radial collateral ligament; PIP, proximal interphalangeal joint.

Quick fact The borders of the "anatomical snuffbox" are made up by the abductor pollicis longus, extensor pollicis longus, and extensor pollicis brevis tendons.

 Use the DVD or visit the website at http://thePoint.lww.com/Long for additional materials about soft tissue palpations of the upper extremity.

GONIOMETRY

Shoulder Flexion
- Patient Position: Supine
- Fulcrum: Lateral aspect of greater tubercle of humerus
- Movement Arm: Midline of humerus (lateral epicondyle)
- Stationary Arm: Parallel to midaxillary line of thorax
- Normal ROM: 150 to 180 degrees

Shoulder Extension
- Patient Position: Supine
- Fulcrum: Lateral aspect of greater tubercle of humerus
- Movement Arm: Midline of humerus (lateral epicondyle)
- Stationary Arm: Parallel to midaxillary line of thorax
- Normal ROM: 50 to 60 degrees

Shoulder Abduction

- Patient Position: Supine
- Fulcrum: Anterior aspect of acromion process
- Movement Arm: Midline of humerus (medial epicondyle)
- Stationary Arm: Parallel to midline of anterior sternum
- Normal ROM: 180 degrees

Shoulder External Rotation

- Patient Position: Supine
- Fulcrum: Olecranon process
- Movement Arm: Midline of ulna (olecranon process and ulnar styloid)
- Stationary Arm: Perpendicular to floor
- Normal ROM: 90 degrees

Shoulder Internal Rotation

- Patient Position: Supine
- Fulcrum: Olecranon process
- Movement Arm: Midline of ulna (olecranon process and ulnar styloid)
- Stationary Arm: Perpendicular to floor
- Normal ROM: 70 to 90 degrees

> Use the DVD or visit the website at http://thePoint.lww.com/Long for additional materials about shoulder functional norms.

Elbow Flexion

- Patient Position: Supine
- Fulcrum: Lateral epicondyle of humerus
- Movement Arm: Midline of radius (radial head and radial styloid process)
- Stationary Arm: Midline of humerus (center of acromion process)
- Normal ROM: 140 to 150 degrees

Elbow Extension

- Patient Position: Supine
- Fulcrum: Lateral epicondyle of humerus
- Movement Arm: Midline of radius (radial head and radial styloid process)
- Stationary Arm: Midline of humerus (center of acromion process)
- Normal ROM: 0 degrees

> **Quick fact** Normal carrying angle for the elbow is 5 to 10 degrees in men and 10 to 15 degrees in women. Increased carrying angle is cubital valgus and a decreased carrying angle is cubital varus.

Forearm Pronation

- Patient Position: Sitting
- Fulcrum: Laterally and proximally to ulnar styloid process
- Movement Arm: Dorsal aspect of forearm, just proximal to styloid processes
- Stationary Arm: Midline of humerus
- Normal ROM: 80 degrees

Forearm Supination

- Patient Position: Sitting
- Fulcrum: Center medially and proximally to ulnar styloid process
- Movement Arm: Ventral aspect of forearm, just proximal to styloid processes
- Stationary Arm: Midline of humerus
- Normal ROM: 80 degrees

Wrist Flexion

- Patient Position: Sitting
- Fulcrum: Lateral aspect of wrist over triquetrum
- Movement Arm: Midline of fifth metacarpal
- Stationary Arm: Midline of ulna (olecranon and ulnar styloid)
- Normal ROM: 60 to 80 degrees

Wrist Extension

- Patient Position: Sitting
- Fulcrum: Lateral aspect of wrist over triquetrum
- Movement Arm: Midline of fifth metacarpal
- Stationary Arm: Midline of ulna (olecranon and ulnar styloid)
- Normal ROM: 60 to 70 degrees

Wrist Radial Deviation

- Patient Position: Sitting
- Fulcrum: Dorsal aspect of wrist over capitate
- Movement Arm: Midline of third metacarpal
- Stationary Arm: Midline of forearm (lateral epicondyle)
- Normal ROM: 20 degrees

Wrist Ulnar Deviation

- Patient Position: Sitting
- Fulcrum: Dorsal aspect of wrist over capitate
- Movement Arm: Midline of third metacarpal
- Stationary Arm: Midline of forearm (lateral epicondyle)
- Normal ROM: 30 degrees

> Use the DVD or visit the website at http://thePoint.lww.com/Long for additional materials at *goniometry of the upper extremity*.

MANUAL MUSCLE TESTS

Lower Trapezius

- Patient Position: Prone, elbow fully extended, arm abducted diagonally overhead, humerus externally rotated, thumb toward ceiling
- Stabilization: Contralateral scapula
- Patient Cue: "Maintain position as pressure is applied"
- Force Direction: Distal forearm—downward

Middle Trapezius

- Patient Position: Prone, elbow fully extended, shoulder abducted 90 degrees, humerus externally rotated, thumb toward ceiling
- Stabilization: Contralateral scapula
- Patient Cue: "Maintain position as pressure is applied"
- Force Direction: Distal forearm—downward

Rhomboid Major and Minor

- Patient Position: Prone, elbow flexed, humerus adducted in slight extension, humerus slightly externally rotated
- Stabilization: None
- Patient Cue: "Maintain position as pressure is applied"
- Force Direction: inner elbow—scapular abduction and downward rotation; shoulder— depression

> **Quick fact** Rhomboid major and minor have the exact same muscle actions.

Supraspinatus

- Patient Position: Sitting or standing, arm at side, neck extended and laterally flexed to ipsilateral side, face rotated toward contralateral side
- Stabilization: None
- Patient Cue: "Lift arm away from side of body"
- Force Direction: Forearm—adduction

> **Quick fact** The supraspinatus tendon travels through the subacromial space, making it prone to being impinged during overhead activities.

Infraspinatus

- Patient Position: Prone, arm resting on table, shoulder abducted 90 degrees, elbow flexed 90 degrees
- Stabilization: Under distal upper arm
- Patient Cue: "Rotate arm backward"
- Force Direction: Forearm—internal rotation

Teres Minor

- Patient Position: Supine, arm resting on table, elbow flexed 90 degrees
- Stabilization: Inner distal humerus
- Patient Cue: "Rotate arm away from body"
- Force Direction: Forearm—internal rotation

Subscapularis

- Patient Position: Supine, arm resting on table, elbow flexed 90 degrees
- Stabilization: Outer distal humerus
- Patient Cue: "Rotate arm toward body"
- Force Direction: Forearm—external rotation

> **Quick fact** The subscapularis muscle is the only member of the rotator cuff group that is a shoulder internal rotator.

Teres Major

- Patient Position: Prone, hand resting on posterior iliac crest, humerus internally rotated
- Stabilization: None
- Patient Cue: "Move arm backward and away from body"
- Force Direction: Distal upper arm—abduction and flexion

Pectoralis Minor

- Patient Position: Supine, arms at side
- Stabilization: None
- Patient Cue: "Lift shoulder off table"
- Force Direction: Anterior shoulder—downward

> **Quick fact** Although the pectoralis major muscle inserts on the humerus, the pectoralis minor does not attach to the humerus.

Anterior Deltoid

- Patient Position: Sitting, elbow flexed 90 degrees, shoulder abducted in slight horizontal flexion, humerus in slight external rotation
- Stabilization: Scapula
- Patient Cue: "Lift arm above head"
- Force Direction: Distal humerus—adduction and extension

Middle Deltoid

- Patient Position: Sitting, elbow flexed 90 degrees, shoulder abducted
- Stabilization: None
- Patient Cue: "Lift arm above head"
- Force Direction: Distal humerus—adduction

Posterior Deltoid

- Patient Position: Sitting, elbow flexed 90 degrees, shoulder abducted in slight horizontal extension, humerus in slight internal rotation

- Stabilization: Scapula
- Patient Cue: "Lift arm above head"
- Force Direction: Distal humerus—adduction and flexion

Coracobrachialis

- Patient Position: Sitting or supine, shoulder externally rotated, elbow fully flexed, forearm supinated
- Stabilization: None
- Patient Cue: "Lift arm above head"
- Force Direction: Upper arm—extension and slight abduction

Biceps Brachii and Brachialis

- Patient Position: Sitting or supine, elbow slightly less than or flexed 90 degrees, forearm supinated
- Stabilization: Under elbow to cushion
- Patient Cue: "Bend lower arm up toward shoulder"
- Force Direction: Forearm—extension

Triceps Brachii and Anconeus

- Patient Position: Supine, elbow slightly less than full extension, shoulder flexed 90 degrees
- Stabilization: Upper arm
- Patient Cue: "Straighten elbow out"
- Force Direction: Forearm—flexion

Quick **fact** The anconeus muscle assists the triceps brachii in extending the elbow.

Brachioradialis

- Patient Position: Sitting or supine, elbow flexed, forearm neutral
- Stabilization: Under elbow to cushion
- Patient Cue: "Bend lower arm up toward shoulder"
- Force Direction: Distal forearm—extension

Supinator

- Patient Position: Supine, shoulder flexed 90 degrees, elbow fully flexed
- Stabilization: Elbow against side
- Patient Cue: "Rotate forearm outward"
- Force Direction: Distal forearm—pronation

Pronator Teres

- Patient Position: Sitting or supine, elbow partially flexed, forearm pronated
- Stabilization: Elbow against the side
- Patient Cue: "Rotate forearm inward"
- Force Direction: Distal forearm—supination

Pronator Quadratus

- Patient Position: Sitting or supine, elbow fully flexed, forearm pronated

- Stabilization: Elbow against the side
- Patient Cue: "Rotate forearm inward"
- Force Direction: Distal forearm—supination

Quick **fact** The pronator quadratus is located between the radius and ulna in the distal aspect of the forearm.

Flexor Carpi Radialis

- Patient Position: Sitting or supine, forearm almost fully supinated
- Stabilization: Posterior forearm
- Patient Cue: "Bend wrist down and toward thumb side"
- Force Direction: Thenar eminence—extension and ulnar deviation

Flexor Carpi Ulnaris

- Patient Position: Sitting or supine, forearm fully supinated
- Stabilization: Under forearm
- Patient Cue: "Bend wrist down and toward little finger side"
- Force Direction: Hypothenar eminence—extension and radial deviation

Palmaris Longus

- Patient Position: Sitting or supine, forearm supinated
- Stabilization: Forearm on table
- Patient Cue: "Cup palm and fingers of hand and bend wrist toward body"
- Force Direction: Thenar and hypothenar eminences—palm flattening and wrist extension

Flexor Digitorum Superficialis

- Patient Position: Sitting or supine, wrist neutral
- Stabilization: Metacarpophalangeal (MCP) joint
- Patient Cue: "Bend middle joints of four fingers with far joints extended"
- Force Direction: Palmar aspect of middle phalanx—extension

Flexor Digitorum Profundus

- Patient Position: Sitting or supine, wrist slightly extended
- Stabilization: Proximal and middle phalanges
- Patient Cue: "Bend end joint of your finger"
- Force Direction: Volar aspect of distal phalanx—extension

Extensor Digitorum

- Patient Position: Sitting or supine
- Stabilization: Wrist

- Patient Cue: "Straighten knuckle joints of four fingers with middle joints relaxed"
- Force Direction: Dorsal aspect of proximal phalanges—flexion

Quick fact A rupture of an extensor digitorum tendon at the distal phalanx of the finger is known as *mallet finger*.

Extensor Carpi Radialis Longus

- Patient Position: Sitting, elbow flexed 30 degrees, forearm almost fully pronated
- Stabilization: Forearm on table
- Patient Cue: "Straighten wrist up and toward thumb side while allowing fingers to bend"
- Force Direction: Dorsum of second and third metacarpals—flexion and ulnar deviation

Extensor Carpi Ulnaris

- Patient Position: Sitting or supine, forearm fully pronated
- Stabilization: Under forearm
- Patient Cue: "Bend wrist down and toward little finger side"
- Force Direction: Dorsum of fifth metacarpal—flexion and radial deviation

Flexor Pollicis Longus

- Patient Position: Sitting or supine, thumb extended
- Stabilization: Metacarpal and proximal phalanx of the thumb
- Patient Cue: "Bend the middle joint of thumb"
- Force Direction: Volar aspect of distal phalanx—extension

Flexor Pollicis Brevis

- Patient Position: Sitting or supine
- Stabilization: Hand
- Patient Cue: "Bend the knuckle joint of thumb without bending middle joint"
- Force Direction: Volar aspect of proximal phalanx—extension

Extensor Pollicis Longus

- Patient Position: Sitting or supine
- Stabilization: Hand
- Patient Cue: "Straighten middle joint of thumb"
- Force Direction: Dorsal aspect of interphalangeal (IP) joint of thumb—flexion

Extensor Pollicis Brevis

- Patient Position: Sitting or supine
- Stabilization: Wrist

- Patient Cue: "Straighten knuckle joint of thumb while pulling thumb away from palm"
- Force Direction: Dorsal aspect of proximal phalanx—flexion

Use the DVD or visit the website at http://thePoint.lww.com/Long for additional materials about *manual muscle tests of the upper extremity*.

LIGAMENTOUS AND SPECIAL TESTS

Apley Scratch Test

- Patient Position: Sitting or standing
- Hand Position: None
- Maneuver: First maneuver—actively place hand on contralateral shoulder; second maneuver—actively externally rotate arm overhead and touch the midline of the back as far down as possible; third maneuver—actively internally rotate arm and touch midline of the back as far up as possible
- Positive Test: Decreased ROM in comparison to contralateral shoulder
- Indication: Shoulder complex immobility

Drop Arm (Codman) Test

- Patient Position: Sitting or standing, elbow extended, palm facing floor
- Hand Position: Distal forearm
- Maneuver: Passively or actively abduct shoulder to 90 degrees, actively and slowly lower arm to side
- Positive Test: Shoulder pain and/or inability to slowly lower arm
- Indication: Rotator cuff pathology

Empty Can (Supraspinatus) Test

- Patient Position: Sitting or standing; shoulder abducted 90 degrees, horizontally adducted 30 degrees, and internally rotated; thumb facing floor
- Hand Position: One hand on distal forearm
- Maneuver: Actively abduct shoulder, resist shoulder abduction
- Positive Test: Pain and/or weakness
- Indication: Supraspinatus muscle/tendon pathology

Gerber Lift-Off Test

- Patient Position: Standing, shoulder internally rotated, dorsum of hand against center of lumbar spine
- Hand Position: None
- Maneuver: Actively lift hand off lumbar spine while maintaining position of shoulder
- Positive Test: Inability to lift hand from lumbar spine
- Indication: Subscapularis muscle tear and/or weakness

Quick fact
It is important that when performing the Gerber Lift-Off test the patient does not extend the shoulder joint, as this could result in a false-negative test.

Yergason Test

- Patient Position: Sitting or standing, shoulder adducted at side, elbow flexed 90 degrees, forearm pronated or neutral
- Hand Position: One hand on distal forearm above wrist, other hand on upper arm with thumb close to intertubercular groove
- Maneuver: Actively supinate forearm and externally rotate shoulder, resist supination and external rotation
- Positive Test: Pain and/or "snapping" sensation within bicipital groove, pain within bicipital groove
- Indication: Pain and/or "snapping" sensation within bicipital groove indicates long head of the biceps tendon subluxation and transverse humeral ligament damage, pain within bicipital groove indicates long head of the biceps tendinitis

Speed Test

- Patient Position: Sitting or standing, shoulder flexed 90 degrees, elbow extended, forearm supinated
- Hand Position: One hand on volar aspect of distal forearm, other hand over the intertubercular groove
- Maneuver: Actively flex shoulder, resist shoulder flexion
- Positive Test: Pain within bicipital groove
- Indication: Bicipital tendinitis

Ludington Test

- Patient Position: Sitting or standing, interlocked hands on posterosuperior aspect of head
- Hand Position: Both hands palpating each long head of the biceps tendon
- Maneuver: Actively contract both biceps brachii muscles
- Positive Test: Pain and/or decrease in biceps brachii tendon tension, absence of biceps brachii tendon tension
- Indication: Pain and/or decrease in biceps brachii tendon tension indicates bicipital tendinitis, absence of biceps brachii tendon tension indicates long head of the biceps brachii muscle/tendon rupture

Hawkins-Kennedy Impingement Test

- Patient Position: Sitting or standing
- Hand Position: One hand holds elbow, other hand holds wrist
- Maneuver: Passively flex shoulder 90 degrees, flex elbow 90 degrees, internally rotate shoulder
- Positive Test: Shoulder pain and/or apprehension
- Indication: Shoulder impingement syndrome

Sternoclavicular Joint Stress Test

- Patient Position: Sitting
- Hand Position: Fingers on sternal end of clavicle, other hand on scapular spine
- Maneuver: Apply easy inferior and posterior stress to clavicle
- Positive Test: Clavicle pain and/or translation
- Indication: Sternoclavicular ligament sprain

Quick fact
Before performing the sternoclavicular joint stress test, assure that there is no obvious deformity of the sternoclavicular joint, as this would be an indication of gross ligamentous instability in which performing the test is contraindicated.

Acromioclavicular Joint Distraction (Traction) Test

- Patient Position: Sitting or standing, elbow extended or flexed 90 degrees
- Hand Position: Fingers over acromioclavicular joint, other hand on distal aspect of upper arm
- Maneuver: Apply downward traction force to upper arm
- Positive Test: Shoulder pain and/or inferior translation of acromion process
- Indication: Acromioclavicular joint and/or coracoclavicular joint sprain

Anterior Drawer Test for Shoulder

- Patient Position: Supine
- Hand Position: One hand within axilla around proximal humerus, other fingers on scapular spine, and thumb over coracoid process for stabilization
- Maneuver: Passively abduct shoulder 70 to 80 degrees, flex shoulder 0 to 10 degrees, externally rotate shoulder 0 to 10 degrees, apply anterior force and slight distraction to glenohumeral joint
- Positive Test: Increased anterior translation of humeral head
- Indication: Anterior glenohumeral joint instability

Anterior Apprehension Test

- Patient Position: Supine, shoulder abducted 90 degrees, elbow flexed 90 degrees
- Hand Position: One hand supports upper arm proximal to elbow, other hand at holding distal forearm
- Maneuver: Passively externally rotate shoulder
- Positive Test: Shoulder pain and/or apprehension
- Indication: Anterior glenohumeral joint instability and/or glenoid labrum tear

Quick fact
A patient who experiences a positive anterior apprehension test may have suffered an anterior dislocation of the glenohumeral joint.

Jobe Relocation Test

- Patient Position: Supine, shoulder abducted 90 degrees and externally rotated, elbow flexed 90 degrees
- Hand Position: One hand over the anterior aspect of humeral head, other hand at holding distal forearm
- Maneuver: Apply posterior force over anterior aspect of humeral head
- Positive Test: Decrease in pain and/or apprehension, increased ability to passively externally rotate shoulder
- Indication: Anterior glenohumeral joint instability and/or glenoid labrum tear

Quick **fact** The Jobe relocation test can be utilized immediately following a positive anterior apprehension test in an effort to reduce pain/apprehension, thereby assisting in confirmation of anterior glenohumeral joint instability.

Posterior Drawer Test for Shoulder

- Patient Position: Supine
- Hand Position: One hand holds flexed elbow, other fingers on scapular spine and thumb over coracoid process for stabilization
- Maneuver: Passively abduct shoulder 90 degrees, horizontally flex shoulder 20 to 30 degrees, apply anterior force to glenohumeral joint
- Positive Test: Increased posterior translation of humeral head
- Indication: Posterior glenohumeral joint instability

Posterior Apprehension Test

- Patient Position: Supine with shoulder just off side of table, shoulder flexed 90 degrees, elbow flexed 90 degrees
- Hand Position: One hand over posterior elbow, other hand supports posterior shoulder
- Maneuver: Apply posterior force to humeral shaft
- Positive Test: Shoulder pain and/or apprehension
- Indication: Posterior glenohumeral joint instability and/or glenoid labrum tear

Load and Shift Test

- Patient Position: Sitting
- Hand Position: One hand stabilizes clavicle and scapula, other hand over humeral head
- Maneuver: Apply axial load to humeral shaft, apply anterior force to humeral head, apply posterior force to humeral head
- Positive Test: Increased anterior translation of humeral head, increased posterior translation of humeral head
- Indication: Anterior glenohumeral joint instability, posterior glenohumeral joint instability

Sulcus Sign Test

- Patient Position: Sitting, elbow extended or flexed 90 degrees
- Hand Position: One hand stabilizing scapula, other hand holding elbow or distal forearm
- Maneuver: Apply downward traction force to upper arm
- Positive Test: Increased translation of humeral head from glenoid fossa and/or sulcus below acromion process
- Indication: Inferior glenohumeral joint instability

Inferior Drawer (Feagin) Test

- Patient Position: Sitting or standing, shoulder abducted 90 degrees, elbow fully extended, distal forearm rests on examiner's shoulder
- Hand Position: Clasp both hands around middle of upper arm
- Maneuver: Apply an anterior and inferior force to upper arm
- Positive Test: Increased inferior translation of humeral head
- Indication: Anterior and/or inferior glenohumeral joint instability

Glenohumeral Glide Test

- Patient Position: Supine, shoulder off edge of table
- Hand Position: One hand over superior shoulder to stabilize scapula, other hand around proximal upper arm
- Maneuver: Anterior glide—apply anterior and distraction force to humeral head; posterior glide—apply posterior and distraction force humeral head; inferior glide—apply inferior and distraction force to humeral head
- Positive Test: Pain and/or increased translation of humeral head
- Indication: Anterior, posterior, and/or inferior glenohumeral joint instability

Clunk Test

- Patient Position: Supine
- Hand Position: One hand on posterior humeral head, other hand on distal humerus
- Maneuver: Passively abduct shoulder, apply anterior force to humeral head, externally rotate shoulder, rotate humeral head around within glenoid fossa
- Positive Test: Grinding and/or clunking sensation/sound
- Indication: Glenoid labrum tear

Active Compression (O'Brien) Test

- Patient Position: Sitting or standing; shoulder flexed 90 degrees, horizontally adducted 10 to 15 degrees, and internally rotated; forearm pronated; thumb facing floor; followed by shoulder external rotation with forearm supinated
- Hand Position: One hand at distal forearm, other hand at elbow or shoulder

- Maneuver: Actively flex and horizontally adduct shoulder, apply resistance to motion, repeat test with shoulder external rotated with forearm supinated
- Positive Test: Pain and/or clicking with shoulder internally rotated, but decreased or absent pain and/or clicking with shoulder externally rotated
- Indication: Glenoid labrum, including superior labral anterior posterior (SLAP) lesion

Adson (Maneuver) Test

- Patient Position: Sitting or standing, shoulder abducted 30 degrees, elbow extended, forearm supinated
- Hand Position: One hand at elbow or shoulder, other fingers palpate radial pulse
- Maneuver: Passively extend and externally rotate shoulder, actively extend and rotate neck toward ipsilateral side, take a deep breath and hold
- Positive Test: Weak or absent radial pulse
- Indication: Thoracic outlet syndrome

Allen Test

- Patient Position: Sitting or standing, shoulder abducted 90 degrees and externally rotated 90 degrees, elbow flexed 90 degrees
- Hand Position: One hand at elbow or shoulder, other fingers palpate radial pulse
- Maneuver: Actively rotates neck toward contralateral side
- Positive Test: Weak or absent radial pulse
- Indication: Thoracic outlet syndrome

> **Quick fact**
> Causes of thoracic outlet syndrome may include a tight pectoralis minor muscle, tight anterior/middle scalene muscles, and/or an accessory cervical rib.

Resistive Tennis Elbow (Cozen) Test

- Patient Position: Sitting, forearm neutral and supported on table, closed-fist hand
- Hand Position: One hand stabilizes elbow with thumb over lateral epicondyle, other hand over closed fist
- Maneuver: Actively pronate forearm, extend wrist, radially deviate wrist, apply resistance to motion
- Positive Test: Pain over lateral epicondyle and/or muscle weakness
- Indication: Lateral epicondylitis of elbow

Pinch Grip Test

- Patient Position: Sitting or standing
- Hand Position: None
- Maneuver: Actively pinch tip of index finger and thumb together
- Positive Test: Inability to pinch tips of index finger and thumb together
- Indication: Anterior interosseous nerve (median nerve branch) pathology

Valgus Stress Test of Elbow

- Patient Position: Sitting or standing, elbow flexed 25 degrees
- Hand Position: One hand at distal forearm, other hand over lateral elbow
- Maneuver: Apply valgus force at elbow
- Positive Test: Medial elbow pain and/or laxity
- Indication: Ulnar collateral ligament complex tear and/or epiphyseal plate injury

Varus Stress Test of Elbow

- Patient Position: Sitting, standing, elbow flexed 25 degrees
- Hand Position: One hand at distal forearm, other hand over medial elbow
- Maneuver: Apply varus force at elbow
- Positive Test: Lateral elbow pain and/or laxity
- Indication: Radial collateral ligament complex tear and/or epiphyseal plate injury

Finkelstein Test

- Patient Position: Sitting or standing, thumb inside closed-fist hand
- Hand Position: One hand holds distal forearm, other hand around fist
- Maneuver: Passively or actively ulnarly deviate wrist
- Positive Test: Pain over extensor pollicis brevis and abductor pollicis longus tendons
- Indication: Tenosynovitis of extensor pollicis brevis and abductor pollicis longus tendons

> **Quick fact**
> A positive Finkelstein test is indicative of de Quervain disease.

Phalen (Wrist Flexion) Test

- Patient Position: Sitting or standing, wrists fully flexed
- Hand Position: None
- Maneuver: Actively push dorsum of hands against each for 1 minute
- Positive Test: Radiating pain, numbness, and/or tingling of the palmar aspect of thumb, index finger, middle finger, and radial half of ring finger
- Indication: Carpal tunnel syndrome

> **Quick fact**
> Carpal tunnel syndrome is due to compression of the median nerve.

Murphy Sign

- Patient Position: Sitting or standing
- Hand Position: None
- Maneuver: Actively make a fist with hand
- Positive Test: Third metacarpal is at equal level with second and fourth metacarpals
- Indication: Lunate dislocation

Tap (Percussion) Test

- Patient Position: Sitting or standing, finger extended
- Hand Position: One hand supporting finger, other finger at tip of patient's finger
- Maneuver: Tap tip of finger
- Positive Test: Pain at injury site
- Indication: Phalanx fracture

Valgus Stress Test of the Wrist

- Patient Position: Sitting, elbow flexed 90 degrees, forearm pronated
- Hand Position: One hand stabilizes distal forearm, other hand stabilizes patient's hand
- Maneuver: Apply valgus force to wrist
- Positive Test: Ulnar wrist pain and/or laxity
- Indication: Wrist ulnar collateral ligament sprain

Varus Stress Test of the Wrist

- Patient Position: Sitting, elbow flexed 90 degrees, forearm pronated
- Hand Position: One hand stabilizes distal forearm, other hand stabilizes patient's hand
- Maneuver: Apply varus force to wrist
- Positive Test: Radial wrist pain and/or laxity
- Indication: Wrist radial collateral ligament sprain

Valgus Stress Test of the Fingers

- Patient Position: Sitting or standing, digit extended
- Hand Position: Fingers stabilize proximal phalanx, other fingers stabilize distal phalanx
- Maneuver: Apply valgus force to finger

- Positive Test: Ulnar aspect of finger pain and/or laxity
- Indication: Finger ulnar collateral ligament sprain

Varus Stress Test of the Fingers

- Patient Position: Sitting or standing, digit extended
- Hand Position: Fingers stabilize proximal phalanx, other fingers stabilize distal phalanx
- Maneuver: Apply varus force to finger
- Positive Test: Radial aspect of finger pain and/or laxity
- Indication: Finger radial collateral ligament sprain

Thumb Ulnar Collateral Ligament Test

- Patient Position: Sitting or standing, slightly abduct and extend thumb
- Hand Position: One thumb stabilizes lateral aspect of first metacarpal, other thumb stabilizes lateral aspect of first proximal phalanx
- Maneuver: Apply valgus force to MCP joint
- Positive Test: MCP joint pain and/or laxity
- Indication: Thumb ulnar collateral ligament sprain

> *Quick fact* Damage to the ulnar collateral ligament of the thumb is known as *gamekeeper's thumb*.

 Use the DVD or visit the website at http://thePoint .lww.com/Long for additional materials about *ligamentous and special tests of the upper extremity.*

P A R T 4 — Examination of the Lower Extremity

KEY TERMS

- Angle of retroversion
- Angle of torsion
- Antalgic gait
- Anteversion
- Coxa valga
- Coxa vara
- Cenu recurvatum
- Genu valgum
- Genu varum
- Hindfoot valgus
- Hindfoot varus
- Q-angle
- Retroversion
- Synovial membrane

PALPATIONS

Bony Palpations

See Table 4.13.

 Use the DVD or visit the website at http://thePoint .lww.com/Long for additional materials about *bony palpations of the lower extremity*.

> **Quick fact**
> Gerdy tubercle is the distal insertion point of the iliotibial band.

Table 4.13 Bony Palpations of the Lower Extremity

Pelvis, Hip, and Thigh	Knee	Lower Leg, Ankle, and Foot
Iliac crest	Medial femoral condyle	Tibial crest
Posterior superior iliac spine (PSIS)	Medial femoral epicondyle	Medial malleolus
Posterior inferior iliac spine (PIIS)	Adductor tubercle	Fibular head
Anterior superior iliac spine (ASIS)	Lateral femoral condyle	Fibular shaft
Anterior inferior iliac spine (AIIS)	Lateral femoral epicondyle	Lateral malleolus
Ischial tuberosity	Patellofemoral joint	Calcaneus
Greater trochanter of femur	Superior patellar pole	Sustentaculum tali
	Inferior patellar pole (apex)	Peroneal tubercle
	Medial tibiofemoral joint line	Medial calcaneal tubercle
	Medial tibial plateau	Talar dome
	Lateral tibiofemoral joint line	Talar head
	Lateral tibial plateau	Talar neck
	Medial tibial condyle	Medial talar tubercle
	Lateral tibial condyle	Sinus tarsi
	Gerdy tubercle	Navicular
	Tibial tuberosity	Navicular tuberosity
		Medial cuneiform
		Intermediate cuneiform
		Lateral cuneiform
		Cuboid
		First to fourth metatarsal bases
		Fifth metatarsal base (styloid process)
		First to fifth metatarsal shafts
		First to fifth metatarsal heads
		First to fifth MTP joints
		Proximal phalanx of great toe
		IP joint of great toe
		Distal phalanx of great toe
		Second to fifth phalanges
		Sesamoids of great toe

MTP, metatarsophalangeal joint; IP, interphalangeal.

> **Quick fact**
> The lateral collateral ligament of the knee can be more easily palpated by flexing the knee and resting the lower leg on top of the contralateral thigh.

Soft Tissue Palpation

See Table 4.14.

> **Quick fact**
> The calcaneonavicular (Spring) ligament is located between the sustentaculum tali and the navicular tubercle.

> **Quick fact**
> The extensor digitorum brevis muscle can be palpated just distal to the sinus tarsi of the ankle.

> **Quick fact**
> The deltoid ligament complex is composed of the anterior tibiotalar, tibionavicular, tibiocalcaneal, and posterior tibiotalar ligaments.

 Use the DVD or visit the website at http://thePoint .lww.com/Long for additional materials about soft tissue palpations of the lower extremity.

Goniometry

> **Quick fact**
> The angle of inclination (approximately 125 degrees) of the hip is viewed in the frontal plane and is slightly increased in women. Coxa valga is an increased angle of inclination and coxa vara is a decreased angle of inclination.

FLASH BOX ***Hip Flexion***
- Patient Position: Supine
- Fulcrum: Greater trochanter
- Movement Arm: Midline of femur (lateral epicondyle)
- Stationary Arm: Midline of pelvis
- Normal ROM: 100 to 120 degrees

FLASH BOX ***Hip Extension***
- Patient Position: Prone
- Fulcrum: Greater trochanter
- Movement Arm: Midline of femur (lateral epicondyle)
- Stationary Arm: Midline of pelvis
- Normal ROM: 20 to 30 degrees

> **Quick fact**
> Abnormal angles of inclination may result in genu valgum or genu varum of the knee.

Table 4.14 Soft Tissue Palpations of the Lower Extremity

Pelvis, Hip, and Thigh	Knee	Lower Leg, Ankle, and Foot
Inguinal ligament	Quadriceps tendon	Tibialis anterior
Femoral artery	Medial collateral	Tibialis anterior
Iliopsoas	ligament (MCL)	tendon
Pectineus	Medial meniscus	Extensor digitorum
Sartorius	Lateral collateral	longus
Adductor longus	ligament	Extensor digitorum
Adductor magnus	Lateral meniscus	longus tendons
Vastus medialis	Patellar tendon	Extensor hallucis
Vastus medialis	Biceps femoris tendon	longus
oblique	Semimembranosus	Extensor hallucis
Rectus femoris	tendon	longus tendon
Vastus lateralis	Semitendinosus tendon	Extensor digitorum
Gluteus medius	Pes anserine	brevis
Tensor fascia latae	Popliteal fossa	Superior extensor
Iliotibial band	Medial gastrocnemius	retinaculum
Trochanteric bursa	head	Inferior extensor
Gluteus maximus	Lateral gastrocnemius	retinaculum
Biceps femoris	head	Dorsalis pedis
Semimembranosus		artery
Semitendinosus		Common peroneal
Gracilis		nerve
		Peroneus longus
		Peroneus brevis
		Peroneus longus
		and brevis
		tendons
		Peroneus tertius
		tendon
		Superior peroneal
		retinaculum
		Inferior peroneal
		retinaculum
		Soleus
		Achilles tendon
		Subcutaneous
		calcaneal bursa
		Tibialis posterior
		tendon
		Posterior tibial
		artery
		Plantar fascia
		Anterior tibiofibular
		ligament
		Crural interosseus
		ligament
		Posterior tibiofibular
		ligament
		Anterior talofibular
		ligament (ATF)
		Calcaneofibular
		ligament (CF)
		Posterior talofibular
		ligament (PTF)
		Deltoid ligament
		complex
		Calcaneofibular
		("Spring") ligament
		Bifurcate ligament

❶ FLASH BOX Hip Internal Rotation
- Patient Position: Sitting
- Fulcrum: Anterior patella
- Movement Arm: Midline of lower leg (tibial crest)
- Stationary Arm: Perpendicular to floor
- Normal ROM: 40 to 45 degrees

❶ FLASH BOX Hip External Rotation
- Patient Position: Sitting
- Fulcrum: Anterior patella
- Movement Arm: Midline of lower leg (tibial crest)
- Stationary Arm: Perpendicular to floor
- Normal ROM: 45 to 50 degrees

> **Quick fact**
> Angle of torsion (angulation) of the hip is viewed in the transverse plane and is approximately 15 degrees. Anteversion (toes in appearance) represents an increased angle of torsion and retroversion (toes out appearance) represents a decreased angle of torsion.

Use the DVD or visit the website at http://thePoint.lww.com/Long for additional materials about *hip functional norms.*

❷ FLASH BOX Knee Flexion
- Patient Position: Supine
- Fulcrum: Lateral epicondyle of femur
- Movement Arm: Midline of fibula (fibular head)
- Stationary Arm: Midline of femur (greater trochanter)
- Normal ROM: 135 to 150 degrees

> **Quick fact**
> *Genu* is the Latin term for knee. Genu valgum is "knocked knee" and genu varum is "bow-legged", whereas genu recurvatum implies hyperextension at the knee joint.

❷ FLASH BOX Knee Extension
- Patient Position: Supine
- Fulcrum: Lateral epicondyle of femur
- Movement Arm: Midline of fibula (fibular head)
- Stationary Arm: Midline of femur (greater trochanter)
- Normal ROM: 0 to 10 degrees

Use the DVD or visit the website at http://thePoint.lww.com/Long for additional materials about *knee functional norms.*

❸ FLASH BOX Ankle Dorsiflexion
- Patient Position: Sitting
- Fulcrum: Lateral malleolus
- Movement Arm: Parallel to fifth metatarsal
- Stationary Arm: Midline of fibula (fibular head)
- Normal ROM: 20 degrees

Ankle Plantar Flexion
- Patient Position: Sitting
- Fulcrum: Lateral malleolus
- Movement Arm: Parallel to fifth metatarsal
- Stationary Arm: Midline of fibula (fibular head)
- Normal ROM: 40 to 50 degrees

 Use the DVD or visit the website at http://thePoint.lww.com/Long for additional materials about *ankle functional norms*.

Use the DVD or visit the website at http://thePoint.lww.com/Long for additional materials about *goniometry of the lower extremity*.

MANUAL MUSCLE TESTS OF THE LOWER EXTREMITY

Iliopsoas (Psoas Major and Iliacus)
- Patient Position: Supine, slight thigh abduction and external rotation, knee extended
- Stabilization: Contralateral iliac crest
- Patient Cue: "Lift leg toward ceiling"
- Force Direction: Distal lower leg—extension and slight abduction

Rectus Femoris, Vastus Intermedius, Vastus Medialis, and Vastus Lateralis
- Patient Position: Sitting
- Stabilization: Thigh
- Patient Cue: "Straighten knee"
- Force Direction: Distal lower leg—flexion

Sartorius
- Patient Position: Supine; hip externally rotated, abducted, and flexed
- Stabilization: None
- Patient Cue: "Rotate thigh outward, push thigh away from side, and pull thigh toward chest"
- Force Direction: Distal thigh—hip extension, adduction, and internal rotation; distal lower leg; knee—extension

Tensor Fascia Latae
- Patient Position: Supine
- Stabilization: None
- Patient Cue: "Rotate thigh inward, push thigh away from side, pull thigh toward chest"
- Force Direction: Lateral aspect of distal lower leg—extension and adduction

Gluteus Medius, Gluteus Minimus, and Tensor Fascia Latae
- Patient Position: Sitting
- Stabilization: Distal medial thigh

- Patient Cue: "Rotate upper thigh inward toward body"
- Force Direction: Lateral aspect of distal lower leg—external rotation

Piriformis, Obturator Internus/Externus, Gemellus Superior/Inferior, and Quadratus Femoris
- Patient Position: Sitting
- Stabilization: Distal lateral thigh
- Patient Cue: "Rotate upper thigh outward toward body"
- Force Direction: Medial aspect of distal lower leg—internal rotation

Gluteus Maximus
- Patient Position: Prone, knee flexed 90 degrees
- Stabilization: Pelvis
- Patient Cue: "Push thigh up toward ceiling"
- Force Direction: Distal posterior thigh—hip flexion

Biceps Femoris
- Patient Position: Prone, knee flexed 50 to 70 degrees, thigh and lower leg laterally rotated
- Stabilization: Thigh
- Patient Cue: "Pull lower leg toward buttocks"
- Force Direction: Distal lower leg—extension

Semitendinosus and Semimembranosus
- Patient Position: Prone, knee flexed 50 to 70 degrees, thigh and lower leg medially rotated
- Stabilization: Thigh
- Patient Cue: "Pull lower leg toward buttocks"
- Force Direction: Distal lower leg—extension

Pectineus, Gracilis, Adductor Magnus, Adductor Longus, and Adductor Brevis
- Patient Position: Sidelying
- Stabilization: Upper leg
- Patient Cue: "Pull bottom leg upward toward opposite leg"
- Force Direction: Medial aspect of distal thigh—abduction

Tibialis Anterior
- Patient Position: Sitting or supine
- Stabilization: Distal lower leg
- Patient Cue: "Pull foot upward and inward"
- Force Direction: Dorsal and medial aspect of foot—plantar flexion and eversion

Extensor Digitorum Longus and Brevis
- Patient Position: Sitting or supine, foot/ankle slightly plantar flexed
- Stabilization: Foot
- Patient Cue: "Straighten four lesser toes"
- Force Direction: Toes—flexion

Extensor Hallucis Longus and Brevis

- Patient Position: Sitting or supine, foot/ankle slightly plantar flexed
- Stabilization: Foot
- Patient Cue: "Straighten great toe"
- Force Direction: Distal and proximal phalanges of great toe—flexion

Peroneus Longus and Brevis

- Patient Position: Sitting or supine, leg internally rotated
- Stabilization: Distal lower leg
- Patient Cue: "Push foot down and outward"
- Force Direction: Plantar and lateral aspect of foot—inversion and dorsiflexion

Tibialis Posterior

- Patient Position: Supine, leg externally rotated
- Stabilization: Distal lower leg
- Patient Cue: "Push foot down and inward"
- Force Direction: Plantar and medial aspect of foot—dorsiflexion and eversion

Gastrocnemius and Plantaris

- Patient Position: Standing
- Stabilization: None
- Patient Cue: "Rise up on toes"
- Force Direction: Gravity—inferior

Soleus

- Patient Position: Prone, knees flexed 90 degrees
- Stabilization: Distal lower leg
- Patient Cue: "Push foot upward toward ceiling"
- Force Direction: Calcaneus—dorsiflexion

Flexor Digitorum Longus

- Patient Position: Sitting or supine, foot/ankle neutral
- Stabilization: Metatarsals
- Patient Cue: "Bend four lesser toes downward"
- Force Direction: Distal phalanges of four lesser toes—extension

Flexor Hallucis Longus

- Patient Position: Sitting or supine, foot/ankle neutral
- Stabilization: Metatarsophalangeal joints
- Patient Cue: "Bend middle joint of great toe downward"
- Force Direction: Distal phalanx of great toe—extension

Flexor Hallucis Brevis

- Patient Position: Sitting or supine, foot/ankle neutral
- Stabilization: Metatarsophalangeal joints
- Patient Cue: "Bend great toe downward"
- Force Direction: Proximal phalanx of great toe—extension

 Use the DVD or visit the website at http://thePoint .lww.com/Long for additional materials about *manual muscle tests of the lower extremity.*

LIGAMENTOUS AND SPECIAL TESTS OF THE LOWER EXTREMITY

Thomas Test

- Patient Position: Supine, hips and knees flexed to chest
- Hand Position: Hand under lumbar curve
- Maneuver: Actively lower hip into extension
- Positive Test: Limited hip extension and normal knee flexion, normal hip extension and limited knee flexion, limited hip extension and limited knee flexion, hip abduction and/or external rotation
- Indication: Limited hip extension and normal knee flexion indicates iliopsoas muscle tightness; normal hip extension and limited knee flexion indicates rectus femoris muscle tightness; limited hip extension and limited knee flexion indicates iliopsoas and rectus femoris muscle tightness; hip abduction and/or external rotation indicates iliotibial band tightness

> **Quick fact**
> There are a variety of methods in which the Thomas test can be performed. For example, starting with both knees bent over the end of the table and then flexing one knee to the chest.

Ely Test

- Patient Position: Prone
- Hand Position: One hand stabilizing pelvis, other hand at distal lower leg
- Maneuver: Passively flex knee
- Positive Test: Ipsilateral hip flexes when knee is passively flexed
- Indication: Rectus femoris muscle tightness

Ober Test

- Patient Position: Sidelying on uninvolved side, hips extended, knees extended
- Hand Position: One hand stabilizes hip/pelvis, other hand around lower leg
- Maneuver: Passively abduct and extends hip, allows leg to lower toward table
- Positive Test: Leg will not completely lower to table
- Indication: Tensor fascia latae/Iliotibial band tightness

Trendelenburg Test

- Patient Position: Single-leg stance
- Hand Position: None
- Maneuver: Maintain single-leg stance for 10 seconds, repeat maneuver with other leg
- Positive Test: Increased pelvic drop on side contralateral to standing leg
- Indication: Gluteus medius muscle weakness on standing leg

Piriformis Test

- Patient Position: Sidelying on uninvolved side, involved hip flexed 60 degrees, knee flexed
- Hand Position: One hand stabilizes hip/pelvis, other hand over lateral knee
- Maneuver: Apply downward force at lateral knee
- Positive Test: Buttock muscle tightness, buttock and/or posterior thigh pain
- Indication: Buttock muscle tightness indicates piriformis muscle tightness, buttock and/or posterior thigh pain indicates sciatic nerve pathology

> **Quick fact** Sciatic nerve pain that is elicited by the piriformis test indicates compression of the sciatic nerve due to a tight piriformis muscle.

90-90 Straight Leg Raise Test

- Patient Position: Supine, both hips flexed 90 degrees, knees flexed, hands behind knees for stabilization
- Hand Position: None
- Maneuver: Actively extend one knee, repeat maneuver with other knee
- Positive Test: Knee flexion greater than 20 degrees
- Indication: Hamstring muscle tightness

Noble Compression Test

- Patient Position: Supine, knee flexed
- Hand Position: Thumb over lateral femoral condyle, other hand around ankle
- Maneuver: Apply pressure over lateral femoral condyle, passively extend and flex knee
- Positive Test: Pain at lateral femoral condyle at approximately 30 degrees of knee flexion
- Indication: Iliotibial band friction syndrome

Patellar Grind Test

- Patient Position: Supine, knee extended
- Hand Position: Hand cupped above superior patella pole
- Maneuver: Apply downward and inferior pressure with hand, actively contract quadriceps muscles
- Positive Test: Pain, apprehension, or inability to complete test
- Indication: Chondromalacia patella

> **Quick fact** Pain and/or apprehension experienced with the patellar grind test is known as *Clarke sign*.

Patella Apprehension Test

- Patient Position: Supine, knee extended
- Hand Position: Both thumbs along medial patella
- Maneuver: Gently move patella in lateral direction
- Positive Test: Apprehension or muscle guarding of quadriceps
- Indication: Patellar dislocation or subluxation

Bounce Home Test

- Patient Position: Supine, knee extended
- Hand Position: One hand supports heel of foot, other hand's fingers over medial and lateral joint lines of the knee
- Maneuver: Passively flex knee, allow knee to drop into extension
- Positive Test: Lack of knee extension and/or "rubbery" end-feel
- Indication: Medial and/or lateral meniscus tear

McMurray Test

- Patient Position: Supine, knee flexed
- Hand Position: One hand holds heel of foot, other thumb and fingers palpate medial and lateral joint lines of tibiofemoral joint
- Maneuver: Externally rotate tibia and extend knee, internally rotate tibia and extend knee
- Positive Test: Joint line pain and/or clicking sound
- Indication: Medial and/or lateral meniscus tear

> **Quick fact** The Apley Compression Test is another method that can be used to assess for meniscal pathology.

Anterior Lachman Test

- Patient Position: Supine, knee flexed 20 to 30 degrees
- Hand Position: One hand holds distal lateral thigh, other hand holds proximal medial tibia
- Maneuver: Apply anterior force to tibia while stabilizing thigh
- Positive Test: Increased anterior translation of tibia
- Indication: Anterior cruciate ligament tear

Anterior Drawer Test

- Patient Position: Supine, hip flexed 45 degrees, knee flexed 90 degrees, tibia in neutral
- Hand Position: Both hands around proximal tibia, fingers palpating hamstring tendons, thumbs just inferior to joint lines, sitting on foot for stabilization
- Maneuver: Apply anterior force to proximal tibia
- Positive Test: Increased anterior translation of tibia
- Indication: Anterior cruciate ligament tear

> **Quick fact** Palpation of the hamstring tendons during the anterior drawer test helps to insure that the hamstring muscles are relaxed, thereby decreasing the chance of a false-negative test.

Slocum Anteromedial Rotary Instability Test

- Patient Position: Supine, hip flexed 45 degrees, knee flexed 90 degrees, tibia externally rotated 15 degrees
- Hand Position: Both hands around proximal tibia, fingers palpating hamstring tendons, thumbs just inferior to joint lines, sitting on foot for stabilization
- Maneuver: Apply anterior force to proximal tibia
- Positive Test: Increased anterior translation of medial tibia
- Indication: Anteromedial rotary instability from anterior cruciate ligament, posterior oblique ligament, medial collateral ligament, and/or posteromedial capsule

Slocum Anterolateral Rotary Instability Test

- Patient Position: Supine, hip flexed 45 degrees, knee flexed 90 degrees, tibia internally rotated 30 degrees
- Hand Position: Both hands around proximal tibia, fingers palpating hamstring tendons, thumbs just inferior to joint lines, sitting on foot for stabilization
- Maneuver: Apply anterior force to proximal tibia
- Positive Test: Increased anterior translation of lateral tibia
- Indication: Anterolateral rotary instability from anterior cruciate ligament, arcuate ligament complex, lateral collateral ligament, posterolateral capsule, and/or iliotibial band damage

Lateral Pivot Shift Test

- Patient Position: Supine, hip flexed 30 degrees, abducted 30 degrees, and internally rotated 20 degrees
- Hand Position: One hand holding foot, other hand at the proximal fibula
- Maneuver: Flex knee while applying valgus force to lateral knee, maintain internal rotation
- Positive Test: Backward reduction of tibia
- Indication: Anterolateral rotary instability from anterior cruciate ligament, arcuate ligament complex, lateral collateral ligament, and/or posterolateral capsule damage

> **Quick fact** The pivot shift test is also known as the *MacIntosh test*.

Posterior Drawer Test

- Patient Position: Supine; hip flexed 45 degrees, knee flexed 90 degrees, tibia in neutral
- Hand Position: Both hands around proximal tibia, fingers palpating hamstring tendons, thumbs just inferior to joint lines, sitting on foot for stabilization
- Maneuver: Apply posterior force to proximal tibia
- Positive Test: Increased posterior translation of tibia
- Indication: Posterior cruciate ligament tear

Godfrey 90-90 Test

- Patient Position: Supine, both hips flexed 90 degrees, both knees flexed 90 degrees
- Hand Position: One arm under both the distal lower legs

- Maneuver: Maintain hips and knees in position, observe tibial tuberosities
- Positive Test: Posterior displacement of tibia
- Indication: Posterior cruciate ligament tear

Posterior Sag (Gravity Drawer) Test

- Patient Position: Supine, hip flexed 45 degrees, knee flexed 90 degrees
- Hand Position: None
- Maneuver: Actively contract quadriceps muscles
- Positive Test: Posterior displacement of tibia
- Indication: Posterior cruciate ligament tear

Valgus Stress Test

- Patient Position: Supine; knee extended 0 degrees; followed by knee flexed 20 to 30 degrees
- Hand Position: One hand on medial lower leg, other hand over lateral knee
- Maneuver: Apply valgus force to knee with knee extended 0 degrees, apply valgus force to knee with knee flexed 20 to 30 degrees
- Positive Test: Medial knee pain and/or laxity at 0 degree extension, medial knee pain and/or laxity at 20 to 30 degrees flexion
- Indication: Medial knee pain and/or laxity at 0 degree extension indicates medial collateral ligament, anterior/posterior cruciate ligament, and/or posteromedial joint capsule tear; medial knee pain and/or laxity at 20 to 30 degrees flexion indicates medial collateral ligament tear

Varus Stress Test

- Patient Position: Supine; knee extended 0 degrees; followed by knee flexed 20 to 30 degrees
- Hand Position: One hand on lateral lower leg, other hand over medial knee
- Maneuver: Apply varus force to knee with knee extended 0 degrees, apply varus force to knee with knee flexed 20 to 30 degrees
- Positive Test: Lateral knee pain and/or laxity at 0 degree extension, lateral knee pain and/or laxity at 20 to 30 degrees flexion
- Indication: Lateral knee pain and/or laxity at 0 degree extension indicates lateral collateral ligament, anterior/posterior cruciate ligament, and/or posterolateral joint capsule tear; lateral knee pain and/or laxity at 20 to 30 degrees flexion indicates lateral collateral ligament tear

Anterior Drawer Test for the Ankle

- Patient Position: Sitting, foot plantar flexed 20 degrees
- Hand Position: One hand around and stabilizing distal tibia and fibula, other hand beneath calcaneus, forearm supports plantar aspect of foot
- Maneuver: Apply anterior force to the calcaneus and talus
- Positive Test: Pain, laxity, and/or "clunking" sensation
- Indication: Anterior talofibular ligament sprain

Care should be taken when performing the anterior drawer test for the ankle because of the possibility of dislocating the talus on an ankle with severe instability.

Inversion Stress (Talar Tilt) Test

- Patient Position: Sitting, supine, or sidelying; ankle in neutral
- Hand Position: One hand around distal tibia and fibula for stabilization, other hand around calcaneus with thumb on calcaneofibular ligament
- Maneuver: Apply inversion stress to ankle
- Positive Test: Pain and/or laxity
- Indication: Calcaneofibular ligament sprain

Eversion Stress (Talar Tilt) Test

- Patient Position: Sitting, supine, or sidelying; ankle in neutral
- Hand Position: One hand around distal tibia and fibula for stabilization, other hand around calcaneus with thumb on deltoid ligament complex
- Maneuver: Apply eversion stress to ankle
- Positive Test: Pain and/or laxity
- Indication: Deltoid ligament complex sprain

Kleiger Test (External Rotation Test)

- Patient Position: Sitting
- Hand Position: One hand around distal tibia and fibula for stabilization, other hand around calcaneus and supporting plantar aspect of foot
- Maneuver: Passively externally rotate foot in neutral position, passively externally rotate foot in full ankle dorsiflexion
- Positive Test: Foot in neutral—medial joint pain and/or talar translation away from medial malleolus; foot in full dorsiflexion—distal tibiofibular syndesmosis complex pain
- Indication: Foot in neutral—deltoid ligament complex sprain; foot in full dorsiflexion—distal tibiofibular syndesmosis complex sprain

Quick fact An individual with a distal tibiofibular syndesmosis complex sprain will experience pain with weight bearing as the talus is forced into the ankle mortise, resulting in a spreading of the tibia and fibula.

Homan Sign

- Patient Position: Sitting or supine, knee extended
- Hand Position: One hand on plantar aspect of foot, other hand under posterior calf
- Maneuver: Passively dorsiflex foot, squeeze calf muscle

- Positive Test: Calf pain
- Indication: Deep vein thrombophlebitis (DVT)

Quick fact The presence of a DVT is a medical emergency because a thrombus can potentially break free from the vascular wall and result in a pulmonary embolism.

Thompson Test

- Patient Position: Prone, feet hanging off table
- Hand Position: One hand on calf muscle
- Maneuver: Squeeze calf muscle
- Positive Test: Absence of foot plantar flexion
- Indication: Achilles tendon rupture

Percussion (Bump) Test

- Patient Position: Supine or sitting, knee extended, ankle/foot off table
- Hand Position: One hand grasps forefoot, palm of other hand at heel
- Maneuver: Passively dorsiflex ankle fully, apply firm bump to plantar aspect of heel, use progressively more force as symptoms allow
- Positive Test: Pain at injury site
- Indication: Calcaneus, talus, tibia, or fibular fracture

Squeeze (Compression) Test

- Patient Position: Supine, knee extended, ankle/foot off table
- Hand Position: One hand on medial tibia, other hand on lateral fibula, both hands away from injury site
- Maneuver: Squeeze tibia and fibula together, gradually increase pressure as symptoms allow, move hand toward injury site
- Positive Test: Pain at injury site
- Indication: Tibia and/or fibula fracture, distal tibiofibular syndesmosis sprain

Long Bone Compression Test

- Patient Position: Sitting, knee extended
- Hand Position: Thumb over dorsal aspect of metatarsal or phalanx, finger over plantar aspect of same metatarsal or phalanx
- Maneuver: Apply compression force on long axis of bone
- Positive Test: Pain at injury site and/or false joint movement
- Indication: Metatarsal or phalanx fracture

 Use the DVD or visit the website at http://thePoint.lww.com/Long for additional materials about *manual muscle tests of the lower extremity.*

1. Which of the following contribute to glenohumeral joint instability?
   a. Labral pathology
   b. Capsular instability
   c. Muscular weakness
   d. Ligamentous pathology
   e. All of the above

2. Which of the following rotator cuff muscles is an internal rotator?
   a. Subscapularis
   b. Infraspinatus
   c. Supraspinatus
   d. Teres minor
   e. All of the above

3. Which of the following special tests is the best one to use to identify a SLAP lesion?
   a. The Gerber lift off test
   b. The Grind test
   c. The O'Brien test
   d. The Clunk test
   e. The Feagin test

4. The military brace position assesses which of the following structures?
   a. Supraspinatus tendon
   b. Subclavian artery
   c. Long thoracic nerve
   d. Subdeltoid bursa
   e. None of the above

5. What is the normal range of motion for shoulder complex internal rotation?
   a. 120 degrees
   b. 90 degrees
   c. 60 degrees
   d. 45 degrees
   e. 20 degrees

6. Which of the following is *true* regarding a type III acromioclavicular joint sprain?
   a. Rupture of acromioclavicular and coracoclavicular ligaments
   b. Tearing of acromioclavicular ligament
   c. Tearing of only the coracoclaviclar ligaments

   d. Rupture of the coracoclaviclar ligaments
   e. None of the above

7. Which of the following terms best describes a defect of the posterior humeral head's articular cartilage?
   a. SLAP lesion
   b. Hill-Sachs lesion
   c. Bankart lesion
   d. Little leaguer shoulder
   e. Reverse SLAP lesion

8. Which of the following most accurately determines the severity of glenohumeral joint instability?
   a. The amount of displacement of the humeral head in relationship to the glenoid fossa
   b. The range of motion of the glenohumeral joint
   c. The amount of labral pain associated with performing a clunk test
   d. The amount of measurable strength of the rotator cuff muscle complex
   e. None of the above

9. A subluxating long head of the biceps tendon could indicate damage to which of the following?
   a. Transverse humeral ligament
   b. Inferior glenohumeral ligament
   c. Coracoclavicular ligament
   d. Sternoclavicular ligament
   e. Superior glenohumeral ligament

10. The drop arm test is performed to assess for what type of pathology?
    a. Cervical nerve root compression
    b. Tight pectoralis major muscle
    c. Rotator cuff tear
    d. Brachial plexus damage
    e. Weak serratus anterior

11. Upon evaluation of an athlete you determine that he or she has unilateral scapular winging. This is an indication of weakness of which of the following muscles?
    a. Teres minor
    b. Subscapularis
    c. Upper trapezius

d. Serratus anterior
e. None of the above

12. A positive piano key sign is indicative of what type of injury?
a. Glenoid labrum tear
b. Scapular fracture
c. Inferior glenohumeral instability
d. Humeral fracture
e. Acromioclavicular joint injury

13. Which of the following is *true* regarding rotator cuff tendinitis?
a. One of the commonly involved structures is the subscapularis tendon
b. It does not heal well because of the relatively poor vascularization of the tendons
c. The injury is typical due to a single acute rotary force of the shoulder
d. Pain commonly refers down the side of the thorax
e. All of the above

14. Which of the following tests would decrease the symptoms that were produced by the shoulder anterior apprehension test?
a. Posterior apprehension test
b. Active compression test
c. Shoulder abduction test
d. Jobe relocation test
e. Speed test

15. Which of the following is a test that assesses for inferior glenohumeral instability?
a. Feagin test
b. Allen test
c. Posterior apprehension test
d. AC joint compression test
e. Roo test

16. Which of the following ligaments is referred to as the *arch* ligament of the shoulder?
a. Coracoclavicular ligament
b. Acromioclavicular ligament
c. Conoid ligament
d. Trapezoid ligament
e. Coracoacromial ligament

17. What is a positive sign when performing the Gerber lift-off test?
a. Inability to lift the hand off the lumbar spine
b. Significant weakness when attempting to lift the arm away from the side
c. Inability to slowly lower the arm
d. Significant weakness when performing active forward flexion against resistance
e. Pain when actively abducting the arm from the side against resistance

18. The empty can test assesses for what type of pathology?
a. Subdeltoid bursitis
b. Short head of the biceps tear
c. Acromioclavicular ligament tear
d. Glenoid labrum tear
e. Supraspinatus muscle weakness

19. Which of the following best describes a type III acromion shape?
a. Irregular shaped
b. "Beak" shaped
c. Curved shape
d. Round shaped
e. None of the above

20. Tingling and/or numbness over the deltoid region of the shoulder would indicate damage to what spinal nerve root?
a. C3
b. C4
c. C5
d. C6
e. C7

21. Which of the following best defines Sprengel deformity?
a. A posteriorly dislocated sternoclavicular joint
b. Atrophy of the deltoid muscle
c. A congenitally undescended scapula
d. Atrophy of the upper trapezius muscle
e. An exostosis at the acromioclavicular joint

22. A positive clunk test is indicative of what type of shoulder pathology?
a. Long head of the biceps tendinitis
b. Glenoid labrum tear
c. Thoracic outlet syndrome
d. Impingement syndrome
e. Long thoracic nerve damage

23. The brachial artery is a continuation of what artery?
a. Axillary
b. Internal carotid
c. Subclavian
d. Sternocleidomastoid
e. External carotid

24. Which of the following tests can be used to determine range of motion deficits in shoulder internal external rotation?
a. Grind test
b. AC joint sheer test
c. Yergason test
d. Posterior drawer test
e. Apley scratch test

25. At what age does the medial epiphysis of the clavicle completely fuse?
    a. 10 years
    b. 15 years
    c. 20 years
    d. 25 years
    e. 30 years

26. Which of the following is the most common type of sternoclavicular dislocation?
    a. Posterior
    b. Anterior
    c. Inferior
    d. Superior
    e. None of the above

27. Which of the following tests can be used to determine a posterior glenohumeral dislocation?
    a. Anterior apprehension test
    b. Hawkins-Kennedy test
    c. Feagin test
    d. Lippman test
    e. None of the above

28. What structures can be involved with shoulder impingement syndrome?
    a. Glenohumeral joint capsule
    b. Humeral head
    c. Supraspinatus tendon
    d. Long head of the biceps brachii
    e. All of the above

29. What muscle is primarily responsible for eccentrically contracting in order to decelerate the arm during the follow-through phase of the throwing motion?
    a. Teres major
    b. Supraspinatus
    c. Infraspinatus
    d. Biceps brachii
    e. Latissimus dorsi

30. What is a positive sign when performing the Ludington test?
    a. Excessive posterior translation of the humeral head
    b. Clunking sensation when externally rotating the humerus
    c. Diminished radial pulse
    d. Changes in sensory and/or motor function in the involved extremity
    e. Decreased tension of the long head of the biceps tendon

31. What muscle is primarily involved with "tennis elbow?"
    a. Extensor digiti minimi
    b. Extensor carpi ulnaris
    c. Extensor carpi radialis longus

    d. Extensor digitorum
    e. Extensor carpi radialis brevis

32. What is the normal carrying angle of the elbow for females?
    a. 0 to 5 degrees
    b. 5 to 10 degrees
    c. 10 to 15 degrees
    d. 15 to 20 degrees
    e. 20 to 25 degrees

33. Which of the following muscles are located across the distal interosseus space between the radius and the ulna?
    a. Dorsal interossei
    b. Extensor carpi radialis longus
    c. Flexor carpi ulnaris
    d. Pronator quadratus
    e. Brachialis

34. The pinch grip test assesses for damage to which of the following nerves?
    a. Median nerve
    b. Ulnar nerve
    c. Musculocutaneous nerve
    d. Deep radial nerve
    e. Anterior interosseus nerve

35. What is the term for a growth plate injury to the medial humerus in an adolescent?
    a. Bennett fracture
    b. Little league elbow
    c. Nightstick fracture
    d. Tennis elbow
    e. Golfer's elbow

36. A positive valgus stress test at 25 degrees of elbow flexion would be indicative of what injury?
    a. Ulnar collateral ligament sprain
    b. Anconeus strain
    c. Annular ligament sprain
    d. Radial head subluxation
    e. Radial collateral ligament sprain

37. How would you best describe the Monteggia fracture?
    a. Proximal ulna fracture and radial head dislocation
    b. Distal ulna fracture and radial head dislocation
    c. Distal radius fracture and radial head dislocation
    d. Proximal radius fracture and radial head dislocation
    e. None of the above

38. Which of the following tests assesses for medial epicondylitis of the elbow?
    a. Passive elbow extension test
    b. Resistive tennis elbow test
    c. The Cozen test
    d. Golfer's elbow test
    e. Hyperextension test

39. The radial artery is a branch of which of the following blood vessels?
    a. Brachial artery
    b. Ulnar artery
    c. Axillary artery
    d. Subclavian artery
    e. Carotid artery

40. What test would assess for cubital tunnel syndrome?
    a. The hyperextension test
    b. The elbow flexion test
    c. The pinch grip test
    d. The Cozen test
    e. The Brachioradialis test

41. Trauma to the radial nerve of the elbow and forearm can result in which of the following?
    a. Bishop deformity
    b. Volkmann ischemic contracture
    c. Wrist drop
    d. Claw hand
    e. Dupuytren contracture

42. Which of the following would be a positive sign for chronic elbow instability when performing the posterolateral rotary instability test?
    a. The elbow subluxates when extended and relocates when flexed
    b. The elbow subluxates when flexed and relocates when extended
    c. The elbow subluxates when applying a varus force
    d. The elbow subluxates when applying a varus force
    e. None of the above

43. The pronator teres syndrome test evaluates for compression of which of the following nerves?
    a. Radial nerve
    b. Axillary nerve
    c. Musculocutaneous nerve
    d. Median nerve
    e. Ulnar nerve

44. Which of the following is *true* regarding the cubital fossa?
    a. Its medial border is formed by the brachioradialis muscle
    b. Its superior border is formed by the pronator quadratus muscle
    c. Its lateral border is formed by the flexor carpi ulnaris muscle
    d. The axillary artery passes through this area
    e. None of the above

45. What type of mechanism most often causes injuries at the elbow region?
    a. Falling on the outstretched hand
    b. Repetitive, low-load stresses
    c. Forceful, direct blows

    d. Single, high tensile forces
    e. Acute, varus forces

46. Radiocapitellar chondromalacia will most likely result in symptoms in what region of the elbow?
    a. Posterior
    b. Medial
    c. Lateral
    d. Anterior
    e. All of the above

47. What type of pathology may be mistaken for radial tunnel syndrome?
    a. Distal biceps tendinitis
    b. Flexor carpi ulnaris tendinitis
    c. Ulnar collateral ligament sprain
    d. Medial epicondylitis
    e. Lateral epicondylitis

48. What type of nerve pathology could potentially accompany a UCL sprain of the elbow?
    a. Brachial
    b. Subclavian
    c. Axillary
    d. Ulnar
    e. Radial

49. In which of the following groups does Panner disease develop?
    a. Children younger than 10 years
    b. Children older than 15 years
    c. Adult males younger than 25 years
    d. Adult males older than 25 years
    e. Females older than 10 years

50. What is a positive sign when performing Cozen test?
    a. Tingling and/or numbness along the lateral aspect of the forearm
    b. Increased laxity of the radial collateral ligament complex
    c. Pain at the lateral epicondyle of the elbow
    d. Grinding sensation at the humeroulnar joint
    e. Weakness of the flexor digitorum superficialis

51. What test would you perform to rule out carpal tunnel syndrome?
    a. The Froment test
    b. The Phalen test
    c. The Finkelstein test
    d. The long finger flexor test
    e. The Wrinkle test

52. The Watson test assesses for a subluxation of what carpal bone?
    a. Scaphoid
    b. Trapezium
    c. Lunate
    d. Triquetrum
    e. Capitate

53. Mallet finger is a rupture of the extensor tendon at what joint?
    a. Metacarpophalangeal joint
    b. Distal interphalangeal joint
    c. Proximal interphalangeal joint
    d. Interphalangeal joint
    e. Carpometacarpal joint

54. The absence of the hand's palmar crease is indicative of which of the following conditions?
    a. Fracture
    b. Swelling
    c. Nerve injury
    d. Vascular deficiency
    e. Ligament damage

55. Which of the following tendons forms the anatomical "snuffbox"?
    a. Adductor pollicis longus, flexor carpi ulnaris, and extensor pollicis longus
    b. Adductor pollicis longus, extensor pollicis brevis, and extensor pollicis longus
    c. Abductor pollicis longus, extensor pollicis brevis, and opponens pollicis
    d. Abductor pollicis longus, extensor pollicis brevis, and extensor pollicis longus
    e. Abductor pollicis longus, flexor carpi ulnaris, and extensor pollicis longus

56. What is Kienbock disease?
    a. An avascular necrosis of the lunate bone
    b. A scaphoid fracture that involves its distal pole
    c. A degeneration of the triangular fibrocartilage
    d. A tenosynovitis condition of the extensor pollicis longus
    e. A degeneration of the ulnar nerve in the hand

57. Which of the following is *true* regarding the pathological hand/finger posture known as *Benediction deformity*?
    a. It is due to radial nerve damage
    b. It causes a hyperextension deformity of the interphalangeal joints
    c. The ability to oppose the thumb is lost
    d. It is also known as *Dupuytren contracture*
    e. The deformity is more pronounced in the fourth and fifth digits

58. Guyon canal is located between what two structures?
    a. The trapezoid and trapezium
    b. The scaphoid and the lunate
    c. The pisiform and hook of the hamate
    d. The scaphoid tuberosity and the capitate
    e. The triquetrum and the lunate

59. What is the indication of a positive test when assessing for Murphy sign of the hand?
    a. The presence of a divot over the lunate when the hand is in a neutral position

b. Pain when passively deviating the wrist in an ulnar direction
    c. Tingling and/or numbness of the fifth digit and ulnar half of the fourth digit
    d. The inability to oppose the thumb toward the hypothenar eminence
    e. The third metacarpal is at equal level with second and fourth metacarpals

60. Pathology of which of following structures would result in the deformity known as *ape hand*?
    a. Palmar fascia
    b. Ulnar nerve
    c. Median nerve
    d. Radial nerve
    e. Central slip of extensor tendon mechanism

61. A rupture of the flexor digitorum profundus tendon is termed which of the following?
    a. Mallet finger
    b. Swan neck finger
    c. Baseball finger
    d. Trigger finger
    e. Jersey finger

62. Which of the following would indicate capsular tightness of the proximal interphalangeal (PIP) joint when performing the Bunnel Littler test?
    a. Inability to flex DIP joint with PIP joint extended
    b. Inability to flex DIP joint with PIP joint flexed
    c. Inability to flex PIP joint with MCP joint extended
    d. Inability to flex PIP joint with MCP joint flexed
    e. None of the above

63. Which of the following would be indicative of median nerve pathology?
    a. Numbness over the volar aspect of the index finger
    b. Numbness over the volar aspect of the pinky
    c. Numbness over the dorsal aspect of the middle finger at the PIP joint
    d. Numbness over the dorsal aspect of the index finger at the MCP joint
    e. Numbness over the dorsal aspect of the hand

64. What test can be used to assess for de Quervain tenosynovitis?
    a. The digital Allen test
    b. The wrinkle test
    c. The Tinel test
    d. The Finkelstein test
    e. The long finger flexor test

65. Damage to the triangular fibrocartilage complex can also result in an avulsion fracture of what structure?
    a. Radial styloid process
    b. Ulnar styloid process
    c. Scaphoid bone
    d. Lunate bone
    e. Lister tubercle

66. What is the mechanism of injury for gamekeeper's thumb?
    a. Forceful thumb flexion
    b. Forceful thumb extension
    c. Forceful thumb adduction
    d. Forceful thumb abduction
    e. None of the above

67. Which of the following structures are involved in Preiser disease?
    a. Volar plate of the PIP joint
    b. Median nerve
    c. Extensor pollicis brevis tendon
    d. Lunate bone
    e. None of the above

68. Bennett fracture involves which of the following structures?
    a. Radius
    b. Thumb
    c. Ulna
    d. Lunate
    e. Ring finger

69. Which of the following is a positive sign when assessing for Froment sign?
    a. Extension of the DIP joint of the index finger
    b. Extension of the PIP joint of the index finger
    c. Flexion of the IP joint of the thumb
    d. Flexion of the DIP joint of the ring finger
    e. Abduction of the MCP joint of the thumb

70. Which of the following is a positive sign for trigger finger?
    a. Finger becomes locked in flexion
    b. Inability to extend the DIP joint of finger
    c. Weakness of the opponens pollicis muscle
    d. Inability to flex the MCP joint of finger when wrist is flexed
    e. None of the above

71. When performing a manual muscle test for the biceps femoris you determine that the athlete cannot perform the test against manual resistance, but he or she is able to move it through the full range of motion against gravity. What type of numerical grade would you give this muscle?
    a. 1
    b. 2
    c. 3
    d. 4
    e. 5

72. Extension of the metacarpophalangeal joints of the fingers is an example of what type of end-feel?
    a. Pathological hard end-feel
    b. Physiological firm end-feel
    c. Physiological hard end-feel
    d. Physiological soft end-feel
    e. Pathological hard end-feel

73. Which of the following movements occur in the sagittal plane of motion?
    a. Shoulder abduction
    b. Cervical lateral flexion
    c. Ankle dorsiflexion
    d. Trunk rotation
    e. Forearm pronation

74. A football player had his neck laterally flexed forcefully in combination with depression of his shoulder when being tackled during a game, which resulted in a brachial plexus injury. Which of the following types of forces best describes the mechanism of injury?
    a. Tensile force
    b. Shearing force
    c. Compressive force
    d. Axial force
    e. None of the above

75. Which of the following bones make up the subtalar joint?
    a. Talus and tibia
    b. Fibula and tibia
    c. Calcaneus and tibia
    d. Fibula and talus
    e. Calcaneus and talus

76. Which of the following muscles is responsible for ankle dorsiflexion and inversion?
    a. Peroneus tertius
    b. Peroneus brevis
    c. Anterior tibialis
    d. Posterior tibialis
    e. Flexor digitorum brevis

77. The spring ligament of the foot is also known as which of the following?
    a. Posterior tibiotalar ligament
    b. Bifurcate ligament
    c. Calcaneonavicular ligament
    d. Posterior talofibular ligament
    e. Anterior tibiofibular ligament

78. Numbness over the dorsum of the great toe could be an indicator of damage to which of the following spinal nerve roots?
    a. L3
    b. L4
    c. L5
    d. S1
    e. S2

79. Which of the following tests can assess the integrity of the anterior talofibular ligament?
    a. The anterior drawer test
    b. The talar tilt inversion stress test

c. The Kleiger test
d. The Intermetatarsal glide test
e. The side-to-side test

80. What does the Fairbank apprehension test **assess** for?
    a. Patella plica syndrome
    b. Chondromalacia patella
    c. Patella subluxation
    d. Iliotibial band friction syndrome
    e. Pes anserine bursitis

81. The Lachman test for the knee assesses for which of the following types of instabilities?
    a. Straight posterior instability
    b. Straight anterior instability
    c. Valgus instability
    d. Varus instability
    e. Multidirectional instability

82. What does the patella tendon length test assess for?
    a. The presence of patella alta or patella baja
    b. To what degree the Q-angle is affecting the function of the patellofemoral joint
    c. The severity of Osgood-Schlatter disease
    d. The severity of chondromalacia patella
    e. A patella retinaculum tear

83. A deterioration of the articular cartilage of the patella is termed which of the following?
    a. Patellofemoral stress syndrome
    b. Chondromalacia patella
    c. Nonunion apophysitis
    d. Osteochondral fracture
    e. Myositis ossificans

84. Which of the following can be used to test for iliopsoas muscle tightness?
    a. The Bowstring test
    b. The bilateral straight leg raise test
    c. The unilateral straight leg raise test
    d. The Thomas test
    e. The Ober test

85. Which of the following bones make up the innominate bone?
    a. Ischium, ilium, and sacrum
    b. Pubis, coccyx, and sacrum
    c. Coccyx, ischium, and sacrum
    d. Sacrum, ilium, and coccyx
    e. Ischium, ilium, and pubis

86. The angle of torsion can be viewed on which of the following planes of motion?
    a. Transverse
    b. Oblique
    c. Frontal
    d. Sagittal
    e. Coronal

87. Which of the following muscles internally rotate the hip?
    a. Piriformis
    b. Obturator internus
    c. Gluteus minimus
    d. Gemellus inferior
    e. Quadratus femoris

88. What does the Gaenslen test access for?
    a. Piriformis syndrome
    b. Hamstring tightness
    c. Sacroiliac joint dysfunction
    d. Gastrocnemius tightness
    e. Lumbar disc pathology

89. Which of the following special tests is used to determine cervical nerve root compression?
    a. The Chvostek test
    b. The Spurling test
    c. The palpation test
    d. The loading test
    e. The swallowing test

90. Upon evaluation you find that the patient has unilateral weakness with elbow flexion and wrist extension. On the basis of this finding, which of the following cervical nerve roots could potentially be involved?
    a. C6
    b. C7
    c. C4
    d. C8
    e. C5

91. Which of the following special tests is utilized in an attempt to relieve the symptoms of a cervical nerve root impingement?
    a. The cervical compression test
    b. The Spurling test
    c. The Valsalva test
    d. The loading test
    e. The shoulder abduction test

92. Which of the following special tests would be the best to perform to rule out an upper motor neuron lesion?
    a. The Babinski test
    b. The Romberg test
    c. The stork standing test
    d. The tandem walking test
    e. The Chvostek test

93. Concentration is assessed, during the standardized assessment of concussion (SAC) tool, by doing which of the following?
    a. Repeating five words at the end of the test that were given at beginning of the test by the examiner
    b. Performing the Romberg test for the examiner
    c. Repeating multiple strings of digits to the examiner in reverse order

d. Providing the month, date, day of the weak, year, and time to the examiner

e. Repeating five words provided by the examiner in three successive trials

94. Which of the following tests would be the most difficult to perform on the sidelines, during an athletic event, if you needed to assess an athlete for a concussion?

a. The standard assessment of concussion test

b. The tandem walk test

c. The Romberg test

d. The balance error scoring system

e. The pupillary reaction test

95. The tongue blade test is used to assess for what type of injury?

a. Zygoma fracture

b. Mandible fracture

c. TMJ subluxation

d. Laryngospasm

e. Tooth fracture

96. The Weber test is used to help assess for which of the following types of conditions?

a. Nasal fracture

b. Epidural hematoma

c. Hyphema

d. TMJ dysfunction

e. Otitis media

97. An athlete reports to you that he or she has been seeing "floaters" and are gradually losing the field of vision. Which of the following types of injuries is most likely the cause of the symptoms?

a. Traumatic iritis

b. Detached retina

c. Intracranial injury

d. Corneal laceration

e. None of the above

98. What is the medical term for a posterior displacement of the eyes?

a. Hyphema

b. Presbyopia

c. Enophthalmos

d. Exophthalmos

e. Nystagmus

99. At what location can the McBurney point be palpated?

a. One third of the way between the ASIS and the umbilicus

b. Upper left quadrant just below the ribcage

c. Between the left shoulder and the manubrium

d. Lower left quadrant just above the inguinal area

e. None of the above

100. Which of the following structures can be palpated in the left upper quadrant when enlarged?

a. Liver

b. Spleen

c. Colon

d. Appendix

e. Urinary bladder

Use the DVD or visit the website at http://thePoint.lww.com/Long to take the online examination.

✓ STUDY CHECKLIST

- ☐ Clinical Examination Process
- ☐ Documentation Procedures
- ☐ Palpations for the Head, Neck, Spine, and Thorax
- ☐ Goniometry for the Head, Neck, Spine, and Thorax
- ☐ Manual Muscle Testing for the Head, Neck, Spine, and Thorax
- ☐ Ligamentous and Special Tests for the Head, Neck, Spine, and Thorax

- ☐ Palpations for the Upper Extremity
- ☐ Goniometry for the Upper Extremity
- ☐ Manual Muscle Testing for the Upper Extremity
- ☐ Ligamentous and Special Tests for the Upper Extremity
- ☐ Palpations for the Lower Extremity
- ☐ Goniometry for the Lower Extremity
- ☐ Manual Muscle Testing for the Lower Extremity
- ☐ Ligamentous and Special Tests for the Lower Extremity

SECTION 4

SUPPLEMENTAL READING

1. Anderson MK, Parr GP, Hall SJ. *Foundations of athletic training: prevention, assessment, and management,* 4th ed. Philadelphia: Lippincott Williams & Wilkins; 2009.

2. Bahr R, Machlum S. *Clinical guide to sports injuries: an illustrated guide to the management of injuries in physical activity.* Champaign: Human Kinetics; 2004.

3. Bernier J. *Quick reference dictionary for athletic training.* Thorofare: Slack Inc; 2005.

4. Binkley HM, Beckett J, Casa DJ, et al. National Athletic Trainers' Association position statement: Exertional heat illnesses. *J Athl Train.* 2002;347(3):329–343.

5. Booher JM, Thibodeau GA. *Athletic injury assessment,* 4th ed. Boston: McGraw-Hill; 2000.

6. Hillman SK. *Introduction to athletic training,* 2nd ed. Champaign: Human Kinetics; 2005.

7. Hoppenfeld S. *Physical examination of the spine and extremities.* Norwalk: Prentice Hall; 1976.

8. Kendall FP, McCreary EK, Provance PG, et al. *Muscles testing and function with posture and pain,* 5th ed. Baltimore: Lippincott Williams & Wilkins; 2005.

9. Konin JG, Wikston DL, Isear JA Jr, et al. *Special tests for orthopedic examination,* 3rd ed. Thorofare: Slack Inc; 2006.

10. Magee DJ. *Orthopedic physical assessment,* 4th ed. Philadelphia: WB Saunders; 2002.

11. Malone TR, McPoil T, Nitz AJ. *Orthopedic and sports physical therapy,* 3rd ed. St. Louis: Mosby; 1997.

12. National Athletic Trainers' Association. *Athletic training educational competencies,* 4th ed. Dallas: National Athletic Trainers' Association; 2006.

13. Norkin CC, White DJ. *Measurement of joint motion a guide to goniometry,* 3rd ed. Philadelphia: FA Davis Co; 2003.

14. Prentice WE. *Arnheim's principles of athletic training: a competency-based approach.* New York: McGraw-Hill; 2006.

15. Reese NB, Bandy WD. *Joint range of motion and muscle length testing.* Philadelphia: WB Saunders; 2002.

16. Shultz SJ, Houglum PA, Perrin DH. *Examination of musculoskeletal injuries,* 2nd ed. Champaign: Human Kinetics; 2005.

17. Starkey C, Johnson G. *AADS athletic training and sports medicine,* 4th ed. Sudburg: Jones and Bartlett; 2006.

18. Starkey C, Ryan J. *Evaluation of orthopedic and athletic injuries,* 2nd ed. Philadelphia: FA Davis Co; 2002.

5

Medical Conditions and Disabilities

Part 1   General Medical Assessment

Part 2   Medical Conditions

Section 5 Examination

OVERVIEW

Medical disorders are common among active participants. The athletic trainer must have an understanding of general medical conditions in order to direct care. With dedicated practice, the athletic trainer can become quite skilled at assessing general medical conditions and referring the athlete to the appropriate medical specialists.

CLINICAL PROFICIENCIES

Demonstrate a general and specific (e.g., head, torso, and abdomen) assessment for the purpose of (a) screening and referral of common medical conditions, (b) treating those conditions as appropriate, and (c) when appropriate, determining a patient's readiness for physical activity. Effective lines of communication should be established to elicit and convey information about the patient's status and the treatment program. While maintaining confidentiality, all aspects of the assessment, treatment, and determination for activity should be documented using standardized record-keeping methods. (Reproduced with permission of the National Athletic Trainers' Association.)

KEY TERMS

- Adenopathy
- Adventitious
- Adventitious lung sounds
- Auscultation
- Blood pressure
- Blumberg sign
- Bowel sounds
- Breath sounds
- Bronchoscopy
- Cardiac assessment
- Crackle
- Dehydration
- Diphtheria
- Dipstick
- First heart sound (S_1)
- Fremitus
- Glucometer
- Guarding
- *In vitro*
- *In vivo*
- Insidious
- Korotkoff sounds
- Latex sensitivity
- Lethargy
- Light reflex
- Malaise
- Mammography
- Manometer
- Morbidity
- Mortality
- Nosocomial
- Ophthalmoscope
- Orthopnea
- Orthostatic
- Otoscope
- Paralysis
- Paresthesia
- Peak flowmeter
- Pedometer
- Percussion
- Prognosis
- Prone
- Puberty

- Pulse oximeter
- Rale
- Rebound tenderness
- Red reflex
- Refractometer
- Resonance
- Rhonchus, rhonchi
- Second heart sound (S_2)
- Sinus rhythm
- Sphygmomanometer
- Stethoscope
- Tactile fremitus
- Tanner stage
- Tragus
- Tuberculin test
- Tympanic thermometer
- Urinalysis
- Vaccination
- Vocal fremitus

PERCUSSION

- Tapping/striking used for depths up to 5 cm
- Determine size/location organs
- Identify abnormal masses
- Recognize structure density
- Elicit deep tendon reflexes
- Determine present pain

Types of Percussion

- Indirect
  - Most common
  - Use both hands
  - Dominant hand strikes nondominant hand
- Direct
  - Striking hand contacts body

Indirect Percussion

- Stationary hand
  - Usually nondominant hand
  - Hyperextend third phalanx
  - Place third phalanx firmly against patient's skin
  - Do not percuss over bone
  - Do not allow remainder of stationary hand to contact body—halts vibration

- Striking hand
  - Usually dominant hand
  - Tap DIP joint of stationary hand
  - Contact right angle of tip of stationary hand
  - Tap twice and move
  - Obese/muscular patients require more percussion force

Percussion Sound

- Amplitude
  - Loudness
  - Dependent on structural ability for vibration
- Pitch
  - Frequency (cycles per second)
  - Increase vibrations = increase tone pitch
  - Decrease vibrations = decrease tone pitch
- Duration
  - Length of tone
- Quality
  - Distinction between similar tones, for example, organs versus muscle

Percussion Notes

- Flat—muscle, bone tumor
- Dull—spleen, liver
- Tympany—stomach, intestines
- Resonant—lung tissue
- Hyper-resonant—adult lung with emphysema

ABDOMINAL QUADRANTS

Upper Right Quadrant

- Gall bladder
- Kidney
- Liver
- Lung
- Pancreas

Lower Right Quadrant

- Appendix
- Bladder
- Colon
- Gonads
- Ureter

Upper Left Quadrant

- Heart
- Kidney
- Lung
- Spleen
- Stomach

Lower Left Quadrant

- Bladder
- Colon
- Gonads
- Ureter

AUSCULTATIONS

- Listening to body sounds with ears or stethoscope (see Fig. 5.1)
- Done after palpations except for abdomen

Stethoscope Parts

- Ear pieces
  - Should be comfortable
  - Slope toward nose
- Tubing
  - 1/8″ or 4 mm thick
  - 30 to 36 cm long (if too long, sound distorted)
- End piece
  - Diaphragm
    - Flat edges
    - Most frequently used
    - Identify normal breath, heart, and bowel sounds
    - Hold firmly against skin (leave imprint on patient)
    - Clean after each use
  - Bell
    - Hollow cup (smaller of two)
    - Hear abnormal heart sounds
    - Hold lightly against skin (just seal edges against skin)
    - Bell turns into diaphragm if held too tightly
    - Clean after each use

Auscultations of Heart

- Aorta semilunar valves—right second intercostal space
- Pulmonary semilunar valve—left second intercostal space at sternal border
- Pulmonary semilunar valve—left third intercostal space at sternal border
- Tricuspid valve—left fourth intercostal space at sternal border
- Bicuspid (mitral) valve—left fifth intercostal space at apex of the heart

OTOSCOPE

- Look at ear, tympanic membrane, and nares
- Five specula sizes
  - Use largest that will fit comfortably
  - Short, broad speculae used for nares
- Hold otoscope upside down
- Pinna position
  - Pull up/back in adult or larger children (decreases ear canal curve)
  - Pull down in infant up to 3 years old
  - Maintain firm traction on pinna throughout entire examination
- Dominant hand holds otoscope with fifth digit/dorsum of hand on patient's cheek
- Never jab speculae into ear

TESTING HEARING ACUITY

- Voice test

Locations for percussion and auscultation

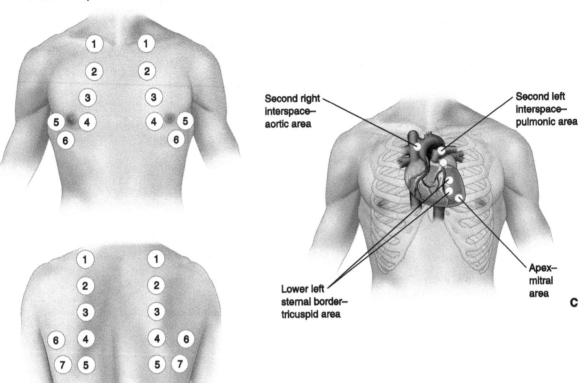

Figure 5.1 Auscultation Locations.

- Tuning fork test
  - Weber test
  - Rinne test

Voice Test

- Push tragus into and out of auditory meatus
- Simultaneously, whisper two-syllable word, for example, softball, nineteen
- Ask patient to repeat word
- Normal—repeats word correctly
- Abnormal—unable to recount word

Tuning Fork Tests

- Measure hearing through bone or air conduction
- Tuning fork of 500 to 1, 000 Hz mimics normal speech
- Air conduction
  - Tympanic membrane → stapes embedded in oval window → basilar membrane of cochlea containing corti hair cells
- Bone conduction
  - Bones of skull vibrate → vibration transfers to inner ear and cranial nerve VIII
- Weber test
  - Used when patient reports hearing better from one ear than other
  - Stem of vibrating tuning fork placed on midline of skull
  - Identify if hearing equally from both ears

- Rinne test
  - Compares air and bone conduction
  - Place stem of tuning fork on mastoid process
  - Then invert and ask patient to identify when sound leaves
  - Place vibrating end near ear canal
  - Ask patient to identify when sound leaves
  - Normal air conduction hearing is two times longer than bone conduction
  - Air conduction greater than bone conduction

OPHTHALMOSCOPE

- Assess internal eye
- Five apertures
- Diopter
  - Lens numbers to compensate for examiner's vision
  - Positive number 0 to +40 (black numbers)
    - Hyperopia (farsighted)—see far not close
    - Diopter is convex
  - Negative numbers 0 to −20 (red numbers)
    - Myopia (nearsighted)—see close not far away
    - Diopter is concave shape

Ophthalmoscope Apertures

- Large—dilated pupils
- Small—undilated pupils
- Red-free filter (green)—optic disc hemorrhage (black) and melanin (gray)

- Slit—assess anterior eye and fundus position
- Grid—assess size of fundus

Using Ophthalmoscope

- Take glasses off (patient/examiner) but leave contacts in (examiner)
- Scope to eye of examiner—brace against cheek and brow
- Index finger adjusts lens
- Keep both eyes open
- Dark room (dilates pupils)
- Patient fixed look on distant object
  - Dilates pupils
  - Hold retina still
- Right hand and eye (examiner) → evaluate right eye (patient)
- Left hand and eye (examiner) → evaluate left eye (patient)
- Begin 10 in. away and 15 degrees lateral to line of vision
- Red reflex—reflection of light off inner retina
  - If you lose this reflex, light is not in correct location
- Adjust lens to +6 and look for opaque black dots or shadows (cataracts)
- Move forward until foreheads almost touch
  - Adjust diopter to see ocular fundus
  - Move inward from 15-degree lateral line to see structures of ocular fundus

FOUR EYE QUADRANTS

- Superior
- Inferior
- Nasal
- Temporal

Six Cardinal Positions of Gaze

See Figure 5.2.

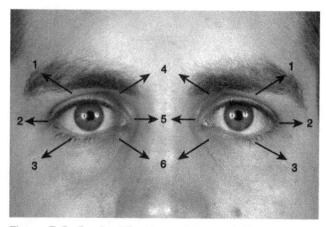

Figure 5.2 Cardinal Positions of Gaze. *1,* Superior Rectus Muscle (Cranial Nerve III); *2,* Lateral Rectus Muscle (Cranial Nerve VI); *3,* Inferior Rectus Muscle (Cranial Nerve III); *4,* Inferior Oblique Muscle (Cranial Nerve III); *5,* Medial Rectus Muscle (Cranial Nerve III); and *6,* Superior Oblique Muscle (Cranial Nerve IV).

STRUCTURES OF OCULAR FUNDUS

- Optic disc
  - Follow vessels from each of four quadrants to disc if difficult to see
  - Creamy yellow-orange to pink color
  - Round or slightly oval shape
  - Distinct edges to disc
  - Edges may be fuzzy along nasal margin
- Retinal vessels
  - Directly view blood vessels (only place in body)
  - Assess for systemic disease
  - Paired artery and vein pass through each quadrant
  - Arteries brighter red than veins
- General background
  - Varies with patient skin color
  - Light red to dark brown-red
  - View should be clear with no lesions
- Macula
  - Located temporal to optic disc
  - Inspect last (may cause pupil constriction)
  - Darker in color compared to remaining fundus

EYE TESTS

- Visual acuity
- Confrontation test
- Corneal light reflex (Hirschberg test)
- Cover test
- Diagnostic positions test

Visual Acuity Far Vision

- Snellen alphabet or E chart
  - Read 20 ft from chart
  - Opaque card to cover one eye
  - Documentation
    - Which eye
    - Numeric fraction on chart
    - Number of missed items
    - With or without glasses/contacts
  - Snellen E chart for 3- to 6-year-olds (direction of table legs)
  - Snellen alphabet chart 7- to 8-year-olds to adult
  - If largest letters cannot be read, shorten distance to 10 ft
- Allen test (picture cards)
  - 2 years 6 months to 2 years 11 months
  - Test at 15 ft
  - Child identifies 3/7 pictures within three to five trials

Visual Acuity Near Vision

- Jaegar or Rosenbaum cards
- Test people older than 40 years old
- Test people with reading difficulty
- Handheld card
- Hold card 15 in. from eye with glasses on
- 14/14 normal
- Test each eye separately

Understanding Normal Visual Acuity

- 20/20 far vision
- 14/14 near vision
- Numerator (first 20) is distance standing from chart
- Denominator (second 20) is what a normal eye could have read that line

Confrontation Tests

- Gross peripheral vision test
- Compares patient with examiner's peripheral vision
- Patient/examiner eye level—2 ft from each
- Cover eye with opaque card and look at each
  - Examiner covers right eye → patient covers left eye
  - Examiner covers left eye → patient covers right eye
- Move pencil or finger through range of peripheral vision
- Cannot do this with temporal visual field

Corneal Light Test (Hirschberg Test)

- Patient stares straight ahead
- Hold light 12 in. away from eyes
- Reflection of light on corneas should be the same on each eye (normal symmetry)
- Assess parallel alignment of eyes

Cover Test

- Patient stares straight ahead at the examiner's nose
- Cover one eye
- Normal: Uncovered eye stays fixed and steady
- Abnormal: Eye weakness causing covered eye to realign itself once uncovered

Diagnostic Positions and Test

- Six cardinal positions of gaze
- Object is held 12 in. from patient
- Test by moving object from center → to test position and hold → return object to center
- Normal: Parallel tracking of both eyes
- Abnormal: Nystagmus (fine oscillations around iris; asymmetrical tracking; lid lag)

TEMPERATURE

- Patients with increased oral temperature above 100 °F should not be allowed to participate
- Oral temperature
  - Normal 96.4°F to 99.1°F
  - Normal 35.8°C to 37.3°C
  - Shake mercury to 96°F (35.5°C)
  - Place in posterior sublingual pocket → close lips/mouth
  - Three to four minutes to check temperature
- Rectal temperature
  - Normal 0.7°F to 1°F higher than oral
  - Normal 0.4°C to 0.5°C higher than oral
  - Place patient on side with hip flexed
  - Apply lubrication (petroleum jelly) to thermometer
  - Insert into anal canal 1 in. (2 to 3 cm) toward umbilicus
- Tympanic temperature
  - Normal 1.4°F higher than oral temperatures

BLOOD PRESSURE

- Measured with sphygmomanometer and stethoscope
- 2.5 cm above antecubital crease
- Inflate cuff to 220 mm per Hg
- Deflate 2 to 3 mm Hg per second
- Cuff too small = increased blood pressure (BP)
- Crossed legs = increased BP
- Patient supports own arm = increased diastolic pressure
- Failure to wait 1 to 2 minutes before retaking BP = increased diastolic BP

Korotkoff Sounds

- Phase I: Systolic pressure
  - First sound
  - Blood enters artery
- Phase II
  - Partially occluded artery
- Phase III
  - Artery closes briefly
- Phase IV
  - Muffling of sound
- Phase V: Diastolic pressure
  - Disappearance of sound
  - Streamlined blood flow

Factors Controlling Blood Pressure

- Volume
- Cardiac output
- Vascular resistance
- Viscosity
- Elasticity of arterial walls

Blood Pressure Levels

Normal	<120/<80 mm Hg
Prehypertension	120–139/80–89 mm Hg
Mild hypertension	140–159/90–99 mm Hg
Moderate hypertension	≥160/≥100 mm Hg
Severe hypertension	>180/>110 mm Hg

PULSE

- Assess rhythm, rate, and force
- Take for 15 seconds and multiply by 4
- Rate: Pulses per minute
  - Bradycardia = <60 beats per minute
  - Tachycardia = >100 beats per minute

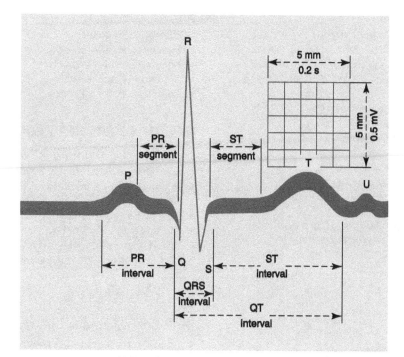

Figure 5.3 Electrocardiogram.

- Rhythm: Tempo of heart beat
  - Normal = even tempo
  - Sinus arrhythmia—common when heart rate varies with respiratory cycle
    - Increases with inspiration
    - Decreases with expiration
- Force: Strength of heart beat
  - Common assessment tools
    - 4+ = bounding
    - 3+ = increased
    - 2+ = normal
    - 1+ = weak, thready
    - 0 = absent
    - 3+ = full, bounding
    - 2+ = normal
    - 1+ = weak, thready
    - 0 = absent

Palpable Pulses

- Brachial
- Carotid
- Dorsalis pedis
- Popliteal
- Posterior tibial
- Radial
- Femoral

RESPIRATIONS

- Assess rate and rhythm
- Normal 12 to 20 breaths per minute
- Assess in quiet, relaxed atmosphere without patient knowing
- Assess for 30 seconds and multiply by 2

ELECTROCARDIOGRAM OF THE HEART

- P = atrial depolarization
- QRS = ventricular depolarization (atrial repolarization occurs here but is not noticed because of the more powerful ventricular action)
- T = ventricular repolarization
- Total cardiac cycle takes 0.8 seconds (see Fig. 5.3)

URINALYSIS

- Hydration status is assessed using refractometer or chemstrips
- Can be used as a screen to determine needs for further assessment, for example, diabetes
- Urine specific gravity levels
  - Well hydrated = <1.010
  - Minimal dehydration = 1.010–1.020
  - Significant dehydration = 1.021–1.030
  - Serious dehydration = >1.030
- pH = acidic
- Color = light yellow—can be affected by some medications, nutraceuticals, and foods
- Proteins, glucose, keytones, nitrates, hemoglobin = negative results for these when using chemstrips

BLOOD ANALYSIS

- Hematocrit
  - Volume percentage of red blood cell (RBC) in whole blood
  - Normal in adult men—42% to 54%
  - Normal in adult women—36% to 46%

- Hemoglobin test
  - Amount of hemoglobin in blood
  - Color chart measures for comparison
  - Normal in adult men—14 to 179/100 mL blood
  - Normal in adult women—12 to 159/100 mL blood
- Red cell count
  - Normal 4.5 to 5.5 million per μL (mm^3)
  - Polycythemia—increased RBC count
  - Anemia—decreased RBC count
- White blood cell (WBC) count
  - Normal 5,000 to 10,000 cells per μL (mm^3)
  - Leukopenia—WBC count below 5,000
  - Leukocytosis—WBC count above 10,000
- Thrombocyte count
  - Normal 150,000 to 450,000 per μL of blood
  - Thrombocytopenia—decreased platelets
- Complete blood count (CBC)
  - Analysis of the following blood components
    - Size
    - Shape
    - Color
    - Number

PEAK FLOW METER

- Identifies normal and abnormal pulmonary function
- Stoplight assessment of pulmonary function
  - Green—within 80% to 100% of normal peak flow readings
  - Yellow—within 50% to 80% of normal peak flow readings
  - Red—below 50% of normal peak flow readings

INOCULATION SCHEDULE (CHILDHOOD)

- Diphtheria, tetanus, pertussis (DPT)
  - 2 doses
  - 15 to 18 months
  - 11 to 16 years
- Hepatitis B
  - 3 doses
  - Birth to 2 months
  - 1 to 4 months
  - 6 to 18 months
- Influenza B—12 to15 months
- Poliovirus—6 to 18 months
- Measles, mumps, rubella (MMR)
  - 12 to 15 months
  - 11 to 12 years
- Varicella—12 to 18 months

INOCULATION SCHEDULE (ADULT)

- Diphtheria—every 10 years
- Hepatitis A—travelers at risk

- Influenza—adult to 65 years; health care workers; third trimester pregnancy
- Meningococcal—college students
- Pneumococcal—adults to 65 years; populations of various disease states
- Tetanus—every 10 years

HEALTH SCREENING RECOMMENDATIONS

- Papanicolaou (Pap) smear—annual at age 18 or when becoming sexually active
- Mammogram—annually at age 40
- Breast self-examination—monthly
- Testicular self-examination—monthly
- Digital rectal examination—annually at age 40
- Prostate-specific antigen (PSA)—annually at age 50
- Colonoscopy—every 5 years at age 50

BIRTH CONTROL

Birth Control versus Contraception

- Birth control—methods preventing childbirth
- Contraception—methods preventing fertilization of egg

Normal Menstrual Cycle Fertility Risk

- Days 1 to 5: Relatively low risk of pregnancy
- Days 6 to 8: Medium risk of pregnancy
- Days 9 to 16: Highest risk of pregnancy with unprotected sex
- Days 17 to 18: Medium risk of pregnancy
- Days 19 to 28: Relatively low risk of pregnancy

Birth Control Methods

- Barrier
- Hormonal
- Natural
- Surgical

Barrier Methods of Birth Control

- Diaphragms
- Male condom
- Female condom
- Sponge
- Vaginal spermicide
- Cervical cap
- Intrauterine device (IUD)
- FemCap
- The Lea shield

Hormonal Methods of Birth Control

- Oral contraceptives
- Contraceptive implants
- Contraceptive patch

- Injectables
- Vaginal ring
- Emergency contraception

Natural Methods of Birth Control

- Abstinence
- Fertility awareness
- Withdrawal

Surgical Methods of Birth Control

- Vasectomy
- Tubal sterilization
- Ovariectomy
- Hysterectomy
- Abortion

DERMA, HEAD, AND FACE

Danger Signs of Pigmented Lesions

- A—asymmetry of lesion
- B—border irregularity
- C—color variation in single lesion
- D—diameter >6 mm
- E—elevation and enlargement

Common Benign Pigmented Lesions

- Birthmarks—tan to brown
- Freckles—small and flat; brown
- Nevus (mole)—flat or raised; tan to brown

Skin Assessment

- Temperature
  - Hypothermia
  - Hyperthermia
- Moisture
  - Diaphoresis
  - Dehydration
- Texture—even, smooth, firm
- Thickness—callus
- Edema—intercellular fluid accumulation
- Mobility—movement of skin
- Turgor—return to original position after movement
- Vascularity—bruising
- Lesions

Four-Point Pitting Edema Scale

- 1+ = Mild—cannot see swelling
- 2+ = Moderate—indent with pressure but subsides rapidly

- 3+ = Deep—leg looks swollen; indent with pressure and stays a short time
- 4+ = Very deep—leg very swollen; indent with pressure remains a long time

Assessing Lesions

- Exudate (odor and color)
- Size
- Location
- Shape or pattern
- Elevation
- Color

Primary versus Secondary Lesions

- Primary lesions
  - Initial lesion on previously normal skin
- Secondary lesions
  - Results from primary lesion but caused by scratching or infection

Primary Skin Lesions

- Bulla
- Cyst
- Macule
- Nodule
- Papule
- Patch
- Plaque
- Pustule
- Tumor
- Urticaria
- Vesicle
- Wheal

Secondary Skin Lesion

- Atrophic scar
- Crust
- Erosion
- Excoriation
- Fissure
- Keloid
- Lichenification
- Scale
- Scar
- Ulcer

Stages of Ecchymosis Color Change

- First stage—red-blue or purple (immediate to 24+ hours)
- Second stage—blue to purple
- Third stage—blue to green
- Fourth stage—yellow
- Fifth stage—brown to disappear

KEY TERMS

- Auricle hematoma
- Melanoma
- Rubor
- Short-term memory (STM)
- Tremor
- Ulcerative
- Lacrimal gland
- Strabismus
- Vertigo
- Allergen
- Aneurysm
- Angina pectoris
- Angioedema
- Aortic stenosis
- Aphasia
- Arteriosclerosis
- Ataxia
- Atherosclerosis
- Athlete's heart
- Aura, aurae
- Benign
- Biopsy
- Cardiac murmur
- Cardiac output
- Cardiac tamponade
- Cellulitis
- Cerumen
- Cheilosis, chilosis
- Communicable disease
- Complex partial seizure
- Diabetes
- Diabetic coma
- Dyslipidemia
- Gallstone
- Glycosuria
- Group A streptococal (GAS) necrotizing fasciitis
- Hemarthrosis
- Hematocrit (Hct)
- Hematuria
- Hemiplegia
- Hemothorax
- Hepatitis B virus (HBV)
- High-density lipoprotein cholesterol (HDL-C)
- Hirsutism
- Hypercalcemia
- Hyperglycemia
- Hyperkalemia
- Hypernatremia
- Hyperthermia
- Hypertrophic cardiomyopathy
- Hyperventilation
- Hyphema
- Hypocalcemia
- Hypocapnia
- Hypoglycemia
- Hypokalemia
- Hyponatremia
- Immunodeficiency
- Insulin
- Insulin shock
- Leukoplakia
- Lymphedema
- Macula, maculae
- Malacia
- Malignant
- Menarche
- Meningitis, meningitides
- Menstrual cycle
- Metastasis
- Mumps virus
- Myocardial infarction (MI)
- Myocarditis
- Myositis
- Natremia, natriemia
- Necrosis
- Neoplasm
- Osteopenia
- Osteoporosis
- Pandemic
- Petechiae
- Phlebitis
- Polydipsia
- Polyuria

- Postprandia
- Proteinuria
- Pruritus
- Pulmonary embolism (PE)
- Purpura
- Purulent
- Reflux
- Rubella
- Rubeola
- Sarcopenia
- Secondary amenorrhea
- Seizure
- Sepsis, sepses
- Septic shock
- Tetanus
- Varicella

SKIN CONDITIONS

Abrasion: A superficial wound on skin
Acne Vulgaris: Pimples resulting from clogged pores
Allergic Contact Dermatitis: A skin inflammation
Alopecia: A complete or partial hair loss
Athlete's Foot: Tinea pedis fungal infection of the foot
Blister: Fluid accumulation under skin
Burn: An injury to superficial to progressively deeper tissues resulting in bulla, charring, and/or redness
Callus: Thickened skin common on feet and hands
Candidiasis (Cutaneous): Yeast infection of skin and mucous membranes
Carbuncle: A cluster of boils
Cellulitis: An inflammation of connective tissue because of infection
Chilblain: Pernio
Cold Urticaria: Itching wheals from exposure to cold temperatures
Corn: A thick callus over prominence
Dermatitis: An inflammation of outer layer of skin
Eczema: Superficial skin inflammations with varied specific definitions
Exercise-Induced Urticaria: Similar to cholinergic urticaria (hives)
Folliculitis: An infected hair, shaft of hair grows inward and becomes infected
Frostbite: Freezing of skin—layers superficial to deep based on exposure
Furunculosis: Complicating condition of folliculitis
Furuncle: A boil
Herpes Gladiatorum: Herpes infection transmitted by close athletic contact
Herpes Simplex: A recurrent skin infection caused by virus
Herpes Zoster: A viral infection called *shingles*
Hives: Raised patches on the skin

Hyperhidrosis: Sweat gland overproduction; usually found on feet and hands
Impetigo: Superficial skin infections
Incision: A wound caused by sharp cutting, no jagged edges
Intertrigo: Superficial dermatitis from friction and maceration
Irritant Contact Dermatitis: Skin inflammation because of friction
Laceration: A jagged-edged wound
Miliaria Profunda: Occluded sweat glands which follow prickly heat
Miliaria Rubra: Heat rash or prickly heat
Molluscum Contagiosum: Skin-colored papules with centralized umbilication
Onychia: Infection of nail matrix
Paronychia: Infection of nail bed
Pediculosis: Infestation of lice on hair shafts
Pernio: Chilblains
Petechiae: Hemorrhagic spots on the skin
Pityriasis Rosea: Skin infection looking like ringworm
Prickly Heat: Skin irritation from retained perspiration
Psoriasis: Scaling like eczema but not deep; crusting areas
Puncture: A piercing wound
Rosacea: A chronic inflammatory disorder of face in middle-age/older adults
Ringworm: Topical fungal infection
Scabies: Topical parasite
Sebaceous Cysts: Slow-growing cysts; benign in nature
Striae Distensae: Stretch marks
Sunburn: An inflammatory response to ultraviolet light
Tinea Barbae: Topical fungal infection of beard or back of neck
Tinea Capitis: Topical fungal infection of the scalp
Tinea Corporis: Topical fungal infection of body or face
Tinea Cruris: Topical fungal infection of the groin area
Tinea Pedis: Topical fungal infection of the feet
Tinea Unguium: Fungal infection to nails (feet/hands)
Tinea Versicolor: Patches of skin often called *sun spots*
Verruca Plantaris: Plantar's wart
Verruca Vulgaris: Common wart
Vitiligo: Depigmented skin patches
Xerotic Skin: Dry skin

 Use the DVD or visit the website at http://thePoint.lww.com/Long for additional information about the *identification, etiology, signs/symptoms, and management of skin conditions.*

THORAX AND ABDOMEN

Appendicitis: An inflammation of the appendix
Cardiac Tamponade: Laceration of coronary arteries and rupture of myocardium
Celiac Plexus Syndrome (Solar Plexus Contusion): Wind knocked out
Clavicle Contusion: Bruised clavicle
Clavicle Fracture: Broken clavicle
Costochondral Fracture: Separation with fracture of cartilage between ribs

Costochondral Sprain: Slipping rib syndrome
Costovertebral Sprain: Ligament stretch between ribs and vertebrae
Hematuria: Blood in urine
Hemorrhoids: Distended veins through anus
Hemothorax: Blood in pleural space
Hernia: Protrusion of internal tissues through abdominal/inguinal wall
Hydrocele: Fluid in tunica vaginalis of scrotum or along spermatic cord
Hyperventilation: Rapid breathing
Kidney Contusion: Bruised kidney
Kidney Laceration: Kidney tear
Kidney Stones: Urinary calculi; urolithiasis
Liver Contusion: Liver bruise
Liver Laceration: Liver tear
Peritonitis: Inflamed peritoneum
Pneumothorax: Collapsed lung—air trapped in pleural space
Proteinuria: Excessive urine protein
Pulmonary Contusion: Bruised lung
Rib Contusion: Rib bruise
Rib Fracture: Discontinuation of a rib bone
Solar Plexus Contusion (Celiac Plexus Syndrome): Wind knocked out
Spermatic Cord Torsion: Twisted spermatic cord and vascular pedicle
Spleen Contusion: Spleen bruise
Spleen Laceration: Spleen tear
Sternal Contusion: Sternal bruise
Sternal Fracture: Broken sternum
Tension Pneumothorax: Air in pleural space compromises lung, heart, and surrounding organs
Testicular Contusion: Testicle bruise
Traumatic Asphyxia: Impaired breathing from massive trauma
Ulcer: Open sore in mucous membrane or skin
Varicocele: Dilation of pampiniform venous plexus and internal spermatic vein

 Use the DVD or visit the website at http://thePoint .lww.com/Long for additional information about the *identification, etiology, signs/symptoms, and management of thorax and abdomen conditions.*

EYES, EARS, NOSE, HEAD, FACE, AND THROAT

Anisocoria: Unequal pupil size may be caused by head injury
Astigmatism: Blurred vision at all distances
Auricular Hematoma: Contused ear auricle (cauliflower ear)
Cauliflower Ear: Auricular hematoma or contused ear auricle
Cerebral Contusion: Traumatic brain injury; bruising of brain
Chalazion: Cyst in eyelid; meibomian gland lipogranuloma
Concussion: Brain injury causing disrupted electrical activity

Conjunctivitis: Pink eye; inflammation of conjunctiva
Corneal Abrasions: Scratches to the cornea
Corneal Laceration: Cut to the cornea
Coryza: Nasal airway mucous membrane inflammation
Dental Caries: Tooth decay and cavity
Detached Retina: Retina separation from epithelium
Deviated Septum: Disrupted nasal septum
Diplopia: Double vision
Endophthlamos: Sunken eyes
Epidural Hematoma: Ruptured middle meningeal artery/vein, bleed between skull and dura mater
Epistaxis: Nose bleed
Exophthalmos: Protruding eyes
Gingivitis: An inflammation of gums
Hordeolum: An infection of the sebaceous gland around the eye (stye)
Hyperopia: Farsightedness
Hyphema: Hemorrhage in anterior eye chamber
Impacted Cerumen: Excessive wax build up in external auditory canal
Intracranial Hematoma: Ruptured blood vessels between skull and brain
Intraparenchymal Hematoma (intracerebral hematoma): Blood in brain damaging white matter
Keratitis: An inflamed cornea
Malignant Brain Edema Syndrome: Clot increases swelling and intracranial pressure
Mandibular Fracture: Fracture to the lower jaw; usually bilateral or in conjunction with dislocation
Maxillary Fracture: LeFort fracture; fracture to upper jaw or middle face
Myopia: Nearsightedness
Nasal Fracture: Nose fracture
Orbital "Blowout" Fracture: Increased intraorbital pressure causes orbital floor fracture
Otitis Externa: Swimmer's ear; infection affects lining of external auditory canal
Otitis Media: Middle ear infection
Pericoronitis: Inflamed gums around molar teeth
Peridontitis: An inflammation of deep gum tissue
Periorbital Ecchymosis: Black eye
Postconcussion Syndrome: Cognitive impairments resulting from concussion
Presbyobia: Unaccommodating eye with aging
Ruptured Globe: Rupture to eyeball
Scleral Trauma: Injury to white portion of eye
Second Impact Syndrome: Life-threatening condition with increased pressure on brain stem following previous head injury
Skull Fracture: Discontinuation of a bone in the skull
Stye: Infection of the sebaceous gland around the eye (hordeolum)
Subarachnoid Hematoma: Bleeding between arachnoid mater and pia mater
Subconjunctival Hemorrhage: Small capillary ruptures in eye sclera
Subdural Hematoma: Bleed between dura mater and arachnoid mater; vein rupture
Temporomandibular Dislocation: Luxation with probable fracture of the temporomandibular joint (TMJ)
Temporomandibular Dysfunction: TMJ disorder secondary to arthritis trauma or other joint changes

Tooth Abscess: Infected tooth at root of gum and tooth

Tooth Extrusion: Partially displaced tooth

Tooth Fracture: Visible fracture to enamel, dentin, pulp, and/or root of tooth

Tooth Intrusion: Impacted tooth

Tooth Luxation: Dislocated tooth

Tympanic Membrane Rupture: Ruptured eardrum

Zygomatic Fractures: Fracture to cheek bone with flattened/depressed cheek

 Use the DVD or visit the website at http://thePoint.lww.com/Long for additional information about the *identification, etiology, signs/symptoms, and management of eyes, ears, nose, head, face, and throat conditions.*

COMMON ILLNESSES AND DISEASE

Absence Seizure (Petit Mal): Type of generalized seizure in children

Acquired Immunodeficiency Syndrome (AIDS): Chronic life-threatening disease caused by human immunodeficiency virus (HIV)

Acute Mountain Sickness: Altitude sickness manifesting from decreased oxygen in the blood

Amenorrhea: Failure or absence of menstruation for 3 months

Amyotrophic Lateral Sclerosis (Lou Gehrig Disease): Voluntary muscle nerve destruction

Anorexia Nervosa: Eating disorder characterized by failure to maintain body weight

Arthritis: An inflammation of the joints

Asthma: Airway inflammation with excessive mucus production and muscle spasm

Bacterial Vaginosis: Vulvovaginal bacterial infection

Breast Cancer: Neoplasm of the breast

Bronchitis: Mucous thickening in bronchial tubes from infection or inflammation

Bulimia Nervosa: Eating disorder characterized by binge and purging activities

Candidiasis: Yeast infection of oral or vaginal cavities

Cerebral Palsy: Chronic neurologic disorder caused by brain lesions

Cerebral Vascular Accident (CVA): Ischemic or hemorrhagic nature, decreased oxygen to brain (stroke)

Charcot Marie Tooth Disease: Hereditary motor and sensory neuropathy

Chickenpox: Communicable viral infection common in childhood

Chlamydia: Sexually transmitted disease (oral, vaginal, or anal)

Chronic Fatigue Syndrome: Persistent, severe fatigue

Chronic Obstructive Pulmonary Disease (COPD): Decreased inspiratory and expiratory lung function

Claudication: Cramping in lower leg secondary to decreased circulation

Coccidioidomycosis (San Juan or Valley fever): Benign self-limiting respiratory disease

Colitis: Inflamed rectal or colon lining

Common Cold: Respiratory viral infection

Commotio Cordis: Sudden cardiac death due to interruption of electrical impulses

Complex Partial Seizure: Type of focal seizure with loss of consciousness

Complex Regional Pain Syndrome (Reflex Sympathetic Dystrophy): Overactivity of the sympathetic nervous system

Congestive Heart Failure: Inefficient heart pumping resulting in edema

Constipation: Decreased fecal fluid content causing hard stools

Coronary Artery Disease: Blocked coronary arteries

Coryza: Nasal airway mucous membrane inflammation

Cryptorchidism (Cryptorchism): Undescended testicle(s)

Cushing Syndrome: Adrenal hyperplasia

Cystic Fibrosis: Life-threatening disorder affecting mucous, sweat, and digestive cells

Deep Vein Thrombosis (DVT): Clot in deeper veins

Diabetes Mellitus: Glucose metabolism disorder

Diarrhea: Decreased absorbability of large intestines; frequent bowel movements

Diphtheria: Acute contagious disease affecting the respiratory, myocardial, and neural tissues

Down Syndrome: Intellectual disability with chromosomal abnormality

Dysmenorrhea: Painful and/or exaggerated menstruation

Encephalitis: An inflammation of the brain

Endometriosis: Ectopic endometrial tissue

Epilepsy: Seizure disorder with episodic symptoms

Esophageal Reflux: Stomach acid regurgitation through esophageal sphincter muscle

Exercise-Iinduced Bronchospasm: Asthma-like symptoms initiated by exercise

Fibromyalgia: Chronic noninflammatory condition

Food Poisoning: Gastroenteritis

Frostbite: Freezing of tissues

Gastritis: Inflamed stomach lining because of acid production

Gastroenteritis (Food Poisoning/Stomach Flu): Inflamed gastrointestinal (GI) tract

Gastroesophageal Reflux Disease (GERD): Recurrent epigastric or retrosternal pain from malfunctioning lower esophageal sphincter muscle

Genital Herpes: Viral infection of the genitalia considered a sexually transmitted disease

Genital Warts: Sexually transmitted viral disease linked to cervical cancer

Gonorrhea: Sexually transmitted bacterial disease

Gout: Recurrent inflammation of peripheral joints secondary to uric acid hypersaturation

Group A Streptococcus (GAS): Necrotizing fasciitis (flesh eating bacteria)

Guillian-Barré Syndrome: Acute, diffuse demyelination of spinal and peripheral nerves

Gynecomastia: Overdevelopment of male breast

Haemophilis Influenza Type B (Hib): Bacteria found in upper respiratory tract; common cause of many diseases, for example, meningitis, sinusitis, otitis media, and so on.

Hay Fever: Allergic reaction to airborne allergens

Heart Murmur: Abnormal heart valve functions that may or may not be significant

Heat Exhaustion: Failure of body's thermoregulatory system with increased body temperature, sweating, and dehydration

Heat Stroke: Life-threatening failure of body's thermoregulatory system

Heat Syncope: Fainting following heat exposure

Hemophilia: Blood coagulation disorder

Hemorrhoids: Varicose veins in anus

Hepatitis A: An inflammation of the liver secondary to infectious virus through fecal material

Hepatitis B: An inflammation of the liver secondary to infectious serum virus through body fluids or sexual contact

Hepatitis C: An inflammation of the liver secondary to infectious serum virus

Hepatitis D: An inflammation of the liver (combination with hepatitis B virus [HBV])

Hepatitis E: An inflammation of the liver caused by a virus (waterborne in nature)

Herpes Zoster (Shingles): An infection involving the dorsal root ganglia

Hodgkin Disease: Malignant tumors found in lymphatic system (lymphoma)

HIV: An infection with wide range of symptoms culminating in AIDS

Hyperglycemia: Abnormally high blood glucose levels

Hyperthyroidism (Grave Disease): Metabolic condition with enlarged thyroid gland

Hyperventilation: Rapid breathing with reduced blood carbon dioxide

Hypertrophic Cardiomyopathy: Hypertrophied, nondilated left ventricle causing sudden death

Hypoglycemia: Abnormally low blood glucose levels

Hypotension: Abnormally low blood pressure

Hypothermia: Decreased body temperature

Hypothyroidism: Metabolic condition with thyroid hormone deficiency

Indigestion: Heartburn

Infectious Mononucleosis: Contagious infection involving the lymphatic cells of the throat

Influenza: Contagious viral infection associated with specific categories

Insulin Shock: Severe hypolycemia

Iron-Deficiency Anemia: Abnormally low concentrations of iron in the body

Irritable Bowel Syndrome: GI disorder with muscle contraction and relaxation

Laryngitis: Edema of vocal cords

Lyme Disease: Tick-borne illness

Marfan Syndrome: Connective tissue disorder

Meningitis: An inflammation of the brain and spinal cord meninges

Methicillin-Resistant *Staphylococcus Aureus* (MRSA): Antibiotic-resistant staphylococcal infection

Migraine Headache: Idiopathic headaches

Mitral Valve Prolapse: Ballooning of mitral valve

Monorchidism: Absent or undescended testicle

Multiple Sclerosis: Chronic neurodegenerative disease

Mumps: Contagious viral disease primarily in children

Muscular Dystrophy: Progressive muscle disorder

Myasthenia Gravis: Antibodies attach to the synaptic junction

Oligomenorrhea: Scanty or infrequent menstruation

Osteoporosis: Decreased bone mass density

Ovarian Cancer: Malignant neoplasm in the ovaries

Pancreatitis: Acute or chronic inflammation of the pancreas

Parkinson Disease: Progressive, degenerative neurologic disease

Pelvic Inflammatory Disease: Acute or chronic inflammation in the female pelvic cavity

Pertussis: Acute bacterial infection (whooping cough)

Pharyngitis: An inflammation of pharynx; sore throat

Pneumonia: Lung infection with multiple classifications

Poliomyelitis (Polio): Flaccid weakness of muscles from viral infection

Post Polio Syndrome: Deterioration of muscle function in people previously diagnosed with poliomyelitis

Pregnancy: Period of gestation from contraception to termination

Pubic Lice (Crabs): Sexually transmitted parasite infestation

Raynaud Syndrome (Raynaud Phenomenon): Spasm of digital arteries causing color and sensation changes

Reflex Sympathetic Dystrophy (Complex Regional Pain Syndrome): Overactivity of the sympathetic nervous system

Reye Syndrome: An illness causing inflammation of brain and fat accumulation in liver

Rhabdomyolysis: Destruction of skeletal muscle with potential fatal effects

Rhinitis: An inflammation of the nasal membranes

Rocky Mountain Spotted Fever: Bacterial infection transmitted by tick bite

Rubella (German Measles): Acute viral infection

Rubeola (Measles): Acute viral infection

Scabies: Sexually transmitted parasitic infection

Seasonal Affective Disorder: Depressive mood disorder in fall and winter

Second Impact Syndrome: Second head injury following a previous unresolved injury

Shock: Collapse of the cardiovascular system

Sickle Cell Anemia: Hemolytic anemia with sickle-shaped RBCs

Sickle Cell Trait: Inherited disorder with sickle-shaped RBCs

Simple Partial Seizure: Focal seizures without impaired consciousness

Sinusitis: An inflammation of the sinus membranes

Spina Bifida: Neural tube defect

Syncope: Fainting

Syphilis: Parasitic sexually transmitted disease with three distinct stages

Testicular Cancer: Neoplasm of the testicle

Tetanus: Bacterial infection (lock jaw)

Tonic Clonic Seizure: Grand mal seizure with impaired consciousness

Tonsilitis: An inflammation of the tonsils

Trichomoniasis: Sexually transmitted vaginal mucosa infection

Ulcerative Colitis: Chronic disease causing rectal and colon ulcerations

Upper Respiratory Infection: Infections of the sinuses, pharynx, and/or bronchi

Urethritis: An inflammation of the urethra

Urinary Tract Infection: An infection of the urinary tract (bladder, kidneys, urethra, or ureters)

Vaginitis: An inflammation of the vagina

Vancomycin Resistant Enterococci (VRE): Bacterial infection resistant to vancomycin

Varicella: Chickenpox

Whooping Cough: Acute bacterial infection (pertussis)

Wolf-Parkinson-White Syndrome: Heart problem with early depolarization and potential progression to sudden heart failure

 Use the DVD or visit the website at http://thePoint .lww.com/Long for additional information about the *identification, etiology, signs/symptoms, and management of common illnesses and disease.*

1. What term defines the process of blood formation?
   a. Hematopoiesis
   b. Hematoprovision
   c. Leukocoagulation
   d. Hematocrit
   e. Thrombopoetic

2. Which component of blood is most used in the clotting process?
   a. Erythrocytes
   b. Thrombocytes
   c. Leukocytes
   d. Albumins
   e. Globulins

3. Which layer of the heart is considered the thickest and contains intercalated discs?
   a. Epicardium
   b. Visceral layer
   c. Myocardium
   d. Endocardium
   e. Pericardium

4. Hair follicles are made from which type of cells?
   a. Ceruminous
   b. Epithelial
   c. Epididymal
   d. Stratum lucidum
   e. Stratum corneum

5. Which portion of the pericardium is anatomically the same as the epicardium?
   a. Fibrous endocardium
   b. Serous endocardium
   c. Fibrous pericardium
   d. Serous pericardium
   e. Myocardium

6. What is the name given to unique dermal projections identifying individuals?
   a. Piloerections
   b. Dermal papillae
   c. Meibomian cells
   d. Erector pili
   e. Lunala

7. What are the two types of sudoriferous glands?
   a. Ceruminous and cilliary glands
   b. Endocrine and exocrine glands
   c. Eccrine and apocrine glands
   d. Sebaceous and meibomian glands
   e. Lucidium and corneum glands

8. Which item identifies normal pathway for systemic circulation?
   a. Right ventricle → pulmonary vein → lungs → pulmonary artery → right atrium
   b. Left ventricle → pulmonary artery → lungs → pulmonary vein → left atrium
   c. Right ventricle → aorta → body → superior/inferior vena cava → left atrium
   d. Left ventricle → aorta → body → systemic veins → superior/inferior vena cava → right atrium
   e. Right ventricle → pulmonary artery → lungs → pulmonary veins → left atrium

9. Which does not contribute to blood pressure increases?
   a. Low blood volume
   b. Vessel diameter
   c. Arterial elasticity
   d. Viscosity of blood
   e. Blood doping with packed red blood cells

10. Which cardiovascular issue is not increased with exercise?
    a. Arterial blood pressure
    b. Cardiac rate
    c. Cardiac output
    d. Stroke volume
    e. Total peripheral resistance

11. Which segment is not uniquely identified on an electrocardiogram?
    a. O segment
    b. P segment
    c. QRS segment
    d. ST segment
    e. T segment

12. Which is not considered a function of the skin?
    a. Manufacturing calcium ions
    b. Excreting electrolytes

c. Preventing infection
d. Controlling body temperature
e. Providing sensory information

13. Which is a skin accessory structure?
    a. Epidermis
    b. Hypodermis
    c. Sudoriferous glands
    d. Dermis
    e. Subcutaneous

14. Which is not a component of the integumentary system?
    a. Nails
    b. Nerves
    c. Glands
    d. Thrombocytes
    e. Skin

15. Which electrocardiogram segment identifies ventricular depolarization?
    a. O segment
    b. P segment
    c. QRS segment
    d. ST segment
    e. T segment

16. Which portion of the epidermis is closest to the dermis?
    a. Stratum lucidum
    b. Meibomian lucidium
    c. Dermal papillae
    d. Stratum germinativum
    e. Stratum basalosus

17. What term identifies the ratio of packed erythrocytes to total blood volume?
    a. Hematopoietic
    b. Hematocrit
    c. Hemostatic
    d. Hemoanastomoses
    e. Hemoglobin

18. What are the formal blood type groups?
    a. A, B, C, O
    b. A, B, AB, O
    c. A, B, AB, D, O
    d. AB, BO, O
    e. A, B, O

19. Which does not identify the Rh factor of blood?
    a. Rh positive contains no D antigen
    b. Rh name given for rhesus monkey in which it was first identified
    c. Rh factor contributes to complications with transfusions

d. Rh factor contributes to complications with pregnancy
e. Rh factor implies there is a D antigen

20. Which is not a characteristic of erythrocytes?
    a. A flattened biconcave disc
    b. Destroyed by liver and spleen
    c. Move through diapedesis
    d. Shape important for oxygen carrying capacity
    e. Live 120 days

21. Which white blood cell fights parasites?
    a. Eosinphils
    b. Neutrophils
    c. Basophils
    d. Monocytes
    e. Lymphocytes

22. What term is given to a group of boils connected together?
    a. Onychia
    b. Paronychia
    c. Folliculitis
    d. Furuncle
    e. Carbuncle

23. Which electrocardiogram segment identifies the timing of atrial repolarization but does not record the process?
    a. O segment
    b. P segment
    c. QRS segment
    d. ST segment
    e. T segment

24. Which is the pathway for pulmonary circulation?
    a. Right ventricle → pulmonary vein → lungs → pulmonary artery → right atrium
    b. Left ventricle → pulmonary artery → lungs → pulmonary vein → left atrium
    c. Right ventricle → aorta → body → superior/inferior vena cava → left atrium
    d. Left ventricle → aorta → body → systemic veins → superior/inferior vena cava → right atrium
    e. Right ventricle → pulmonary artery → lungs → pulmonary veins → left atrium

25. Which is considered false regarding plasma proteins?
    a. γ-Globulins are antibodies produced by erythrocytes
    b. β-Globulins are formed by liver
    c. α-Globulins transport lipids and fat-soluble vitamins in blood
    d. Fibrinogen is produced by liver and converts to fibrin
    e. Albumins draw water from surrounding tissue through osmotic pressure

26. Which portion of the skin contains no blood vessels?
    a. Endodermis
    b. Epidermis
    c. Dermis
    d. Hypodermis
    e. Subcutaneous layer

27. Which microorganism is very small, lacking independent metabolism and reproduction capabilities?
    a. Bacteria
    b. Staphylococci
    c. Streptococci
    d. Virus
    e. Tinea

28. Which cells comprise the epidermis?
    a. Leukocytes and thrombocytes
    b. Keratinocytes and melanocytes
    c. Bacillicytes and erythrocytes
    d. Spirochetes and corneocytes
    e. Comdomes and macules

29. Which term identifies an infection to the nail bed?
    a. Hordeolum
    b. Hyphema
    c. Onychia
    d. Paronychia
    e. Hidradenitis

30. Cardiac output is measured by:
    a. Stroke volume × forced vital capacity
    b. Vital capacity/cardiac output
    c. Arterial blood pressure × cardiac output
    d. Cardiac rate × stroke volume
    e. Vital capacity × stroke volume × cardiac rate

31. Which condition does not result in an increase in blood pH?
    a. Hyperventilation
    b. Decrease in carbon dioxide
    c. Metabolic alkalosis
    d. Loss of bicarbonate
    e. Respiratory alkalosis

32. Which answer appropriately identifies the steps to blood clotting?
    a. Prothrominase attaches to Na^+ → converts prothrombin to thrombin → converts to fibrin → clot forms
    b. Thrombin converts fibrinolysin to fibrin → forms clot
    c. Calcium and prothrombinase converts prothrombin to thrombin → converts fibrinogen to fibrin → adds to plasma to form clot
    d. Platelets convert fibrinogen to fibrin → fibrinolysin breaks down fibrin to thrombin → mixes with plasma and clot forms
    e. Neutrophils neutralize calcium to form fibrin and fibrin mixes with mast cells to form clot

33. Which electrocardiograph segment identifies atrial depolarization?
    a. O segment
    b. P segment
    c. QRS segment
    d. ST segment
    e. T segment

34. Which type of shock identifies the type seen with an upper spinal cord injury?
    a. Cardiogenic
    b. Anaphylactic
    c. Axonogenic
    d. Hypovolemic
    e. Neurogenic

35. Why doesn't diastolic blood pressure rise with exercise?
    a. Skin warms, increasing blood flow to decrease heat
    b. Blood flow to heart more increased than to periphery
    c. Decreased peripheral resistance
    d. Visceral blood flow needs decrease so extremities can have more flow
    e. Brain prevents blood pressure increase by releasing antidiuretic hormone

36. Which autonomic nervous system decreases heart rate?
    a. Sympathetic nervous system
    b. Peripheral nervous system
    c. Visceral nervous system
    d. Parasympathetic nervous system
    e. Central nervous system

37. Which muscle prevents the atrioventricular valves from inverting with increased pressure?
    a. Mitral muscle
    b. Tricuspid muscle
    c. Trabeculae carnae
    d. Chordae tendineae
    e. Papillary muscle

38. Where should one place a stethoscope when auscultating tricuspid closing?
    a. Right second intercostal space
    b. Left second intercostal space
    c. Right fifth intercostal space close to the sternal border
    d. Left fifth intercostal space close to the sternal border
    e. Manubrium

39. How does the autonomic nervous system act on the heart to maintain rate?
    a. Acts to increase filling capabilities of the right atrium
    b. Acts on the atrioventricular and sinoatrial nodes

c. Triggers more forceful contraction from the left ventricle

d. Triggers cranial nerve VI to pace the heart

e. Dilates blood vessels to increase muscle pump rate

40. Which comment is true of the cardiac cycle?
    a. Diastole is when AV valves close
    b. Systole is when AV valves open
    c. Diastole is when blood goes to the ventricle
    d. Systole is the phase of relaxation
    e. Systole plus diastole equals two heart beats

41. Pathologic softening of muscle is called:
    a. Fibromyalgia
    b. Mycoplasma
    c. Myofibrosis
    d. Myomalacia
    e. Myoedema

42. Pathological hardening of muscle is called:
    a. Fibromyalgia
    b. Myosclerosis
    c. Myofibrosis
    d. Myomalacia
    e. Myoedema

43. A myositis that is caused by a parasitic worm *Trichinella spiralis* and occurs from eating undercooked pork is called:
    a. Bovine mysositis
    b. Polymyalgia rheumatica
    c. Trichinosis
    d. Granulomatosis
    e. Ankylosing spondylitis

44. What is a glioma?
    a. A star-shaped nerve cell
    b. A tumor of neuroglia
    c. A myelinated neuron
    d. An inflammation of a glial cell
    e. A form of leukemia

45. What term identifies an accumulation of lymph fluid resulting in subcutaneous swelling?
    a. Lymphedema
    b. Lymphostasis
    c. Lymphoma
    d. Lymphadenopathy
    e. Lymphangiomyomatosis

46. What is the cessation of lymph flow?
    a. Lymphedema
    b. Lymphostasis
    c. Lymphoma
    d. Lymphadenopathy
    e. Lymphangiomyomatosis

47. What is an enlarged spleen?
    a. Hypersplenism
    b. Gaucher disease
    c. Splenomegaly
    d. Splenadenopathy
    e. Splenostasis

48. What is a tumor within a lymphatic tissue?
    a. Lymphedema
    b. Lymphostasis
    c. Lymphoma
    d. Lymphadenopathy
    e. Lymphangiomyomatosis

49. What is Kaposi sarcoma?
    a. Bone marrow tumor
    b. A common tumor caused by pelvic inflammatory disease
    c. An inflamed connective tissue
    d. A deadly form of skin cancer—prevalent in AIDS
    e. A side effect of rheumatoid arthritis

50. What is the inflamed lymph node caused by an infection called?
    a. Lymphedema
    b. Lymphomegaly
    c. Adenitis
    d. Lymphadenopathy
    e. Lymphitis

51. What term identifies a heart rate of 100 beats per minute or less?
    a. Dyscardia
    b. Bradycardia
    c. Normocardia
    d. Tachycardia
    e. Hypercardia

52. What pulse rhythm abnormality occurs in children and young adults where heart rate varies with respiratory cycle?
    a. Sinus arrhythmia
    b. Mitral valve prolapse
    c. Premature ventricular contractions
    d. Atrial fibrillation
    e. Ventricular hypertrophy

53. What condition is identified by a drop of systolic pressure >20 mm Hg and/or pulse increases of 20 beats per minute with a change in standing position?
    a. Recumbent hypotension
    b. Idiosyncranous hypotension
    c. Orthostatic hypotension
    d. Etiological hypotension
    e. Hypersensitivity hypotension

54. What is considered to be hypotension in regularly normotensive adults?
    a. <95/60 mm Hg
    b. <100/65 mm Hg

c. <110/56 mm Hg
d. <115/70 mm Hg
e. <120/65 mm Hg

55. Why does hypotension occur during an acute myocardial infarction?
 a. Increased heart rate
 b. Decreased cardiac output
 c. Increased stroke volume
 d. Decreased respiratory rate
 e. Decreased oxygen

56. Why does hypotension occur with shock?
 a. Increased heart rate
 b. Decreased cardiac output
 c. Increased stroke volume
 d. Decreased respiratory rate
 e. Decreased oxygen

57. Why does hypotension occur with hemorrhage?
 a. Decreased oxygen exchange
 b. Decreased thrombocytes
 c. Decreased blood volume
 d. Increased internal inflammation
 e. Respiratory acidosis

58. Which is not a sign of hypotension caused by decreased cardiac output?
 a. Low blood pressure
 b. Increased pulse rate
 c. Diaphoresis
 d. Hypocalcemia
 e. Blurred vision

59. What referral recommendations should be given to someone with stage 3 hypertension (≥180/≥100)?
 a. Wait 1 month and recheck blood pressure
 b. Refer immediately or wait not more than 1 week
 c. Place patient on immediate bed rest
 d. Refer within 1 month
 e. Confirm reading within 2 months

60. What referral recommendation should be given to someone with stage 2 hypertension (160 to 179/100 to 109)?
 a. Wait 1 month and recheck blood pressure
 b. Refer immediately or wait not more than 1 week
 c. Place patient on immediate bed rest
 d. Refer within 1 month
 e. Confirm reading within 2 months

61. What referral recommendation should be given to someone with stage 1 hypertension (140 to 159/90 to 99)?
 a. Wait 1 month and recheck blood pressure
 b. Refer immediately or wait not more than 1 week
 c. Place patient on immediate bed rest
 d. Refer within 1 month
 e. Confirm reading within 2 months

62. What is optimal adult blood pressure?
 a. 110/65 mm Hg
 b. <120/<80 mm Hg
 c. 130/70 mm Hg
 d. <135/<85 mm Hg
 e. 140/90 mm Hg

63. What is considered normal adult blood pressure?
 a. 110/65 mm Hg
 b. <120/<80 mm Hg
 c. 130/70 mm Hg
 d. <130/<85 mm Hg
 e. 140/90 mm Hg

64. What do the letters in the mnemonic ABCDE mean to identifying dangerous skin lesions?
 a. Anovulation, Boggy, Crimson, Density, Examination
 b. Asymmetry, Border irregularity, Color, Diameter, Elevation
 c. Ascription, Braun, Capsular, Dimensions, Erythema
 d. Abscess, Border, Cytopenia, Density, Edema
 e. Anemia, Boggy, Color, Diameter, Examination

65. What is a benign tan or brown-pigmented area that has accompanied a patient since birth called?
 a. Nevus
 b. Birthmark
 c. Hemaginoma
 d. Macule
 e. Lichenification

66. What are benign flat macules of melanin that occur with sun exposure called?
 a. Nevus
 b. Birthmark
 c. Hemaginoma
 d. Freckles
 e. Lichenification

67. What term is given to a proliferation of melanocytes that are macular or popular?
 a. Nevus
 b. Birthmark
 c. Hemaginoma
 d. Macule
 e. Lichenification

68. What acquired condition is represented by the absence of melanin pigment and light (white) patchy areas on the face, hands, feet, neck, orifices, and folds?
 a. Intertrigo
 b. Psoriasis
 c. Vitiligo
 d. Tinea versicolor
 e. Petichiae

69. What is profuse perspiration?
    a. Gynecomastia
    b. Diaphoresis
    c. Hirsutism
    d. Aphasia
    e. Dysphagia

70. Which syndrome is associated with febrile aspirin use in children during acute viral conditions?
    a. Marfan syndrome
    b. Hemophilia
    c. Wolf-Parkinson-White syndrome
    d. Miliaria rubra
    e. Reye syndrome

71. What is an ordinary name for an upper respiratory viral infection?
    a. Coccidioidomycosis
    b. Common cold
    c. Influenza
    d. Sinusitis
    e. Pharyngitis

72. What families of viruses cause the common cold?
    a. Epstein-Barr virus
    b. Rhinovirus or corona virus
    c. Influenza A virus
    d. Human papillomavirus
    e. Human parvovirus

73. What are the types of influenza?
    a. Types A, B, and C (A is most common)
    b. Types A, B, C, and D (D is most common)
    c. Types I, II, and III (III is most common)
    d. Types α, β, and δ (β is most common)
    e. Types α, β, δ, and γ (α is most common)

74. How is influenza most often spread?
    a. Airborne
    b. Bloodborne
    c. Water vapor and droplet
    d. Improperly prepared food
    e. Sexually transmitted

75. How long does the typical viral upper respiratory infection last?
    a. 3 to 5 days
    b. 7 to 10 days
    c. 10 to 14 days
    d. 14 to 21 days
    e. 21 to 28 days

76. How long does influenza (uncomplicated by secondary infection) last?
    a. 3 to 5 days
    b. 7 to 10 days
    c. 1 to 2 weeks
    d. 2 to 3 weeks
    e. 3 to 4 weeks

77. What are the two common types of measles?
    a. Miliaria profunda and miliaria rubra
    b. Rubeola and rubella
    c. Pertussis and diphtheria
    d. Tetanus and petichiae
    e. Russian and German

78. Which form of measles is less infectious than the other?
    a. Rubella
    b. Russian
    c. Rubeola
    d. Pertussis
    e. Diphtheria

79. How is rubeola spread?
    a. Bloodborne
    b. Water vapor and droplet
    c. Improperly prepared food
    d. Sexually transmitted
    e. Mouth-to-mouth (direct/indirect) and airborne droplets

80. What organism genus causes rubeola?
    a. *Paramyxovirus* (morbillivirus)
    b. *Pseudomonas aeruginosa*
    c. *Legionella pneumophila*
    d. *Clostridium tetani*
    e. *Salmonella*

81. What complications may arise in first trimester pregnant women exposed to rubella?
    a. Miscarriage or birth defects
    b. Eclampsia
    c. Premature rupture of the membranes
    d. Amniotic fluid leakage
    e. Gestational diabetes

82. Which type of measles is referred to as the 9-day measles?
    a. Rubella
    b. Russian
    c. Rubeola
    d. Pertussis
    e. Diphtheria

83. Which type of measles is known commonly as German measles?
    a. Rubella
    b. Russian
    c. Rubeola
    d. Pertussis
    e. Diphtheria

84. Where is the predominant swelling associated with mumps located?
    a. Maxilla and mandible
    b. Mandible and cheeks
    c. Cheeks and neck

d. Neck and shoulder
e. Axilla and upper arm

85. Which sexually transmitted disease is the most common in the United States?
a. Gonorrhea
b. Syphilis
c. Chlamydia
d. Genital herpes
e. Genital warts

86. What is the standard course of treatment of Chlamydia patients?
a. Antifungals
b. Oral antibiotics
c. Antimalarials
d. Antivirals
e. Topical medications

87. Which sexually transmitted disease is referred to as the *clap*?
a. Gonorrhea
b. Syphilis
c. Chlamydia
d. Genital herpes
e. Genital warts

88. What type of organism causes gonorrhea?
a. Bacteria
b. Virus
c. Fungus
d. Protozoa
e. Piron

89. What are the most common types of hepatitis?
a. Types A, B, and C
b. Types A, B, C, and D
c. Types I, II, and III
d. Types α, β, and δ
e. Types α, β, δ, and γ

90. Which hepatitis types are considered to be sexually transmitted diseases?
a. A and B
b. B and C
c. I and II
d. II and III
e. β and δ

91. What name is given to the metabolic disorder that affects the body's production of insulin?
a. Metabolic alkalosis
b. Metabolic acidosis
c. Diabetes mellitus
d. Ketoacidosis
e. Hypoglycemia

92. Which is not a responsibility of insulin?
a. Regulating carbohydrate metabolism
b. Protein synthesis
c. Fat storage
d. Decreasing blood sugar levels
e. Receptor antagonism

93. What condition does glucose levels below 70 mg per dL represent?
a. Hyperglycemia
b. Hypoglucoma
c. Hyperglucoma
d. Hypoglycemia
e. Ketoacidosis

94. What are malignant tumors interfering with the blood-cell producing function of bone marrow and causes anemia called?
a. Carcinoma
b. Neuroma
c. Myelomas
d. Sarcoma
e. Glioma

95. What type of injury or illness presents with hidden or unapparent cause?
a. Fastidious
b. Insidious
c. Etiological unspecific
d. Unintentional
e. Ambiguous

96. What identifies a size decrease in cells with subsequent wasting of tissue?
a. Hypoplasia
b. Hypotrophy
c. Atrophy
d. Sarcopenia
e. Myopenia

97. What is excessive growth of hair in females and children often related to higher than normal androgen levels?
a. Gynecomastia
b. Diaphoresis
c. Hirsutism
d. Aphasia
e. Dysphagia

98. What are abnormal amounts of earwax in the external auditory canal called?
a. Otitis media
b. Otitis external
c. Pericornitis
d. Impacted cerumen
e. Cauliflower ear

99. What gives blackheads their color?
    a. Melatonin and dirt
    b. Melanin and oxidized oil
    c. Impacted dirt and oil
    d. Macrophages and dirt
    e. Mesoderm and oil

100. What is a common over-the-counter application for tinea versicolor?
    a. Calamine lotion
    b. Selsun shampoo (selenium sulfide)

c. Tinactin
d. Lotrimin
e. Hydrocortisone

Use the DVD or visit the website at http://thePoint.lww.com/Long to take the *online examination*.

STUDY CHECKLIST

I have studied:
- [ ] Auscultation and Percussion
- [ ] Hearing and Vision Assessment
- [ ] Vital Sign Assessment
- [ ] Inoculations
- [ ] Health Screenings

- [ ] Birth Control
- [ ] Derma, Head, and Face Assessment
- [ ] Skin Conditions
- [ ] Thorax and Abdomen Conditions
- [ ] Eyes, Ears, Nose, Head, Face, and Throat Conditions
- [ ] Common Illnesses and Diseases

SECTION 5

SUPPLEMENTAL READING

1. American Cancer Society. www.cancer.org. 2007.

2. American Heart Association. www.americanheart.org. 2007.

3. Anderson MK, Parr GP, Hall SJ. *Foundations of athletic training: prevention, assessment, and management*, 4th ed. Philadelphia: Lippincott Williams & Wilkins; 2009.

4. Beers MH, Berkow R, eds. *The Merck manual*, 17th ed. Whitehouse Station: Merck Research Laboratories; 1999.

5. Bernier J. *Quick reference dictionary for athletic training*. Thorofare: Slack Inc; 2005.

6. Binkley HM, Beckett J, Casa DJ, et al. National Athletic Trainers' Association Position Statement: exertional heat illnesses. *J Athl Train*. 2002;347(3):329–343.

7. Cuppett K, Walsh KM. *General medical conditions in the athlete*. St. Louis : Elsevier Science, Mosby; 2005.

8. Follin SA. *Professional guide to signs and Symptoms*, 5th ed. Baltimore: Lippincott Williams & Wilkins; 2007.

9. Howard TM, Butcher JD. *The little black book of sports medicine*, 2nd ed. Sudbury: Jones and Bartlett Publishers; 2006.

10. Jarvis C. *Physical examination and health assessment*, 4th ed. St. Louis: WB Saunders; 2004.

11. Landing GL, Bernhardt DT. *Essentials of primary care sports medicine*. Champaign: Human Kinetics; 2003.

12. National Athletic Trainers' Association. *Athletic training educational competencies*, 4th ed. Dallas, TX: National Athletic Trainers' Association; 2006.

13. Prentice WE. *Arnheim's principles of athletic training: a competency-based approach*. New York: McGraw-Hill; 2006.

14. Skinner JS. *Exercise testing and exercise prescription for special cases theoretical basis and clinical applicator*, 3rd ed. Baltimore: Lippincott Williams & Wilkins; 2005.

15. *Steadman's Medical Dictionary for the Health Professions and Nursing*, 5th ed. Philadelphia: Lippincott Williams & Wilkins; 2005.

16. Thomas CL, ed. *Taber's cyclopedic medical dictionary*. Philadelphia: FA Davis; 1993.

Acute Care of Injuries and Illnesses

Part 1 Responding to Emergencies

Part 2 Skin and Musculoskeletal Injuries

Part 3 Head, Face, Spine, and Thorax Injuries

Part 4 Respiratory and Cardiac Emergencies

Part 5 Environmental Injuries and Illnesses

Part 6 Other Medical Emergencies

Part 7 Ambulation and Moving Patients

Section 6 Examination

OVERVIEW

Evaluating and treating acute injuries is a critical component of an athletic trainer's job, and is the one that athletic trainers are most identified with in regard to the general public. The athletic trainer should possess the ability to quickly evaluate an emergency situation and implement the appropriate techniques for treating the acutely injured or ill patient. Bandaging an open wound, splinting a fracture, treating heat exhaustion, and performing cardiopulmonary resuscitation (CPR) are just a few examples of the knowledge and skills that athletic trainers must possess to perform their job. In addition, having a sound emergency action plan and having readily available appropriate emergency supplies and equipment is also the responsibility of the athletic trainer. The overwhelming majority of injuries and illnesses the athletic trainer will treat will not be life or limb threatening, but the athletic trainer must be prepared at any moment to act in an emergency situation.

CLINICAL PROFICIENCIES

Demonstrate the ability to manage acute injuries and illnesses. This will include surveying the scene, conducting an initial assessment, utilizing universal precautions, activating the emergency action plan, implementing appropriate emergency techniques and procedures, conducting a secondary assessment, and implementing appropriate first aid techniques and procedures for non–life-threatening situations. Effective lines of communication should be established and the results of the assessment, management, and treatment should be documented. (Reproduced with permission of the National Athletic Trainers' Association.)

Responding to Emergencies

KEY TERMS

- Acute compression triad
- Advanced cardiac life support (ACLS)
- Advanced life support (ALS)
- Ambu bag
- Anoxia
- Automatic external defibrillator (AED)
- Beck triad
- Biot respiration
- Blood-borne pathogens
- Gag reflex
- Head-tilt/chin-lift maneuver
- Hemostat
- Occlude
- Occlusion
- Personal protective equipment
- Symptom
- Universal precautions

- EAP locations
  - Posted at each athletic location
- Access to athletic locations
  - Ability to unlock doors/gates
  - Physical addresses for EMS
  - Driving directions for EMS
- Emergency supplies and equipment
  - Location—easily accessible
  - Checked regularly to assure that it works properly
- Communication
  - Prior planning with personnel and EMS
  - Radio, cell phones, and landline phones
  - Parent/guardian notification
  - Administration notification
- Transportation
  - Who transports?
  - Who travels to hospital with athlete?
  - Where will they be transported?
- Rehearsal frequency
  - At the very least annually
  - Additional rehearsal on a regular basis is preferable
- Documentation
  - Training and rehearsal
  - Maintenance of equipment
  - Full description of emergency event and actions taken

PREPARING FOR EMERGENCIES

Emergency Action Plan

- Personnel
  - Certified athletic trainers (ATCs), athletic training students (ATSs), physicians, emergency medical service (EMS), coaches, administrators
  - Educated in emergency action plan (EAP) procedures
  - Trained in first aid, cardiopulmonary resuscitation (CPR), AED, and universal precautions
- Roles and responsibilities
  - Predetermined in EAP
  - Clearly stated
  - Rehearsed on a regular basis
- Policies and procedures
  - In writing
  - Athletic location and sport specific
  - Emergency removal of protective equipment (e.g., football and/or lacrosse helmets)
  - Environmental considerations
  - Athletes versus spectators
  - Emergency transportation
  - Evaluated on a regular basis

> **Quick fact** Emergency action plan education and rehearsal should ideally take place before each athletic season and allow enough time for staff members and other personnel to feel confident about their roles and responsibilities.

 Use the DVD or visit the website at http://thePoint .lww.com/Long for additional information about *emergency supplies and equipment*.

Consent to Treat Patients in an Emergency

- Written consent
  - Obtained from patient before participation
  - Younger than 18—parent/guardian consent
  - Signed document that states the athletic training (AT) staff has permission to treat emergency injuries and/or illnesses
- Verbal consent
  - Patient verbally gives ATC permission to treat in an emergency

- Implied consent
  - In an emergency, if patient is unable to verbally consent to treatment, then it is implied that he or she would want assistance

Emergency Information of Athletes

- Name, social security number, home address, and phone number
- Parent/guardian names, address, and phone number
- Name of emergency contact person, address, and phone number
- Health insurance agency and policy/group number
- Primary care physician, address, and phone number
- Medical conditions
- Allergies
- Family history
- Written consent to treatment in an emergency

PRIMARY ASSESSMENT

Components of the Primary Assessment

- Scene assessment
- Universal (body substance isolation [BSI]) precautions
- Initial impression
- Establish level of (consciousness) responsiveness
- Airway assessment
- Breathing assessment
- Circulation and external bleeding assessment

Scene Assessment

- Safe to approach the patient?
  - Assess situation before providing assistance
- Does patient need to be moved due to immediate danger?
  - Do not move unless it is absolutely necessary
  - If patient must be moved, do so without exacerbating injury

Universal (Body Substance Isolation) Precautions

- Protect against transmission of infectious diseases
  - Examples—Blood-borne pathogens, tuberculosis, meningitis
- Blood-borne pathogens
  - Examples—human immunodeficiency virus (HIV), hepatitis B virus (HBV), hepatitis C virus (HCV)
- Universal (BSI) precautions
  - Personal protective equipment (PPE), handwashing, equipment disinfection
- PPE (see Fig. 6.1)
  - Gloves, gowns, goggles, masks, resuscitation masks

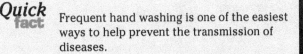

Quick fact Frequent hand washing is one of the easiest ways to help prevent the transmission of diseases.

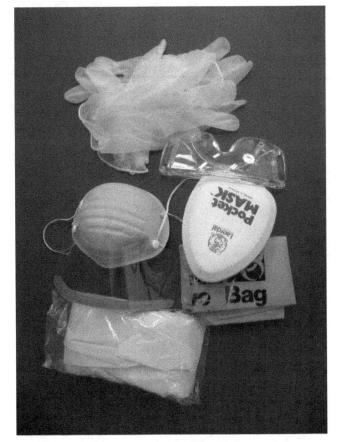

Figure 6.1 Personal Protective Equipment.

Initial Impression

- Observe for multiperson incident
  - If multiple persons are involved, start thinking about priority of care
- What appears to be the nature of the injury or illness?
- Unusual posture of body
  - Decorticate rigidity—extension of legs and flexion of elbow, wrist, and fingers
  - Decerebrate rigidity—extension of arms and legs
  - Gross malalignment of joints
  - Self-splinting of extremities

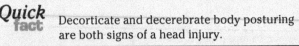

Quick fact Decorticate and decerebrate body posturing are both signs of a head injury.

Establish Level of (Consciousness) Responsiveness

- Determines mental status
- Gently squeeze patient's shoulder (use caution if head and/or spine injured is suspected)
- Loudly ask if they are all right or if they can hear you
- AVPU
  - Alert (A)—awake, responsive, and oriented
  - Verbal (V)—disoriented, response to verbal stimulus

- Pain (P)—eyes closed, no response to verbal stimulus, does respond to painful stimulus (sternal rub or pinch skin)
- Unresponsive (U)—no response to verbal or painful stimulus

> **Quick fact** Always suspect a head and/or spine injury in a patient who is unresponsive.

> **Quick fact** Never use any type of inhalant, such as an ammonia capsule, when attempting to arouse an unconscious patient who could potentially have a head and/or spine injury.

Airway Assessment
- Is airway open and clear?
  - Visible foreign object, blood, and/or vomit
- Clear airway if necessary (gloved hand or portable suction unit if available)
- Establish and manage the airway
  - If no head or spine injury is suspected, perform head-tilt/chin-lift method to open airway
  - If suspecting potential head and/or spine injury, perform jaw-thrust maneuver to open airway
- What if patient is wearing protective sports headgear?
  - Face mask must be removed as soon as possible if airway cannot be established and managed due to face mask

Breathing Assessment
- Is patient breathing?
  - Look—chest to rise/fall?
  - Listen—breath sounds?
  - Feel—breath on your cheek?
  - If not breathing, follow procedures for management of respiratory arrest
- Is the airway obstructed?
  - If so, follow procedures for management of an obstructed airway
  - Causes of obstructions—anatomic (e.g., tongue) or mechanical (e.g., food)
  - Partial obstruction—some type of breath sound is heard (e.g., wheezing, coughing)
  - Complete obstruction—no breath sound is heard
- What if patient is wearing protective sports headgear?
  - Face mask must be removed as soon as possible if (i) breathing cannot be assessed due to face mask, (ii) patient is experiencing difficulty breathing, (iii) patient is unconscious, or (iv) there is suspicion of a spine injury

> **Quick fact** It is very important to maintain an open airway, even for patients who are breathing, because the tongue can easily relax to the back of throat and cause an airway obstruction.

Circulation and External Bleeding Assessment
- Unconscious patient
  - Check carotid pulse (no longer than 10 seconds)
  - If no pulse, follow procedures for management of patient in cardiac arrest
- Conscious patient
  - Check radial pulse
- External bleeding
  - Any significant external bleeding needs to be treated immediately
  - Follow procedures for management of external bleeding

SECONDARY ASSESSMENT

Components of the Secondary Assessment
- Vital signs
- Medical history
- Scalp, skull, and face
- Eyes and ears
- Nose, mouth, and jaw
- Neck and cervical spine
- Clavicles and chest
- Lung sounds
- Abdomen and pelvis
- Lower extremities
- Upper extremities
- Spine and scapula

> **Quick fact** All life-threatening conditions must be addressed before continuing on to the secondary assessment.

> **Quick fact** The secondary assessment is also referred to as a *head-to-toe examination*.

Vital Signs
- Pulse
- Respirations
- Blood pressure
- Skin temperature, moisture level, and color
- Pupillary appearance and response
- Core body temperature
- Blood oxygen saturation level

> **Quick fact** Vital signs should be assessed every 5 minutes.

Pulse
- Palpate carotid artery (at neck) or radial artery (at wrist)
- Count number of beats in 1 minute (30 seconds × 2) (15 seconds × 4)
- Determine rate, strength, and rhythm
  - Rate—rapid or slow?

- ○ Strength—strong or weak?
- ○ Rhythm—regular or irregular?
- Normal pulse rates
  - ○ Adult: 60 to 100 bpm
  - ○ Adolescents: 60 to 105 bpm
  - ○ Child (5 to 12 Years Old): 70 to 110 bpm
  - ○ Child (up to 5 Years Old): 80 to 140 bpm
  - ○ Newborn Infants: 120 to 160 bpm
- Abnormal adult pulse rates
  - ○ <60 bpm = bradycardia
  - ○ >100 bpm = tachycardia
- Abnormal rate and character of pulse
  - ○ Rapid and weak—shock, blood loss, heat exhaustion, diabetic emergency
  - ○ Rapid and strong—heatstroke, high blood pressure
  - ○ Slow and strong—brain injury, skull fracture, stroke
  - ○ No pulse—cardiac arrest

Quick fact An athlete who is well conditioned may have a resting heart rate that is lower than that of the average person.

Respirations
- Observe and feel chest for breathing
- Count number of breaths in 1 minute (30 seconds × 2) (15 seconds × 4)
- Rate of respirations
  - ○ Rapid versus slow
- Character of respirations
  - ○ Rhythm—regular versus irregular
  - ○ Depth—shallow versus deep
  - ○ Sound—wheezing, gurgling, coughing, gasping, and so on
  - ○ Ease—labored, painful, and so on
- Normal respiratory rates
  - ○ Adult: 12 to 20 bpm
  - ○ Child: 15 to 30 bpm
  - ○ Infant: 25 to 50 bpm
- Abnormal respiratory rates
  - ○ Adult: <8 bpm or >28 bpm
  - ○ Child (1 to 5 Years Old): <20 bpm or >30 bpm
  - ○ Child (6 to 10 Years Old): <15 bpm or >30 bpm
- Abnormal rate and character of respirations
  - ○ Rapid and shallow—shock, diabetic emergency
  - ○ Labored, deep, or gasping—myocardial infarction, diabetic emergency
  - ○ Slow—head injury, stroke, chest injury
  - ○ Wheezing—asthma, obstructed airway
  - ○ Gurgling—obstructed airway, lung pathology
  - ○ Snoring—skull fracture, partially obstructed airway

Blood Pressure
- Stethoscope and sphygmomanometer (blood pressure cuff)
- Systolic pressure—pressure in arteries when heart is contracting
- Diastolic pressure—pressure in arteries when heart is relaxed
- Measured in millimeters of mercury (mm Hg)

- Normal adult blood pressure (American Heart Association)
  - ○ <120 systolic and <80 diastolic
- Abnormal adult blood pressure (American Heart Association)
  - ○ Prehypertension: 120 to 139 systolic and/or 80 to 89 diastolic
  - ○ Hypertension: >139 systolic and/or >89 diastolic

Quick fact A drop in normal blood pressure could be an indication of a medical emergency such as severe bleeding, shock, or myocardial infarction.

Skin Temperature, Moisture Level, and Color
- Relative skin temperature
  - ○ Assess with back of hand
  - ○ Hot—heatstroke, inflammation, infection, fever
  - ○ Cool—shock, heat exhaustion, hypothermia, frostbite
- Moisture level
  - ○ Assess with back of hand
  - ○ Dry—heatstroke
  - ○ Diaphoretic (moist)—shock, heat exhaustion
- Skin color
  - ○ Bluish (cyanosis)—choking, hypoxia, respiratory arrest
  - ○ Paleness—shock, hypoxia, heat exhaustion
  - ○ Blackish/bluish—contusion, infection, gangrene
  - ○ Reddish—inflammation, infection, hypertension, increased body temperature, heatstroke
  - ○ Yellowish—hepatitis

Quick fact Cyanosis can be observed in the skin, lips, tongue, and/or nail beds.

Pupillary Appearance and Response
- Observation and penlight assessment
- Normal pupillary responses
  - ○ Constricted—in bright environment
  - ○ Dilated—in dark environment
  - ○ Pupils should be equal in size
  - ○ PEARL—pupils are equal and reactive to light
- Abnormal pupillary responses
  - ○ Constricted (in dark environment)—central nervous system (CNS) damage, drug use
  - ○ Dilated (in bright environment)—unconsciousness, head injury, cardiac arrest
  - ○ Unequal (anisocoria)—head injury, stroke
  - ○ Slow to respond—head injury

Quick fact A small percentage of people may present with anisocoria without any type of injury.

Core Body Temperature
- Methods of assessment
  - Sublingual—under tongue
  - Axillary—within armpit
  - Tympanic—within ear
  - Rectal—within rectum
- Normal core body temperature
  - 98.6° F
- Abnormally high temperature—illness, infection, hyperthermia
- Abnormally low temperature—hypothermia

> **Quick fact** The rectal method of assessing body temperature will provide the most accurate representation of core body temperature.

Blood Oxygen Saturation (SpO₂)
- Amount of hemoglobin (thereby oxygen) in blood
- Measured with a pulse oximeter (noninvasive)
- Normal percentage of oxygen-saturated hemoglobin
  - 90% to 100%
- Abnormal percentage of oxygen-saturated hemoglobin
  - Below 90% = hypoxia

> **Quick fact** With some injuries/illnesses, pulse oximeter readings may not be completely accurate.

Medical History
- Patient information
  - Name and age
  - Other pertinent information
- Chief complaint
  - What hurts?
  - Level and type of pain
  - Symptoms
- Mechanism of injury
  - How did the injury occur?
- Past injury/illness history
  - Has this happened before?
- Major medical conditions
  - Examples—asthma, diabetes
- Allergies
  - Examples—medications, foods, insects
- Medications
  - Currently taking and for what purpose?
- Medical alert identification
  - Bracelet, necklace, or I.D. card
  - Alerts of serious medical conditions
- Time of last meal and liquid consumption
  - May indicate pathology of illness

> **Quick fact** It is important to know the last time a patient has had anything to eat or drink in the event that he or she would require surgery.

SCALP, SKULL, AND FACE

- Observation
  - Lacerations
  - Ecchymosis
  - Battle sign—bruising of mastoid process (indicates skull fracture)
  - Bony deformities and depressions—face and/or skull fracture
  - Facial symmetry—fracture, nerve injury
- Palpation
  - Bony deformities and depressions—face and/or skull fracture
  - Bony crepitus and false movement—fracture
  - Soft tissue structures

> **Quick fact** Lacerations often look worse than what they actually are because of the high vascularity of the scalp.

EYES AND EARS

- Observation
  - Eyelids—lacerations
  - Pupils—size and equality
  - Abnormal pathology—hyphema, subconjuctival hemorrhage
  - Outer ear
  - External auditory canal (using penlight)—cerebrospinal fluid (CSF) or blood
- Halo effect on guaze-indicates presence of CSF

> **Quick fact** Presence of CSF or blood in the ear and/or nose is an indication of a potential facial or skull fracture.

NOSE, MOUTH, AND JAW

- Observation
  - Ecchymosis
  - Deviated septum
  - Nose (with penlight)—CSF and/or blood
  - Unusual odors on breath—fruity or acetone smell (diabetic coma)
  - Cyanosis of lips—lack of oxygen
  - Tongue and lip lacerations
  - Tooth fractures and luxations
  - Blood in mouth
  - Bony deformities of jaw—mandibular fracture
- Palpation
  - Teeth
  - Bony deformities of mandible—mandibular fracture
  - Bony crepitus and false movement—fracture
  - Temporomandibular joint (TMJ)
  - Soft tissue structures

NECK AND CERVICAL SPINE

- Observation
  - Ecchymosis or swelling
  - Distended neck veins—cardiac and/or thoracic condition
  - Deviated trachea—pneumothorax ("collapsed lung")
  - Thyroid cartilage ("Adam's apple")
  - Deformities—damaged trachea, vertebral fracture
- Palpation
  - Thyroid cartilage
  - Bony deformities of cervical vertebra—vertebral fracture/dislocation
  - Bony crepitus and false movement—fracture
  - Subcutaneous emphysema—crepitus sensation with palpation (e.g., trachea injury)
  - Soft tissue structures

> **Quick fact** Subcutaneous emphysema is the presence of air bubbles underneath the skin due to the leaking of air from the trachea or lungs.

CLAVICLES AND CHEST

- Inspection
  - Ecchymosis or swelling
  - Deformities—fractures, dislocations
  - Scars—pacemaker
  - Flail chest injury
  - Unequal chest movement
  - Paradoxical breathing—chest moves outward during inspiration and inward during expiration
- Palpation
  - Clavicle
  - Ribs
  - Bony deformities—fractures, dislocations
  - Bony crepitus and false movement—fracture
  - Subcutaneous emphysema—lung injury
  - Soft tissue structures

LUNG SOUNDS

- Auscultate (listen) using stethoscope
- Presence of unusual or diminished sounds
  - Examples—absent, wheezing, stridor, gurgling, rales, and so on

ABDOMEN AND PELVIS

- Auscultate (listen) abdomen using stethoscope
- Inspection
  - Ecchymosis
  - Abdominal distension—abdominal bleeding, air in stomach
  - Deformities—fractures, dislocations
  - Genital trauma—keep privacy in mind
- Palpation
  - Abdominal quadrants (right upper quadrant [RUQ], left upper quadrant [LUQ], right lower quadrant [RLQ], and left lower quadrant [LLQ])
  - Percussion—tap over region of internal organs
  - Abdominal tenderness, guarding, and/or rigidity
  - Rebound test—pain occurs when releasing pressure
  - Compress iliac crests and pelvis from the sides—instability, false movement, tenderness, and/or crepitus (any of these could indicate fracture)
  - Soft tissue structures

> **Quick fact** A positive rebound test is an indication of an internal injury within the abdomen.

LOWER EXTREMITIES

- Inspection
  - Ecchymosis, lacerations, swelling
  - Deformities—fractures, dislocations
- Palpation
  - Bony deformities—fracture, dislocation
  - Bony crepitus, false movement, pain/tenderness—fracture
  - Soft tissue structures
- Circulation
  - Posterior tibialis pulse—behind medial malleolus
  - Dorsalis pedis pulse—dorsum of foot
- Sensory function
  - Sensation of toes
- Motor function
  - Wiggle toes (as long as it does not exacerbate injury)

UPPER EXTREMITIES

- Inspection
  - Ecchymosis, lacerations, swelling
  - Deformities—fractures, dislocations
- Palpation
  - Bony deformities—fracture, dislocation
  - Bony crepitus, false movement, pain/tenderness—fracture
  - Soft tissue structures
- Circulation
  - Radial pulse—located on thumb side of wrist
- Sensory function
  - Sensation of fingers
- Motor function
  - Wiggle fingers (as long as it does not exacerbate injury)

> **Quick fact** A more thorough neurologic screen can be performed during the secondary assessment in the event that a patient presents with signs and/or symptoms of a neurologic injury.

SPINE AND SCAPULA

- If head and/or spine injury is suspected, patient should be carefully log rolled to inspect back
  - Cervical spine control must be maintained at all times
- Inspection
  - Ecchymosis, lacerations, deformities
- Palpation
  - Bony crepitus, false movement, and pain/tenderness—fracture
  - Soft tissue structures

PART 2
Skin and Musculoskeletal Injuries

SKIN INJURIES

Types Of Open Skin Injuries

- Abrasion—scraped against rough surface
- Avulsion—partially or completely torn away
- Incision—sharply cut
- Laceration—irregularly torn
- Puncture—sharp object penetration

Management of External Bleeding

- Direct pressure
  - Apply sterile gauze or nonadherent dressing
- Elevation
  - Elevate limb above heart level
  - Consider if fracture and/or dislocation is present
- Indirect pressure
  - Upper extremity—brachial artery (upper arm)
  - Lower extremity—femoral artery (groin)
- Splint (if fracture and/or dislocation)
  - Limits movement to prevent exacerbation of injury and additional bleeding
- Tourniquet
  - Last resort method—only used if all other methods are unsuccessful
  - Must be prepared to sacrifice limb in order to save life

Management of Open Wounds

- Apply gloves
- Universal precautions
- Cut away clothing to expose site (if necessary)
- Control bleeding
- Contact EMS, treat for shock, and assess vital signs if bleeding cannot be controlled
- Clean with sterile saline or other appropriate solution
- Debride with sterile gauze pad
- Apply antibiotic ointment (if appropriate)
- Close with superficial skin closures if required
- Dress and bandage

- Refer to physician or hospital if sutures are required or if patient has not received a tetanus booster in last 5 years
- Disinfect equipment used and discard disposable items in biohazardous waste receptacle or sharps container
- Wash hands
- Change dressings (as needed)
- Check wound regularly for signs of infection
- Refer to a physician if wound shows signs of infection or is not healing appropriately

> **Quick fact** Signs of an infection include redness, red streaks, swelling, pain, purulent discharge, increased warmth, and/or elevated core body temperature.

Application of Superficial Skin Closures for Open Wounds

- Select appropriate superficial skin closures
- Apply an appropriate skin adhesive
- Approximate lacerated edges
- Apply the first skin closure strip in the center of the laceration in an inferior to superior direction (for horizontal lacerations)
- Apply the second strip to the right of the first strip in an inferior to superior direction
- Apply the third strip to the left of the first strip in an inferior to superior direction
- Continue procedure until laceration is secured

MUSCULOSKELETAL INJURIES

Initial Treatment of Closed Soft Tissue Injuries

- Rest
  - Stay off injured limb, crutches, sling
- Ice
  - Ice pack or ice bag

- Compression
  - Elastic bandage
- Elevation
  - Above heart level
- Protection
  - Air cast brace, custom splint

 Use the DVD or visit the website at http://thePoint.lww.com/Long for additional material about *types of musculoskeletal injuries.*

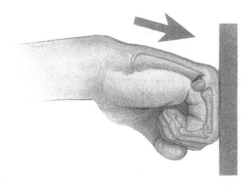

Figure 6.2 Boxer's Fracture. (Asset provided by Anatomical Chart Co.)

Types of Fractures

- Blowout—wall of ocular orbit
- Comminuted—multiple fragments
- Contrecoup—trauma to opposite side of impact site
- Depressed—fracture of skull that appears depressed towards brain
- Greenstick—incomplete fracture to adolescent bone
- Impacted—caused by compressive forces
- Longitudinal—along the length of bone
- Oblique—occurs at an angle
- Serrated—jagged, sharp-edged fracture
- Spiral—due to rotational force
- Transverse—straight line across bone

Quick **fact** A common non–athletic-related cause of a boxer's fracture is directly punching a wall with a closed fist (see Fig. 6.2).

Splinting of Fractures and Dislocations

- Contact EMS if necessary
- Expose injury site

- Manually stabilize the joints proximal and distal to injury
- Stabilize in position found
- Assess circulation (pulse points)
- Assess motor function (fingers or toes)
- Assess sensory function (stroking finger on skin)
- Select appropriate splint
- Splint the joints proximal and distal to injury
- Splint in position found
- Reassess circulation, motor, and sensory function
- Treat for shock and assess vital signs if necessary
- Refer patient to physician or hospital emergency room

Quick **fact** Motor function should not be assessed before and after splinting if it could potentially exacerbate the injury.

P A R T **3** Head, Face, Spine, and Thorax Injuries

KEY TERMS

- Abdominal guarding
- Acromegaly
- Concussion
- Decerebrate rigidity
- Decorticate rigidity
- Epidural hematoma

- Flail chest
- Nystagmus
- Stupor
- Subdural hemorrhage
- Traumatic brain injury (TBI)

HEAD AND FACE INJURIES

Skull Fracture

- Contact EMS
- Manually stabilize head and cervical spine
- Control any external bleeding (avoid additional pressure)
- Maintain open airway and monitor breathing
- If conscious—position supine with upper body/head elevated (if no sign of head/spine injury or shock)
- Treat for shock
- Monitor vital signs
- Transport to hospital by EMS

> **Quick fact**
> If the patient has a potential skull fracture, do not attempt to stop a nosebleed due to the fact that it can increase intracranial pressure.

Cerebral Contusion, Epidural Hematoma, or Subdural Hematoma

- Contact EMS (see Fig. 6.3)
- Maintain open airway and monitor breathing
- Treat for shock
- Monitor vital signs
- Transport to hospital by EMS

> **Quick fact**
> Epidural and subdural hematomas are life-threatening injuries that require prompt management and transportation to a hospital.

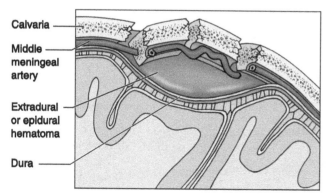

Calvaria

Middle meningeal artery

Extradural or epidural hematoma

Dura

Figure 6.3 An Epidural Hematoma Caused By a Skull Fracture. (From Moore KL, Dalley AF. *Clinical oriented anatomy*, 4th ed. Baltimore: Lippincott Williams & Wilkins; 1999.)

Concussion

- Remove from activity
- If unconscious, you must suspect a head and/or spine injury—patient should be treated appropriately and transported to hospital by EMS
- Question athlete on concussion symptoms
- Perform neurologic screen
- Administer neuropsychological screen (e.g., Standardized Assessment of Concussion test)
- Withdrawal or return to activity is dependent on duration of symptoms, concussion severity, and management protocol of sports medicine team
- Refer to physician or hospital as needed

> **Quick fact**
> If an athlete who has experienced a concussion has been cleared by the sports medicine team, exertional testing should be performed before return to play.

 Use the DVD or visit the website at http://thePoint.lww.com/Long for additional material about *standard assessment of concussion (SAC) testing*.

Second Impact Syndrome

- Contact EMS
- Maintain open airway and monitor breathing
- Treat for shock
- Monitor vital signs
- Transport to hospital by EMS

> **Quick fact**
> Second impact syndrome occurs when an athlete suffers a second concussion before the resolution of symptoms from a prior concussion.

Zygomatic Fracture

- Contact EMS (if necessary)
- Control any bleeding
- Cold application (avoid additional pressure)
- Maintain open airway and monitor breathing
- Treat for shock
- Monitor vital signs
- Refer to physician or transport to hospital by EMS

Maxillary Fracture

- Contact EMS (see Fig. 6.4)
- Control any bleeding
- Maintain open airway and monitor breathing
- Cold application (avoid additional pressure)
- If conscious—position upright and leaning slightly forward

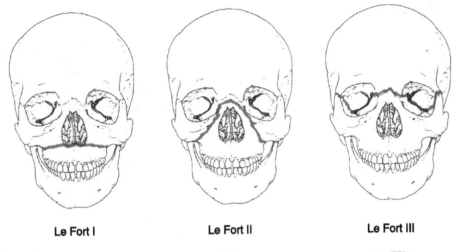

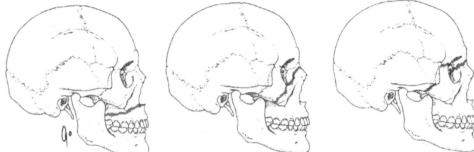

Le Fort I   Le Fort II   Le Fort III

Figure 6.4 LeFort Maxillofacial Fracture Classifications. (From Snell RS. *Clinical anatomy*, 7th ed. Lippincott Williams & Wilkins; 2003.)

- Treat for shock
- Monitor vital signs
- Transport to hospital by EMS

> *Quick* **fact** A patient with a maxillary fracture may present with numbness in the region of the cheek and/or lip, and is a sign of additional nerve trauma.

Mandible Fracture

- Contact EMS (if necessary)
- Control any bleeding
- Maintain open airway and monitor breathing
- Cold application
- Treat for shock
- Monitor vital signs
- Immobilize with bandage that spans under jaw and over head (before applying—ensure that this will not compromise the patient's airway)
- Refer to physician or transport to hospital by EMS

> *Quick* **fact** In the absence of an obvious deformity of the mandible, the tongue blade test can be used to assess for a mandibular fracture.

Auricular Hematoma

- Cold application and compression
- Refer to physician for potential drainage and compression dressing

> *Quick* **fact** Appropriate management of an auricular hematoma is important to prevent the formation of "cauliflower ear."

Tympanic Membrane (Eardrum) Rupture

- Control any bleeding
- Refer to physician or hospital

> *Quick* **fact** Tympanic membrane ruptures will typically heal on their own within a few weeks.

Corneal Abrasion or Laceration

- Instruct patient not to rub the eye
- Patch eye (patching of both eyes may be necessary to limit eye movement)
- Refer to physician or hospital

Quick fact
A hallmark sign of a corneal laceration is a "teardrop"-shaped pupil.

Quick fact
An eye examination that includes the administration of fluorescein dye and viewing with a blue cobalt light or slit-lamp.

Detached Retina
- Patch eye (patching of both eyes may be necessary to limit eye movement)
- Refer to physician or hospital

Hyphema
- Contact EMS (see Fig. 6.5)
- Patch eye (patching of both eyes may be necessary to limit eye movement)
- Position in seated or semireclining position
- Transport to hospital by EMS

Quick fact
A hyphema is due to an accumulation of blood within the anterior chamber of the eye.

Orbital Blowout Fracture or Globe Rupture
- Contact EMS
- Control any bleeding (avoid additional pressure)
- Patch eye (patching of both eyes may be necessary to limit eye movement)
- Transport to hospital by EMS

Quick fact
A hallmark sign of an orbital blowout fracture is the inability to look in an upward direction with the involved eye.

Foreign Bodies in Eye
- Instruct patient not to rub the eye
- Use cotton applicator stick to fold upper eyelid upward
- Use cotton swab or moist sterile gauze to remove the foreign body
- Flush eye with sterile eye wash (ideally with an eye cup)
- If needed, patch both eyes and refer to physician or hospital

Epistaxis (Nosebleed)
- Apply gloves
- Follow universal precautions
- Control bleeding
- Place sterile gauze under nostrils
- Pinch nostrils (if it will not exacerbate injury)
- Tilt head slightly forward
- Cold application
- Maintain open airway
- Do not blow nose
- Cotton nasal plug may be used for return to competition (be careful not to force the plug too far up into the nose)
- Refer to physician or hospital if bleeding cannot be controlled

Quick fact
Blowing the nose during or shortly after a nosebleed has stopped may disrupt the clotting process and therefore is not recommended.

Nasal Fracture or Septal Deviation
- Control any bleeding
- Cold application (avoid additional pressure)
- Maintain open airway
- Do not blow nose
- Refer to physician or hospital

Tooth Extrusion
- Control any bleeding (see Fig. 6.6)
- Attempt to reposition tooth (do not force)
- Refer to dentist or hospital

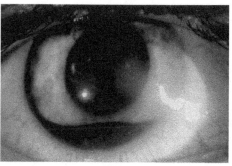

Hyphema

Figure 6.5 Hyphema of the Eye. (From Moore KL, Dalley AF. *Clinical oriented anatomy*, 4th ed. Baltimore: Lippincott Williams & Wilkins; 1999.)

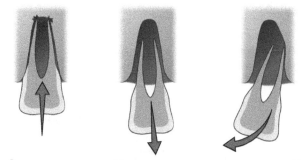

A   B   C

Figure 6.6 Tooth Injuries. **A:** Intrusion. **B:** Extrusion. **C:** Avulsion.

Tooth Intrusion

- Control any bleeding
- Do not attempt to reposition tooth
- Refer to dentist or hospital

Tooth Fracture

- Control any bleeding (Fig. 6.6)
- Refer to dentist or hospital

Tooth Avulsion (Luxation)

- Control any bleeding (Fig. 6.6)
- Handle tooth by the crown only
- Rinse tooth off with saline or milk (do not rub)
- Transport tooth in prepared "tooth-saving" solution, saline, milk, or between cheek and gum
- If care by a dentist will not be available within 30 minutes, attempt to replace tooth within the socket
- Refer to dentist or hospital

Quick fact Handling the tooth by the crown or rubbing it to clean it off can result in damage to the periodontal ligament, and decrease the chance for successful replantation.

SPINE INJURIES

Emergency Management of Head and/or Spine Injury

- Establish manual stabilization of head/neck
- Establish level of consciousness
- Airway assessment
- Breathing assessment
- Circulation and external bleeding assessment
- Activate EMS
- Chief complaint
- Vital signs
- Secondary survey
- Neurologic screen
- Apply cervical collar
- Transfer to spine board
- Apply cervical immobilization device (CID)
- Secure patient to spine board with straps
- Transport to hospital by EMS

Football Helmet and Shoulder Pads Removal for a Spine-Injured Athlete (Inter-Association Task Force for Appropriate Care of the Spine-Injured Athlete)

- Remove face mask (as soon as possible)—using appropriate tool to cut all face mask loop-straps

- One person manually stabilizes head, neck, and helmet
- Cut jersey and other garments of the torso for removal
- Cut all pad straps and laces
- Cut any pad accessories straps/laces (e.g., neck rolls, cowboy collars)
- Other persons appropriately position their hands under athlete in preparation for patient lift
- Another person cuts chinstrap
- Remove cheek pads (using tongue depressor or other stiff, flat instrument)
- Another person manually stabilizes the chin and back of neck for cervical spine stabilization, then person who was stabilizing head, neck, helmet relinquishes control
- Lift patient as one unit using six-person lift
- Slightly rotate helmet forward and slide off of the occiput; if helmet does not move, slight traction can be applied to helmet (do not spread the helmet apart by the ear holes)
- Immediately remove shoulder pads and any pad accessories—spread apart front panels and pull around the head
- Lower patient as one unit
- Cervical spine control at the head and neck is then reestablished, and person who was stabilizing chin and back of neck relinquishes control

Quick fact Removal of the helmet or shoulder pads alone will result in flexion or extension of the cervical spine, therefore they must be removed in conjunction with each other.

Circumstances That Warrant Football Helmet and Shoulder Pads Removal (Inter-Association Task Force for Appropriate Care of the Spine-Injured Athlete)

- Football helmet
  - If face mask cannot be removed in a reasonable period of time in order to access airway
  - If airway cannot be controlled or accessed for ventilation due to design of helmet or chinstrap
  - If head is not securely held in place by helmet and chinstraps thereby preventing appropriate immobilization of head
  - If helmet prevents appropriate immobilization for athlete transport to hospital
- Shoulder pads
  - If the helmet has been removed
  - If there are multiple injuries that require full access to shoulder region
  - If shoulder pads are ill-fitting thereby causing the inability to maintain spinal immobilization

Tools Commonly Used to Remove Football Helmet Face Masks

- FMXtractor
- Trainer's Angel

- Anvil pruner
- Electric screwdriver

> **Quick fact** ATCs should be proficient in removing a football helmet face mask in a safe, efficient, and quick manner.

THORAX INJURIES

Pneumothorax and Hemothorax

- Activate EMS
- Maintain open airway and monitor breathing
- Position seated (unless in shock)
- Treat for shock
- Monitor vital signs
- Transport to hospital by EMS

Pulmonary Contusion and Traumatic Asphyxia

- Activate EMS
- Maintain open airway and monitor breathing
- Treat for shock
- Monitor vital signs
- Transport to hospital by EMS

Hyperventilation

- Instruct patient to breathe in through the nose and out through the mouth
- Calm and reassure patient
- Maintain open airway and monitor breathing
- Monitor vital signs
- Transport to hospital by EMS if necessary

> **Quick fact** In severe cases of hyperventilation, breathing into a paper bag may be effective.

Heart Contusion

- Activate EMS
- Have AED ready if needed
- Maintain open airway and monitor breathing
- Treat for shock
- Monitor vital signs
- Transport to hospital by EMS

Flail Chest Injury

- Activate EMS
- Splint with a pillow
- Maintain open airway and monitor breathing
- Treat for shock
- Monitor vital signs
- Transport to hospital by EMS

> **Quick fact** A hallmark sign of a flail chest injury is when the flail rib segments intrude with inhalation and protrude with exhalation.

Solar (Celiac) Plexus Contusion

- Remove/loosen restrictive equipment and clothing
- Position supine with knees flexed
- Instruct patient to take slow, deep breath
- Maintain open airway and monitor breathing
- Monitor vital signs
- Transport to hospital by EMS if needed

Abdominal Organ Contusion, Laceration, or Rupture

- Activate EMS
- Maintain open airway and monitor breathing
- Supine with knees flexed
- Treat for shock
- Monitor vital signs
- Transport to hospital by EMS

> **Quick fact** If the spleen has been injured, a patient can lose a significant amount of blood in a short period of time due to its high vascularity.

Acute Appendicitis

- Activate EMS
- Treat for shock
- Nothing to eat or drink
- Monitor vital signs
- Transport to hospital by EMS

PART 4

Respiratory and Cardiac Emergencies

KEY TERMS

- Bradycardia
- Bradypnea
- Cheyne-Stokes respiration
- Cyanosis
- Dyspnea
- Hypercapnia
- Hyperpnea
- Hypopnea
- Hypovolemic
- Hypoxemia
- Hypoxia
- Pulmonary edema
- Suffocation
- Tachycardia
- Tachypnea
- Traumatic asphyxia

RESPIRATORY EMERGENCIES

Respiratory Distress

- Activate EMS
- Determine if airway obstruction exists
- If conscious, place in position that makes breathing easier
- Maintain open airway and monitor breathing
- Treat for shock
- Monitor vital signs
- Transport to hospital by EMS

Respiratory Arrest and Rescue Breathing (American Red Cross)

- Unconscious and no breathing, but pulse present
- Treat with rescue breathing using a breathing barrier
- Provide two initial rescue breaths
- If two rescue breaths do not go in, reposition head and attempt two breaths again; if they still do not go in, follow procedures for treating airway obstructions

- Rescue breathing
  - Adult: One breath every 5 seconds
  - Child: One breath every 3 seconds
  - Infant: One breath every 3 seconds
- Each breath—breathe slowly until chest clearly rises (approximately 1 second)
- After approximately 2 minutes, recheck for movement, breathing, and pulse (for no more than 10 seconds)

Quick fact If available, use an oropharyngeal airway and bag-valve mask (BVM) to deliver rescue ventilations to a patient who is not breathing.

Quick fact Gastric distension, due to air within the stomach, is a sign that rescue ventilations are being delivered too long or too forcefully.

Airway Obstructions (American Red Cross)

- Management of conscious patient
  - Adult: Five back blows followed by five abdominal thrusts
  - Child: Five back blows followed by five abdominal thrusts
  - Infant: Five back blows followed by five chest thrusts
- Management of unconscious patient
  - Adult: Five chest thrusts (depth = 1.5 to 2 in.)
  - Child: Five chest thrusts (depth = 1 to 1.5 in.)
  - Infant: Five chest thrusts (depth = 0.5 to 1 in.)
- Foreign object check/removal
  - After five chest thrusts, perform a foreign object check, but only attempt to remove (sweep) it if it is visible
- Hand placement for unconscious patient chest thrusts
  - Adult: Center of chest (both hands)
  - Child: Center of chest (both hands)
  - Infant: Center of chest just below nipple line (two to three fingers)

Quick fact If an adult patient is pregnant or their abdomen is too large to reach around, then use the chest-thrust technique for a conscious choking adult instead of an abdominal thrust.

CARDIAC EMERGENCIES

Angina Pectoris (Chest Pain) or Heart Attack

- Activate EMS
- Have AED ready if needed
- Remove protective equipment and/or restrictive clothing
- Place the patient in a comfortable position (e.g., semisitting)
- Maintain open airway and monitor breathing
- Calm and reassure patient
- Treat for shock
- Monitor vital signs
- Question patient about nitroglycerin use
- Transport to hospital by EMS

Cardiac Arrest and Cardiopulmonary Resuscitation (American Red Cross)

- Unconscious, no breathing, and no pulse
- CPR—combination of rescue breaths and chest compressions
  - Compression rate—100 per minute
- Circulation assessment
  - Adult: Carotid pulse
  - Child: Carotid pulse
  - Infant: Brachial pulse
- One-person CPR (chest compressions and breaths)
  - Adult: 30 compressions and 2 breaths
  - Child: 30 compressions and 2 breaths
  - Infant: 30 compressions and 2 breaths
- Two-person CPR (chest compressions and ventilations)
  - Adult: 30 compressions and 2 breaths
  - Child: 15 compressions and 2 breaths
  - Infant: 15 compressions and 2 breaths
- Hand placement for chest compressions
  - Adult: Center of chest (both hands)
  - Child: Center of chest (one or both hands)
  - Infant: Center of chest just below nipple line (two to three fingers)
- Chest compression depth
  - Adult: 1.5 to 2 in.
  - Child: 1 to 1.5 in.
  - Infant: 0.5 to 1 in.
- Cardiac "chain of survival"
  - Early access: Recognition of cardiac emergency and contacting EMS
  - Early CPR: Start CPR as soon as possible
  - Early defibrillation: The sooner an AED is used, the better chance of survival
  - Early ALS: Provided by emergency medical technicians (EMTs)

Cardiac Arrest and Automated External Defibrillation (American Red Cross)

- Automated external defibrillators (AEDs) assess heart rhythm and defibrillate patients to correct abnormal heart rhythms

- Common abnormal heart rhythms (arrhythmias)
  - Ventricular fibrillation—disorganized electrical activity
  - Ventricular tachycardia—very rapid heart rhythm
- Asystole—no electrical activity of heart
- When warranted, AEDs should be utilized as soon as they are available
- Rapid AED use increases chance of survival for cardiac arrest victims
- Chest should be dry before applying AED pads
- AED pad locations
  - One pad: Upper right chest
  - Other pad: Lower left side
- Using AEDs on children
  - If AED is equipped with pediatric pads, then use them if child is 1 to 8 years old or if the child weighs <55 lb
  - If pediatric pads are not available, you can use adult pads
- Protocol
  - If shock advised: One shock followed by five cycles of CPR (2 minutes) followed by analysis
  - If no shock advised: Five cycles of CPR (2 minutes) followed by analysis
- Precautions for AED use
  - Do not dry patient's chest with alcohol
  - Assure that other persons and resuscitation equipment are not in contact with patient before analyzing or shocking
  - Do not use AED and/or pads manufactured for adults on a child younger than 8 years or weighing <55 lb, unless pediatric pads are not available
  - Do not use pediatric pads on adult patients
  - Do not use if patient is in contact with water
  - Do not use in a moving vehicle
  - Do not use in the presence of flammable or combustible materials
  - Do not use on patient wearing any type of medicated patch on chest (patch must be removed first)
  - Do not use within 6 ft of mobile phones or radios

 Use the DVD or visit the website at http://thePoint.lww.com/Long for additional information about *algorithm for management of cardiorespiratory emergencies.*

Quick fact AEDs will not defibrillate a patient who has no electrical activity of the heart.

PART 5

Environmental Injuries and Illnesses

KEY TERMS

- Relative humidity
- Acclimatization, acclimation
- Altitude sickness
- Frostbite
- Heat cramps
- Heat exhaustion
- Heat stroke, heatstroke
- Acute coronary syndrome
- Cholecystitis

HEAT-RELATED ILLNESSES

Dehydration

- Move to cool environment
- Ingestion of water and/or electrolyte drinks
- Check weight and urine specific gravity (Usg)
- Monitor vital signs
- Transport to hospital if intravenous (IV) fluids are required

Heat Syncope

- Move to cool environment
- Lie down and elevate legs
- Maintain open airway and monitor breathing
- Monitor vital signs
- Ingestion of water and/or electrolyte drinks
- Transport to hospital if necessary

Heat Cramps

- Move to cool environment
- Ingestion of water and/or electrolyte drinks
- Mild stretching
- Ice massage
- Rest
- Transport to hospital if IV fluids are required

Exertional Heat Exhaustion

- Move to cool environment
- Remove any equipment and unnecessary clothing
- Assess rectal core body temperature

- Cool patient until rectal body temperature is approximately 101°F
  - Sponge down with cool water and fan with towels
  - Ice pack or ice towel application over pulse points
- Ingestion of water and diluted electrolyte drink
- If conscious, position supine with legs elevated
- If unconscious, position sidelying on left side
- Maintain open airway and monitor breathing
- Monitor vital signs and CNS status
- Monitor core body temperature (every 5 to 10 minutes)
- Transport to hospital by EMS if necessary

> **Quick fact**
> If a patient is unable to keep down fluids due to nausea and vomiting, they must be transported to the hospital for intravenous (IV) fluids.

Exertional Heatstroke

- Activate EMS
- Move to cool environment, but do not delay cooling
- Remove any equipment and unnecessary clothing
- Assess rectal core body temperature
- Cool patient until rectal body temperature is approximately 101°F to 102°F
  - Full-body cool water immersion (35°F to 59°F)
  - If immersion is not available: ice pack or ice towel application over the body or sponge down with cool water and fan with towels
- Maintain open airway and monitor breathing
- Monitor core body temperature (every 5 to 10 minutes)
- Monitor vital signs and CNS status
- Transport to hospital by EMS

> **Quick fact**
> In the event that a patient is suffering from heat stroke, his or her core body temperature must be lowered as soon as possible.

> **Quick fact**
> Heatstroke involves the inability of the thermoregulatory mechanism to maintain a normal body temperature.

Exertional Hyponatremia

- Activate EMS
- Maintain open airway and monitor breathing
- Monitor vital signs and CNS status
- Transport to hospital by EMS

> **Quick fact**
> Exertional hyponatremia is due to a decrease in sodium levels and an excessive amount of water in the body.

COLD-RELATED INJURIES AND ILLNESSES

Hypothermia

- Activate EMS
- Remove from cold environment
- Assess rectal core body temperature
- Remove wet clothing and apply dry clothing
- Place blanket above and below patient and cover top of head
- If mild hypothermia
  - Apply hot packs to back of neck, armpits, and groins
  - If able, drink warm fluids (avoid drink with stimulants—e.g., coffee)
- If moderate to severe hypothermia
  - Do not attempt to rewarm on-site (this is best performed at hospital)
- Maintain open airway and monitor breathing
- Monitor vital signs and CNS status
- Transport to hospital by EMS

> **Quick fact**
> When assessing the pulse of a patient who is suffering from hypothermia, check the carotid pulse for a longer period of time.

Superficial (Early) Frostbite

- Activate EMS
- Remove from cold environment
- Remove wet clothing and jewelry
- Dry the skin
- Gradually rewarm body part
  - Wrap extremity in blanket and slightly elevate
  - If hands, additionally place hands under axilla
- Monitor for hypothermia
- Transport to hospital by EMS (if transport will be delayed, immerse body part in water (100 °F to 105 °F)

Deep (Late) Frostbite

- Activate EMS
- Remove from cold environment
- Remove wet clothing and jewelry
- Dry off skin
- Apply sterile dressing (if fingers/toes are involved, place sterile dressing between each digit)
- Do not actively rewarm area (this is best performed at hospital)
- Monitor for hypothermia
- Transport to hospital by EMS

OTHER ENVIRONMENTAL INJURIES

Lightning Strike

- Activate EMS
- If scene is unsafe due to environmental conditions, move patient to a safe location for treatment
- Perform primary assessment
- Administer rescue breathing, CPR, and/or AED as necessary
- Transport to hospital by EMS

PART 6 — Other Medical Emergencies

SHOCK

Types of Shock

- Anaphylactic shock—severe allergic reaction
- Cardiogenic shock—heart cannot effectively pump blood
- Hemorrhagic shock—loss of blood due to internal/external bleeding
- Hypovolemic shock—loss of blood/plasma due to injury/illness
- Metabolic shock—excessive loss of body fluid due to illness
- Neurogenic shock—blood vessels dilate
- Psychogenic shock—syncope (fainting)
- Respiratory shock—lungs are unable to supply adequate oxygen to blood
- Septic shock—blood vessels dilate due to infection

Management of Shock

- Activate EMS
- Maintain open airway and monitor breathing
- Control any external bleeding
- Lay patient supine (unless another position is necessary due to injury)

- Elevate legs above heart (8 to 12 in.) unless position will exacerbate injury
- Splint all fractures and/or dislocations
- Maintain normal body temperature
- Do not give anything to eat or drink
- Monitor vital signs
- Transport to hospital by EMS

DIABETIC EMERGENCIES

Hyperglycemia and Diabetic Coma

- Activate EMS
- Place in recovery position
- Treat for shock
- Maintain open airway and monitor breathing
- Monitor vital signs
- Measure blood glucose level with glucometer
- Transport to hospital by EMS

Quick fact Untreated hyperglycemia can progress to diabetic coma, and untreated hypoglycemia can progress to insulin shock—both can lead to death if not treated appropriately.

Hypoglycemia and Insulin Shock

- Activate EMS
- Measure blood glucose level with glucometer
- If responsive and has a gag reflex, administer oral glucose, sugar, candy, orange juice, or soda that has sugar in it
- Treat for shock
- Maintain open airway and monitor breathing
- Monitor vital signs
- Transport to hospital by EMS

Quick fact If you are unsure if a person is suffering from hypoglycemia or hyperglycemia, go ahead and administer oral glucose or other food/drink with sugar as long as the person is conscious and has a gag reflex.

ASTHMA AND ALLERGIC REACTIONS

Asthma Attack

- Remove patient from area (if caused by environmental trigger)
- Position seated with arms above head
- Control breathing rate
- Calm and reassure
- Use emergency inhaler (if one has been prescribed)
- Give water
- Maintain open airway and monitor breathing
- Monitor vital signs
- Activate EMS if necessary

Quick fact If baseline measurements have been obtained, a peak flow meter can be used to assess an athlete's ability to return to competition after experiencing an asthma attack.

Using an Emergency Inhaler

- Remove cap
- Shake inhaler
- Completely exhale through mouth
- Position inhaler in mouth so that it is upright and the lips create a good seal
- Press down on inhaler while slowly breathing in
- Hold breath for as long as possible
- Remove inhaler from mouth
- Repeat dose as directed by physician

Insect Stings for Nonallergic Patients

- Remove stinger—scrape away from skin (plastic credit card works well)
- Clean site with soap and water
- Apply insect sting/bite medication
- Place ice pack over the area
- Patient may administer an over-the-counter (OTC) antihistamine (if not allergic to antihistamine)
- Refer to physician or hospital if necessary

Quick fact Insect stings in patients who are allergic can lead to anaphylactic shock.

Anaphylactic Shock and Using an Epinephrine Autoinjector (EpiPen)

- Remove autoinjector from case
- Remove safety cap from autoinjector
- Hold autoinjector with black tip pointing toward outer thigh
- Swing autoinjector and jab firmly into outer thigh at a 90-degree angle (see Fig. 6.7)
- Hold against thigh for 10 seconds
- Remove autoinjector from outer thigh
- Massage thigh at site of injection for 10 seconds
- Activate EMS
- Maintain open airway and monitor breathing
- Treat for shock
- Monitor vital signs
- Transport to hospital by EMS

POISONINGS

Poisonous Spider Bite (Black Widow or Brown Recluse)

- Activate EMS
- Position patient supine

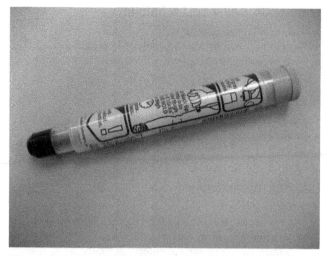

Figure 6.7 The EpiPen Trainer can be Used to Help Instruct an Individual on How to Administer Epinephrine.

- Remove any jewelry from hands and fingers
- Clean site with soap and water
- Keep extremity immobilized and below level of heart
- Maintain open airway and monitor breathing
- Treat for shock
- Monitor vital signs
- Find the spider (if you can do so safely) and send to hospital (dead or alive)
- Transport to hospital by EMS

Poisonous Snakebite

- Activate EMS
- Position patient supine
- Remove any jewelry from hands and fingers
- Clean site with soap and water
- Keep extremity immobilized and below level of heart
- Treat for shock
- Maintain open airway and monitor breathing
- Monitor vital signs
- Transport to hospital by EMS

OTHER EMERGENCIES

Seizures

- Activate EMS
- Place patient on floor/ground
- Do not force any object between teeth or into mouth
- Loosen restrictive clothing
- Protect patient from injury but do not attempt to hold the person still
- Place in recovery position after seizure has stopped
- Maintain open airway and monitor breathing
- Monitor vital signs
- Transport to hospital by EMS

PART 7 Ambulation and Moving Patients

CRUTCHES AND CANES

Crutch Fitting

- Assure crutches are in safe working condition
- Shoes on
- Crutch tips 6 in. from outer margin of shoe
- Crutch tips 2 in. in front of shoe
- Underarm crutch brace 1 in. below axilla
- Elbow flexed approximately 30 degrees

Crutch Walking Instruction

- Three-point gait (tripod method)
  - Stand on uninjured foot
  - Place crutch tips 12 to 15 in. ahead
  - Lean forward and straighten elbows
  - Pull upper cross-piece against thorax
  - Swing injured extremity between crutches
  - Avoid applying pressure on axilla
- Four-point gait
  - Stand on both feet
  - Move one crutch forward while opposite foot steps forward
  - Move crutch on the other side forward while opposite foot steps forward
- Going up the stairs
  - Move uninvolved extremity up one step
  - Transfer body weight to uninvolved extremity
  - Crutch tips and involved extremity move up one step
- Going down the stairs
  - Crutch tips and involved extremity move down one step
  - Move uninvolved extremity down one step

> **Quick fact**
> Placing excessive pressure within the axilla with crutches can potentially cause damage to the nerves and blood vessels within the upper arm.

> **Quick fact**
> If a handrail is available, use the three-point gait, with both crutches in outside hand.

Cane Fitting

- Shoes on
- Cane should span from superior aspect of greater trochanter down to floor

Cane Walking Instruction

- Assure that cane is in safe working condition
- Hold cane in hand on uninvolved side
- Move cane forward simultaneously with involved extremity

MOVING PATIENTS

Ambulatory Assistance

- Walking assist technique
- Patient is able to walk but requires some assistance
- Ideally, a person on each side of the patient is needed to assist

Manual Conveyance Technique

- Two-person seat carry
- Patient may not be able to walk with assistance
- Two persons carry patient with support under each leg

Stretcher Carry

- Patient moved using stretcher
- Safest and most of the time easiest way to move patient

Log Roll Technique

- When is it used?
  - Patient needs to be in a supine position to assess airway, breathing, and circulation properly and/or to administer appropriate emergency care
  - Patient needs to be transferred onto a spine board for EMS transport
- How many people are needed?
  - A minimum of two persons needed
  - Ideally, a minimum of four persons to limit movement of head and spine

Six-Person Lift Technique

- When is it used?
  - When the patient needs to be transferred onto a spine board for EMS transport
  - When it is necessary to remove the football helmet and shoulder pads of a patient in order to provide appropriate care

1. Which would best describe an abnormal respiratory rate?
   a. 6 bpm
   b. 10 bpm
   c. 12 bpm
   d. 20 bpm
   e. 26 bpm

2. Within what period of time do you have to place a luxated tooth back into its socket in order to give the tooth the best chance of survival?
   a. Within 30 minutes
   b. Between 30 minutes and 1 hour
   c. Within 2 hours
   d. Between 2 and 3 hours
   e. Within 3.5 hours

3. Which of the following is best described as a harsh vibrating sound heard during lung auscultation?
   a. Rales
   b. Stridor
   c. Gurgle
   d. Wheezing
   e. Bronchi

4. What medical specialist would you refer an athlete to if he or she has a deviated septum?
   a. An orthopaedist
   b. ENT
   c. An ophthalmologist
   d. A neurologist
   e. A maxillofacial specialist

5. What technique would you use to open the airway of an unconscious athlete who may have a potential head and/or neck injury?
   a. Head tilt-chin lift
   b. Foreign object finger sweep
   c. Abdominal thrusts
   d. Look, listen, and feel
   e. Jaw thrust maneuver

6. When examining the pupil you notice that it appears to have a "teardrop" shape to it. This is an indication of what type of injury?
   a. Traumatic iritis
   b. Detached retina
   c. Intracranial injury
   d. Corneal laceration
   e. Blepharoptosis

7. A rapid and weak pulse in a patient would be an indication of which of the following conditions?
   a. Heatstroke
   b. Shock
   c. Cardiac arrest
   d. Severe external bleeding
   e. Severe internal bleeding

8. Which is *false* regarding blood pressure?
   a. Systolic pressure is the pressure exerted on the arterial walls when the heart is relaxed
   b. A systolic blood pressure of 140 mm Hg is considered to be hypertensive
   c. Low blood pressure could be a sign of shock
   d. A diastolic blood pressure of 85 mm Hg is considered to be prehypertensive
   e. Is measured as diastolic over systolic

9. What does the term *tachypnea* mean in regard to an adult patient?
   a. The patient has a systolic blood pressure that is greater than the diastolic blood pressure
   b. The patient has a respiration rate that is >20 breaths per minute
   c. The patient has a heart rate that is <60 beats per minute
   d. The patient demonstrates an irregular heart rate when the pulse is assessed at the radial artery
   e. The patient demonstrates an abnormal pupillary response when you shine a penlight in the eyes

10. A reddish discoloration of the skin is a sign of what condition?
    a. Shock
    b. Hypoxia
    c. Hypertension
    d. Contusion
    e. Hepatitis

11. Which of the following is NOT a sign or symptom of shock?
    a. Moist, cool skin
    b. Vomiting
    c. Rapid pulse

d. Slow breathing

e. Loss of consciousness

12. What is the proper positioning of the stethoscope on the diaphragm when assessing lung sounds on the back?
    a. Below the inferior angle of the scapula
    b. Directly over the top of the xiphoid process
    c. Just above the clavicle
    d. Directly over the scapula
    e. Just below the acromion process of the scapula

13. Which of the following types of injuries can be potentially life threatening if not treated properly?
    a. Radioulnar joint dislocation
    b. Acute glenohumeral joint subluxation
    c. Talocrural joint dislocation
    d. Chronic glenohumeral joint dislocation
    e. Posterior sternoclavicular joint dislocation

14. Battle sign is an indication of what type of injury in a patient?
    a. Damaged trachea
    b. Deviated septum
    c. Skull fracture
    d. Stroke
    e. Fractured nose

15. What is the cause of commotio cordis?
    a. An obstruction of the coronary arteries
    b. Marfan syndrome
    c. Hypertrophic cardiomyopathy
    d. A blunt force chest trauma over the heart region between contractions
    e. Dangerous arrhythmia due to a lightning strike

16. A cross-country runner comes to you in the athletic training room saying he or she may have been bitten on the leg by something when stretching before practice 2 days ago. There is a clearly noticeable area on the calf that appears bluish in color with white edges, which is surrounded by a red halo. The bite of what creature is most likely responsible for this type of skin lesion?
    a. A black widow spider
    b. A brown recluse spider
    c. A mosquito
    d. A hornet
    e. A coral snake

17. A field hockey athlete was stung by a yellow jacket at practice. He or she reports to you about feeling sick, that the throat feels like it is swelling up, and also tells you that he or she is allergic to bees. What type of shock is this athlete experiencing?
    a. Septic
    b. Hypovolemic
    c. Anaphylactic

d. Neurogenic

e. None of the above

18. Which of the following is FALSE regarding injuries to the throat?
    a. Severe neck lacerations could potentially lead to an air embolism in the bloodstream
    b. Peak swelling due to throat contusions occurs approximately 2 hours post injury
    c. Bloody sputum that is coughed up after a throat contusion warrants activation of EMS
    d. Trauma-induced laryngospasm warrants activation of EMS
    e. Subcutaneous crepitus in the neck is an indication of air escaping from the trachea

19. Where do you place the thermometer to assess a person's core body temperature tympanically?
    a. Beneath the tongue
    b. Within the armpit
    c. Within the ear
    d. Within the groin
    e. Within the rectum

20. Which pulse is the most appropriate to assess when determining the circulation status of the lower extremity?
    a. Radial pulse
    b. Posterior tibial pulse
    c. Brachial pulse
    d. Femoral
    e. Carotid

21. What piece of stabilizing equipment should be applied around the neck of a spine-injured athlete before placing him or her on the backboard?
    a. Towel rolls
    b. A rigid cervical collar
    c. A cervical immobilization device
    d. An air splint
    e. A SAM splint

22. What is the purpose of conducting a secondary survey on a patient?
    a. To check the status of the airway and circulation
    b. To perform a complete check of the neurologic status
    c. To assess for any severe external bleeding
    d. To perform a complete head-to-toe evaluation for any injuries
    e. To determine if the patient needs to be removed immediately away from the scene of the accident

23. What is the appropriate number of chest compressions per cycle when performing two-person CPR on an adult patient?
    a. 5 compressions
    b. 10 compressions
    c. 15 compressions

d. 20 compressions

e. 30 compressions

24. How long should an EpiPen be held in place after being injected into the thigh?

a. 5 seconds

b. 10 seconds

c. 30 seconds

d. 1 minute

e. 2 minutes

25. The tongue blade test is used to assess for what type of injury?

a. Zygoma fracture

b. Mandible fracture

c. TMJ subluxation

d. Laryngospasm

e. Tooth fracture

26. How long can the bloodborne pathogen known as *HBV* live outside the body?

a. 24 hours

b. 72 hours

c. For at least 7 days

d. It dies immediately once it is in a dry state

e. It cannot survive outside the body in a dry state or a liquid state

27. What organ of the body is responsible for secreting the hormone known as *insulin*?

a. Liver

b. Stomach

c. Kidney

d. Spleen

e. Pancreas

28. What type of splint should you ideally use to immobilize an obvious fracture of the tibia and fibula bones of the lower leg?

a. A SAM splint

b. An air splint

c. A stax splint

d. A rapid form vacuum splint

e. A half-ring traction splint

29. In the event that you need to remove the football helmet of an athlete with a spine injury, in what direction should you slightly rotate the helmet as you remove it?

a. Forward

b. Backward

c. To the right side

d. To the left side

e. You do not rotate it at all

30. In what position should you transport a patient with a potential skull fracture?

a. Supine, with upper body and head elevated

b. Prone, with the legs elevated

c. Sidelying, with the knees bent

d. Supine, with the legs elevated

e. Prone, with the upper body and head elevated

31. Which of the following would be an indication of an internal thoracic injury in a patient?

a. A deviated trachea

b. CSF fluid leaking from the nose

c. Crepitus when palpating the pelvis

d. Unequal pupil size

e. Battle sign

32. What should you do if both direct pressure and elevation are not helping to control the bleeding of a moderate-to-severe open wound of the lower leg that does not involve a fracture?

a. Immobilize the leg with a vacuum splint

b. Apply pressure over the radial pulse with your hand

c. Apply a tourniquet just above the open wound

d. Apply pressure over the femoral artery with your other hand

e. Continue with direct pressure and elevation and wait for EMS to arrive

33. What is the appropriate ratio when performing rescue breathing for a child?

a. One breath every 3 seconds

b. One breath every 5 seconds

c. Two breaths every 3 seconds

d. Two breaths every 5 seconds

e. None of the above

34. What works best for removing a wasp stinger from a person's skin?

a. Fingernail clippers

b. Tweezers

c. A fingernail

d. Miniature forceps

e. A plastic credit card

35. Which of the following is a sign or symptom of hypoglycemia?

a. Dry, red, warm skin

b. Breath that smells like fingernail polish

c. Intense hunger and drooling

d. Dry mouth and intense thirst

e. Gradual onset over a period of days

36. What is the term used to describe a condition in which the heart's ventricle chambers contract at an extremely rapid rate?

a. Ventricular fibrillation

b. Diastole

c. Ventricular tachycardia

d. Ventricular defibrillation

e. Asystole

37. What is a scoop stretcher used for?
    a. To transport an athlete from the ground into an ambulance
    b. To transfer a patient from the ground onto a spine board
    c. To transport a patient off the athletic field to the sidelines
    d. To transfer an athlete from a spine board to a treatment table
    e. To transfer an athlete from a spine board into an ambulance

38. What is the best location to assess for a pulse in an unconscious adult patient?
    a. Dorsal pedal pulse
    b. Femoral pulse
    c. Brachial pulse
    d. Carotid pulse
    e. Ulnar pulse

39. You are examining an unconscious athlete, and during the secondary survey you discover that CSF is leaking from the ear. This would indicate an injury to which of the following structures?
    a. Nose
    b. Sinuses
    c. Brain
    d. Throat
    e. Eye

40. What should your chest compression depth be when performing CPR on an adult?
    a. 0.5 to 1 in.
    b. 1 to 1.5 in.
    c. 1.5 to 2 in.
    d. 2 to 2.5 in.
    e. 2.5 to 3 in.

41. When performing palpation of a patient's arm, which of the following would be the best indication of a potential fracture?
    a. Pain
    b. Swelling
    c. Bruising
    d. Increased skin temperature
    e. False movement

42. What is the term for pupils that are unequal in size?
    a. Enophthalmos
    b. Anisocoria
    c. Diplopia
    d. Exophthalmos
    e. PEARL

43. What is the sign of a positive rebound test when palpating the abdomen?
    a. The patient experiences nausea when palpation is conducted

b. The patient experiences pain with palpation but none with release
c. The patient experiences dizziness with palpation
d. The patient experiences pain when palpation is released
e. The patient does not experience any pain at all with palpation

44. Which type of shock can occur due to loss of blood?
    a. Metabolic
    b. Septic
    c. Hypovolemic
    d. Psychogenic
    e. Neurogenic

45. What is the term for the process of removing foreign material from an open wound?
    a. Extortion
    b. Debridement
    c. Scrubbing
    d. Extraction
    e. Excision

46. Which of the following should NOT be performed if an athlete is suffering from moderate epistaxis?
    a. Pinching of the nostrils
    b. Tilting of the head slightly backward
    c. Application of a cold pack
    d. Instructing the athlete to sit down
    e. Inserting of a cotton nasal plug

47. Over what artery would you apply pressure to help control severe bleeding of a lower leg wound?
    a. Carotid
    b. Aortic
    c. Radial
    d. Femoral
    e. Brachial

48. What specific ocular structure should you look at when assessing an athlete for a possible hyphema?
    a. Sclera
    b. Cornea
    c. Pupil
    d. Conjunctiva
    e. Iris

49. Exertional hyponatremia is due to excessive levels of water and low levels of which of the following minerals?
    a. Sodium
    b. Potassium
    c. Calcium
    d. Iron
    e. Zinc

50. What would be the ideal way of handling a spine-injured athlete who starts to vomit

after he or she has already been secured onto a spine board?
a. Remove spider-straps and log roll athlete onto side
b. Log roll athlete and spine board to the side
c. Provide the athlete with an emesis (vomit) basin
d. Use an automatic suction unit
e. Remove spider-straps and let the athlete sit up to vomit

51. What is the most ideal technique for resuscitating a spine-injured athlete who is not breathing but has a pulse?
a. Rescue breathing using a bag-valve mask
b. CPR using mouth-to-mouth technique
c. CPR using a resuscitation mask
d. Rescue breathing using a resuscitation mask
e. CPR using a bag-valve mask

52. Which of the following tools should NOT be used to remove the face mask of a spine-injured football player?
a. A bolt cutter
b. An FM extractor
c. Ratchet pruners
d. An electric screwdriver
e. The Trainer's Angel

53. Which of the following is NOT an indication of increasing intracranial pressure?
a. Decreasing blood pressure
b. Irregular tracking of the eyes
c. Severe headache
d. Irregular respirations
e. Nausea

54. Tinnitus is best described as which of the following?
a. Temporary confusion
b. Dizziness
c. Nausea
d. Unsteady balance
e. Ringing of the ears

55. How would you treat an athlete who has suffered a tooth intrusion?
a. Rinse off the tooth and place it back into the socket
b. Attempt to move the tooth back to its normal position
c. Instruct the athlete to put the tooth underneath the tongue
d. Put the tooth in a glass of whole milk
e. Refer the athlete to a dentist immediately

56. Which of the following would best describe a decorticate posture?
a. Extension of the arms and flexion of the knees
b. Extension of both the arms and legs
c. Flexion of both the knees and elbows

d. Extension of legs and the arms in the position of being crossed
e. Extension of the legs with flexion of the elbows, wrists, and fingers

57. Which technique should NOT be used to arouse an unconscious spine-injured athlete?
a. Sternal rub
b. Verbal stimuli
c. Ammonia capsule
d. Painful stimuli
e. Pinching the skin

58. Which of the following is FALSE regarding facial lacerations?
a. A facial laceration that is 1.5 in. long and quarter inch deep should be closed with wound closure strips
b. The wound should be cleaned with either sterile saline or an antiseptic solution
c. If the laceration requires sutures, the athlete should be referred to a physician within 10 hours
d. Sterile gauze should be used to control bleeding before wound closure
e. A tetanus shot is always required when an athlete sustains a facial laceration

59. Pain at the location of the McBurney point indicates an injury to which structure?
a. The spleen
b. The urinary bladder
c. The appendix
d. The kidney
e. The large intestine

60. How would you treat a dislocation of the proximal interphalangeal joint of the index finger of an athlete who is participating in a baseball game?
a. Reduce the dislocation, buddy-tape to third digit, and allow athlete to return to game
b. Splint in the position found and refer to hospital emergency department immediately
c. Splint the athlete with an aluminum splint, allow athlete to return to game, and refer to hospital emergency room after the game
d. Buddy-tape the finger to the first digit and allow the athlete to return to play
e. Reduce the dislocation, and refer athlete directly to hospital emergency department

61. What treatment measure would be contraindicated for an athlete who has suffered a severe quadriceps contusion?
a. A massage
b. Range of motion
c. Ice
d. Compression
e. NSAIDs

62. Which of the following can be utilized to assess for internal bleeding in the abdominal cavity?
    a. Refractometry
    b. The rib compression test
    c. Lung auscultations
    d. Abdominal percussion
    e. The Kehr test

63. In what position do you want to place an unconscious athlete suffering from heat exhaustion?
    a. Prone
    b. Supine with legs elevated
    c. Lying on left side
    d. Supine
    e. Lying on right side with knees bent toward chest

64. What is the most common cause of airway obstruction in unconscious patients?
    a. Vomit
    b. Mucus
    c. Foreign object
    d. Tongue
    e. Blood

65. What is the fracture called when two bony fragments have a "saw tooth" appearance?
    a. Serrated
    b. Comminuted
    c. Spiral
    d. Greenstick
    e. Oblique

66. Which of the following can be administered to an athlete to assess for a concussion?
    a. AVPU
    b. SAC
    c. PEARL
    d. BVM
    e. CAD

67. An athlete who has experienced a splenic rupture would report Kehr sign at which location?
    a. The right groin
    b. The right lower abdominal quadrant
    c. The right lower back
    d. The left shoulder
    e. The manubrium of the sternum

68. What is the term used to describe a condition in which a patient experiences difficulty breathing?
    a. Dyspnea
    b. Subcutaneous emphysema
    c. Laryngospasm
    d. Cyanosis
    e. Vocal cord spasm

69. What medical specialist would you refer an athlete to if he or she has hyphema?
    a. A periodontist
    b. A dentist
    c. ENT
    d. An orthodontist
    e. An ophthalmologist

70. At what point should the face mask be removed in the event of a spine-injured football player?
    a. After the player has been secured to the spine board
    b. As soon as possible
    c. After a rigid cervical collar has been applied
    d. The face mask should never be removed unless artificial ventilation is necessary
    e. After the shoulder pads have been removed

71. A rapid and weak pulse is a sign of which of the following conditions?
    a. Heat exhaustion
    b. Hypertension
    c. Skull fracture
    d. Heat stroke
    e. Brain injury

72. What is the best technique to use in order to splint an athlete with a fractured mandible?
    a. Apply a rigid cervical collar
    b. Apply a CID
    c. Apply a flexible aluminum splint under the jaw
    d. Apply a bandage that spans around the jaw and head
    e. Apply a bandage that spans under the jaw and over the head

73. The inability of a patient to look upward after being hit in the eye with a racquetball is an indication of what type of injury?
    a. Hyphema
    b. Orbital blowout fracture
    c. Corneal laceration
    d. Auricular hematoma
    e. Detached retina

74. What is the name of the lightweight, aluminum, flexible splint that can be conformed to a body part?
    a. SAM splint
    b. Thermoplastic splint
    c. Air splint
    d. Board splint
    e. Vacuum splint

75. Which is the most appropriate technique to use in order to remove a foreign object from an unconscious patient's airway?
    a. Chest compressions
    b. Heimlich maneuver
    c. Back blows
    d. Chest thrusts
    e. Back blows and chest thrusts

76. A bluish discoloration of the skin, lips, and fingernail beds is termed as which of the following?
   a. Hyperemia
   b. Hypoxia
   c. Cyanosis
   d. Diaphoretic
   e. Erythema

77. What test would be the best to perform to rule out an upper motor neuron lesion in a patient?
   a. The Oppenheim test
   b. The Romberg test
   c. The stork standing test
   d. The tandem walking test
   e. The Chvostek test

78. You are treating a spine-injured football player and determine that you have to remove the football helmet. Why do you need to additionally remove the shoulder pads?
   a. To assess the thoracic spine for fractures
   b. To maintain in-line stabilization of the spine
   c. To be prepared to perform CPR if necessary
   d. To assess the posterior thorax for injury
   e. To allow the athlete to breathe more effectively

79. Which of the following is TRUE regarding a flail chest injury?
   a. It only involves the first four ribs of the thoracic cage
   b. It occurs when a single rib is fractured in multiple locations
   c. A pneumothorax is not a potential complication
   d. Exhalation causes the flail segment to protrude out
   e. It usually occurs during a violent twisting of the thoracic spine

80. What structure can be palpated in the left upper quadrant of the abdomen?
   a. The liver
   b. The urinary bladder
   c. The gall bladder
   d. The appendix
   e. The spleen

81. Which of the following tests would be the most difficult to perform on the sidelines, during an athletic event, if you needed to assess an athlete for a concussion?
   a. The SAC test
   b. The tandem walk test
   c. The Romberg test
   d. The balance error scoring system (BESS) test
   e. The pupillary reaction test

82. What technique should be used to move a potential spine-injured patient from a prone position to a supine position to assess breathing?
   a. A manual conveyance
   b. A four-person lift

   c. An ambulatory assist
   d. A six-person lift
   e. A log roll

83. Which of the following should NOT be performed if you suspect that a person has been bitten by a poisonous spider on the forearm?
   a. Keep the arm immobilized and below the level of heart
   b. Apply ice to the area
   c. Treat for shock
   d. Clean area with soap and water
   e. Remove any jewelry from the hand

84. Untreated hypoglycemia can progress into what type of condition if not treated in a prompt manner?
   a. Insulin shock
   b. Hyponatremia
   c. Diabetic coma
   d. Hypotension
   e. Neurogenic shock

85. Which of the following is TRUE regarding crutch fitting?
   a. The crutch tips should be 4 in. from the outer margin of the shoe
   b. The elbow should be flexed approximately 15 degrees
   c. The shoes should not be on the feet during fitting
   d. The underarm crutch brace should be 2 in. below the anterior axillary fold
   e. The crutch tips should be 2 in. in front of the shoe

86. Which of the following should NOT be performed in the event an athlete is suffering from deep frostbite of the toes?
   a. Dry the feet and toes
   b. Immerse the feet in hot water
   c. Take the athlete to a warmer environment
   d. Apply a sterile dressing between the toes
   e. Monitor the athlete for hypothermia

87. Which of the following is TRUE regarding AED use for a patient in cardiac arrest?
   a. Pediatric AED pads can effectively be used on adults
   b. AED pads are placed on the upper right chest and lower left side
   c. An AED can effectively analyze when moving the patient
   d. After one shock has been delivered, perform three minutes of CPR
   e. The patient's chest can be dried with alcohol before applying AED pads

88. What type of equipment should be used to stabilize an acute femur fracture?
   a. A half-ring traction splint
   b. A spine board
   c. A rapid-form vacuum splint

d. An air splint
e. A full-leg padded board splint

89. What should a patient avoid doing when attempting to warm the fingers if he or she has a frostnip?
    a. Placing the fingers in warm water
    b. Rubbing the fingers together
    c. Placing the fingers under the axilla
    d. Applying firm pressure to the fingers
    e. Blowing on the fingers

90. Dilated pupils in an unconscious patient are a sign of what condition?
    a. Cocaine overdose
    b. Epidural hematoma
    c. Subdural hematoma
    d. Heat stroke
    e. Stroke

91. In what position would the leg be in if an athlete suffered a hip dislocation?
    a. Flexed and internally rotated
    b. Neutral and internally rotated
    c. Extended and internally rotated
    d. Extended and externally rotated
    e. Adducted and externally rotated

92. Which injury is considered to be a medial emergency?
    a. Biceps brachii tendon rupture
    b. Acute compartment syndrome
    c. Anterior cruciate ligament rupture
    d. Acromioclavicular joint separation
    e. Patella subluxation

93. Which of the following is a "hallmark" sign of an extensor tendon rupture?
    a. The inability to flex the DIP joint
    b. The inability to oppose the thumb across the palm
    c. Pain with palpation within the anatomic snuff box
    d. The inability to extend the DIP joint
    e. Gross deformity of the distal carpal row

94. Which would be a sign of trauma or disease to the kidneys?
    a. Hydrocele
    b. Hernia
    c. Hematuria
    d. Hyperhydrosis
    e. Hemiplegia

95. Which is TRUE regarding the use of an air splint to immobilize a fractured extremity?
    a. It can take an extended amount of time to inflate
    b. It can place compression over the fracture site

c. It is classified as a rigid type of splint
d. It is opaque, and therefore you cannot see the injury site
e. It can only be used once

96. A slit lamp and fluorescein dye are diagnostic tools that are used to diagnose which of the following types of injuries?
    a. Hyphema
    b. Detached retina
    c. Corneal abrasion
    d. Keratitis
    e. Chalazion

97. What is the medical term for the inability to speak?
    a. Dysphasia
    b. Dysphagia
    c. Dysnomia
    d. Aphagia
    e. Aphasia

98. Tingling and/or numbness over the medial epicondyle of the elbow would indicate damage at what spinal nerve root level?
    a. C3
    b. C4
    c. T1
    d. C6
    e. L1

99. What is the first step you should take in treating a non–spine-injured athlete whose eyes are closed when you arrive at the scene?
    a. Check breathing
    b. Establish level of consciousness
    c. Assess the blood pressure
    d. Open the airway
    e. Assess the carotid pulse

100. What type of medication should an athlete have with them at practice in the event of an asthma attack?
    a. Albuterol
    b. Loperamide
    c. Diphenhydramine
    d. Epinephrine
    e. Pseudoephedrine

Use the DVD or visit the website at http://thePoint.lww.com/Long to take the *online examination*.

![checkmark] **STUDY CHECKLIST**

I have studied:
- ☐ Responding to Emergencies
- ☐ Skin and Musculoskeletal Injuries
- ☐ Head, Face, Spine, and Thorax Injuries

- ☐ Respiratory and Cardiac Emergencies
- ☐ Environmental Injuries and Illnesses
- ☐ Medical Conditions
- ☐ Ambulation and Moving Patients

SECTION 6

SUPPLEMENTAL READING

1. American Red Cross. *CPR/AED for the professional rescuer.* Yardley: StayWell; 2006.

2. Andersen JC, Courson RW, Kleiner DM, et al. National Athletic Trainers' Association. National Athletic Trainers' Association position statement: Emergency planning in athletics. *J Athl Train.* 2002;37(1):99–104.

3. Anderson MK, Parr GP, Hall SJ. *Foundations of athletic training: prevention, assessment, and management,* 4th ed. Philadelphia: Lippincott Williams & Wilkins; 2009.

4. Bergeron JD, Bizjak G, Krause GW, et al. *First responder.* Upper Saddle River: Pearson Prentice Hall; 2005.

5. Binkley HM, Beckett J, Casa DJ, et al. National Athletic Trainers' Association position statement: Exertional heat illnesses. *J Athl Train.* 2002;37(3):329–343.

6. Hillman SK. *Introduction to athletic training,* 2nd ed. Champaign: Human Kinetics; 2005.

7. Kleiner DM, Almquist JL, Bailes J, et al. *Prehospital care of the spine-injured athlete Inter-Association Task Force for the spine-injured athlete.* Dallas: National Athletic Trainers' Association; 2001.

8. Limmer D, Karren KJ, Hafen BQ. *First responder: a skills approach.* Upper Saddle River: Pearson Prentice Hall; 2007.

9. National Athletic Trainers' Association. Inter-Association Task Force on exertional heat illnesses consensus statement. *NATA News.* 2003;6:24–29.

10. National Athletic Trainers' Association. *Athletic training educational competencies,* 4th ed. Dallas: National Athletic Trainers' Association; 2006.

11. National Athletic Trainers' Association. *Inter-Association Task Force on exertional heat illnesses consensus statement.* Online: www.nata.org/consumer/heatillness/index.htm. 2003.

12. NCAA. *2006–07 NCAA sports medicine handbook,* 18th ed. Indianapolis: NCAA; 2006.

13. Prentice WE. *Arnheim's principles of athletic training: a competency-based approach.* New York: McGraw-Hill; 2006.

SECTION
7
Therapeutic Modalities

Part 1   Science of Modalities

Part 2   Pain

Part 3   Modalities

Section 7 Examination

OVERVIEW

Providing the optimal environment for the body to heal itself following injury is the premise of modality treatment. Modalities are often applied for pain control and reduction of swelling, thereby improving return to function following injury. A skilled athletic trainer continually refers to evidence-based practice criteria when determining the efficacy of modality treatment. Applications of modalities place stress on the body that may be helpful, harmful, or benign in nature during the treatment process. Understanding the indications, contraindications, and treatment parameters will assure the treating professional is selecting the best care for the patient's dysfunction.

CLINICAL PROFICIENCIES

Synthesize information obtained in a patient interview and physical examination to determine the indications, contraindications, and precautions for the selection, patient set-ups, and evidence-based application of therapeutic modalities for acute and chronic injuries. The student will formulate a progressive treatment and rehabilitation plan and appropriately apply the modalities. Effective lines of communication should be established to elicit and convey information about the patient's status and the prescribed modality(s). While maintaining confidentiality, all aspects of the treatment plan should be documented using standardized record-keeping methods. (Reproduced with permission of the National Athletic Trainers' Association.)

PART 1

Science of Modalities

KEY TERMS

- Alternating current (AC)
- Anion (A)
- Anode
- Cathode (C)
- Cation
- Chronaxie
- Conductance
- Coupling agent
- Direct current (DC)
- Hertz (Hz)
- Megavolt
- Rarefaction
- Refraction
- Refractory period
- Rheobase
- Sherrington law
- Sine wave
- Threshold
- Velocity (v)
- Voltage
- Watt (W)
- Wavelength (λ)

METHODS OF HEAT TRANSFER

- Conduction
- Convection
- Conversion
- Radiation
- Evaporation

Conduction

- Direct collision
- Transfer from higher to lower temperature
- Transfer ends when equal temperature
- Higher temperature increases heat transfer speed
- Tissue thickness dictates rate of temperature rise
- Examples: Hot and cold packs

Convection

- Direct contact
- Motion of treatment medium
- Increasing medium motion increases heat transfer rate
- Examples: Fluidotherapy and whirlpools

 Quick fact Thermoregulation is an example of convection form heat transfer found in the body.

Conversion

- Changing nonthermal energy to thermal energy
- Rate of transmission depends on power
- Modality temperature does not affect energy transfer
- Examples: Ultrasound and diathermy

Quick fact Metabolism is an example of conversion form heat transfer found in the body.

Radiation

- Direct energy transfer
- No medium
- Depends on intensity, size, distance, and angle
- Example: Infrared lamp

Quick fact The sun provides a natural form of radiant energy.

Evaporation

- Change between liquid to gas state
- Example: Vapocoolant spray

 Quick fact Sweating is an example of radiant heat transfer found in the body.

WAVELENGTH

- Distance between one point on a wave to the successive point on the next wave

- Wavelength increases, then frequency decreases
- Often measured in kilometers, meters, or angstroms

FREQUENCY

- Wave oscillations in a second
- Reported as cycles per second (cps) or pulses per second (pps)
- Frequency increases, then wavelength decreases
- Expressed in Hertz (Hz) or Megahertz (MHz)

> *Quick* **fact** There is an inverse relationship between wavelength and frequency. As frequency increases, wavelength decreases.

ELECTROMAGNETIC RADIATION

- Falls within the electromagnetic spectrum
- Visible and nonvisible refracted light (colors)
- Produces radiant energy
- Radiant energy travels through space and is emitted from all matter
- Chemical or electrical forces can generate electron movement

Electromagnetic Modalities

- Electrical stimulation
- Biofeedback
- Iontophoresis
- Diathermy
- Infrared modalities
- Ultraviolet
- Low-power light amplification by the stimulation of emitted radiation (LASER)

Specific Infrared Modalities

- Cold packs
- Cold whirlpool
- Hot whirlpool
- Paraffin
- Hydrocollator
- Luminous infrared lamp
- Nonluminous infrared lamp

Acoustic Modalities

- Transmit energy through sound waves

- Above audible sound
- Ultrasonography

Characteristics of Electromagnetic Radiation

- Reflect—bend back from surface
- Transmit—penetrate to deeper tissue
- Refract—change direction or bend away
- Absorb—infiltrate deeper tissue (see Fig. 7.1)

Scientific Premises of Electromagnetic Radiation

- Arndt-Schultz principle
- Law of Grotthus-Draper
- Cosine law
- Inverse square law

Arndt-Schultz Principle

- Absorbed energy must be sufficient to initiate a physiological effect
- Example: Tepid hot packs will have no effect because energy transfer does not occur.

Law of Grotthus-Draper

- Unabsorbed energy is transmitted deeper
- Example: If the frequency of ultrasound is low enough, the sound waves will penetrate deeper tissue.

Cosine Law

- Based on the angle of treatment
- Cosine of the treatment angle dictates significance of heating
- Heating perpendicular to the treatment surface (90 degrees) implies 100% heating effect
- Heating at 45 degrees to the treatment surface implies 71% heating effect (cosine of 45 = 0.71)
- Example: Treating with a diathermy unit, perpendicular to treatment area assures better heating than one that is set at 45 degrees to the treatment area.

Inverse Square Law

- Based on the distance of treatment
- Decreases distance and increases intensity of treatment
- Decreases distance by 1/3: inverse is 3/1 or 3; $3^2 = 9$; treatment intensity increases nine times
- Example: Applying an infrared lamp closer to patient is more intense than placing it farther away from patient (see Fig. 7.2).

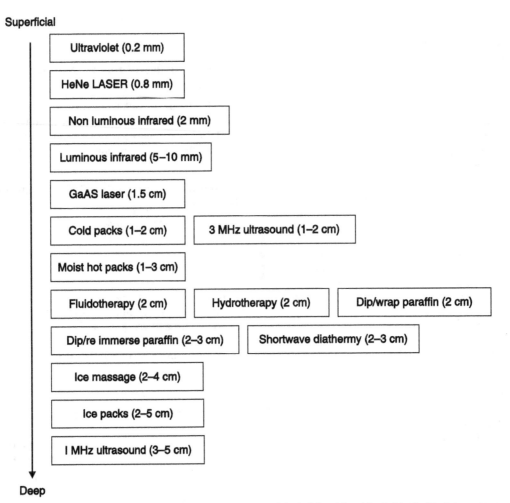

Superficial

Ultraviolet (0.2 mm)

HeNe LASER (0.8 mm)

Non luminous infrared (2 mm)

Luminous infrared (5–10 mm)

GaAS laser (1.5 cm)

Cold packs (1–2 cm) | 3 MHz ultrasound (1–2 cm)

Moist hot packs (1–3 cm)

Fluidotherapy (2 cm) | Hydrotherapy (2 cm) | Dip/wrap paraffin (2 cm)

Dip/re immerse paraffin (2–3 cm) | Shortwave diathermy (2–3 cm)

Ice massage (2–4 cm)

Ice packs (2–5 cm)

I MHz ultrasound (3–5 cm)

Deep

Figure 7.1 Depth of Penetration for Pertinent Modalities Used in Athletic Training. LASER, Light Amplification by Stimulated Emossion of Radiation.

PART **2**   Pain

KEY TERMS

- Epicrisis
- Epicritic, epicritic sensibility
- Gate control theory
- Golgi tendon organ (GTO)
- Golgi-Mazzoni corpuscle
- Krause end bulb
- Nociceptor
- Pain
- Pain-spasm-pain cycle
- Palliative

- Protopathic
- Radicular pain
- Radiculopathy

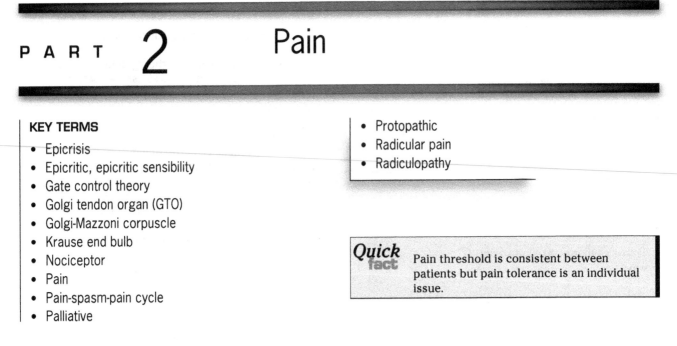

Quick fact   Pain threshold is consistent between patients but pain tolerance is an individual issue.

- Proprioceptors (tension)—muscle spindles and Golgi tendon organs
- Thermoreceptors (temperature)—Ruffini corpuscles and Krause end bulbs

PAIN TRANSMISSION

- Afferent pathway—periphery to brain (dorsal horn)
- Efferent pathway—brain to periphery (ventral horn)
- First-order neurons—periphery to dorsal root ganglion
- Second-order neurons—spinal cord connecting to thalamus
- Third-order neurons—thalamus connecting to cerebral cortex

SELECTED NERVE FIBERS

- A-β fibers—fast size and speed; myelinated
- A-δ fibers—moderate size and speed; myelinated
- C-fibers—small, slow, and unmyelinated

> **Quick fact** Myelinated nerve fibers transmit impulses faster than unmyelinated nerve fibers. Larger diameter nerve fibers transfer impulses faster than small diameter nerve fibers.

PAIN TRANSMISSION AND CONTROL CONCEPTS

- Ascending pathways—gate control theory
- Descending pathways—central biasing theory; ß-endorphin and dynorphin theory (endogenous opioid theory)

Gate Control Theory

Synopsis
- A-β fibers travel faster than A-δ and C-fibers to dorsal horn and stimulate inhibitory neurons (I neurons).
- Substantia gelatinosa activity determines whether pain or other sensation moves to second-order afferents
- Enkephalin (endogenous opioid) may be in substantia gelatinosa
- T cell (second-order afferent) takes sensory information to the brain
- Key is to "close the gate" by stimulating enough A-β fibers to block the A-δ and C-fiber transmission (see Fig. 7.3).

Affected nerves: A-β, A-δ, and C-fibers

Pathway: Ascending

Selected modalities: Sensory level transcutaneous electrical nerve stimulation (TENS), moist heat packs, whirlpools, ice treatments, and some massage

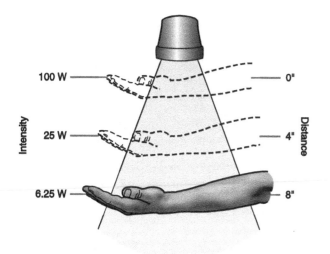

Figure 7.2 Inverse Square Law. (From Anderson MK, Parr GP, Hall SJ, et al. *Foundations of athletic training: prevention, assessment, and management*, 4th ed. Baltimore: Lippincott Williams & Wilkins; 2009.)

COMPLEXITY OF PAIN RESPONSE

- Behavioral
- Cognitive
- Cultural
- Emotional
- Sensory

DIFFERING FORMS OF PAIN

- Acute
- Chronic
- Radiating
- Referred
- Sclerotomic
- Somatic
- Trigger point
- Visceral

ASSESSING PAIN

- Activity Pattern Indicator Pain Profile
- Brief Pain Inventory
- Faces Pain Scale
- Graphic Rating Scale
- McGill Pain Questionnaire
- Neuropathic Pain Scale
- Numerical Rating Scale
- P-Q-R-S-T (Provocation, Quality, Refer/Radiate, Severity, Timing)
- Simple Descriptor Scale
- Visual Analog Scale

SELECTED SENSORY RECEPTORS

- Mechanoreceptors (pressure)—Meissner, Pacinian, and Merkel corpuscles
- Nociceptors (pain)—free nerve endings

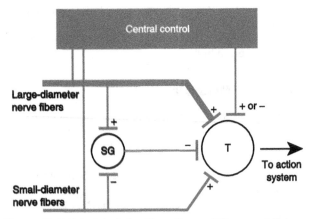

Figure 7.3 Model of the Gate Control Theory of Pain Control. SG, Substantia Gelatinosa. (From Knight KL, Draper DO. *Therapeutic modalities: the art and science.* Baltimore: Lippincott Williams & Wilkins; 2008.)

Central Biasing Theory

Synopsis
- Brain impulses (thalamus) are carried to dorsal horn

- "Close the gate" to painful stimulus
- Influenced by past experiences, emotions
- Midbrain (periaqueductal gray [PAG]) and pons/medulla (raphe nucleus) stimulate release of enkephalin in dorsal horn

Affected nerves: A-β, A-δ, and C-fibers
Pathway: Descending
Selected modalities:Accupressure, TENS, point stimulators, and strong motor electrical stimulation

ß-Endorphin and Dynorphin Theory (Endogenous Opioid Theory)

Synopsis
- Not clearly understood
- Hypothalamus influences PAG in brainstem
- ß-Endorphin released from brainstem
- Dynorphin found in PAG

Affected nerves: A-δ and C-fibers
Pathway: Descending
Selected modalities: Noxious electrical stimulation, acupuncture, and electroacupuncture

PART 3 Modalities

KEY TERMS

- Contraindication
- Erythema dose
- High TENS
- Hunting response
- Indication
- Interferential current (IFC)
- Intermittent compression
- Laser
- Lead
- Microcurrent
- Mottling
- Ohm law
- Paraffin bath
- Physical agent
- Piezoelectric ultrasonic device
- Polarity
- Power
- Russian current
- Tender point
- Trigger point

COLD

Depth of Penetration of Cold Application

- 2 to 5 cm (ice bag)

Commercial Cold Storage Units

- Temperature of unit 12°F (not lower than 0°F)
- Require insulating medium

Ice Massage (Conduction)

- Do not apply to area larger than 4 × 4 cm
- Treatment Duration: 5 to 15 minutes
- Initially colder than ice bag but long term same effects

Ice Immersion (Convection)

- Temperature Range: 50°F to 60°F
- Increases temperature as body area immersed increases
- Treatment Duration: 10 to 15 minutes
- Increases temperature duration as adipose tissue increases

Cryostretch (Spray and Stretch)

- Products: Ethyl chloride and fluoromethane
- Treatment Position: Treatment area on stretch; nozzle 12 to 24 in. away and strike skin at 30- to 45-degree angle with spray

Cold Whirlpools (Convection)

- Treatment Duration: 20 to 30 minutes and increased for larger adipose tissue quantities
- Temperature Range: 50°F to 65°F—temperature is increased as the proportion of the body area treated increases
- Depth of Penetration: 2 cm

HEAT

Temperature Increases from Baseline

- Mild heating (1.8°F change)—mild inflammation, accelerates metabolic rate
- Moderate heating (3.6°F to 5.4°F)—decreasing muscle spasm, pain, and chronic inflammation; increases blood flow
- Vigorous heating (5.4°F to 9.0°F)—tissue elongation, scar reduction, inhibition of sympathetic activity

Depth of Penetration of Heat Application

- Superficial agents—1 to 2 cm
- Deep-heating agents—2 to 5 cm

Moist Heat Packs (Conduction)

- Temperature at Storage: 160°F to 166°F
- Treatment Duration: 20 to 30 minutes—increase duration over structures with high adipose tissue
- Apply insulation to comfort
- Depth of Penetration: 1 to 3 cm

Paraffin Bath (Conduction)

- Temperature Range: 118°F to 126°F
- Treatment Duration: 15 to 20 minutes
- Wax-to-Mineral Oil Ratio: 7:1
- Can be used as immersion or glove method (assure first submersion is highest on arm to avoid burns)
- Depth of Penetration: Dip/wrap—2 cm; dip/reimmersion—2 to 3 cm

Fluidotherapy (Conduction)

- Temperature Range: 110°F to 125°F
- Treatment Duration: 20 minutes
- Depth of Penetration: 2 cm

Hot Whirlpool (Convection)

- Treatment Range: 90°F to 110°F
- Treatment Duration: 20 to 30 minutes
- Depth of Penetration: 2 cm

Contrast Whirlpool (Convection)

- Treatment Range: *Cold* (50°F to 60°F) and *hot* (105°F to 110°F)
- Treatment Duration: 20 to 30 minutes; *hot immersion* (3 to 4 minutes); *cold immersion* (1 to 2 minutes)

SHORTWAVE DIATHERMY (CONVERSION)

Thermal Effects of Shortwave Diathermy

- Deep heating
- Increased blood flow
- Increased cell metabolism
- Increased extensibility of collagen-rich tissues
- Muscular relaxation
- Possible changes in some enzyme reactions

Nonthermal Effects of Shortwave Diathermy

- Edema reduction
- Healing of superficial wounds
- Lymphedema reduction

Depth of Penetration

- 2 to 3 cm

Treatment Parameters

- Inductive Drum: Position 0.5 to 1 in. above toweling
- Capacitive Plate: 3 cm from the skin (both plates have to be at the same distance)
- Pulsed or continuous

ELECTRICAL STIMULATION

See Figures 7.4 to 7.7.
See Tables 7.1 to 7.4.

Frequency

- AC current = Hertz (Hz)
- DC current = N/A
- Pulsatile current = pulses per second (pps)
- Carrier frequencies
  - Associated with "Russian" current and interferential current
  - Low frequency → <1,000 Hz
  - Medium frequency → 1,000 to 10,000 Hz
  - High frequency → >10,000 Hz

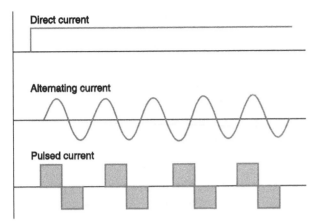

Figure 7.4 Method of Current Flow. (From Knight KL, Draper DO. *Therapeutic modalities: the art and science*. Baltimore: Lippincott Williams & Wilkins; 2008.)

Phase Duration

- A measure of time (microseconds [μs])
- Monophasic: Phase duration and pulse duration synonymous
- Biphasic: Phase duration = Half pulse duration if wave is symmetrical or phases are divided equally in half
- Polyphasic: Determined by carrier wave frequency

Phase Charge

- The electrical charge delivered during a phase of pulsatile current
- Phase duration and amplitude are the determinants of phase charge
- The electrical charge in the first phase of each pulse (or series of pulses with polyphasic waveforms)

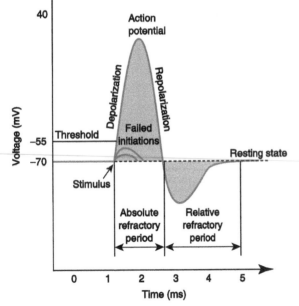

Figure 7.5 Nerve Refractory Periods. (From Knight KL, Draper DO. *Therapeutic modalities: the art and science*. Baltimore: Lippincott Williams & Wilkins; 2008.)

determines the physiological response, for example, nerve fiber depolarization
- Phase charge and nerve capacitance—key concept
- Phase charge = intensity × phase duration
- Measured in microcoulombs
- Commercially available units range in maximum phase charge from 12 to 40 microcoulombs
  - 12 to 15 microcoulombs = weak
  - 20 to 30 microcoulombs = moderate
  - 30 to 40 microcoulombs = intense

Duty Cycle

- Only applies to neuromuscular stimulation (NMS)
- Provides time for muscle recovery through replenishment of adenosine triphosphate (ATP)
- Also, called *phosphate repletion*

Ramp Time

- A series of pulses of gradually increasing phase charge used in NMS
- Build force of contraction over a period of 3 to 5 seconds

Polarity

- Applies to iontophoresis
- Positive charge is used to drive "repel" positively charged ions and negative charge for negatively charged ions
- TENS units, either polarity depolarizes a nerve
  - Monopolar (monophasic currents only)
    - One polarity over treatment site and one polarity over remote site
    - Usually large dispersive pad
  - Bipolar (monophasic currents only)
    - Positive and negative leads are placed over the treatment site
  - For biphasic and polyphasic waveforms, the treatment electrodes are placed over the target area

Choice of Electrodes

- Area to be treated: Quads → large electrodes
- Purpose of treatment: Trigger point → small electrode
- Current density: Different size electrode → different "feel" of stimulation → spread same current over large or small area

Electrode Information

- Placement for pain
  - "Art form"
  - Over site of pain
  - Within dermatome
  - Over nerve root related to dermatome experiencing pain
  - Same area on contralateral limb
  - Trigger point → stimulate directly
  - NMS → stimulate motor point
- Application
  - Bipolar technique—surface area from each lead is equal → equal current density (you could have each

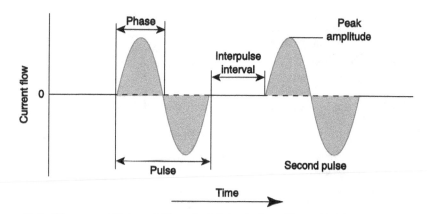

Figure 7.6 Phase and Pulse of Electrical Stimulation. (From Knight KL, Draper DO. *Therapeutic modalities: the art and science.* Baltimore: Lippincott Williams & Wilkins; 2008.)

lead to bifurcate accepting two electrodes from each lead)
- Monopolar technique—active electrode(s) over target tissue and dispersive electrode to complete circuit
- Quadripolar technique—two sets of electrodes operating with two independent channels

- Depth of stimulation
  - Increased distance between electrodes → increased depth of penetration
- Neuromuscular Electrical Muscle Stimulation (NMES)
  - Depolarization of α motor neurons → the more neurons depolarized the stronger the contraction

Direct (galvanic) wave form

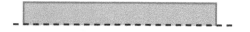

Interrupted DC wave form

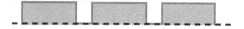

Sinusoidal wave form

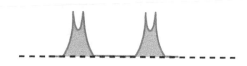

Faradic wave form

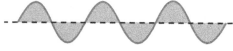

Rectangular

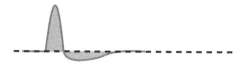

Biphasic

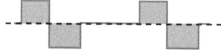

Twin pulse wave form

Interferential wave form

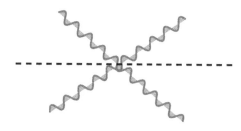

Russian wave form

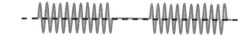

Figure 7.7 Electrical Stimulation Waveforms. (From Knight KL, Draper DO. *Therapeutic modalities: the art and science.* Baltimore: Lippincott Williams & Wilkins; 2008.)

Table 7.1 Differences between Physiological and Electrical Induced Muscle Contraction

Physiologically Induced Contractions	Electrical Stimulation Induced Contraction
Slow-twitch muscle fibers (first)	Fast-twitch muscle fibers (first)
Asynchronous recruitment	Synchronous recruitment
Golgi tendon organs protect muscles	Golgi tendon organs cannot protect muscle
Slow fatigue	Quick fatigue

- ○ Strength of contraction is directly proportional to phase charge
  - ■ ↑ phase charge → ↑ number of motor units fired → ↑ force of contraction
  - ■ Recruitment not hypertrophy
- ○ 12/12 duty cycle may be appropriate, for example, 12s contraction (5s ramp) followed by 12s rest
- ○ 30 to 40 repetitions with volitional assistance, for example, Straight leg raise (SLR)

Stimulation Levels

- Subsensory level—first discrete electrical sensation
- Sensory level—only sensory nerves; slight twitch, then decrease the output by approximately 10%
- Motor level—visible muscle contraction without pain
- Noxious level—stimulates pain fibers

Pulse Frequency Ranges

- Low—<15 pps; twitch; individual muscle contractions
- Medium—15 to 40 pps; summation; blending contractions result in increased tone
- High—>40 pps; tonic; steady or constant contraction

Sensory Level Pain Control

- Target Nerves: A-β
- Phase Duration: 60 to 100 μs
- Pulse Frequency: 80 to 200 pps
- Intensity: Submotor

Motor Level Pain Control

- Target Nerves: Motor nerves (A-δ)
- Phase Duration: 150 to 300 μs
- Pulse Frequency: 50 to 70 pps
- Intensity: Strong contraction

Noxious Level of Pain Control

- Target Nerves: A-δ and C-fibers
- Phase Duration: 250 μs to 1 ms
- Pulse Frequency: 1 to 5 pps
- Intensity: As painful as can be tolerated

INFRARED LAMPS (RADIANT)

Treatment Parameters of Infrared Lamps

- Treatment Duration: 20 to 30 minutes as needed
- Distance from Lamp:
  - ○ Luminous lamp—24 in.
  - ○ Nonluminous lamp—32 in.

Table 7.2 Electrical Stimulating Currents

Type	Use	Parameter
TENS	Gate theory pain control	80–200 pps; 60–100 μs
	β-Endorphin pain control	1–5 pps; 150–250 μs
	Enkephalin pain control	Varied pps; under 250 μs
NMES	Muscle reeducation	50–70 pps; duty cycle 10/50
	Edema	30–50 pps; duty cycle 5/5 or 10/10
	Muscle spasm	50–70 pps; duty cycle 10/10
HVPC	Edema	120 pps
	Wound care	100 pps
	β-Endorphin pain control	1–5 pps
	Muscle reeducation	50–70 pps—not ideal modality but can be used
Interferential	Gate theory pain control	80–150 pps
	Edema	50 pps
	Muscle spasm	4 pps
	Bone healing	100 pps
Russian	Muscle reeducation	50–70 bps
	Edema	50–70 bps
Iontophoresis	Scar remodeling	Sterile saline
	Medication delivery	Dependent on ion charge of medication

TENS, transcutaneous electrical nerve stimulation; HVPC, high-voltage pulsed direct current.

Table 7.3 Therapeutic Modality Indications

Modality Type / Indication	Acute Injury	Acute Inflammation	Acute Pain	Chronic Pain	Neuralgia or Neuroma	Muscle Spasms	Superficial	Decreased	Hematoma	Joint	Chronic Inflammation	Fractures	Osteoarthritis	Peripheral Nerve Injury	Wound	Drug	Skin Infections or Disorders	Myositis	Trigger Points	Scar	Vertebral Disc Pathology	Nerve Root Compression	Muscle Re-Education	Impaired Circulation	Lymphedema
Cold whirlpool	X	X	X	X				X	X		X														
Contrast bath				X				X	X	X	X													X	
Cryostretch				X				X											X						
Fluidotherapy				X		X		X	X	X	X														
HVPC	X	X	X	X		X		X		X	X				X				X					X	
Ice bag	X	X	X	X			X	X	X																
Ice massage			X	X		X					X								X						
Infrared lamps											X			X	X										
Interferential stimulation	X	X	X	X		X					X	X													X
Intermittent compression											X														X
Iontophoresis				X							X					X				X					
LASERS				X							X	X	X		X										
Massage				X		X					X								X	X				X	X
Mechanical traction	X		X	X		X		X		X		X									X	X			
Moist heat packs				X		X		X	X	X	X														
NMES	X	X	X	X		X		X	X	X	X												X		
Paraffin				X		X		X	X	X	X														
Russian stimulation			X	X		X		X		X	X														
Shortwave diathermy			X	X		X		X			X	X													
TENS	X		X	X															X		X				
Ultrasound (continuous)				X		X		X		X	X								X						
Ultrasound (pulsed)	X	X	X		X										X	X		X		X					
Ultraviolet																X	X								
Warm whirlpool[a]				X		X		X	X	X	X				X										

[a]Whirlpool must be cleaned after every patient and cultured if using for debridement in wound care. Not typical of athletic training facilities.
HVPC, high-voltage pulsed direct current; LASER, light amplification by stimulated emission of radiation; TENS, transcutaneous electrical nerve stimulation.

Table 7.4 Therapeutic Modality Contraindications

Modality Type \ Indication	Malignancy	Pregnancy	Sensory Loss	Open Wounds	Circulatory Insufficiency	Osteoporosis	Raynaud's Phenomenon	Peripheral Vascular Disease	Cold Sensitivity	Advanced Diabetes	Acute Injury	Acute Inflammation	Thrombophlebitis	Poor Thermal Regulation	Sensitive Areas[a]	Spinal Cord/Nerve Plexus	Infection or Fever	Epiphyseal Plate	Metal Implants or Piercing	Hemorrhage	Pacemaker	Sunburns or Sensitivity to UV	Fracture	Scar Tissue	Systemic Disease[b]	Polyphyria	Radiation Therapy	Birth Control (specific types)	Compartment Syndrome	Unstable Segment	Significant Disc Disease or Fragments
Cold whirlpool	X	X	X	X	X		X	X	X	X					X										X					X	
Contrast bath	X	X	X	X	X		X	X	X	X					X										X					X	
Cryotherapy	X		X		X										X										X						
Fluidotherapy	X	X									X				X										X						
HVPC	X	X	X		X		X	X		X			X		X				X	X	X		X		X					X	
Ice bag	X		X	X	X		X	X	X	X					X										X						
Ice massage	X		X	X			X	X	X	X					X										X						
Infrared lamps	X	X	X							X	X				X							X		X	X						
Interferential stimulation	X	X													X		X		X	X	X		X		X					X	
Intermittent compression	X	X			X								X		X		X			X	X		X		X					X	
Iontophoresis	X	X													X										X				X	X	
LASERS	X	X													X		X	X							X		X				
Massage	X	X		X								X	X		X		X			X			X		X					X	
Mechanical traction	X	X				X						X	X		X				X	X	X		X		X					X	X
Moist heat packs	X	X	X		X							X			X		X								X						
NMES	X	X	X		X							X	X	X	X		X	X	X	X	X		X		X					X	
Paraffin	X	X	X		X							X	X		X				X	X	X		X		X						
Russian stimulation	X	X											X		X		X		X	X	X		X		X					X	
Shortwave diathermy	X	X			X			X				X	X		X		X	X	X	X	X		X		X						
TENS	X	X	X										X		X		X		X		X	X			X					X	
Ultrasound (continuous)	X	X	X									X	X		X		X	X	X	X	X		X	X	X		X				
Ultrasound (pulsed)	X	X	X		X								X		X			X	X	X	X		X		X				X		
Ultraviolet	X	X	X							X					X							X		X	X	X	X	X			
Warm whirlpool	X	X	X		X							X	X		X										X						

[a] Sensitive areas include heart, face, head, eyes, neck (carotid artery), skull, and genitals.
[b] Systemic disease includes diabetes mellitus, rheumatoid arthritis, tuberculosis, hyperthyroidism, lupus, herpes virus, albinism, congestive heart failure, arteriosclerosis, meningitis, or other diseases. Please refer specifically to modality resources for these contraindications.
HVPC, high-voltage pulsed direct current; LASER, light amplification by stimulated emission of radiation; TENS, transcutaneous electrical nerve stimulation.

Depth of Penetration

- Luminous: 0.5 to 1 cm (5 to 10 mm)
- Nonluminous: 2 mm

ULTRAVIOLET (RADIANT)

Treatment Parameters of Ultraviolet

- Treatment Duration: Based on minimal erythema dose (MED); every other day
- Depth of Penetration: 0.2 mm

LIGHT AMPLIFICATION BY THE STIMULATION OF EMITTED RADIATION

Treatment Parameters of Light Amplification by the Stimulation of Emitted Radiation

- Depends on type of LASER
- Depth of Penetration: 0.8 to 15 mm

ULTRASOUND (CONVERSION)

Local Effects of Thermal Ultrasound

- Increased sensory nerve conduction velocity
- Increased motor nerve conduction velocity
- Increased extensibility of collagen-rich structures
- Increased collagen deposition
- Increased blood flow
- Reduction of muscle spasms
- Increased macrophage activity
- Enhanced adhesion of leukocytes to damaged endothelial cells

Local Effects of Nonthermal Ultrasound

- Increased cell membrane permeability
- Changes diffusion across the cell membrane
- Increased vascular permeability
- Increased blood flow
- Increased fibroblastic activity
- Stimulation of phagocytosis
- Production of healthy granulation tissue
- Synthesis of protein
- Synthesis of collagen
- Reduction of edema
- Diffusion of ions
- Tissue regeneration
- Formation of stronger, more deformable connective tissue

Treatment Parameters

- Treatment Area: Two to three times the effective radiating area (ERA)
- Coupling Methods:
  - Direct coupling
    - 0.44 to 1.32 lb of pressure
  - Immersion
  - Bladder

- Treatment Duration: 3 to 12 minutes depending on area
- Treatment Length: Not more than 10 to 14 treatments because of risk to red blood cell (RBC)
- Frequency: 1 to 3.3 MHz (1 MHz deepest penetration; 3 MHz more superficial)
- Duty Cycle: 20% to 100%
- Beam Nonuniformity Ratio (BNR): Not greater than 8:1 according to U.S. Food and Drug Administration (FDA) mandate

Depth of Penetration

- 1 MHz: 3 to 5 cm
- 3 MHz: 1 to 2 cm

Phonophoresis

- Preheat area treated
- Direct coupling method recommended
- Common Medication Classifications Used: Corticosteroids, salicylates, and anesthetics
- Common Examples of Medication Names: Hydrocortisone, dexamethasone, chlorzoxazone (Myoflex), and lidocaine

INTERMITTENT COMPRESSION

Treatment Parameters

- Temperature: Some devices have this option 50°F to 55°F
- Duty Cycle: 3 on 1 off 3:1
- Treatment Duration: 20 minutes to several hours
- Inflation Pressure: Upper extremity (40 to 60 mm Hg)
- Inflation Pressure: Lower extremity (60 to 100 mm Hg)
- Do not exceed blood pressure reading

THERAPEUTIC MASSAGE

Basic Strokes of Massage

- Effleurage—stroking of the skin
- Petrissage—lifting or kneading
- Friction—deep pressure
- Tapotment—tapping or pounding
- Vibration—rapid shaking

 Quick **fact** Pressure over sensitive areas such as the popliteal and cubital spaces should be avoided.

MANUAL THERAPY TECHNIQUES

 Quick **fact** Fascia is geared toward separating structures and holding structures together.

Muscle Energy Technique

- Malalignments occur because of injury, weakness, or muscle spasm
- Muscle contraction can realign structures
- Patient controls magnitude of submaximal contraction
- Place patient in position of restriction and contract muscle
- End result of contraction is improved motion and relaxation
- Contraction: 5 to 10 seconds
- Repetitions: Three to five

Myofascial Release Techniques

- Active and latent trigger points
- Work superficial from skin progressing to deeper levels
- Long-duration stretching of superficial to deep fascial restrictions

Strain–Counterstrain

- Abnormal neuromuscular reflex correction
- Tender points
- Position of comfort key to treatment

Feldenkrais

- Self-awareness movement program
- No mind–body separation—learning encompasses both

TRACTION

Cervical Traction Treatment Parameters

- Angle of Pull: 25 to 30 degrees of flexion
- Treatment Duration: Muscle spasm (20 minutes); facet joint pathology (25 minutes); disc protrusion (8 to 10 minutes); degenerative disc disease (DDD) (10 minutes)
- Pathology Guidelines:
  - Facet Joint: Cervical (flexion); intermittent pull
  - Intervertebral Space, e.g., DDD: Cervical (flexion); sustained pull
  - Nerve Root Impingement: Bilateral (neutral); unilateral (neutral with opposite side lateral flexion); sustained pull
  - Disc Protrusion: Cervical (extension, neutral of flexion based on symptoms); intermittent pull
  - Muscle Spasm: Position to elongate spasm structures; sustained pull
- Duty Cycle: On–Off 3:1 or 4:1 (for intermittent traction)
- Traction Amounts: 10 lb or 7% of body weight

Lumbar Traction Treatment Parameters

- Angle of Pull:
  - L5-S1—hips flexed 45 to 60 degrees
  - L4-5—hips flexed 60 to 75 degrees
  - L3-4—hips flexed 75 to 90 degrees
  - Posterior intervertebral space—hips flexed at 90 degrees
  - Upper lumbar and lower thoracic spine facet joints—extension
  - Lower lumbar—prone
- Treatment Duration: Muscle spasm (20 minutes); facet joint pathology (25 minutes); disc protrusion (8 to 10 minutes); DDD (10 minutes)

Pathology Guidelines

- Facet Joint: Lumbar (extension); intermittent pull
- Intervertebral Space, e.g., DDD: Lumbar (neutral); sustained pull
- Nerve Root Impingement: Bilateral (neutral); unilateral (neutral with opposite side lateral flexion); sustained pull
- Disc Protrusion: Cervical (extension, neutral of flexion based on symptoms); intermittent pull
- Muscle Spasm: Position to elongate spasm structures; sustained pull
- Duty Cycle: On–Off 3:1 or 4:1 (for intermittent traction)
- Traction Amounts: 25% to 60% of body weight

1. What type of massage is identified as stroking?
   a. Petrissage
   b. Friction
   c. Effleurage
   d. Tapotment
   e. Vibration

2. What type of massage is identified as kneading or compression?
   a. Petrissage
   b. Friction
   c. Effleurage
   d. Tapotment
   e. Vibration

3. What type of massage is deep pressure against underlying tissues?
   a. Petrissage
   b. Friction
   c. Effleurage
   d. Tapotment
   e. Vibration

4. Which term identifies the return of a cell to its resting potential?
   a. Depolarization
   b. Apolarization
   c. Refractory period
   d. Saltatory conduction
   e. Repolarization

5. What term identifies a change in a cell's permeability evoking an action potential?
   a. Depolarization
   b. Apolarization
   c. Refractory period
   d. Saltatory conduction
   e. Repolarization

6. What is the approximate resting potential of a nerve cell?
   a. −70 mV
   b. −50 mV
   c. −120 mV
   d. −90 mV
   e. −20 mV

7. Which ions are present in high concentration within a normal resting nerve cell?
   a. Sodium
   b. Potassium
   c. Calcium
   d. Magnesium
   e. Chlorine

8. Which ions are present in high concentration outside of a normal resting nerve cell?
   a. Sodium and chlorine
   b. Calcium and magnesium
   c. Sodium and potassium
   d. Zinc and fluorine
   e. Iron and niacin

9. What name is given to the fatty myelin sheath covering some nerve cells?
   a. Astrocytes
   b. Microglia
   c. Schwann cells
   d. Cook cells
   e. Nodes of Ranvier

10. What are the gaps where the cell membrane is exposed in a myelinated nerve cell?
    a. Astrocytes
    b. Microglia
    c. Schwann cells
    d. Cook cells
    e. Nodes of Ranvier

11. What identifies a time when even higher than normal stimulus cannot further depolarize a nerve?
    a. A relative refractory period
    b. An absolute refractory period
    c. Saltatory conduction
    d. A depolarization period
    e. A repolarization period

12. What identifies a time when higher than normal stimulus can further depolarize a nerve?
    a. A relative refractory period
    b. An absolute refractory period
    c. Saltatory conduction
    d. A depolarization period
    e. A repolarization period

13. Which afferent peripheral nerves have the slowest conduction velocity?
    a. A-fibers
    b. B-fibers
    c. C-fibers
    d. D-fibers
    e. Type IIb fibers

14. Which afferent peripheral nerves have the fastest conduction velocity?
    a. A-α
    b. A-β
    c. A-δ
    d. A-γ
    e. C-fibers

15. Where is acetylcholine located?
    a. Myofibrils
    b. Motor nerves and central nervous system
    c. Cerebellum
    d. Brocca area
    e. Peripheral nerves

16. Which neurotransmitter transmits motor impulses?
    a. Dopamine
    b. Acetylcholine
    c. Seratonin
    d. Epinephrine
    e. Norepinephrine

17. What is the main function of acetylcholine?
    a. Saltatory conduction
    b. Inhibits hormone production
    c. Transmits motor impulses
    d. Facilitates mast cell production
    e. Increases heart rate

18. Where is dopamine located?
    a. Brainstem
    b. Cerebellum
    c. Cerebrum
    d. Frontal cortex
    e. Occipital lobe

19. Where is epinephrine located?
    a. Brainstem
    b. Cerebellum
    c. Cerebrum
    d. Frontal cortex
    e. Occipital lobe

20. What is the space and fluid found between the tissues?
    a. Plasma
    b. Exudate
    c. Interstitial
    d. Leukocytic
    e. Granulation

21. What is the resistance to tearing and the ability to withstand a longitudinal force?
    a. Shearing
    b. Torsion
    c. Compression
    d. Approximation
    e. Tensile strength

22. What is the resistance of fluid to flow?
    a. Density
    b. Buoyancy
    c. Colloid pressure
    d. Viscosity
    e. Pascal law

23. Which modality uses electricity to introduce ions into the body?
    a. Electrophoresis
    b. Phonophoresis
    c. Iontophoresis
    d. Calciumphoresis
    e. Photophoresis

24. What are nociceptors?
    a. Motor neurons
    b. Pain transmitters
    c. Thermoreceptors
    d. Proprioceptors
    e. Mechanoreceptors

25. What type of heat is lost or gained through indirect energy transmission?
    a. Ultraviolet heat
    b. Infrared heat
    c. Indirect heat
    d. Conductive heat
    e. Radiant heat

26. When multiple stimuli can activate a receptor it is termed as:
    a. Polymodal
    b. Antagonistic
    c. Synergistic
    d. Nociceptive
    e. Idiosyncrasy

27. What is the introduction of medication to the body through acoustical media?
    a. Electrophoresis
    b. Phonophoresis
    c. Iontophoresis
    d. Calciumphoresis
    e. Photophoresis

28. What substance opens and closes the gate according to the gate control theory?
    a. White matter
    b. Norepinephrine
    c. Cerebrospinal fluid

d. T cells

e. Substantia gelatinosa

29. What is the transformation of a chemical stimulus into an action potential?
  a. Conduction
  b. Transduction
  c. Reduction
  d. Coagulation
  e. Phagocytosis

30. What phagocyte is released immediately following trauma controlling bacteria and damaging healthy tissue?
  a. Neutrophil
  b. Mast cell
  c. Fibroblasts
  d. Adipocyte
  e. Lymphocyte

31. Which of the following is *not* an indication for cryotherapy application?
  a. Arthritis
  b. Tendinitis
  c. Postsurgical edema
  d. Muscle spasm
  e. Chronic pain

32. Which of the following cannot be modulated with TENS units?
  a. Intensity
  b. Output modulation (mode)
  c. Effective radiating area (ERA)
  d. Pulse duration
  e. Pulse frequency

33. Which does not describe the minimal erythemal dose (MED)?
  a. Redness occurs between 1 and 6 hours following treatment
  b. Used with ultraviolet radiation treatments
  c. Redness disappears within 24 hours
  d. Each generator produces its own MED
  e. MED testing is performed using a template of plastic

34. A field hockey player tells you she twisted her ankle near the very end of practice yesterday. After evaluation, you conclude that she most likely has a second-degree ankle sprain and is showing signs of significant swelling and ecchymosis around the lateral ankle. Which of the following modalities would be the most appropriate to use at this time?
  a. Warm whirlpool
  b. Contrast bath
  c. Cold whirlpool
  d. Diathermy
  e. Ice bag with a compression wrap

35. How long should mechanical traction be applied for facet joint pathology?
  a. 10 minutes
  b. 15 minutes
  c. 20 minutes
  d. 25 minutes
  e. 30 minutes

36. Which is not considered a contraindication of cold treatments?
  a. Neuralgia
  b. Lupus
  c. Peripheral vascular disease
  d. Raynaud phenomenon
  e. Circulatory insufficiency

37. Ice massage application to an injured body part results in a large reactive hyperemia once the treatment has ended. Owing to the hyperemia, which of the following injuries should not be treated with an ice massage?
  a. Tendinitis
  b. Acute muscle contusion
  c. Chronic bursitis
  d. Muscle spasm
  e. Trigger points

38. Which of the following is *not* an effect of cryotherapy?
  a. Analgesia
  b. Inhibits release of inflammatory mediators
  c. Decrease in cell metabolism
  d. Vasodilation
  e. Decrease in cell permeability

39. Which is considered an indication of mechanical cervical traction energy?
  a. An extruded disc fragmentation
  b. A positive vertebral artery test
  c. Spinal cord compression
  d. Meningitis
  e. Capsulitis of the vertebral joints

40. In which of the following orders does an athlete experience these sensations during cryotherapy?
  a. Burning – aching – cold – analgesia
  b. Cold – burning – aching – analgesia
  c. Aching – cold – burning – analgesia
  d. Burning – cold – aching – analgesia
  e. Aching – burning – cold – analgesia

41. In which of the following situations should you *not* use a thermotherapy for an athlete?
  a. To facilitate tissue healing
  b. To reduce acute inflammation
  c. To reduce muscle spasm
  d. To reduce swelling in a subacute injury
  e. To reduce ecchymosis

42. A full-body hot whirlpool should be maintained at what temperature?
    a. 85°F to 90°F
    b. 90°F to 96°F
    c. 98°F to 102°F
    d. 100°F to 110°F
    e. None of the above

43. What term identifies the spreading of a beam or wave?
    a. Convergence
    b. Interferential
    c. Divergence
    d. Conversion
    e. Approximation

44. What term identifies the focalization of a beam or wave?
    a. Convergence
    b. Interferential
    c. Divergence
    d. Conversion
    e. Approximation

45. Which heat transfer occurs when energy is changed from one form to another?
    a. Convection
    b. Conduction
    c. Conversion
    d. Radiation
    e. Magnetism

46. Which heat transfer occurs through a circulating medium?
    a. Convection
    b. Conduction
    c. Conversion
    d. Radiation
    e. Magnetism

47. Which heat transfer occurs when two objects touch each other?
    a. Convection
    b. Conduction
    c. Conversion
    d. Radiation
    e. Magnetism

48. How long will a cold modality remove heat from a body?
    a. Until the modality and skin are the same temperature
    b. Until the modality is colder than the skin
    c. Until temperature changes 1 degree 1 cm below the skin
    d. Until cold penetrates the muscle tissue
    e. When the modality reaches room temperature

49. Which two body structures represent the largest changes in temperature with cold applications?
    a. Muscle and nerve
    b. Skin and synovium
    c. Skin and adipose tissue
    d. Cartilage and bones
    e. Ligaments and tendons

50. How long does it take for decreases in superficial blood flow to level off during cold applications?
    a. 5 minutes
    b. 25 minutes
    c. Approximately 13 minutes
    d. 45 minutes
    e. 60 minutes

51. What skin temperature represents the maximal decrease in local blood flow during cold applications?
    a. 32°F (0° C)
    b. 57°F (13.9° C)
    c. 70°F (21.1° C)
    d. 85°F (29.5° C)
    e. 95°F (35° C)

52. In sedentary treatments, how long will treatments from cold applications remain effective?
    a. 5 to 10 minutes
    b. 10 to 15 minutes
    c. 20 to 60 minutes
    d. 30 to 40 minutes
    e. 60 to 90 minutes

53. Why does compression with cold application enhance the cooling effects?
    a. Makes the ice colder
    b. Prevents the cold from escaping
    c. Increases the contact of the cold application
    d. Increases the depth of ice penetration
    e. Prevents ice migration

54. What substance category causes irritation of superficial sensory nerves in order to reduce pain transmission from underlying nerves?
    a. Analgesic
    b. Antitussive
    c. Anti-inflammatory
    d. Steroids
    e. Counterirritant

55. How does cold application reduce muscle spasm?
    a. Suppress stretch reflex
    b. Increased neural activity
    c. Decreases sarcomere viscosity
    d. Decreases myofibril recruitment
    e. Decreases myofascial compression

56. What is a combination of range of motion exercises with simultaneous application of cold?
    a. Thermokineses
    b. Cryokinetics

c. Isokinetics
d. Plyokinetics
e. Proprioceptive neuromuscular facilitation

57. What capillary bed pressure is reduced when applying compression and elevation?
a. Vascular hydrostatic pressure
b. Plasma osmotic colloid pressure
c. Hydrostatic pressure
d. Viscosity
e. Interstitial lymphatic pressure

58. Which is not a superficial heating agent?
a. An Infrared lamp
b. Moist heat packs
c. Paraffin bath
d. Warm whirlpool (immersion)
e. Diathermy

59. What is the effect on muscle spasm with heat application?
a. Reduced spasm
b. Increased spasm
c. Decreased hypotonicity
d. Increased phosphocreatine uptake
e. Increased lactic acid permeability

60. What is the effect on capillary permeability with heat application?
a. Neutral effect
b. Increased permeability
c. Decreased permeability
d. Slows diffusion rate
e. Increased rate osmosis

61. What depth of penetration occurs with superficial heating modalities?
a. <2 cm
b. 2 to 4 cm
c. 3 to 5 cm
d. 6 to 8 cm
e. 8 cm and more

62. What is mottling?
a. An enhanced skin pigmentation
b. Skin exfoliation
c. A blotchy skin discoloration
d. A macular skin formation
e. Keratosis

63. What happens to hemoglobin when heating the body?
a. Replaces lost iron concentrations
b. Releases oxygen
c. Enhances chemical exchange
d. Metabolic acidosis
e. Rhabdomyolysis

64. At what temperature does protein, cell, and tissue damage occur?
a. 98.6°F (37°C)
b. 104°F (40°C)
c. 107°F (41.6°C)
d. 110°F (43.3°C)
e. More than 113°F (45°C)

65. What method can be used to decrease coldness to the toes and fingers during ice immersion or cold whirlpool treatments?
a. Decrease thermoplane
b. Increase rate of circulating medium
c. Neoprene covers
d. Add sodium chloride
e. Cryokinetics

66. Which is not an indication for using vapocoolant spray ("spray and stretch")?
a. Trigger points
b. Decreased range of motion
c. Neural inflammation
d. Muscle spasm
e. Pain control

67. What are the chemicals used for cryostretch?
a. Sodium chloride
b. Benzyl alcohol and witch hazel
c. Ceytyl alcohol and glycerine
d. Ethyl chloride or fluoromethane
e. Prunius avium

68. How long does a properly heated moist heat pack provide effective treatment?
a. 12 minutes
b. 20 minutes
c. 30 to 45 minutes
d. 60 minutes
e. 60 to 90 minutes

69. What is the ratio of wax to mineral oil in a paraffin bath?
a. 1:1
b. 3:1
c. 5:1
d. 7:1
e. 10:1

70. Why does paraffin bath feel cooler than water at the same temperature?
a. Because of the mineral oil
b. Low specific heat
c. Increased density
d. Decreased viscosity
e. Because of application process

71. Why should paraffin be applied at lower temperatures to the lower extremity?
a. Circulation less efficient than upper extremity
b. Circulation more efficient than upper extremity

c. Larger skin to surface area ratio
d. Increased neural sensitivity
e. Increased resistance to heat transfer

72. What is the optimal length of a paraffin treatment?
    a. 1 to 2 minutes
    b. 5 to 8 minutes
    c. 15 to 20 minutes
    d. 30 to 40 minutes
    e. 60 minutes

73. Why are multiple layers of paraffin desirable with treatment?
    a. Layers act as conductors
    b. Decreases treatment time
    c. Decreases thermogenic response
    d. Layers act as insulator
    e. Increases the surface area coverage

74. Why should a patient be instructed to avoid touching the insides or bottom of a paraffin bath?
    a. Contaminates the paraffin
    b. OSHA standards
    c. Multiple patient treatment device
    d. Burns can occur
    e. Ineffective surface area coverage

75. How often should an extremity be dipped and dried during paraffin bath immersion treatment?
    a. 1 to 2 times
    b. 3 to 4 times
    c. 5 to 6 times
    d. 6 to 12 times
    e. More than 12 times

76. Why is an extremity dipped and dried during paraffin bath immersion treatment?
    a. To increase surface area coverage
    b. To decrease the likelihood of burns
    c. OSHA standards
    d. To maintain thermal effect
    e. To prevent contamination of paraffin

77. Which category of heat transfer does fluidotherapy occupy?
    a. Conduction
    b. Radiation
    c. Convection
    d. Infrared
    e. Conversion

78. Which is not a treatment parameter variable for fluidotherapy application?
    a. Air speed
    b. Phase time
    c. Temperature
    d. Treatment time
    e. Preheat time

79. Which cold modality has a higher chance of producing frostbite?
    a. Cryokinetics
    b. Cold whirlpool
    c. Ice massage
    d. Reusable cold packs
    e. Vapocoolant spray

80. Which conduction modality has the deepest penetration?
    a. Ice bag
    b. Ice massage
    c. Cold whirlpool
    d. Vapocoolant spray
    e. Contrast bath

81. What happens when surface area increases in cold water?
    a. Water depth should decrease
    b. Buoyancy decrease
    c. Water temperature increases
    d. Hydrostatic pressure decreases
    e. Treatment times extend

82. What happens when surface area increases in warm water?
    a. Water depth should decrease
    b. Buoyancy decrease
    c. Hydrostatic pressure decreases
    d. Treatment times extend
    e. Decreased water temperature

83. What is a megahertz (MHz)?
    a. 1,000,000,000 cycles per second
    b. 1,000 cycles per second
    c. 10,000 cycles per second
    d. 10,000,000 cycles per second
    e. 1,000,000 cycles per second

84. Which spectrum defines ultrasound?
    a. Infrared spectrum
    b. Electromagnetic spectrum
    c. Acoustical spectrum
    d. Therapeutic spectrum
    e. Ultraviolet spectrum

85. What is the usual temperature range for fluidotherapy applications?
    a. 88°F to 145°F
    b. 90°F to 100°F
    c. 100°F to 123°F
    d. 120°F to 136°F
    e. 100°F to 150°F

86. What does the beam nonuniformity ratio (BNR) mean?
    a. Uniformity of ultrasound output
    b. Depth of penetration
    c. Increase in temperature per square centimeter

d. Size of treatment area

e. Transducer size

87. What beam nonuniformity ratio (BNR) is considered safe?
   a. <8:1
   b. 9:1
   c. 10:1
   d. 15:1
   e. Any BNR is safe

88. Which modality is used for muscle reeducation?
   a. Low-voltage electrical stimulation
   b. MENS
   c. TENS
   d. Biofeedback
   e. LASER

89. Cosine law states:
   a. For every action, there is an equal and opposite reaction
   b. No changes occur in tissue because the amount of energy is not being absorbed
   c. More energy will be absorbed the closer the energy source is to a right angle
   d. Energy not absorbed superficially will penetrate deeper
   e. Longer wavelength radiation will absorb deeper

90. Which electrical stimulating current helps soft tissue and bone heal by using subsensory microcurrent?
   a. Ultrasound
   b. Direct current
   c. Alternating current
   d. TENS
   e. MENS

91. What identifies the duty cycle of an ultrasound?
   a. Percentage of time energy emitted from ultrasound
   b. Length of treatment time
   c. Effective treatment area
   d. Beam nonexistence ratio
   e. Equation of off to on time

92. A _____ MHz ultrasound can penetrate up to 2 cm.
   a. 1
   b. 2
   c. 3
   d. 4
   e. 5

93. What determines ultrasound penetration?
   a. Beam nonuniformity ratio
   b. Effective radiating area
   c. Frequency
   d. Intensity
   e. Application method

94. What is the frequency range for therapeutic ultrasound in megahertz (MHz)?
   a. 75 to 3.3 MHz
   b. 1 to 2 MHz
   c. 3 to 4 MHz
   d. 5 to 6 MHz
   e. Above 7 MHz

95. What converts alternating current to sound waves in an ultrasound?
   a. Coaxial cable
   b. Electricity
   c. Transducer
   d. Converter box
   e. Sine wave

96. Pulse duration is also called:
   a. Frequency
   b. Interval
   c. Rate
   d. Amplitude
   e. Width

97. Which electrical measurement is identified as volts times amps?
   a. Ohms
   b. Resistance
   c. Watt
   d. Electrical impedance
   e. Potential difference

98. Which is not true of electrically induced muscle contractions?
   a. Large diameter fibers are recruited first
   b. Fast-twitch muscle fibers are recruited first
   c. Contractions are synchronous
   d. GTO cannot protect the structure
   e. Fatigue occurs slowly

99. Which is *true* regarding noxious level pain control?
   a. Motor nerves A-β fibers targeted
   b. Phase duration of 100 μs
   c. Variable pulse frequency
   d. Submotor intensity
   e. Delivered with MENS

100. Which is not *true* of motor level pain control?
   a. Motor nerves are targeted
   b. Phase duration is 150 to 250 μs
   c. Pain decreases through muscle inhibition
   d. 2 to 4 pps or 80 to 120 pps
   e. Strong to moderate contraction targeted

 Use the DVD or visit the website at http://thePoint.lww.com/Long to take the *online examination.*

✔ STUDY CHECKLIST

I have studied:
- ☐ Heat Transfer
- ☐ Electromagnetic Radiation
- ☐ Infrared Modalities
- ☐ Acoustic Modalities
- ☐ Pain
- ☐ Electrodes
- ☐ Intermittent Compression
- ☐ Mechanical and Manual Therapy

SECTION 7

SUPPLEMENTAL READING

1. Denegar CR, Saliba E, Saliba S. *Therapeutic modalities for musculoskeletal injuries,* 2nd ed. Champaign: Human Kinetics; 2006.

2. Hayes KW. *Manual for physical agents,* 5th ed. Upper Saddle River: Prentice Hall; 2000.

3. Knight KL, Draper DO. *Therapeutic modalities: the art and science.* Philadelphia: Lippincott Williams & Wilkins; 2008.

4. National Athletic Trainers' Association. *Athletic training educational competencies,* 4th ed. Dallas: National Athletic Trainers' Association; 2006.

5. Prentice WE. *Therapeutic modalities for sports medicine and athletic training,* 5th ed. Boston: McGraw Hill; 2003.

6. Prentice WE. *Arnheim's principles of athletic training: a competency-based approach.* New York: McGraw-Hill; 2006.

7. Starkey C. *Therapeutic modalities,* 3rd ed. Philadelphia: FA Davis Co; 2004.

SECTION

8

Conditioning and Rehabilitative Exercise

Part 1   General Exercise and Rehabilitation
             Parameters

Part 2   Joint Mobilizations

Part 3   Proprioceptive Neuromuscular Facilitation
             (PNF)

Part 4   Aquatic Exercise

Section 8 Examination

OVERVIEW

Assuring that non injured and injured athletes are appropriately prepared for the physical stresses associated with exercise and sports is a critical component to the athletic trainer's job. Implementing training and rehabilitation that is specific, progressive, and challenging while maintaining a positive, fun atmosphere is critical to excellent outcomes. The athletic trainer will be as aggressive with conditioning and rehabilitation to the extent to which knowledge is possessed in the areas of functional anatomy, biomechanics, tissue healing, causes and effects of the injury (or surgical procedure), and the proposed treatment effects. People with extensive knowledge in these areas may act more aggressive with their programming while people with little knowledge tend to be more conservative. Positive outcomes are often proportional to knowledge.

CLINICAL PROFICIENCIES

Synthesize information obtained in a patient interview and physical examination to determine the indications, contraindications, and precautions for the selection, application, and evidence-based design of a therapeutic exercise program for injuries to the upper extremity, lower extremity, trunk, and spine. The student will formulate a progressive rehabilitation plan and appropriately demonstrate and/or instruct the exercises and/or techniques to the patient. Effective lines of communication should be established to elicit and convey information about the patient's status and the prescribed exercise(s). While maintaining patient confidentiality, all aspects of the exercise plan should be documented using standardized record-keeping methods. (Reproduced with permission of the National Athletic Trainers' Association.)

General Exercise and Rehabilitation Parameters

KEY TERMS

- Active range of motion (AROM)
- Aerobic respiration
- Agonist
- Allograft
- Antagonist
- Asymmetry
- Atrophy
- Autogenic inhibition
- Autograft
- Autologous
- Basal metabolic rate (BMR)
- Body mass index (BMI)
- Bohr effect
- Borg scale
- Center of gravity (COG)
- Closed-chain movement
- Concentric contraction
- Continuous passive motion (CPM) machine
- Contracture
- Delayed onset muscle soreness (DOMS)
- Endurance
- Fartlek training
- Flexibility
- Graded exercise test (GXT)
- Hooke law
- Hyperplasia
- Hypertrophy
- Hypotonic
- Imbalance
- Inspiratory reserve volume
- Interval training
- Ipsilateral
- Isometric
- Isotonic
- Karvonen method
- Kinetic energy
- Krebs cycle
- Lactacid oxygen debt
- Lactate threshold
- Lactic acid oxygen debt
- Maximal oxygen consumption
- Non–weight bearing exercise
- Open-chain movement
- Open-packed position
- Overload principle
- Oxygen debt
- Pelvic tilt
- Peak expiratory flow rate (PEFR)
- Periodization
- Plyometric training
- Potential energy
- Preload
- Progressive-resistance exercise (PRE)
- Proprioception
- Psychomotor
- Pulmonary function test (PFT)
- Pulmonary insufficiency
- Rating of perceived exertion (RPE)
- Reaction time
- Recumbent
- Recurrence
- Repetition maximum (RM)
- Resting energy expenditure (REE)
- Retrograde
- Scaption
- Sherrington law
- Specialization
- Strength
- Stroke volume
- Synchronous
- Target heart rate
- Tidal volume
- Torque (T)
- Variable resistance training
- Weight-bearing exercise
- Wellness

LIMITS TO MOBILITY

- Skin
- Adipose tissue
- Bony structures
- Contractures in connective tissue

- Muscles and tendons
- Fascia
- Age
- Gender
- Activity level
- Muscle size

> **Quick fact** Decreased flexibility and range of motion will lead to decreased force generation at a muscle.

RANGE OF MOTION AND FLEXIBILITY

- Active range of motion (AROM)—dynamic flexibility
- Passive ROM—static flexibility

STRETCHING TECHNIQUES

- Ballistic stretching—quick and bouncing
- Static stretching—slow and progressive
- Proprioceptive neuromuscular facilitation—concentric, isometric, and passive stretch; partner stretching
- Dynamic stretching—sport-specific movement patterns

> **Quick fact** Current controversy exists regarding the value of preparticipation stretching. Established guidelines encourage stretching before and after exercise.

EXERCISE PRESCRIPTION

- Frequency—number of exercise sessions times per week
- Intensity—overload to the cardiovascular system (THR, $\dot{V}O_2max$, $\dot{V}O_{2R}$) for training
- Duration (time)—length of time per exercise session
- Type (mode)—program of exercise

OVERLOAD

- Body adapts to stress as long as the stress is not too great
- Exercise is a form of stress
- Overloading cardiovascular and muscular systems is followed by adaptation
- Adaptation = improved fitness/strength
- Patterns continue until the body (system or tissue) can no longer adapt
- Fatigue must occur with exercise for adaptation to occur

> **Quick fact** Conversely to the principle of overload, physical gains are easily lost when removing overload. It is much easier to maintain a fitness level than it is to attain it.

SPECIFICITY

- SAID Principle—specific adaptations to imposed demands
- Training must mimic the ultimate task for which preparation is occurring
- Specific muscle fibers and energy systems must be trained to reap benefits of the training
- An upper body ergometer exercise program will have little benefit for an athlete who needs to sprint
- Rehabilitation programs must ultimately prepare the athlete for return to sport; therefore, must attend to specificity

RECOVERY BETWEEN SETS

- Up to 60 seconds recovery between isotonic sets
- At least 60 seconds between isometric sets
- 2 to 4 minutes between isokinetic sets

DETERMINING TARGET HEART RATE

- Target heart rate (THR) and $\dot{V}O_2max$ have a linear relationship in nonsedentary individuals (see Table 8.1)
- Determining exercise intensity prescription can be accomplished through finding THR
- Exercise prescription generally occurs between 60% and 80% of the sum of heart rate reserve (HRR) and resting heart rate (RHR)
- THR depends on exercise goals

> **Quick fact** Heart rate monitors are a relatively inexpensive way to determine how hard an athlete is working during the conditioning and rehabilitation session. Consider getting this device for integration into programming.

ENERGY SYSTEMS FOR EXERCISE

- Phosphagen system—Adenosine Triphosphate Phosphocreatine (ATP-PC) energy systems (e.g., 8 to 10 seconds)

Table 8.1 Karvonen Target Heart Rate (THR) Method for a 41-Year-Old with an RRH of 80 bpm

Karvonen THR Formula	Applied Karvonen THR Method
220 − age = MHR	220 − 41 = 179 MHR
MHR − RHR = Heart rate reserve (HRR)	179 − 80 = 99 HRR
HRR × 60%–80% = HRR value	99 × 70% = 69.3 HRR value
RHR + HRR value = THR	80 + 69.3 = 149.3 THR

MHR, maximum heart rate; HRR, heart rate reserve; RHR, resting heart rate.

- Glycolytic-lactic acid system (e.g., <2 minutes)
- Aerobic respiration (e.g., unlimited time)

STRENGTH TRAINING IN REHABILITATION SETTINGS

- Body weight
- Free weights
- Isokinetic machines
- Isometrics
- Isotonic machines
- Manual resistance
- Rubber bands/tubing

> **Quick fact** Williams flexion exercises (e.g., knee to chest) and McKenzie extension exercises (e.g., quadruped opposite arm leg raises) continue to be used in rehabilitation of spinal region dysfunction.

BODY WEIGHT ACTIVITIES

- Allows for concentric and eccentric training
- Vary repetitions, ROM, resistance, and speed
- Quantify by using body weight scale
- Integrates kinetic chain
- Difficult to isolate segments
- Inexpensive training

> **Quick fact** Changing gravity's effect on the body allows for easier variation of resistance while performing body weight exercises, for example, push-up on the wall versus the floor.

FREE WEIGHTS

- Vary repetitions, ROM, resistance, and speed
- Cuff weights, dumbbells, and barbells
- Instruction and spotting is critical
- Integrate primary and secondary stabilizers
- May be difficult because of stabilization in multiplanes needed

ISOKINETIC MACHINE

- Dynamic muscle activity—fixed speed and variable resistance (accommodating resistance)
- Mostly single-plane activities
- Quantify training in open kinetic chain
- Extremely costly machines
- Does not mimic function in activity or speed
- Testing curve must be avoided before officially measuring strength

ISOMETRICS

- Static muscle activity—vary repetitions but ROM constant
- Fatigue after approximately 5 to 10 seconds to half strength
- Instituted early in rehabilitation program
- Low joint stress
- Institute with very weak muscles
- Isolated strength gain (e.g., 15 degrees from exercise position)
- Caution patients with Valsalva
- Inexpensive exercise

ISOTONIC MACHINES

- Dynamic muscle activity—vary repetitions, ROM, resistance, and speed
- Concentric—muscle shortening contraction
- Eccentric—muscle lengthening contraction

> **Quick fact** When exercising an injured shoulder, consider beginning with scaption exercises (plane of the scapula).

MANUAL RESISTANCE

- Allows for isometric, concentric, and eccentric training
- Vary repetitions, ROM, resistance, and speed
- Difficult to quantify strength gains
- Time consuming for treating professional
- Inefficient
- Allows for interactive work between practitioner and patient
- Inexpensive unless billing for time in a clinic

RUBBER BANDS/TUBING

- Allows for dynamic resistance
- Vary repetition, ROM, resistance, and speed
- Color coded for easy progression
- Easy and cost effective to use
- As band stretches, resistance increases

> **Quick fact** A muscle is capable of generating the most force nearing the middle of joint motion; rubber bands/tubing provide the highest resistance at the end of the range.

AEROBIC ENDURANCE

- Critical component to any exercise or rehabilitation program
- Consider using aquatic environment to train injured athletes
- Attention to heart rate using heart rate monitors

- Minimum 20 minutes three times per week at THR
- Examples of common rehabilitation equipment for aerobic training: upper body ergometer, bike, stairmaster, treadmill, and elliptical

> **Quick fact**
> Get patients performing some form of aerobic endurance exercise as soon as possible in the rehabilitation process. This enhances their self-concept and perceptions, especially critical for athletes.

AGILITY

- Explosive directional change
- Reaction changes in sport
- Requires acceleration, deceleration, and speed
- Improvement must be measured with timing devices
- Examples include T-test and shuttle test

CLOSED VERSUS OPEN KINETIC CHAIN

- Closed chain—when distal segment engaged
- Open chain—when distal segment disengaged
- Functional activities incorporate both types of training
- One joint's function impacts other surrounding joints
- Closed chain activities produce less shear and are safer earlier in rehabilitation
- Open chain activities produce high-velocity stresses—maybe unsafe

CORE STABILITY

- Control of the extremities must be generated by a strongly anchored core
- Core includes neuromuscular control over the lumbar spine, pelvis, and hips

- Located around center of gravity (COG)
- Imbalances in core may precipitate injury in periphery
- Training includes more than abdominal work—approximately 30 muscles attach on and around the core

> **Quick fact**
> Core instability may be one of the culprits causing extremity noncontact injuries. Do not forget during rehabilitation to address the segments proximal and distal to the injury.

NEUROMUSCULAR CONTROL

- Efficient afferent input and efferent response
- Progressive motor control: mobility, stability, controlled mobility, and skill
- Refine and reinforce neural pathways
- Proprioception, static/dynamic muscle ability, reflex integration, and function

> **Quick fact**
> One component of the neuromuscular control system are protection mechanisms within the muscle body and tendons called *muscle spindles* and *golgi tendon* organs.

PLYOMETRICS

- Lengthen, then shorten muscle for increased power
- Contractile and noncontractile elements
- Stretch reflex, muscle spindles (see Fig. 8.1), and golgi tendon organs (GTO) contribute
- Consider 2 days' rest between sessions
- Work-to-rest ratio 1:5 or 1:10

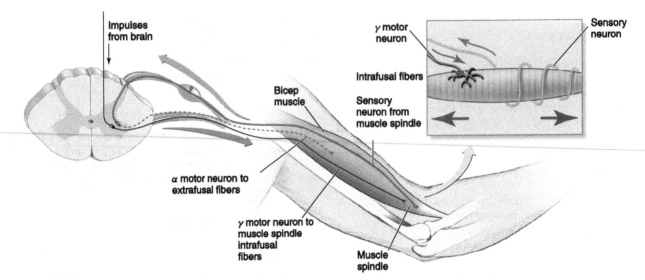

Figure 8.1 Muscle Spindle. (From Premkumar K. *The massage connection anatomy and physiology*. Baltimore: Lippincott Williams & Wilkins; 2004.)

Table 8.2 Training Progressions

Simple exercises to more difficult
Few exercises to more
General exercises to specific
Single plane activities to multiplanar

- Use care in applying high-level plyometrics in athletes weighing more than 220 lb
- Low volume and intensity plyometrics in children (8 to 13 years)
- Phases of plyometrics
  ○ Eccentric (preparation)
  ○ Amortization (transition)
  ○ Concentric (outcome)

> **Quick fact** Decreasing the amortization phase will enhance overall outcome of plyometric exercise.

> **Quick fact** Do not allow athletes to perform plyometric exercises in the absence of enough strength to handle the task.

RESISTANCE TRAINING

- Continuum based on goals
- Strength development—high weight and low repetitions
- Endurance development—low weight and high repetitions
- Machines, free-weights, and cuff weights

 Use the DVD or visit the website at http://thePoint .lww.com/Long for additional materials about *selected resistance training programs and muscle activity in selected weight training.*

SWISS BALLS AND FOAM ROLLERS

- Unstable surface
- Challenges coordination and positional awareness
- Can add resistance to activity
- Size of Swiss ball selected based on athlete's height
- Hips and knees at 90 degrees when sitting on the Swiss ball
- Use care initially with athletes while using these devices

FITNESS EXAMINATION COMPONENTS

- Anthropometric measurements
- Flexibility
- Muscular endurance

- Muscular strength
- Muscular power
- Cardiorespiratory endurance
- Speed
- Agility
- Balance and proprioception

ANTHROPOMETRIC MEASUREMENTS

- Limb girth
  ○ Tape measure (centimeters or inches)
  ○ Assess for muscle atrophy, muscle hypertrophy
- Limb length
  ○ Tape measure (centimeters or inches)
  ○ Assess for arm wing span, leg length discrepancies
- Body composition
  ○ Assessment of body fat percentage
  ○ Methods: Skinfold thickness, bioelectrical impedance analysis (BIA)
- Body type
  ○ Ectomorph—a thin build, low body mass; relatively fragile
  ○ Mesomorph—an athletic build, average body mass; overload bony matrix
  ○ Endomorph—a stocky build, high body mass; hypermobility

FLEXIBILITY

- Apley scratch test
  ○ Shoulder internal and external rotators
  ○ Posterior shoulder capsule
- Sit-and-reach test
  ○ Hamstring complex
  ○ Low back
- V-sit reach test
  ○ Hamstring complex
  ○ Low back
- Thomas test
  ○ Hip flexors
- Groin flexibility test
  ○ Adductors
- Calf muscle flexibility test
  ○ Gastrocnemius
  ○ Soleus

> **Quick fact** The gastrocnemius, soleus, and plantaris muscles make up what is known as the *triceps surae.*

MUSCULAR ENDURANCE

- Push-up test
  ○ Equipment—a stopwatch
  ○ Number of properly performed push-ups in 1 minute
  ○ Involved muscles—pectoralis major, triceps brachii
- Pull-up (chin-up) test
  ○ Equipment—a pull-up bar
  ○ Number of properly performed pull-ups until fatigued
  ○ Involved muscles—latissimus dorsi, biceps brachii

- Flexed arm hang
  - Equipment—a pull-up bar, a stopwatch
  - Length of time athlete is able to properly hold flexed-arm hang position with the chin above the bar until fatigued
  - Involved muscles—latissimus dorsi, biceps brachii
- Abdominal curl-up test
  - Equipment—a stopwatch
  - Number of abdominal curl-ups in 1 minute
  - Involved muscles—rectus abdominus, internal/external obliques
- Wall-sit
  - Equipment—a stopwatch
  - Length of time athlete is able to properly hold wall-sitting position until fatigued
  - Involved muscles—quadriceps, hip flexors

> **Quick fact** Instead of target heart rate being the method for determining intensity, some patients often need the rate of perceived exertion scale to identify how hard they are working.

MUSCULAR STRENGTH

- One repetition maximum (1-RM) bench press test
  - Equipment—bench press

Rating	Description
6	None at all
7	Extremely light
8	
9	Light
10	
11	Light
12	
13	Somewhat hard
14	
15	Hard (heavy)
16	
17	Very hard
18	
19	Extremely hard
20	Maximal

Figure 8.2 Rate of Perceived Exertion Scale. Hall CM, Brody LT. *Therapeutic exercise: moving toward function.* 2nd ed. Lippincott Williams & Wilkins; 2006:100.

- Amount of weight that can be bench pressed for one repetition
  - Involved muscles—pectoralis major, triceps brachii
- Three RM (3-RM) bench press test
  - Equipment—bench press
  - Amount of weight that can be bench pressed for three repetitions
  - Involved muscles—pectoralis major, triceps brachii
- Abdominal strength test
  - Equipment—exercise mat
  - Athlete performs a series of four to seven levels of sit-ups
  - Involved muscles—rectus abdominus, internal/external obliques
- Isometric back strength test
  - Equipment—a padded bench/table, a stopwatch
  - The athlete performs isometric back extension for 45 seconds or until fatigued while prone and torso hanging off end of table
  - Involved muscles—the erector spinae group
- One RM (1-RM) leg press test
  - Equipment—leg press machine
  - Amount of weight that can be leg pressed for one repetition
  - Involved muscles—quadriceps, hip flexors
- Three RM (3-RM) leg press test
  - Equipment—leg press machine
  - Amount of weight that can be leg pressed for three repetitions
  - Involved muscles—quadriceps, hip flexors
- Hand dynamometer grip strength test
  - Equipment—a hand dynamometer
  - Athlete squeezes hand dynamometer as hard as possible, and the results are measured in pounds per square inch (PSI)
  - Involved muscles—forearm flexors, finger flexors

MUSCULAR POWER

- Overhead medicine ball throw
  - Equipment—medicine ball (2 to 5 kg), tape measure
  - Distance ball is thrown using a two-handed overhead throwing technique
  - Upper body power
- Vertical jump (leap) test
  - Equipment—vertical jump measuring apparatus (i.e., Vertec) or height-marked wall
  - Height of vertical jump
  - Lower body power
- Standing broad (long) jump test
  - Equipment—flat jumping surface, tape measure
  - Distance jumped using a 2-ft take-off technique
  - Lower body power

CARDIORESPIRATORY ENDURANCE

- Maximal oxygen consumption (VO_2max) test
  - Equipment—an ergometer, a stopwatch, an apparatus for analyzing VO_2max
  - Direct method—the athlete performs test on an ergometer (i.e., treadmill, cycle) as intensity is gradually increased

- Measured as absolute $\dot{V}O_2$max (liters O_2 per minute or relative $\dot{V}O_2$max) (milliliters O_2/kilogram body weight/minute)
- 1-Mile run/walk test
  - Equipment—track, a stopwatch
  - Length of time taken by the athlete to complete 1-mile run/walk
- 1.5-Mile run test
  - Equipment—track, a stopwatch
  - Length of time taken by the athlete to complete 1.5-mile run
- Cooper 12-minute walk/run test
  - Equipment—track, cones, stopwatch
  - Distance completed in 12-minute walk/run
- 20-M shuttle run (beep) test
  - Equipment—a flat running surface, cones, measuring tape, "beep" recording
  - Athlete runs continuously between two end-lines that are 20 m apart in synchronization with recorded "beeping" sounds, as the time between "beeps" decreases every minute
  - Number of shuttles completed before athlete is unable to keep up with "beep" recording
- Harvard step test
  - Equipment—a box/platform (20 in. height), stopwatch, metronome
  - Athlete steps up/down on box/platform every 2 seconds (30 steps per minute) for 5 minutes or until exhausted
  - Score is calculated using heart rate during specific 30-second intervals

SPEED

- Time to cover a certain distance
- High-velocity activities
- Assisted or resisted sprinting activities
- One of the final components of a rehabilitation program
- 10- to 60-yard/meter sprint (dash) test
  - Equipment—cones, stopwatch

- Athlete runs in a straight line from start to finish line (distance may vary)
- Length of time to finish line

AGILITY

- Shuttle run test
  - Equipment—a flat running surface, wood blocks (two), cones, stopwatch
  - Athlete runs back and forth between two parallel lines (30 ft apart) while retrieving and returning blocks to finish line
  - Length of time taken to complete course
- T-test
  - Equipment—a flat running surface, cones, stopwatch
  - Involves forward/backward running and lateral sliding
  - Length of time taken to complete course
- Illinois agility run test
  - Equipment—a flat running surface, cones, stopwatch
  - Involves cutting and figure-eight movements
  - Length of time taken to complete course
- Zigzag test
  - Equipment—a flat running surface, cones, stopwatch
  - Involves primarily of cutting movements
  - Length of time taken to complete course

BALANCE AND PROPRIOCEPTION

- Standing balance test
  - Equipment—a flat surface, stopwatch
  - Athlete stands on one leg as long as possible
  - Length of time balance can be maintained
- Stork standing test
  - Equipment—a flat surface, stopwatch
  - Athlete stands on one leg with nonsupporting foot resting on inner knee of support leg
  - Ability to maintain balance for 1 minute

P A R T 2   Joint Mobilizations

KEY TERMS

- Capsular pattern
- Close-packed position
- Concave
- Convex
- Loose-packed position
- Manual therapy
- Muscle energy technique (MET)

 Quick *fact* Increasing range of motion calls for two to three treatment times per week.

 Quick *fact* Decreasing pain may be aided by daily joint mobilizations.

Quick **fact** Apply four to five repetitions per treatment session.

JOINT MOBILIZATION AND MANUAL THERAPY TECHNIQUES

- Manual therapy technique
- Passive movements
- Oscillations or sustained stretch
- Increase joint ROM
- Decrease pain—gate control

CATEGORIES OF ACCESSORY MOTION

- Compression
- Distraction
- Glide (slide)
- Roll
- Spin

NORMAL JOINT END-FEELS

- Bony
- Capsular
- Muscular
- Tissue approximation

ABNORMAL JOINT END-FEELS

- Boggy
- Bony
- Internal derangement
- Loose (empty)
- Muscle spasm

CAPSULAR PATTERN

- Abnormal movement pattern because of joint capsule involvement (see Table 8.3)
- Joint specific
- Joint must be controlled by muscles to have capsular pattern

CLOSE-PACKED POSITION

- Maximum joint stability (see Table 8.4)
- Joint structures compressed
- No accessory motion possible
- Ligaments and capsule at maximum tightness

LOOSE-PACKED POSITION

- Resting or open position (see Table 8.5)
- Joint structures have least congruency
- Portions of ligaments and capsule are lax
- Accessory motion is possible

Table 8.3 Capsular Patterns for Selected Joints

Joint	Pattern of Restriction
Glenohumeral	ER → Abd → IR
Humeroulnar	F → E
Radiohumeral	F → E → Supination → Pronation
Wrist	F → E (equally)
MCP	F → E
IP	F → E
Hip	F → Abd → IR (order may vary)
Knee	F → E
Talocrural	PF → DF
Subtalar	Varus
First MTP	F → E

ER, external rotation; Abd, abduction; IR, internal rotation; F, flexion; E, extension; PF, plantar flexion; DF, dorsiflexion; MCP, metacarpophalangeal; IP, interphalangeal; MTP, metatarsophalangeal extension.

 Quick **fact** Joint mobilizations are best completed in loose-packed position. Joint injury may occur if doing them in close-packed position because of maximal joint congruency.

CONCAVE–CONVEX PRINCIPLE

- Determines which direction a joint is mobilized
- Understands joint components and bony surface anatomy
- Concave fixed—convex mobilized → opposite of desired motion

Table 8.4 Close-Packed Position for Selected Joints

Joint	Position
Glenohumeral	Abd/ER
Humeroulnar	Extension
Radiohumeral	90-Degree elbow flexion and 5-degree supination
Wrist	Extension/radial deviation
MCP	Flexion (fingers) opposition (thumb)
IP	Extension
Hip	Extension/IR/Abd
Knee	Extension and tibial ER
Talocrural	Dorsiflexion
Subtalar	Supination
First MTP	Extension

Abd, abduction; ER, external rotation; MCP, metacarpophalangeal; IP, interphalangeal; IR, internal rotation; MTP, metatarsophalangeal extension.

Table 8.5 Loose-Packed Position for Selected Joints

Joint	Position
Glenohumeral	55-Degree Abd and 30-degree horizontal Add
Humeroulnar	70-Degree elbow flexion and 10-degree supination
Radiohumeral	Full extension and full supination
Wrist	Neutral with slight ulnar deviation
MCP	Slight flexion
IP	Slight flexion
Hip	30-Degree flexion and Abd; slight ER
Knee	25-Degree flexion
Talocrural	10-Degree plantar flexion; midway between INV and EV
Subtalar	Midway between supination and pronation
First MTP	Neutral

Abd, abduction; ADD, adduction; MCP, metacarpophalangeal; ER, external rotation; IP, interphalangeal; INV, inversion; EV, eversion; MTP, metatarsophalangeal extension.

- Convex fixed—concave mobilized → direction of desired motion (see Fig. 8.3)

> *Quick* **fact** Common exceptions to concave–convex principle are found in spinal facets, scapulothoracic joint, and proximal tibiofibular joint.

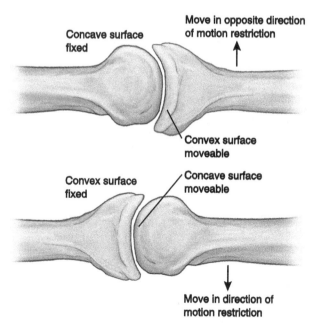

Figure 8.3 Concave–Convex Principle.

LEVER ARMS

- Lever arm length influences surface movement in joint
- Must mobilize close to the target joint
- Mobilizing too far from intended target may change joint motion

TREATMENT PLANE

- Perpendicular to the concave surface
- Moves when concave surface moves
- Stationary when convex surface moves
- Assess joint play or mobilize at right angles to the treatment plane
- Oscillate parallel to treatment plane

> *Quick* **fact** Oscillations are quick thrusts toward or away from the dysfunctional movement based on mobilizing bone shape.

INDICATIONS FOR JOINT MOBILIZATIONS

- Pain
- Joint hypomobility

CONTRAINDICATIONS FOR JOINT MOBILIZATIONS

- Hypermobility
- Malignancy
- Infection
- Acute inflammation
- Bony deformity (including fracture)
- Circulatory insufficiency
- Osteoarthritis
- Neurologic insufficiency
- Rheumatoid arthritis
- Osteoporosis
- Osteoarthritis
- Unstable surgical repair

KALTENBORN'S MOBILIZATION GRADES

- Grade I—joint play
- Grade II—joint separation
- Grade III—joint restriction and beyond (see Fig. 8.4)

MAITLAND'S MOBILIZATION GRADES

- Grade I—joint play
- Grade II—midrange
- Grade III—midrange to joint restriction
- Grade IV—joint restriction (Fig. 8.4)
- Grade V—beyond joint restriction

> *Quick* **fact** Mobilization and traction can be done effectively simultaneously.

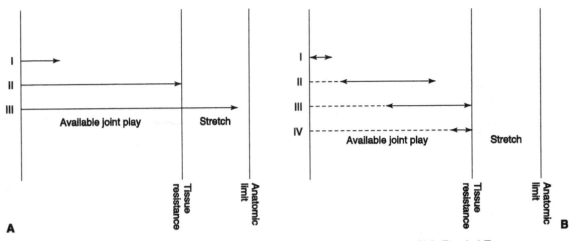

Figure 8.4 Kaltenborn and Maitland Grades of Mobilization. Hall CM, Brody LT. *Therapeutic exercise: moving toward function.* 2nd ed. Lippincott Williams & Wilkins; 2006:129.

LOWER EXTREMITY MOBILIZATIONS

Hip Posterior Glide (Flexion)

Patient Position: Supine with hip near full flexion
Stabilize: Posterior pelvis
Mobilize: Femur (convex)
Force Direction: Opposite to restriction

Hip Anterior Glide (Extension)

Patient Position: Prone with hip near full extension
Stabilize: Anterior pelvis with towel/wedge
Mobilize: Femur (convex)
Force Direction: Opposite to restriction

 Quick **fact** Assure patient and professional are relaxed during mobilizations.

Tibial Glide at 90 Degrees (Flexion/Extension)

Patient Position: Supine, knee 90 degrees, foot on table
Stabilize: Foot under certified athletic trainer's (ATC's) thigh
Mobilize: Tibia (concave)
Force Direction: Same as restriction

Talocrural Glide (Plantarflexion)

Patient Position: Prone, foot over table
Stabilize: Distal tibia/fibula
Mobilize: Talus (convex)
Force Direction: Opposite to restriction

Talocrural Glide (Dorsiflexion)

Patient Position: Supine, foot over table
Stabilize: Distal tibia/fibula
Mobilize: Talus (convex)
Force Direction: Opposite to restriction

Calcaneus-Talus Tibial Glide (Inversion)

Patient Position: Sidelying, medial foot over table
Stabilize: Distal leg
Mobilize: Anterior calcaneus (concave)
Force Direction: Same as restriction

Calcaneus-Talus Tibial Glide (Eversion)

Patient Position: Sidelying, medial foot over table
Stabilize: Distal leg
Mobilize: Posterior calcaneus (convex)
Force Direction: Opposite to restriction

 Quick **fact** Treatment length should be not longer than 1 minute.

Metatarsophalangeal Glide (Flexion/Extension)

Patient Position: Sitting or supine with knee extended
Stabilize: Proximal phalanx
Mobilize: Distal phalanx (concave)
Force Direction: Same as restriction

UPPER EXTREMITY MOBILIZATIONS

Anterior Humeral Glide (Extension/External Rotation)

Patient Position: Prone, shoulder over table on towel/wedge
Stabilize: Scapula
Mobilize: Proximal humerus (convex)
Force Direction: Opposite to restriction

Posterior Humeral Glide (Flexion/Internal Rotation)

Patient Position: Supine, shoulder over table, scapula on towel/wedge
Stabilize: Posterior distal humerus

Mobilize: Proximal humerus (convex)
Force Direction: Opposite to restriction

Ulnar Glide (Flexion/Extension)

Patient Position: Seated, elbow slightly flexed, forearm slightly pronated
Stabilize: Distal forearm
Mobilize: Proximal ulna (concave)
Force Direction: Medial/lateral

Radial Glide (Pronation/Supination)

Patient Position: Seated, forearm pronated, hand off table
Stabilize: Arm against table
Mobilize: Proximal radius (convex)
Force Direction: Anterior/posterior

Radiocarpal Glide (Flexion)

Patient Position: Supine, forearm pronated
Stabilize: Distal radius/ulna

Mobilize: Proximal carpals (convex)
Force Direction: Opposite to restriction

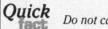 *Do not cause pain* with mobilizations.

Radiocarpal Glide (Extension)

Patient Position: Supine, forearm pronated
Stabilize: Distal radius/ulna
Mobilize: Proximal carpals (convex)
Force Direction: Opposite to restriction

Metacarpophalangeal Joint (Flexion/Extension)

Patient Position: Seated, forearm pronated
Stabilize: Proximal phalanx
Mobilize: Distal phalanx (concave)
Force Direction: Same as restriction

PART 3 Proprioceptive Neuromuscular Facilitation (PNF)

KEY TERMS

- Approximate
- Proprioceptive neuromuscular facilitation (PNF)

 PNF takes advantage of (i) sensory, (ii) motor, and (iii) physiologic processes.

 Brain recognizes gross movement so increased recruitment will facilitate contraction.

PROPRIOCEPTIVE NEUROMUSCULAR FACILITATION POINTS

- Manual contacts
- Resistance
- Muscle overflow
- Succinct, verbal cueing

FACILITATION

- Increases subliminal fringe discharge of motor neuron
- Increases excitation

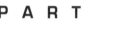 All patterns are identified by the proximal pivot; in the upper extremity it is the glenohumeral joint and in the lower extremity it is the acetabular femoral joint.

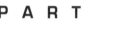 Quick stretch to muscle can increase the force of the contraction through the stretch reflex.

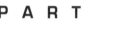 Start motion when muscle is in lengthened position and end in a contracted position.

INHIBITION

- Decreases subliminal discharge of motor neuron
- Decreases excitation

STRETCH REFLEX

- Muscle spindles—reflex contraction so quick stretch causes increased contraction force
- GTO—reflexive relaxation (override muscle spindles) by causing antagonist contraction

TRACTION

- Increased muscular response
- Promotes movement
- Assists isotonic contractions
- Used with flexion and antigravity movements

APPROXIMATION

- Increased muscular response
- Promotes stability
- Assists isometric contractions
- Used with extension gravity-assisted movements

Quick fact Because of overflow (irradiation), energy is channeled from stronger muscles or groups of muscles to weaker ones.

UPPER EXTREMITY PATTERNS

D1 Flexion—Moving from Side to Scratching Opposite Shoulder Blade (Also Sometimes Called the *Feeding Position*)

Fingers—flexion and adduction
Wrist—radial flexion
Forearm—supination
Scapula—protraction and upward rotation
Shoulder—flexion, external rotation, and adduction
Manual resistance—palmar hand and cubital elbow

D1 Extension—Moving from Scratching Opposite Shoulder Blade Toward Same Side (Frisbee Throw)

Fingers—extension and abduction
Wrist—ulnar extension
Forearm—pronation
Scapula—retraction, depression, and downward rotation
Shoulder—extension, abduction, and internal rotation
Manual resistance—dorsum of hand and distal humerus above elbow

D2 Flexion—Hand in Opposite Pocket to Waiter with Tray Position (Removing Sword)

Fingers—extension and abduction
Wrist—radial extension
Forearm—supination
Scapula—retraction, elevation, and upward rotation
Shoulder—flexion, abduction, and external rotation
Manual resistance—dorsum of hand and back of humerus above elbow

D2 Extension—Waiter with a Tray above Head to Opposite Pocket (Sheathing a Sword)

Fingers—flexion and adduction
Wrist—ulnar flexion
Forearm—pronation
Scapula—protraction, depression, and downward rotation
Shoulder—extension, internal rotation, and adduction
Manual resistance—volar surface of hand and cubital elbow

LOWER EXTREMITY PATTERNS

D1 Flexion—Slight Abducted Position to Cross Legs

Toes—extension
Foot—inversion
Ankle—dorsiflexion
Tibia—internal rotation
Knee—flexion
Hip—flexion, adduction, and external rotation
Manual resistance—dorsomedial foot and anteromedial knee

D1 Extension—Uncross Legs Into Abducted Position

Toes—flexion
Foot—eversion
Ankle—plantarflexion
Tibia—external rotation
Knee—extension
Hip—extension, abduction, and internal rotation
Manual resistance—plantarlateral foot and posterolateral knee

D2 Flexion—Adducted to Prepare to Kick a Soccer Ball

Toes—extension
Foot—eversion
Ankle—dorsiflexion
Tibia—external rotation
Knee—flexion
Hip—flexion, abduction, and internal rotation
Manual resistance—dorsolateral foot and anterolateral condyle of the femur

D2 Extension—Kicking Soccer Ball

Toes—flexion
Foot—inversion
Ankle—plantarflexion
Tibia—internal rotation
Knee—extension

Hip—extension, adduction, and external rotation
Manual resistance—plantarmedial foot and posteromedial femoral condyle

Use the DVD or visit the website at http://thePoint.lww.com/Long *Trunk and neck PNF*

FREQUENTLY USED PROPRIOCEPTIVE NEUROMUSCULAR FACILITATION STRENGTHENING PROCESSES

Slow Reversal

- Isometric contraction of agonist
- Isotonic contraction of antagonist
- Facilitates succeeding agonist contraction
- Keys push against resistance using antagonist and pull against resistance using agonist
- Used for AROM and normal timing of agonist/antagonist

Repeated Contraction

- Move isotonically throughout full ROM until fatigue
- Once fatigued, give quick stretch to facilitate weaker muscles
- Used for patient with weakness in specific point of ROM or throughout entire ROM

Slow Reversal Hold

- Isotonic contraction of agonist
- Isometric contraction, hold at the end of each active movement
- No relaxation between switching directions
- Used for developing strength at certain points in a ROM

Rhythmic Initiation

- Progression of Passive Range of motion (PROM)—Active Assisted Range of Motion (AAROM)—AROM through agonist pattern
- Movement is slow so no stretch reflex initiated
- Used for limited ROM and patients who are unable to initiate movement

FREQUENTLY USED PROPRIOCEPTIVE NEUROMUSCULAR FACILITATION STRETCHING PROCESSES

Contract-Relax

- Move body passively in agonist pattern (for hamstrings this is hip flexion with knee straight)
- Contract antagonist (hamstrings) through full ROM
- Relax antagonist (hamstrings) and move back in agonist pattern
- Used for muscle tightness causing limited ROM

Hold-Relax

- Isometric antagonist (hamstrings)
- Concentric contraction of agonist (quadriceps) with ATC pushing toward agonist pattern (for hamstrings this is hip flexion and knee extension)
- Used for: when high tone occurs in either agonist or antagonist side of joint

Slow-Reversal Hold Relax

- Isotonic agonist contraction (quadriceps) into agonist pattern
- Isometric antagonist contraction (hamstrings)
- Antagonist (hamstring) relaxes and agonist contracts (quadriceps) moving toward agonist pattern
- Used for increased ROM when primary limiter is antagonist muscle group

PART 4 — Aquatic Exercise

KEY TERMS

- Archimedes principle
- Hydrostatic
- Maximum expiratory pressure (MEP)
- Maximum inspiratory pressure (MIP)
- Maximum voluntary ventilation (MVV)
- Partial pressure
- Pascal law

Quick fact Center of gravity (COG) usually around L5-S2.

Quick fact Center of buoyancy (COB) usually around T2-T4.

> **Quick fact**
> Floatation devices should be applied between COG and COB.

> **Quick fact**
> A relative density of 0.86 implies that 86% of the structure is submerged while 14% will float. Human relative density generally averages between 0.95 and 0.97.

> **Quick fact**
> Aquatic exercise in patients with low forced vital capacities may not be advisable because of hydrostatic pressure.

> **Quick fact**
> 43 psi for every foot an object is immersed.

> **Quick fact**
> Light refraction makes determining patient positioning in the pool difficult from the deck of a pool. Consider getting in the pool with patients.

> **Quick fact**
> Vertical alignment in the deep water occurs when COG and COB are in line with each other.

PHYSICAL PROPERTIES OF WATER

- Buoyancy
- Hydrostatic pressure
- Viscosity

BUOYANCY

- Upward thrust of water acting opposite to gravity
- Archimedes principle—upward and equal force to amount of displaced fluid
- Relative density (specific gravity)—weight of body compared to equal volume of water

> **Quick fact**
> Because of Archimedes' principle, weight bearing decreases in the lower extremity as water increases its level on the body. Water level at C7 approximately 10%, xiphoid process approximately 25% to 30%, and ASIS approximately 50% of total weight.

> **Quick fact**
> Relative density of >1 will sink and <1 will float. Relative density increases with lean muscle mass so is generally highest in a young adult and less in youth and elderly.

HYDROSTATIC PRESSURE

- Pressure exerted by fluid on a body at rest
- Pascal's law—fluid pressure applied equally on all immersed objects at a given depth
- Pronounced effect on inspiratory muscles
- Hydrostatic pressure increases with depth of water

> **Quick fact**
> Standing in a water level to C7 will exert more than two times the pressure on the calf than an elastic wrap.

VISCOSITY

- Thickness of water
- Resistance that occurs between the molecules of a liquid
- Viscosity of water decreases as temperature increases
- Allows for 3-dimensional resistance with aquatic exercise
- Water is almost 800 times thicker than air
- Movement in the water is resisted because of molecular friction

APPLICATION OF NEWTON'S FIRST LAW

- Law of inertia—objects resist changes in motion unless acted on by an outside force
- Frequent directional changes increase the intensity of aquatic workouts
- Must overcome stationary inertia when initiating movement in water
- Movement inertia (momentum) occurs when energy is required to continue moving
- Inertial lag (drag) is the loss of forward momentum requiring more energy to increase further momentum
  - Form drag
  - Wave drag
  - Frictional drag

> **Quick fact**
> Because of form drag, the larger an object the greater is the drag. Wave drag implies the faster an object moves the greater the resistance. Frictional drag causes water surface tension resistance.

APPLICATION OF NEWTON'S SECOND LAW

- Law of acceleration—object acceleration proportional to the force acting on it and inversely proportional to mass with same direction of resultant force

- Smaller people accelerate quicker and larger people will require more muscle power to attain speed
- Surface area resistance may apply up to 15 psi of pressure against moving objects

APPLICATION OF NEWTON'S THIRD LAW

- Law of action/reaction—for every action there is an equal and opposite reaction
- Aquatic rehabilitation progression increases core stability
- Altering lever arm length, movement patterns, or increasing resistive devices increases difficulty of activity
- Critical point in assuring patient safety with unstable segments, for example, joints

> *Quick* **fact** Because of leverage, shorter things take less energy than longer things to be moved an equal distance in water.

PATIENT POSITIONING CONSIDERATIONS

- Continued interaction between COG and COB
- COG overcomes COB—patient sinks
- Vertical alignment of COG and COB creates pivot for proximal trunk stabilization
- Water assisted movements for hip abduction → exercise in sidelying position
- Water supported movements for hip abduction → exercise in supine position
- Water resisted movements for hip abduction → exercise in vertical position

> *Quick* **fact** Never leave a patient unattended in the pool.

INDICATIONS OF AQUATIC EXERCISE

- Sprains, strains, and contusions
- Preoperative and postoperative conditions
- Complex regional pain syndrome
- Proprioceptive deficits
- Degenerative diseases

- Low endurance and strength patients
- Restricted weight bearing status

CONTRAINDICATIONS OF AQUATIC EXERCISE

- Severe weakness
- Uncovered open wounds
- External fixating device
- Urinary tract infections
- Pool chemical allergies
- Fever and/or contagious disease

EQUIPMENT USED IN AQUATIC EXERCISE PROGRAMS

- Assistive devices
- Resistive devices
- Heat rate monitors
- Underwater exercise equipment, for example, treadmills, bikes, steps

ASSISTIVE DEVICES

- Equipment that assists the patient to increase buoyancy
- Usually placed around abdomen or distal portion of an extremity
- Increases floatation
- Floatation vests, belts, noodles

RESISTIVE DEVICES

- Equipment that increases the normal resistance the body has in water
- Two categories of resistive devices
  - Surface area resistance
    - Flat objects
    - Perpendicular collision of water molecules
    - Speed specific
  - Gravity reversed resistance
    - Foam products
    - Upward resistance to gravity-assisted muscle groups
    - Can be facilitating or inhibiting in nature
- Foam barbells usually provide 2.5 to 5.0 lb of resistance based on surface area (square, triangular, circular, thickness)
- Foam barbells, kick boards, web-gloves

1. Generally harmless muscle soreness that occurs following unaccustomed exertional work is termed:
   a. Fatigue
   b. Delayed-onset muscle soreness
   c. Lactic acid buildup
   d. Stress–strain relationship
   e. Neuromuscular lag

2. How much reduction in strength can be expected with DOMS?
   a. 5% to 10%
   b. 10% to 15%
   c. 15% to 20%
   d. 20% to 25%
   e. 25% to 30%

3. What term is applied to muscles with less than normal tone?
   a. Hypertrophic
   b. Hypoplasia
   c. Flaccid
   d. Dyskinesis
   e. Myoplasia

4. What is the term used to identify a state when muscle decreases in size secondary to progressive loss of myofibrils?
   a. Hypoplasia
   b. Hypertrophy
   c. Flaccid
   d. Myoplasia
   e. Atrophy

5. Aside from disease states, what factors may decrease the strength of a muscle contraction?
   a. Fatigue, lack of nutrients, and lack of oxygen
   b. Sprain, strain, and sarcopenia
   c. Lactic acid, carbon dioxide, and estrogen
   d. Prothombinase, glycotropic, factor, and fibrinolysin
   e. Kallikrein, reticulin, and lack of elastin

6. Which fascicular arrangement is best for muscular power?
   a. Parallel
   b. Pennate
   c. Striated
   d. Fusiform
   e. Spiral

7. Which fascicular arrangement is best for range of motion?
   a. Parallel
   b. Pennate
   c. Sphincter
   d. Fibrous
   e. Multifibrous

8. What is another name for prime mover?
   a. Antagonist
   b. Concentric
   c. Voluntary
   d. Eccentric
   e. Agonist

9. What happens if both the antagonist and agonist muscles contract at the same time?
   a. Stronger muscle will move
   b. Hyperextension at the joint
   c. No motion occurs
   d. Eccentric contraction
   e. Bone fracture

10. What name is given to a structured attempt to contract the agonist and antagonist muscle?
    a. Stabilization
    b. Cocontraction
    c. No motion occurs
    d. Isometric contraction
    e. Isotonic contraction

11. Which systems control balance?
    a. Neuromuscular, ophthalmic, and vestibular
    b. Somatosensory, vestibular, and oculomotor
    c. CNS, motor neurons, and optic
    d. Olfactory, neuromuscular, and oculomotor
    e. Dynamic control, olfactory, and vestibular

12. What happens to the scapula if the glenohumeral joint is unstable?
    a. Moves inferiorly
    b. Moves medially
    c. Moves superiorly
    d. No motion
    e. Compensated at the scapulothoracic joint

13. What properties impact a tissue's reaction to stretch?
    a. Hydration, strength, and lack of nutrients
    b. Creep, fatigue, and stress–strain
    c. Atrophy, nutraceuticals, and glycolysis
    d. Phosphocreatine, lack of calcium, and lactic acid
    e. Neuromuscular dysfunction and hydration status

14. What criteria are used for the selection of Swiss ball size?
    a. Weight of the patient
    b. Patient injury status
    c. Length of arm span
    d. Height of the patient
    e. Patient's shoe size

15. What structure inhibits muscle contraction with slow stretching?
    a. Muscle spindles
    b. Golgi tendon organs
    c. Pacinian corpusles
    d. Lysosomes
    e. Ruffini endings

16. What will happen to an object in water if the specific gravity is 1?
    a. Float
    b. Sink
    c. Horizontal suspension
    d. Vertical placement
    e. Torques

17. What does an extension lag mean?
    a. Inability to fully flex the body part
    b. Inability to perform a cocontraction
    c. Inability to fully extend a body part
    d. Inability of isokinetic movement
    e. Lack of voluntary muscle control

18. What is the proper timing sequence for an upper extremity D2 extension pattern?
    a. Shoulder extension, forearm pronation, finger flexion
    b. Shoulder flexion, forearm supination, finger extension
    c. Shoulder extension, forearm supination, finger extension
    d. Shoulder external rotation, forearm pronation, finger flexion
    e. Shoulder internal rotation, forearm supination, finger extension

19. What conditioning component is needed to perceive the position of the foot as it hits the ground following swing phase of gait?
    a. Vestibular control
    b. Proprioception
    c. Oculomotor control
    d. Neuromuscular stabilization
    e. Axonotemesis

20. What type of muscle contraction is the quadriceps exhibiting when running down hill?
    a. Concentric
    b. Eccentric
    c. Stabilization
    d. Isotonic
    e. Isokinetic

21. When following the DAPRE techniques of progressive resistance, the first set of ten repetitions is performed with what percentage of the weight lifted in the third set?
    a. 25%
    b. 50%
    c. 60%
    d. 75%
    e. 100%

22. Which muscle groups are involved in a bench press?
    a. Triceps, pectoralis minor, and biceps brachii
    b. Anterior deltoid, triceps, pectoralis major, latissimus dorsi
    c. Posterior deltoid, pectoralis major, and biceps femoris
    d. Anterior deltoid, triceps, and serratus anterior
    e. Psoas major, rhomboid major, and pectoralis major

23. Which muscle groups are involved in a full squat?
    a. Quadriceps, hamstrings, erector spinae, gluteus maximus
    b. Quadriceps, hamstrings, popliteus, and hip flexors
    c. Quadratus lumborum, piriformis, and serratus anterior
    d. Hamstrings, rhomboids, iliocostalis, biceps femoris
    e. Piriformis, rectus femoris, psoas major, and tibialis anterior

24. Which muscle groups are involved in a seated military press?
    a. Triceps, pectoralis minor, and biceps brachii
    b. Anterior deltoid, triceps, pectoralis major, latissimus dorsi
    c. Posterior deltoid, pectoralis major, and biceps femoris
    d. Anterior deltoid, triceps, and serratus anterior
    e. Trapezius, pectoralis major, serratus anterior, triceps

25. What words describe the letters SAID?
    a. Sports adaptations to increased demands
    b. Special adjustments to improved demands
    c. Specific adaptation to imposed demands
    d. Sensitivity adjustments to impossible demands
    e. Serious adjustments to integrated demands

26. What are the sensory receptors located in the musculotendinous junction, which monitor active muscle tension during a contraction?
    a. Muscle spindles
    b. Golgi tendon organs
    c. Pacinian corpusles
    d. Lysosomes
    e. Ruffini endings

27. What will happen to a patient in water having a specific gravity of <1?
    a. Float
    b. Sink
    c. Horizontal suspension
    d. Vertical placement
    e. Torques

28. How much body weight is moved in water if the water is located at the patient's xiphoid process?
    a. 10%
    b. 20%
    c. 30%
    d. 50%
    e. 70%

29. What term describes the amount of movement possible at a joint?
    a. Flexibility
    b. Stress–strain
    c. Range of motion
    d. Elasticity
    e. Plasticity

30. What is the maximum frequency recommended for plyometric exercises?
    a. Once per week
    b. Biweekly
    c. Every other day
    d. Twice per day
    e. Once per season

31. What type of drill is a T-drill shuffle test?
    a. Balance
    b. Coordination
    c. Agility
    d. Plyometric
    e. Endurance

32. What category is a cariocca drill?
    a. Balance
    b. Coordination
    c. Agility
    d. Plyometric
    e. Endurance

33. What is the progression for an injured patient to progress with figure 8 running?
    a. Start with longer distance and progress to shorter
    b. Start with shorter distance and progress to longer

    c. Start with shorter distance to intermediate distance
    d. Start maximum speed and reduce jogging
    e. Does not matter

34. What area of the brain assists in controlled movement?
    a. Cerebrum
    b. Brain stem
    c. Cerebellum
    d. Brocca area
    e. Occipital lobe

35. What are the afferent receptors responsible for assisting in limb stability through muscle contraction?
    a. Muscle spindles
    b. Golgi tendon organs
    c. Pacinian corpusles
    d. Lysosomes
    e. Ruffini endings

36. What is the vestibular ocular response?
    a. Cilia triggers anisocoria
    b. Inner ear–triggered response helping with nystagmus
    c. Outer ear triggers strabismus
    d. Cochlear response triggers retinal dysplasia
    e. Brocca area triggers constriction

37. What is an appropriate work-to-rest ratio for plyometric drills?
    a. 1:3
    b. 1:5
    c. 1:10
    d. 1:15
    e. 1:60

38. Which structures detect rapid movement and initiate the stretch reflex?
    a. Muscle spindles
    b. Golgi tendon organs
    c. Pacinian corpusles
    d. Lysosomes
    e. Ruffini endings

39. Where is glycogen stored within a muscle cell for energy production?
    a. Lysosomes
    b. Nucleus
    c. Axon
    d. Mitochondria
    e. Endoplasmic reticulum

40. When does the greatest physiological advantage occur in a muscle?
    a. Close-packed position
    b. On stretch
    c. Resting length

    d. Passive insufficiency
    e. Active insufficiency

41. What is the product of distance and force?
    a. Power
    b. Work
    c. Acceleration
    d. Deceleration
    e. Velocity

42. What is work done in a specific amount of time?
    a. Power
    b. Work
    c. Acceleration
    d. Deceleration
    e. Velocity

43. What is an object's ability to resume its original shape following deformation?
    a. Strain
    b. Stress
    c. Elasticity
    d. Creep
    e. Viscoelasticity

44. What is the capacity to do work?
    a. Velocity
    b. Force
    c. Power
    d. Time
    e. Energy

45. What is the rate of change of position often represented in miles per hour?
    a. Velocity
    b. Force
    c. Power
    d. Time
    e. Energy

46. What is the rate at which velocity changes?
    a. Power
    b. Work
    c. Acceleration
    d. Deceleration
    e. Velocity

47. Which law says the strain of an object is proportional to the stress applied?
    a. Seyle law
    b. Wolfe law
    c. Hooke law
    d. Hick law
    e. Maxwell law

48. What is the resistance between two surfaces?
    a. Abrasion
    b. Viscoelasticity
    c. Friction
    d. Creep
    e. Strain

49. What type of motion within a joint cannot be achieved through active motion but is necessary for normal kinematics?
    a. Passive joint motion
    b. Assisted joint motion
    c. Accessory joint motion
    d. Hypermobility
    e. Hypomobility

50. What is a joint's mobility?
    a. Flexibility
    b. Stress–strain
    c. Range of motion
    d. Elasticity
    e. Plasticity

51. What identifies a musculotendinous unit's ability to lengthen?
    a. Flexibility
    b. Stress–strain
    c. Range of motion
    d. Elasticity
    e. Plasticity

52. What is a failure of a muscle to relax?
    a. Contraction
    b. Dysphagia
    c. Contracture
    d. Hypotonicity
    e. Sarcopenia

53. What is prolonged reflex muscle contraction?
    a. Contraction
    b. Dysphagia
    c. Muscle spasm
    d. Hypotonicity
    e. Sarcopenia

54. What is the main chemical responsible for muscle fatigue?
    a. Glycogen
    b. Hydrochloric acid
    c. Lactic acid
    d. Acetoacetic acid
    e. Seratonin

55. What identifies multiple stimuli arriving at a high frequency initiating a sustained muscle contraction?
    a. Contraction
    b. Dysphagia
    c. Muscle tetany
    d. Hypotonicity
    e. Sarcopenia

56. What situation exists that allows a greater force to be generated within a muscle if additional stimulation produces a twitch in muscle fibers before the initial twitch is completed?
    a. Active insufficiency
    b. Passive insufficiency
    c. Refractory period
    d. All-or-none response
    e. Summation of forces

57. Which skeletal muscle type is more prepared for endurance activities?
    a. Type I
    b. Type II
    c. Type III
    d. Type IV
    e. Type V

58. Which skeletal muscle type has fast acting ATPase?
    a. Type I
    b. Type II
    c. Type III
    d. Type IV
    e. Type V

59. Which skeletal muscle type has a lower recruitment threshold?
    a. Type I
    b. Type II
    c. Type III
    d. Type IV
    e. Type V

60. What are the major components of muscle rehabilitation and function?
    a. Agility, proprioception, and flexibility
    b. Strength, power, and endurance
    c. Coordination, neuromuscular control, and stability
    d. Force, proprioception, and speed
    e. Range of motion, flexibility, and strength

61. What is a muscle's ability to repeatedly contract with submaximal contractions?
    a. Power
    b. Strength
    c. Force
    d. Endurance
    e. Torque

62. What does high repetition, low intensity weight lifting train?
    a. Power
    b. Strength
    c. Force
    d. Endurance
    e. Torque

63. What does low repetition, high intensity weight lifting train?
    a. Power
    b. Strength
    c. Force
    d. Endurance
    e. Torque

64. How many repetitions of an exercise allows for strength emphasis?
    a. 3-9 repetitions
    b. 10-12 repetitions
    c. 20 or more repetitions
    d. 10 repetition max
    e. Does not matter

65. What is the recovery period between sets using isokinetic activities?
    a. 30 seconds
    b. 1 to 2 minutes
    c. 2 to 4 minutes
    d. 8 minutes
    e. 15 minutes

66. What is the recovery period between sets using isometric exercises?
    a. 10 seconds
    b. 30 seconds
    c. 1 minute
    d. 90 seconds
    e. 2 minutes

67. What is the recovery period between sets using isotonic activities?
    a. 15 to 30 seconds
    b. 30 to 60 seconds
    c. 60 to 90 seconds
    d. 90 to 120 seconds
    e. 120 to 180 seconds

68. What is the increase in muscle fiber size secondary to exercise?
    a. Atrophy
    b. Heterotrophic
    c. Hypertrophy
    d. Hyperplasia
    e. Hypotrophy

69. What is the decrease in muscle fiber size secondary to lack of activity?
    a. Atrophy
    b. Heterotrophic
    c. Hypertrophy
    d. Hyperplasia
    e. Hypotrophy

70. What is the rotational force responsible for joint movement?
    a. Power
    b. Strength

c. Force
d. Endurance
e. Torque

71. What defines an isokinetic muscle activity?
    a. Static, no range of motion change
    b. Dynamic contraction at a preselected speed
    c. Consistent resistance and same speed
    d. Dynamic contraction and speed per resistance ratio
    e. Eccentric contraction at varied speed

72. What defines an isotonic muscle activity?
    a. Dynamic contraction with length change
    b. Static, no range of motion change
    c. Consistent resistance and same speed
    d. Dynamic contraction and speed per resistance ratio
    e. Eccentric contraction at varied speed

73. What are the types of isotonic contractions?
    a. Cocontraction and dynamic
    b. Concentric and eccentric
    c. Static and variable
    d. Plyometric and ballistic
    e. Ecconcentric and dynamic

74. What defines an isometric muscle activity?
    a. Static, no range of motion change
    b. Consistent resistance and same speed
    c. Dynamic contraction and speed per resistance ratio
    d. Eccentric contraction at varied speed
    e. Contraction with no length change (static)

75. What are dynamic contractions of a muscle?
    a. Isometric and Isotonic
    b. Concentric and eccentric
    c. Isotonic and isokinetic
    d. Isotropic and ballistic
    e. Ecconcentric and dynamic

76. What is a static contraction of a muscle?
    a. Isotonic
    b. Isokinetic
    c. Isotrophic
    d. Isometric
    e. Isotopic

77. What is a contraction with muscle lengthening?
    a. Dynamic
    b. Static
    c. Eccentric
    d. Concentric
    e. Isometric

78. What is a contraction with muscle shortening?
    a. Dynamic
    b. Static
    c. Eccentric
    d. Concentric
    e. Isometric

79. What allows more force production with eccentric exercise?
    a. Contractile elements
    b. Series eccentric component
    c. Noncontractile elements
    d. Parallel eccentric component
    e. Mechanical unit

80. Which isotonic contraction requires more energy to generate?
    a. Dynamic
    b. Static
    c. Eccentric
    d. Concentric
    e. Isometric

81. Which type of isotonic contraction produces greater incidences of delayed-onset muscle soreness?
    a. Dynamic
    b. Static
    c. Eccentric
    d. Concentric
    e. Isometric

82. What happens to a muscle's ability to generate force as the speed of a concentric contraction increases?
    a. Force increases
    b. Force decreases
    c. Force is static
    d. Force accommodates
    e. Force initially increases and then decreased

83. What is a kinetic chain activity with the distal segment fixed?
    a. An open kinetic chain
    b. Stable kinetic chain
    c. Closed kinetic chain
    d. Static kinetic chain
    e. Transferable kinetic chain

84. What is a device that measures grip strength?
    a. Pinch tensiometer
    b. Grip dynamometer
    c. Isokinetic device
    d. Cable crossover
    e. Sphygmomanometer

85. What happens to a resistance band or tube when a patient performs an exercise with the band stretched progressively further with each set?
    a. The resistance declines
    b. Resistance increases
    c. Resistance accommodates
    d. Resistance remains static
    e. Resistance inverts

86. What exercise technique uses afferent receptors throughout the body to stimulate the desired response?
    a. Muscle energy technique
    b. Strain-counter strain technique
    c. Proprioceptive neuromuscular facilitation
    d. Feldenkrais maneuver

87. What position is the ankle in performing D1 flexion of PNF?
    a. Plantarflexion, eversion
    b. Dorsiflexion, inversion
    c. Flexion, supination
    d. Plantarflexion, subtalar neutral
    e. Extension, pronation

88. Why does a patient exhibit strength improvement very quickly during the early phase of rehabilitation?
    a. Myofibral hypertrophy
    b. Decreased oculomotor response
    c. Improved neural control
    d. Sarcopenia
    e. Increased sarcomere length

89. What principle of exercise requires progressively applying more stress to the system being trained in order to achieve improvement?
    a. Specificity principle
    b. Hooke law
    c. Wolfe law
    d. Hysteresis
    e. Overload principle

90. What exercise principle implies that fitness gains are only achieved in the particular system being trained?
    a. Specificity principle
    b. Hooke law
    c. Wolfe law
    d. Hysteresis
    e. Overload principle

91. What are the three most important components of an exercise program?
    a. Flexibility, strength, endurance
    b. Frequency, intensity, duration
    c. Power, strength, plyometrics
    d. Agility, coordination, proprioception
    e. Range of motion, proprioception, endurance

92. What pyramidal style of strength system is the Oxford technique of strength progression?
    a. Light-to-heavy system
    b. Heavy-to-light system
    c. Single-set system
    d. Compound system
    e. Negative system

93. What pyramidal style of strength system is the DeLorme strength progression?
    a. Light-to-heavy system
    b. Heavy-to-light system
    c. Single-set system
    d. Compound system
    e. Negative system

94. What weight is used in the first set of the DeLorme strength progression?
    a. 75% 10 RM
    b. 50% 10 RM
    c. 25% 3 RM
    d. 100% 10 RM
    e. 90% 1 RM

95. How many repetitions are completed in the first set of the DeLorme strength progression?
    a. 1
    b. 3
    c. 5
    d. 10
    e. 12

96. What weight is used in the second set of the DeLorme strength progression?
    a. 75% 10 RM
    b. 50% 10 RM
    c. 25% 3 RM
    d. 100% 10 RM
    e. 90% 1 RM

97. What weight is used in the first set of the Oxford technique of strength progression?
    a. 75% 10 RM
    b. 50% 10 RM
    c. 25% 3 RM
    d. 100% 10 RM
    e. 90% 1 RM

98. What position is the hip in performing D2 extension of PNF?
    a. Extension, adduction, external rotation
    b. Extension, abduction, internal rotation
    c. Flexion, adduction, external rotation
    d. Flexion, abduction, internal rotation
    e. Circumduction, extension, adduction

99. Which intrafusal fiber is located in muscle and detects the rate and magnitude of muscle contraction?
    a. Golgi tendon organ
    b. Kraus end-bulb
    c. Muscle spindle
    d. Ruffini corpusles
    e. Pacinian corpusles

100. Why might a COPD patient be inappropriate for pool exercises?
    a. Pascal law
    b. Decrease in forced vital capacity
    c. Hydrostatic pressure
    d. A and C
    e. All of the above can contribute

Use the DVD or visit the website at http://thePoint.lww.com/Long to take the *online examination*.

✔ STUDY CHECKLIST

I have studied:
- ☐ General Exercise Parameters
- ☐ Flexibility
- ☐ Strength Training
- ☐ Cardiorespiratory Endurance
- ☐ Neuromuscular Control
- ☐ Agility
- ☐ Fitness Examination
- ☐ Joint Mobilizations
- ☐ Proprioceptive Neuromuscular Facilitation
- ☐ Aquatic Exercise

SECTION 8

SUPPLEMENTAL READING

1. American College of Sports Medicine. *ACSM's guidelines for exercise testing and prescription*, 7th ed. Baltimore: Lippincott Williams & Wilkins; 2006.

2. Baechle TR, Earle RW. *Essentials of strength training and conditioning*, 2nd ed. Champaign: Human Kinetics; 2000.

3. Clover J. *Sports medicine essentials core concepts in athletic training and fitness instruction*, 2nd ed. Clifton Park: Thomson-Delmar Learning; 2007.

4. Hall CM, Brody LT. *Therapeutic exercise moving toward function*, 2nd ed. Philadelphia: Lippincott Williams & Wilkins; 2005.

5. Houglum PA. *Therapeutic exercise for musculoskeletal injuries*. Champaign: Human Kinetics; 2005.

6. Kaltenborn FM. *Manual mobilization of the joints the extremities*, Vol. 1. Minneapolis: OPTP; 1999.

7. National Athletic Trainers' Association. *Athletic training educational competencies*, 4th ed. Dallas: National Athletic Trainers' Association; 2006.

8. Prentice WE, Voight MI. *Techniques in musculoskeletal rehabilitation*. New York: McGraw-Hill; 2001.

9. Prentice WE. *Rehabilitation techniques for sports medicine and athletic training*, 4th ed. Boston: McGraw-Hill; 2004.

10. Prentice WE. *Arnheim's principles of athletic training: a competency-based approach*. New York: McGraw-Hill; 2006.

11. Top End Sports www.topendsports.com. 2007.

12. Voss DE, Ionka MK, Myers BJ. *Proprioceptive neuromuscular facilitation patterns and techniques*, 3rd ed. Philadelphia: Harper & Row; 1985.

SECTION

9

Pharmacology

Part 1   Administrative and Legal Issues

Part 2   Science of Chemical Agents

Section 9 Examination

OVERVIEW

While most athletic trainers are limited by state practice acts in administering and dispensing medications, knowledge about medication uses, effects, and implications on exercise is crucial. This section includes administrative, legal, and scientific components to pharmacology. Online ancillaries give the athletic trainer a brief overview of commonly used prescription and over-the-counter medications as well as dietary supplements commonly used in athletic participation.

CLINICAL PROFICIENCIES

There are no proficiencies assigned by the *Athletic Training Educational Competencies*, 4th edition for this section.

Administrative and Legal Issues

KEY TERMS

- National Formulary
- Pharmacopeia, pharmacopoeia
- t.i.d
- U.S. drug enforcement administration (DEA)
- United states pharmacopeia (USP)

FOOD AND DRUG ADMINISTRATION

- Establishes general safety standards
- Approves and removes products from the marketplace

DRUG ENFORCEMENT AGENCY

- Deals with only controlled substances
- Monitors needs for controlled substance schedule changes
- Enforces drug laws

1906 PURE FOOD AND DRUG ACT

- Established official references for approved drugs
  - United States Pharmacopia (USP)
  - National Formulary (NF)
- Required minimal quality, purity, and strength standards

1938 FEDERAL FOOD, DRUG, AND COSMETIC ACT

- Amended in 1951 and 1965
- Established U.S. Food and Drug Administration (FDA) under Department of Health and Welfare
- Specific antitampering regulations
- Established drug warning labels

1970 CONTROLLED SUBSTANCES ACT

- Established Drug Enforcement Agency (DEA) under Department of Justice
- Controls abuse of legal and illegal substances
- Established five levels of controlled substances
- Prescriber must obtain DEA registration number (Table 9.2)

> **Quick fact** Anabolic steroids were once considered safe and nonscheduled substances.

1988 ANTI-DRUG ABUSE ACT

- Reclassified anabolic steroids
- Moved anabolic steroids to Controlled Substances Schedule III drug

1990 NUTRITIONAL LABELING AND EDUCATION ACT

- Added Daily Value totals to packaged food
- Established dietary supplement definition to include herbs and other substances

Table 9.1 Common Medication Abbreviations

a	Before	PCA	Patient-controlled analgesics	ad lib	As discretion
Ac	Before meals	PO	By mouth	ASA	Aspirin
b.i.d	Twice a day	PRN	Whenever necessary	APAP	Acetaminophen
c	With	qh	Every hour	IBU	Ibuprofen
DC	Discontinue	q2h	Every 2 hours	q.d	Every day
EC	Enteric coated	s	Without	q.o.d	Every other day
Elix	Elixir	subq	subcutaneous	q.i.d	4 times per day
ER	Extended release	stat	Immediately	qwk	Every week
NPO	Nothing by mouth	tab	Tablet	y.o.	Years old
OTC	Over the counter	t.i.d	Three times a day		
P	After	TO	Telephone order		
PC	After meals	VO	Verbal order		

Table 9.2 Controlled Substances Schedules

Schedule Number	Abuse Potential	Legal Limitations	Examples
C-I	High	Used for research No medical use	LSD, heroin, and marijuana
C-II	High	Written prescription only No refills No phone prescriptions	Percocet and morphine
C-III	Limited	Written, fax, and phone prescriptions Refills five times in 6 months	Tylenol with codeine, anabolic steroids
C-IV	Low	Prescription by health care worker and signed by physician	Valium, Ambien, Xanax, and Darvocet
C-V	Low		Paregoric, Phenagran with codeine

LSD, lysergic acid diethylamide.

1994 DIETARY SUPPLEMENT HEALTH AND EDUCATION ACT

- Weakened FDA enforcement of supplements
- Established definitions of dietary supplements
- Developed a safety framework
- Limits the claims manufacturers could make about supplements
- Allowed supplement manufacturers to market, produce, distribute, and inform consumers about dietary supplements

DRUG APPROVAL TIMEFRAME

- Public health threats may expedite FDA review and approval, for example, acquired immunodeficiency syndrome (AIDS)
- Four to eight years to begin clinical trials on less than 100 patients
- Ten to 15 years to get FDA approval for physician prescription of new medications

POISON CONTROL CENTERS

- Dedicated drug information and care for overdose or inappropriate use
- National phone number 1-800-222-1222
- Callers should communicate about the following factors:
  ○ Facts about situation
  ○ Patient information (age, weight, gender, name, and location)
  ○ Ingestion facts (substance and amount)
  ○ Signs and symptoms of the patient

RESOURCE LIST

- American Hospital Formulary Service (AHFS) Drug Handbook
- Drug Facts and Comparisons
- Drug Information Handbook
- Handbook of Nonprescription Drugs
- Health Professional's Drug Guide
- Nursing Drug Reference
- Physicians' Desk Reference (PDR) for prescription, nonprescription and dietary supplements
- Physician's Drug Handbook
- Professional's Handbook of Complementary and Alternative Medicines
- United States Pharmacopia/Dispensing Information

PHYSICIANS' DESK REFERENCE

- Listings of prescription, over-the-counter (OTC), herbal supplements
- Complete information on each drug listed
- Can purchase online portion to assure constantly updated drugs and supplements
- Page colors represent specific information
  ○ White pages—manufacturers' index and product information
  ○ Pink pages—brand and generic name index
  ○ Blue pages—product category index
  ○ Gray pages—product identification guide

REQUIREMENTS FOR PRESCRIPTION LABELS

- Names (patient, prescriber, pharmacy, medication, and dispenser)
- Pharmacy address and telephone number
- Date of filled prescription
- Dose information and directions for use
- Warnings (if any)
- Refills (if any)

REQUIREMENTS FOR OVER-THE-COUNTER MEDICATION LABELS

- Names (product, manufacturer, habit-forming drugs, and active ingredients)

- Contents
- Warnings or cautionary statements
- Directions for effective and safe use
- Quantity of active ingredients
- Address of manufacturer

DOCUMENTATION

- Can be hard-copy or computer program
- Should be easily retrievable
- Include patient date, patient name, drug name, dosage information, and signature of administering professional

DRUG STORAGE

- Keep away from children and pets
- Located in a secure location
- Original container
- Destroy expired medication through biohazardous waste procedures
- Avoid extreme temperatures: store away from direct sunlight, heat, freezing, and damp locations

> **Quick fact** Refrigerators in athletic training facilities must have a lock on them and cannot store food or drink if storing medications.

MEDICATION RELEASE

- Document that allows a health care professional to work with a patient's medications
- Needed for action on behalf of patients:
  - Procuring and retrieving medications from pharmacy
  - Forward prescription orders
  - Secure and store medications
  - Travel with medications
  - Administering medications, for example, inhaler or Epi-Pen

TRAVELING WITH MEDICATIONS

- Keep in original container
- Maintain secure location
- Take original prescription copy
- Travel with enough medication to cover unexpected lay-over or delay in return
- When travelling extensively, contact locations in the area to provide refills
- Check abroad regulations regarding medications to assure legalities
- Assure medication stays with original patient
- Carry-on medications instead of checking them with luggage

BASIC MEDICATION INFORMATION

- Follow directions
- Do not ingest if there is evidence of tampering or discoloration of medication
- Report medication use to prescribing physician, including herbal and nutritional supplements
- Never use medications after the expiry date—potency and toxicity may be issues
- Do not share prescription medications—this practice is illegal

> **Quick fact** Assure that your athletic training facility is updated on current requirements for medication usage. Having standardized policies that mimic requirements for OTC and prescription use will assure practical reinforcement of the legal requirements of medications use.

Quick fact Regulations vary between states regarding most issues related to medication use. Know the law in the state you practice.

- Stimulant
- Street drug
- Suppurative
- Sympathomimetic
- Therapeutic index
- Toxicity
- Tussive

KEY TERMS

- Adverse drug reaction (ADR), adverse drug event
- Androgen
- Angiotensin-converting enzyme (ACE)
- Anticoagulant
- Antihistamines
- Antiseptic
- Bioavailability
- Biotransformation
- Blood doping
- Cholinergic
- Corticosteroid
- Disinfectant
- Enteric coated tablet
- Fungicide
- Fungistatic
- Generic name
- Half-life
- Hydrocortisone
- Intrathecal
- Lethal dose (LD)
- Metered-dose inhaler (MDI)
- Monoamine oxidase inhibitor (MAOI)
- Nebulizer
- Nonsteroidal antiinflammatory drug (NSAID)
- Nutraceutical
- Over the counter (OTC)
- Pharmacodynamic
- Pharmacodynamics
- Pharmacokinetics
- Pharmacology
- Potency
- Prescription
- Proton pump inhibitor
- Runner's high
- Rx
- Selective serotonin reuptake inhibitor (SSRI)
- Side effect

BRAND, GENERIC, AND CHEMICAL NAMES

Brand Name

- Also called the *trade name*
- Proprietary name, for example, Motrin
- Given by the manufacturer
- Brand names can be given to drugs that have been moved into the generic manufacturing phase

Generic Name

- Shorter than the chemical name
- Nonproprietary name of a drug
- All drugs have generic names but may not be generic drugs

Chemical Name

- Drug name with specific chemical structure
- Very long name listing all the chemical components of a drug

GENERIC DRUG

- Drug that is produced after the initial manufacturer's patent has expired
- May be produced under either a generic or brand name, for example, ibuprofen or Advil
- Not all drugs are generic drugs
- Patents usually exist for 20 years for a given manufacturer

FIRST-PASS EFFECT

- Drugs absorbed in small intestine will be transported to liver before going to the body
- Liver may metabolize some of the drug first
- Liver can render drug inactive
- Drugs with high first-pass effect must be administered with higher dosage

> **Quick fact** A milliliter (mL) is equivalent to a cubic centimeter (cc).

FIVE STEPS OF PHARMACOKINETICS

- Administration
- Absorption
- Distribution
- Metabolism
- Excretion

Administration

- Process by which drugs enter the body
- Two general categories of administration
  - Enteral
  - Parenteral

Enteral Administration

- Through the alimentary canal—use the gastrointestinal (GI) tract to introduce the drug
- Most common route
- Medication + vehicle = drug in the body
- Three general routes
  - Oral
  - Sublingual and buccal
  - Rectal

Oral Route to Administration

- Most common and convenient
- Undergo first-pass effect (liver metabolism)
- Possible GI irritation
- Blood concentration levels difficult

Sublingual and Buccal Routes to Administration

- Under the tongue or in the cheek
- Drug blends with oral mucosa
- Rapid onset of action

Rectal Route to Administration

- Mode of administration with upset stomach or patients with limited consciousness
- Absorption is inconsistent
- May cause rectal irritation

Parenteral Administration

- Through nonalimentary canal—does not use the GI tract to introduce drugs to the body
- Varied absorption rate—instantaneous → slow
- Five general routes
  - Intravenous (IV)/intra-arterial
  - Intramuscular/subcutaneous
  - Inhalation
  - Topical
  - Transdermal

Intravenous/Intra-arterial Route to Administration

- Rapid onset—10 to 15 seconds
- Complete absorption
- Controlled administration

Intramuscular/Subcutaneous Route to Administration

- Controlled administration
- Complete absorption
- Absorption rate based on blood flow rate, for example, deltoids faster than glutteals
- Drug volume administration based on size of injection site, for example, glutteals accept larger volume than deltoids

Inhalation Route to Administration

- Rapid onset—<1 minute
- Quick absorption
- Tissue irritation possible

Topical Route to Administration

- Localized effects
- Easy, noninvasive administration

Transdermal Route to Administration

- Localized effects
- Easy, noninvasive administration
- Dependent on skin thickness

Absorption

- Drug movement from administered site to the blood
- ↑ Dissolvability = ↑ drug onset of action
- IV administration has ↑ absorption
- Oral administration has ↓ absorption
- Absorption sites depend on the following:
  - Stomach contents
  - Lipid solubility
  - pH

Common Things Affecting Absorption

- Blood flow
- First-pass effect
- Administration
- Integrity of GI system
- High fatty diet
- Pain and stress level, for example, decreases absorption
- Drug formulation
- Drug interactions
- Absorption occurs primarily through the following:
  - Passive transport
  - Active transport
  - Pinocytosis

Drug Distribution

- Movement of drug from blood into tissues and fluids
- Selective distribution occurs—some drugs prefer certain organs, for example, amphetamines prefer cerebral spinal fluid for distribution
- Common things affecting distribution

Protein Binding

- Drug binds to protein
- Inactivates drug
- Drug has no therapeutic effect

Metabolism

- Biotransformation in the liver
- Drug turned into more water-soluble substance
- Changing drug into another form
- Disease or illness in the liver affects drug metabolism

Excretion/Elimination

- Removal of drug from body
- Usually occurs through the kidneys
- Dependent on half-life and clearance

Half-Life

- Time for drug to decrease by half
- Dependent on metabolism and excretion
- Determined by measuring plasma concentrations
- Plasma concentration = drug concentration at site of action
- ↑ Half-life = ↑ Dose interval
- ↓ Half-life = ↓ Dose interval

Clearance

- The ability of the body to excrete drug
- Dependent on metabolism and excretion
- ↑ Clearance = ↓ half-life
- ↓ Clearance = ↑ half-life

> **Quick fact** Maximum daily safe dose of acetaminophen is 4,000 mg and of ibuprofen is 2,400 mg.

VARIABLES AFFECTING DRUG PROCESSING

- Absorption
- Distribution
- Metabolism
- Excretion
- Weight
- Gender
- Age
- Disease state
- Psychological state

BIOAVAILABILITY

- Ease of a drug being absorbed and reaching systemic circulation
- Opportunity to reach site of action
- ↑ Bioavailability = ↑ rate of absorption
- Affected by
  - Amount of drug absorbed
  - Rate of absorption

BIOEQUIVALENCE

- Similar to bioavailability
- Comparison of two similar drugs, for example, trade versus generic drugs
- Used to demonstrate that generic products are equivalent to brand products

PHARMACODYNAMICS

- Drug's impact on the body
- Mechanism of drug action

RECEPTOR THEORY

- Drugs interact with a receptor usually on the cell membrane
- Reaction causes biochemical changes
- Site of action is defined as the location of interaction between the cell and the drug
- Cells may be specific for a certain interaction
- Lock and key mechanism
- A drug may prevent endogenous substances from binding to receptors or *vice versa*
- Transduction mechanism is the intrinsic ability of a drug receptor to interface and cause a biological response
- Action is either agonist or antagonist

Agonist

- Enhances or stimulates receptors
- Has affinity and efficacy
- Mimics the effects of endogenous compounds
- Intrinsic activity—drug's initiation of response following receptor binding

Antagonist

- Occupies receptor
- Has affinity
- Has no intrinsic activity
- Blocks the effects of endogenous substances
- Two types of antagonists
  - Competitive antagonist
  - Noncompetitive antagonist

Competitive Antagonist

- Compete with agonist for receptor site
- If there is more antagonist drug, the antagonist usually attaches to the receptor site
- Requires increased dosage to overcome

Noncompetitive Antagonist

- Strong almost permanent bond to receptor
- Does not compete with agonist for receptor
- Inhibition of this receptor remains cohesive for days because it may be bound for life of the cell
- Increased dosage does not overcome

ADMINISTERED MEDICATION

- Medications given and consumed within 24 hours
- Minimal label requirements (patient name and directions)

DISPENSED MEDICATIONS

- Medications given in dosages for greater than a 24-hour period

- Extensive labeling (patient name, date of service, physician name, medication name, strength, quantity, expiration date, physician's name and/or initials, lot number, and facility address)

OVER-THE-COUNTER MEDICATIONS

- Purchase without prescription
- Does not include dietary or food supplements
- Recommending OTC medications may exceed the athletic trainers' state scope of practice
- Use unit dose packs—single-dose packs already prelabeled

PRESCRIPTION MEDICATIONS

- Considered potentially harmful or dangerous medications
- Must be labeled "Prescription Only"
- Subject to state and federal laws

DRUG DOSAGE TERMINOLOGY

- Lethal dose—drug level causing death
- Loading dose—high initial dose to elevate blood levels of drug
- Maintenance dose—amount of drug used to maintain steady-state blood level
- Maximum dose—largest amount of drug for desired effect without causing toxicity
- Minimal dose—smallest amount of drug needed for desired effect
- Therapeutic dose—normal dose given to cause desired effect
- Threshold dose—minimal dose required to cause some minimal effect
- Toxic dose—drug levels causing harmful side effects (e.g., poisoning)

ORAL DRUG FORMS

- Capsule—drug inside gelatin container
- Elixir—alcohol-based liquid
- Emulsion—liquid drug with oils and fats in water
- Enteric-coated tablet—tablet with coating to prevent disintegration in GI system
- Lozenge (troche)—tablet with palatable taste
- Solution—liquid with evenly dissolved drug
- Suspension—liquid with drug particles that needs shaking before administration
- Syrup—sweetened, flavored liquid
- Tablet—compressed drug disk
- Timed-release capsule—capsule with various coatings that dissolve at differing times causing dose delivery over extended periods

NEEDLE ANGLES FOR INJECTIONS

- Intramuscular—90 degrees with rapid absorption
- Subcutaneous—45 degrees

- Intradermal—10 to 15 degrees, for example, purified protein derivative (PPD) or allergy testing

NEEDLE GAUGE

- 27-gauge smallest lumen diameter
- 16-gauge largest lumen diameter
- ↑ Gauge number = thinner needle
- ↓ Gauge number = thicker needle

TOPICAL DRUGS

- Cream—dissolves easier
- Dermal patches—skin patches with varied absorption rates for drug applications
- Liniment—counterirritant
- Lotion—Liquid should be patted on, not rubbed
- Ointments—Not water soluble

> **Quick fact** Wet skin → Use cream and Dry skin → use ointment

DRUG STANDARDS

- Rules to assure consumer safety
- Provide drug names
- Uniform purity, strength, and quality

DRUG POTENCY

- Amount of drug required to cause a response
- ↑ Potency = ↓ dosage
- ↓ Potency = ↑ dosage

DOSE–RESPONSE CURVE

- Graphic representation of the response to a specific drug dosage
- Shape is based on number of bound receptors
- Information about appropriate dosage range of drugs
- May provide information on binding characteristics of drugs
- Information about threshold dose and ceiling effect
- ↓ Dose = ↓ drug effect = ↓ bound receptors
- ↑ Dose = ↑ drug effect = ↑ bound receptors

DRUG STORAGE SITES

- May be different than target sites for a drug
- Drug storage may cause toxic effects
- Drug storage may cause localized tissue damage
- Primary sites
  - Adipose tissue—most common
  - Bone—generally toxic agents, for example, lead
  - Muscle
  - Organs—liver and kidneys

PHARMACOTHERAPEUTICS

- Acute therapy—immediate, intensive treatment
- Empirical therapy—based on practical versus scientific data
- Maintenance therapy—chronic condition treatment
- Palliative therapy—treatment based on terminal conditions
- Replacement therapy—supplements endogenous substances
- Supportive therapy—nondisease treatment but treats systems affected by disease and its treatments

THERAPEUTIC INDEX

- Margin of safety in drug application
- Relative term
- Drugs with lower therapeutic index (TI) have narrower safety margins
- Drugs with low TI may require plasma concentration monitoring, for example, blood tests
- TI is a ratio
- TI = median toxic dose/median effective dose

CATEGORIES OF ADVERSE DRUG EFFECTS

- Anaphylaxis
- Dependency
- Hypersensitivity
- Idiosyncrasy
- Teratonic
- Tolerance

DRUG TOLERANCE

- Decreased response over administered time
- Relatively slow process (days → weeks)
- Generally related to liver enzymes and receptor effects
- Not all drugs produce tolerance
- Cross tolerance usually occurs to all drugs in the same classification

DRUG DEPENDENCY

- Physical and/or psychological need for drug

- Produces withdrawal symptoms
- Drug-seeking behaviors

DRUG INTERACTIONS

- Additive effects—summative effects of similarly administered drugs
- Potentiation (synergistic effects)—one drug increases effects of another
- Antagonistic effect—one drug decreases effects of another
- Changed absorption rate
- Changed metabolism rate
- Changed excretion rate

> **Quick fact** Food or herbal supplementation can cause drug interactions.

ADVERSE DRUG EFFECT (SIDE EFFECT)

- Undesirable response
- May be harmful
- Harmful effects range from mild to deadly
- Toxic effects can occur in anyone
- Allergic effects require the patient to previously have taken the same or similar drug in a class
- Some patients are hypersensitive to drugs because of their pharmokinetics
- Overdose = too much medication = toxic reaction
- Iatrogenic effects—mimics pathological disorders, for example, asthma

> **Quick fact** There are too many pharmaceutical and nutraceuticals to remember the nuances of each substance. Know names, dosage recommendations, maximum dose amounts, indications, and contraindications for only the key medications associated with sport.

1. The term most related to a drug's absorption, distribution, metabolism, and excretion is called:
   a. Pharmacology
   b. Pharmacodynamics
   c. Pharmacokinetics
   d. Pharmacotherapeutics
   e. Pharmacomedicatics

2. Changing a drug into a form that can be excreted is termed:
   a. Absorption
   b. Excretion
   c. Metabolism
   d. Mechanical distribution
   e. Pinocytosis

3. The time it takes for half of a drug to be eliminated by the body is called:
   a. Half-time
   b. Half-division
   c. Half-life
   d. Half-kinetics
   e. Half-excretion

4. Which term identifies a drug working in humans?
   a. Adverse reactions
   b. Pharmacodynamics
   c. Pharmacokinetics
   d. Pharmacomedicatics
   e. Pharmacotherapeutics

5. All are documented adverse reactions for NSAIDs except:
   a. Drowsiness
   b. Headache
   c. Bladder infection
   d. Nausea
   e. Hyperactivity
   f. Liver toxicity

6. Drugs that have a high potential for dependency or addiction and some medical value are found in what category?
   a. Schedule I
   b. Schedule II
   c. Schedule III
   d. Schedule IV
   e. Schedule V

7. The ability of a drug to activate the receptor once it is bound is called:
   a. Drug effects
   b. Intrinsic activity of the drug
   c. Potency of the drug
   d. Efficacy of a drug
   e. Inhibition of a drug

8. Drugs that are capable of binding and activating receptors are called:
   a. Lock and key drugs
   b. Intrinsic drugs
   c. Agonist
   d. Potent drugs
   e. Antagonist

9. The type of transportation across membranes that drugs with small molecular weight experience is termed:
   a. Active transport
   b. Filtration
   c. Facilitated diffusion
   d. Facilitated osmosis
   e. Active osmosis

10. The potential reason why patients who have been anesthetized get a "euphoric" feeling during initial aerobic exercise is because of:
   a. Redistribution of drugs
   b. Enzyme-catalyzed conversion
   c. First-order elimination
   d. Clearance
   e. Potency

11. The amount of drug that is actually available and active in the body tissues to exert a therapeutic effect is termed:
   a. Chemical activity
   b. Antagonists
   c. Selective activity
   d. Bioavailability
   e. Conversion appropriation

12. When administering drugs such as Zithromax or in life/death situations, it may become necessary to give more of a medication initially and less during later doses. This process is called:

a. Maintenance dose
b. Beginning dose
c. Primary dose
d. Loading dose
e. Initiation dose

13. Which level of controlled substances includes Valium and Ambien?
    a. I
    b. II
    c. III
    d. IV
    e. V

14. What number must be included with a physician's signature when writing a narcotic prescription?
    a. FDA registration number
    b. Controlled substance registration number
    c. Prescription identification number
    d. DEA registration number
    e. Narcotic control number

15. What name identifies a drug's molecular configuration?
    a. Anatomic name
    b. Medicinal identification name
    c. Trade name
    d. Chemical name
    e. Molecular configuration name

16. What are the cellular changes resulting from drug administration?
    a. Drug effects
    b. Drug actions
    c. Systemic effects
    d. Local effects
    e. None of the above are correct

17. What term identifies two drugs working together to produce an effect not possible independently?
    a. Antagonism
    b. Agonism
    c. Partial agonism
    d. Synergism
    e. Potentiation

18. Which of the following is not an injection route to medication application?
    a. Intravenous
    b. Intramuscular
    c. Subcutaneous
    d. Intragastric
    e. Intrathecal

19. What term identifies a mild immune response to a drug?
    a. Anaphylaxis
    b. Ototoxicity
    c. Hypersensitivity

d. Idiosyncrasy
e. Teratonic

20. Which adverse reaction produces physical and/or psychological symptoms of withdrawal?
    a. Idiosyncrasy
    b. Potentiation
    c. Tolerance
    d. Addiction
    e. Dependency

21. Which of the following is not an adverse drug effect?
    a. Teratonic
    b. Addiction
    c. Idiosyncrasy
    d. Dependency
    e. Anaphylaxis

22. Which is not considered to be an advantage of transdermal drug administration?
    a. Enhanced proportionate distribution
    b. Easy application
    c. Effectiveness
    d. Consistent blood levels
    e. All are advantages of transdermal drug administration

23. Which oral liquid must be shaken before taking as the medication is unevenly distributed?
    a. Syrup
    b. Solution
    c. Suspension
    d. Emulsion
    e. Elixir

24. Which type of injectable medication administration is the tuberculin skin test (PPD)?
    a. Intracardiac
    b. Intrathecal
    c. Intradermal
    d. Intramuscular
    e. Subdermal

25. In which space does intraspinal injections occur?
    a. Epidural space
    b. Pia matter space
    c. Dura matter space
    d. Subarachnoid space
    e. Subdural space

26. Which type of medication alleviates pain while maintaining consciousness?
    a. Narcotic
    b. Opioid
    c. Analgesic
    d. Nonsteroidal anti-inflammatory
    e. Antitussive

27. Which level of controlled substances includes Ritalin and morphine?
    a. I
    b. II
    c. III
    d. IV
    e. V

28. What type of coating is added to aspirin to lessen the effects on the gastrointestinal system?
    a. Gelatinous
    b. Sustained release covering
    c. Enteric coating
    d. Solubility covering
    e. Emulsified coating

29. Corticosteroids function by limiting which chemical?
    a. Cyclooxygenase
    b. Norepinephrine
    c. Phospholipase
    d. Arachadonic acid
    e. Bradykinin

30. Which of the following medications is not an NSAID?
    a. Diclofenac
    b. Ketoprofen
    c. Naproxen
    d. Nabumetone
    e. Prednisolone

31. Which drug interaction has one medication canceling the effects of another?
    a. Antagonism
    b. Agonism
    c. Partial agonism
    d. Synergism
    e. Potentiation

32. Which is not an antibacterial medication class?
    a. Tetracyclines
    b. Sulfonamides
    c. MAO inhibitors
    d. Fluroquinolones
    e. Cephalosporins

33. Which federal drug act controlled the distribution of prescription drug samples to physicians from the manufacturer?
    a. The Federal Anti-Tampering Act
    b. The Humphrey Amendment
    c. The Prescription Drug Marketing Act
    d. The Fair Packaging and Labeling Act
    e. The Federal Food, Drug, and Cosmetic Act

34. Why is the oral dose of morphine much higher than the injectable dose?
    a. Undergoes large first-pass effect in the kidneys
    b. Undergoes large first-pass effect in the liver
    c. Endogenous opioids occur throughout the body

d. Enkephaline is triggered with injection
e. β-Endorphin is triggered by injection

35. Which anatomic structure produces endogenous corticosteroids?
    a. Hypothalamus
    b. Pituitary gland
    c. Adrenal cortex
    d. Gallbladder
    e. Parathyroid gland

36. Which of the following is not considered an opioid withdrawal symptom?
    a. Rhinitis
    b. Diarrhea
    c. Anorexia
    d. Tinnitis
    e. Tremors

37. Which category of controlled substances may lead to limited dependency?
    a. I
    b. II
    c. III
    d. IV
    e. V

38. Traditionally, drug absorption has been referred to as:
    a. Absorption from the muscles to the systemic circulation
    b. Absorption from the gastrointestinal tract to the peripheral circulation
    c. Absorption from the subcutaneous to the systemic circulation
    d. Absorption from the subcutaneous to the peripheral circulation
    e. Absorption from the gastrointestinal tract into systemic circulation

39. Ibuprofen is a generic name for all but which of the following?
    I. Tylenol
    II. Advil
    III. Nuprin
    IV. Motrin
    V. Aspirin
    a. II and III
    b. II, III, and IV
    c. I and V
    d. IV and V
    e. I, II, and III

40. ADME stands for:
    a. Admission, distinction, metabolism, and evaporation
    b. Apocrine, distraction, measured, and exercitation
    c. Absorption, distribution, metabolism, and elimination
    d. Administration, deoxygenation, menochemical, and extraction

41. What term identifies the cause of tinnitus secondary to drug usage?
    a. Anaphylaxis
    b. Hypersensitivity
    c. Ototoxicity
    d. Idiosyncrasy
    e. Ophthalmicity

42. What is the maximum safe dosage of Tylenol in a day?
    a. 2,400 mg
    b. 3,000 mg
    c. 3,200 mg
    d. 4,000 mg
    e. 4,800 mg

43. What is the blue index within the *Physicians' Desk Reference*?
    a. Manufacturers' Index and Product Information
    b. Brand and Generic Name Index
    c. Product Identification Guide
    d. Product Category Index
    e. Adverse Reactions Index

44. Which drug process identifies the physical/chemical changes within the body?
    a. Absorption
    b. Systemic effects
    c. Distribution
    d. Localized effects
    e. Metabolism

45. What drug pH level is best absorbed in the small intestine?
    a. Alkaline
    b. Acidic
    c. Neutral
    d. Makes no difference

46. What are the recommendations for a medication that produces gastric upset?
    a. Take before bed
    b. Take on empty stomach
    c. Take with a glass of clear liquid
    d. Take with food
    e. Take with an antacid

47. Where is the selective distribution for amphetamines?
    a. Heart
    b. Liver
    c. Cerebrospinal fluid (CSF)
    d. Gastrointestinal tract
    e. Lungs

48. What area of the body is usually responsible for biotransformation of a medication?
    a. Lungs
    b. Kidneys
    c. Liver
    d. Pancreas
    e. Large intestines

49. What area of the body is most responsible for drug excretion?
    a. Lungs
    b. Kidneys
    c. Liver
    d. Pancreas
    e. Large intestine

50. What is an increased presence of a drug because of poor excretion and repeated applications?
    a. Cumulative effects
    b. Antagonistic effects
    c. Agonistic effects
    d. Idiosyncrasy
    e. Potentiated effects

51. Which two age-groups have higher risks for cumulative drug effects?
    a. Middle-aged and mentally ill people
    b. Diseased and injured people
    c. Elderly and children
    d. Athletes and the physically active
    e. Infants and teenagers

52. What type of medication has inactive substances as the main ingredient?
    a. Submaximal dose
    b. Placebo
    c. Agonistic
    d. Tetrogenic
    e. Idiosyncrasy

53. Which drug interaction occurs when one medication prolongs the effect of another?
    a. Synergism
    b. Potentiation
    c. Antagonism
    d. Agonistic
    e. Tetrogenic

54. What is the largest amount of a drug given for a therapeutic effect?
    a. Load dose
    b. Maintenance dose
    c. Maximum dose
    d. Lethal dose
    e. Toxic dose

55. What body weight amount is used to calculate standard adult doses of medications?
    a. 110 lb
    b. 135 lb
    c. 150 lb
    d. 175 lb
    e. 200 lb

56. What medication dosage level produces adverse effects or symptoms of poisoning?
    a. Loading dose
    b. Maintenance dose
    c. Lethal dose
    d. Tolerance dose
    e. Toxic dose

57. Which injection is not considered parenteral drug administration?
    a. Sublingual (buccal)
    b. Injection
    c. Topical
    d. Intracardiac
    e. Inhalation

58. Which drug application route has the fastest effects?
    a. Intravenous (IV)
    b. Subcutaneous (SC)
    c. Intramuscular (IM)
    d. Rectal (R)
    e. Oral (PO)

59. What drug term is used when an effect occurs opposite to that desired?
    a. Idiosyncrasy
    b. Teratonic
    c. Hypersensitivity
    d. Dependency
    e. Anaphylaxis

60. Which adverse reaction occurs when increasingly more medication must be administered to achieve desirable effects?
    a. Teratonic
    b. Hypersensitivity
    c. Tolerance
    d. Dependence
    e. Anaphylaxis

61. What is a potentially fatal allergic reaction to a medication?
    a. Idiosyncrasy
    b. Teratonic
    c. Hypersensitivity
    d. Dependency
    e. Anaphylaxis

62. What term identifies a mild immune response to a drug?
    a. Teratonic
    b. Hypersensitivity
    c. Tolerance
    d. Dependence
    e. Anaphylaxis

63. Which federal act established officially approved drug references?
    a. The 1906 Pure Food and Drug Act
    b. The 1938 Federal Food, Drug, and Cosmetic Act

c. The 1952 Durham-Humphrey Amendment
    d. The 1970 Controlled Substances Act
    e. The 1988 Anti-Drug Abuse Act

64. What book defines official U.S. standards for making drugs?
    a. The Pharmacological Basis of Therapeutics
    b. USP/NF United States Pharmacopeia/National Formulary
    c. Drug Facts and Comparisons
    d. American Society of Health-System Pharmacists Drug Handbook
    e. Physicians' Desk Reference

65. What rules assure that medications called by the same name are uniform?
    a. National Formulary
    b. Drug Standards
    c. Drug Identification Program
    d. Drug Facts and Comparisons
    e. Potentiation Standards

66. What do drug standards assure?
    a. Prescription versus over-the-counter medications
    b. Warnings and side-effect labeling
    c. Purity, quality, and uniform strength
    d. Indications and contraindications
    e. Actions of medications

67. What federal act established the Food and Drug Administration (FDA)?
    a. The 1906 Pure Food and Drug Act
    b. The 1938 Federal Food, Drug, and Cosmetic Act
    c. The 1952 Durham-Humphrey Amendment
    d. The 1970 Controlled Substances Act
    e. The 1988 Anti-Drug Abuse Act

68. What federal organization must approve medications before public release?
    a. Controlled Substances Agency
    b. Food and Drug Administration
    c. Narcotic Control Board
    d. Drug Enforcement Administration
    e. Department of Health and Human Services

69. What federal act secures medications with high abuse potential?
    a. The 1906 Pure Food and Drug Act
    b. The 1938 Federal Food, Drug, and Cosmetic Act
    c. The 1952 Durham-Humphrey Amendment
    d. The 1970 Controlled Substances Act
    e. The 1988 Anti-Drug Abuse Act

70. What federal act established the Drug Enforcement Administration (DEA)?
    a. The 1906 Pure Food and Drug Act
    b. The 1938 Federal Food, Drug, and Cosmetic Act
    c. The 1952 Durham-Humphrey Amendment

d. The 1970 Controlled Substances Act
e. The 1988 Anti-Drug Abuse Act

71. How many levels of controlled substances exist?
    a. 3
    b. 4
    c. 5
    d. 6
    e. 7

72. What abuse potential does C-V controlled substances exhibit?
    a. High abuse
    b. Limited dependency
    c. Addiction potential
    d. High dependency
    e. Low abuse

73. What abuse potential does C-I controlled substances exhibit?
    a. High abuse
    b. Limited dependency
    c. Addiction potential
    d. High dependency
    e. Low abuse

74. Which category of controlled substances may lead to limited dependency?
    a. C-I
    b. C-II
    c. C-III
    d. C-IV
    e. C-V

75. Which category of controlled substances generally includes cough suppressants?
    a. C-I
    b. C-II
    c. C-III
    d. C-IV
    e. C-V

76. Which controlled substance categories allow health care workers to call a pharmacy instead of a physician?
    a. C-1 and C-II
    b. C-II and C-III
    c. C-III and C-IV
    d. C-IV and C-V
    e. C-III, C-IV, and C-V

77. Which controlled substance category(s) allow refills up to 5 times in 6 months?
    a. C-1 and C-II
    b. C-II and C-III
    c. C-III and C-IV
    d. C-IV and C-V
    e. C-III, C-IV, and C-V

78. Which controlled substances' schedule houses drugs with limited medical use?
    a. C-I
    b. C-II
    c. C-III
    d. C-IV
    e. C-V

79. Which level of controlled substances includes anabolic steroids?
    a. C-I
    b. C-II
    c. C-III
    d. C-IV
    e. C-V

80. Which level of controlled substances requires a written prescription?
    a. C-I
    b. C-II
    c. C-III
    d. C-IV
    e. C-V

81. Which level of controlled substances includes marijuana and heroin?
    a. C-I
    b. C-II
    c. C-III
    d. C-IV
    e. C-V

82. Which level of controlled substances includes Ritalin and morphine?
    a. C-I
    b. C-II
    c. C-III
    d. C-IV
    e. C-V

83. Which level of controlled substances includes cocaine?
    a. C-I
    b. C-II
    c. C-III
    d. C-IV
    e. C-V

84. Which antibiotic is considered a fluoroquinolone?
    a. Cipro
    b. Zithromax
    c. Biaxin
    d. Augmentin
    e. Erythromycin

85. Which level of controlled substances includes Tylenol with codeine?
    a. C-I
    b. C-II

c. C-III
d. C-IV
e. C-V

86. Which level of controlled substances includes Robitussin-A-C?
    a. C-I
    b. C-II
    c. C-III
    d. C-IV
    e. C-V

87. What federal organization must register persons prescribing controlled substances?
    a. Controlled Substances Agency
    b. Food and Drug Administration
    c. Narcotic Control Board
    d. Drug Enforcement Administration
    e. Department of Health and Human Services

88. Which controlled substance prescriptions may be phoned to a pharmacy?
    a. C-III, IV, and V
    b. C-I, II, and III
    c. C-II, III, IV, and V
    d. C-IV and V
    e. C-V

89. When can C-II substances be phoned to a pharmacy?
    a. Never
    b. Emergency (72 hours to forward written prescription)
    c. At any time
    d. Only if physician calls
    e. Only if emergency room physician calls

90. Which federal agency is concerned with safety standards of cosmetics, drugs, and food?
    a. The Controlled Substances Agency
    b. Food and Drug Administration
    c. Narcotic Control Board
    d. Drug Enforcement Administration
    e. Department of Health and Human Services

91. Which federal agency is responsible for removing or approving cosmetics, food, or drugs for the marketplace?
    a. Controlled Substances Agency
    b. Food and Drug Administration
    c. Narcotic Control Board
    d. Drug Enforcement Administration
    e. Department of Health and Human Services

92. Which federal agency assures that laws are enforced regarding drugs?
    a. Controlled Substances Agency
    b. Food and Drug Administration

c. Narcotic Control Board
d. Drug Enforcement Administration
e. Department of Health and Human Services

93. Which federal agency monitors controlled substance schedules and recommends changes?
    a. Controlled Substances Agency
    b. Food and Drug Administration
    c. Narcotic Control Board
    d. Drug Enforcement Administration
    e. Department of Health and Human Services

94. What term identifies the study of drugs and their effect on living organisms?
    a. Pharmocodynamics
    b. Pharmacokinetics
    c. Pharmacotherapeutics
    d. Pharmacology
    e. Pharmacomedicatics

95. What term identifies a pain relieving classification of medications?
    a. Metabolic agents
    b. Ophthalmic agents
    c. Analgesic agents
    d. Central nervous system agents
    e. Nonsteroidal agents

96. What drug classification reduces fever?
    a. Antiemetics
    b. Antipyretic
    c. Antiflatulent
    d. Antipruritic
    e. Antibiotic

97. What drug name is the commonly referred name and never capitalized?
    a. Generic name
    b. Trade name
    c. Medicinal identification name
    d. Chemical name
    e. Molecular configuration name

98. What name identifies brand of a pharmaceutical company?
    a. Generic name
    b. Trade name
    c. Medicinal identification name
    d. Chemical name
    e. Molecular configuration name

99. Which drug is not considered a narcotic analgesic medication?
    a. Oxycodone
    b. Dilaudid
    c. Meperidine

d. Voltaren
e. Codeine

     d. Side effects or adverse reactions
     e. Hypersensitivity list

100. What list identifies undesired effects of a medication application?
     a. Warnings list
     b. Contraindications list
     c. Actions list

Use the DVD or visit the website at http://thePoint.lww.com/Long to take the *online examination.*

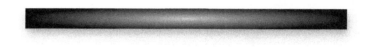

S E C T I O N

10

Psychosocial Intervention and Referral

Part 1   Mental Health and Illnesses

Part 2   Psychosocial Interactions

Section 10 Examination

OVERVIEW

The athletic trainer often is the first person to identify an athlete with emotional or mental distress. Understanding the framework of diagnoses of various mental illnesses allows the athletic trainer to refer the athlete for appropriate care. Recognizing that there are many clinical and subclinical diagnoses within the boundaries of psychosocial issues is critical to efficient care. The athletic trainer should always remember the boundaries presented by the standards of his/her professional practice and never infringe on areas outside the purview of the athletic training profession.

CLINICAL PROFICIENCIES

- Demonstrate the ability to conduct an intervention and make the appropriate referral of an individual with a suspected substance abuse or other mental health problem. Effective lines of communication should be established to elicit and convey information about the patient's status. While maintaining patient confidentiality, all aspects of the intervention and referral should be documented using standardized record-keeping methods.

311

- Demonstrate the ability to select and integrate appropriate motivational techniques into a patient's treatment or rehabilitation program. This includes, but is not limited to, verbal motivation, visualization, imagery, and/or desensitization. Effective lines of communication should be established to elicit and convey information about the techniques. While maintaining patient confidentiality, all aspects of the program should be documented using standardized record-keeping techniques. (Reproduced with permission of the National Athletic Trainers' Association.)

Mental Health and Illnesses

KEY TERMS

- Addiction
- Attention deficit hyperactivity disorder (ADHD)
- Circadian
- Imagery
- Kinesics
- Maslow hierarchy
- Mental image
- Modeling
- Motivation
- Posttraumatic stress disorder (PTSD)
- Rapport
- Somatization disorder
- Stress
- Withdrawal
- Withdrawal syndrome

PSYCHOLOGICAL HEALTH

- Cognitive function that allows for adaptation
- Emotional expression
- Stress-coping strategies
- Dealing with adversity and success

> **Quick fact** Psychological health can influence physical health or illness.

SELF-ESTEEM

- Valuing, respecting, and accepting yourself
- Self-pride
- Can be negative or positive
- Caused by internal and external factors

GENERAL ADAPTATION SYNDROME

- Body's response to stress and relationship to disease
- Alarm stage—activates sympathetic nervous system
- Resistance stage—new homeostasis, disease resistance
- Exhaustion stage—body cannot withstand stress and breaks down
- Stress raises the levels of homeostasis

MASLOW'S HIERARCHY OF NEEDS

- Basic to advanced needs
- Physiological needs → safety and security → belonging and love → esteem needs → self-actualization

PROCHASKA'S STAGES OF CHANGE

- Precontemplation—think about change
- Contemplation—desire to change
- Preparation—believe that change is possible
- Action—implement
- Maintenance—formation of new habits
- Termination—habits entrenched and change over time

> **Quick fact** National Suicide Hotline, 1-800-SUICIDE (1-800-784-2433).

KUBLER-ROSS' STAGES OF DYING

- Denial and isolation
- Anger
- Bargaining
- Depression
- Acceptance

> **Quick fact** Dr. Elizabeth Kubler-Ross' stages of dying are often used to identify stages of loss following a significant injury. Patients often waver between stages.

SEVEN MAJOR CATEGORIES OF ANXIETY DISORDERS

- Generalized anxiety disorder (GAD)
- Social phobia
- Panic disorder
- Specific phobia
- Agoraphobia
- Obsessive compulsive disorder (OCD)
- Post-traumatic stress disorder (PTSD)

Generalized Anxiety Disorder

- Most common anxiety disorder
- Long-lasting state of tension and worry
- Unreasonable worries
- Daily for 6 months
- Restlessness and irritability
- Often tired
- Tension in neck and back
- Difficulties with sleep

Social Phobia

- Fear of public interactions
- Believe themselves inadequate

- Fear is greater than reality
- Anxiety increases during social situations; for example, party and public speaking
- Social avoidance

Panic Disorder

- Periods of intense fear with accompanying anxiety
- Panic attack may mimic heart attack or symptoms
- Trigger avoidance implemented by patient
- Vicious cycle where fear precipitates symptoms and further feeds fear

Specific Phobia (Simple Phobia)

- Fear is exaggerated around specific trigger; for example, snake and spider
- Fear is unreasonable
- Anxiety signs
- Drastic daily behavior changes to avoid fears

Agoraphobia

- Usually begins in adults
- Avoid inescapable situations
- Fears may multiply over time
- Anxiety signs
- Fear avoidance drastically changes life

Obsessive Compulsive Disorder

- Obsessions and/or compulsions
- Obsessions—repetitive thoughts, images, and impulses but no actions
- Compulsions—repetitive actions required to decrease anxiety, difficult to resist actions
- Cycle of obsession may trigger anxiety and compulsion may relieve anxiety

Post-Traumatic Stress Disorder

- Significant trauma causes emotional and/or physical responses
- Responses occur immediately to years after the event
- Common with situations of terror or helplessness
- Patients with PTSD avoid things that remind them of the event
- Common for patient with PTSD to reexperience event through flashbacks or dreams
- Difficulty controlling temper and concentrating
- Sleep disturbance

DEPRESSION

- Signs may be extreme, for example, no sleep → sleep all the time
- Avoid or withdrawing from relationships
- May only have physical signs—increased blood pressure, constipation, and pain

Six Major Depressive Disorders

- Major depressive disorder
- Dysthymia
- Adjustment disorder
- Bipolar disorder
- Seasonal affective disorder (SAD)
- Hormonal-induced depression

Major Depressive Disorders

- Psychosis—out of touch with reality, hear voices, and see visions
- Paranoia—unrealistically distrustful, fear people out to get you
- Delusional—mild to severe unfounded beliefs

Dysthymia

- Less severe than major depressive disorders
- More chronic in nature → >2 years
- May not have physical signs of depression
- Decreased concentration, increased struggles with decision making
- Decreased self-concept, increased guilt, increased death/suicide thoughts

Adjustment Disorder

- Reaction to specific events, for example, divorce
- Decreased ability to work
- Decreased cooperation with others
- Decreased mood
- Increased mood
- Increased crying
- Increased hopelessness
- Depressed mood

Bipolar Disorder

- Called *manic depressive disorder*
- Extreme highs (mania) followed by mild to severe lows (depression)
- Decreased judgment
- Increased risk of suicide because of extreme mood changes

Seasonal Affective Disorder

- Regular depression during fall and winter
- Related to decrease sunlight
- Crave for carbohydrates
- Increased appetite, sleep, and irritability

Schizophrenia

- Mild to severe cases
- Imprecise diagnosis
- Lots of diseases may manifest as schizophrenia
- Perceptions altered hallucinations
- Confusing thoughts
- Decreased socialization
- Delusions
- Disorganized thoughts
- Flat affect

Specific Hormonal-Induced Depression
- Premenstrual dysphoric disorder
- Postpartum depression

Premenstrual Dysphoric Disorder
- Symptoms increase a week before menstruation
- Increased anger and sadness, fatigue, anxiety, bloating, withdrawal, and crying

Postpartum Depression
- Occurs following delivery of child—days or weeks after
- Same symptoms as major depressive disorder

EATING DISORDERS

- Anorexia nervosa
- Bulimia nervosa
- Binge eating disorder
- Anorexia athletica (see Section 11)

 Quick **fact** Eating disorders have multidimensional causes.

 Quick **fact** Subclinical eating disorders, ones that do not fit defined categories, can be very dangerous to athletic participation.

 Quick **fact** Anorexia athletica may be athlete-specific eating disorders.

SUBSTANCE ABUSE

- May be genetically predisposed to abuse problems
- Screening examples include CAGE or F-Q Max questions
- Tolerance—increased substance use for same effect
- Withdrawal—distress with substance revocation
- Dependency—compulsion to use substance
- At-risk use—substance use increases participants' hazardous problems

PSYCHOTHERAPY PROFESSIONALS

- Psychiatrists
  - Medical doctor with 4-year residency program
  - Biological treatment for emotional disorders, for example, medications
  - Licensed
- Clinical psychologists
  - Doctorate in psychology
  - One year of internship
  - May have specialty areas
  - Licensed
- Social worker
  - Various levels and titles
  - Generally Master's degree with 2 years' supervision
  - Pass comprehensive national examination
- Counselor
  - Bachelor's in theology, psychology, or education
  - Master's degree with 2 years' supervision

P A R T **2** # Psychosocial Interactions

COMMUNICATIONS

- Verbal
- Nonverbal

Verbal Communications
- Roles as sender or receiver of communications
- Talk with people
- Understand audience
- Establish and maintain positive environment
- Become skilled at listening
- Give clear and concise instructions

Nonverbal Communications
- Extremely powerful aspect of communications

- Three major components
  - Kinesics—body language
  - Paralanguage—voice characteristics
  - Proxemics—personal space

LISTENING SKILLS

- Active listening—demonstrate concern
- Parroting—repeat words
- Paraphrasing—restate key concepts
- Reflection—focus on emotions
- Be disciplined in attempts to listen

DERAILING COMMUNICATIONS

- Past experiences of sender or receiver of communications

- Clarity of message
- Verbal and nonverbal language
- Using electronic media to communicate when nonverbal language cannot be interpreted

> *Quick* **fact** Treating injuries usually requires encroaching the patient's intimate space. Use care and ask permission.

COMPLEX REGIONAL PAIN SYNDROME

- Reflex sympathetic dystrophy (RSD)
- Disproportionate pain
- Injury may respond normally and then deteriorate
- Hypersensitivity, hyperhydrosis, erythema, edema, and muscle guarding
- Early intervention is key to success
- Possibly permanent disability

MYOFASCIAL PAIN SYNDROME

- Connective tissue and muscles
- Commonly associated with cervical and lumbar musculature
- Bilateral trigger points
- Contributed to by both physical and emotional stress
- Often a diagnosis of exclusion

SOMATIZATION

- Physical symptoms originating from psychological illness
- History of physical illness/injury
- Do not assume somatization—always consider physical complaints
- Patient interactions may become difficult
- Consider counseling
- Often a diagnosis of exclusion

> *Quick* **fact** Clinicians should never assume that causes of chronic pain are unfounded. Patients are often misdiagnosed—search for the answers to the pain puzzle.

ADJUSTMENT TO INJURY

- Stage model
- Cognitive model

Stage Model

- Linear model
- Includes predictable emotional progression and structural factors
- On the basis of Dr. Elizabeth Kubler-Ross' emotional stages

Cognitive Model

- Thought-focused model
- Developed because of perceived differences among patients with similar diagnoses
- Personal and situational factors dictate treatment progression

> *Quick* **fact** Good athletic trainers provide emotional as well as physical first aid.

GOAL SETTING

- Method to focus treatment progression
- Divided into short-term, intermediate, and long-term goals
- Objective
- Measurable
- Attainable
- Realistic
- Devised in cooperation with the athlete to promote compliance
- Constructed with positive wording
- Recorded and monitored with verbal and visual feedback

> *Quick* **fact** Incorporating the injured athlete into team activities enhances psychosocial support throughout the rehabilitation process.

> *Quick* **fact** Each athlete will react differently to an injury. The athletic trainer must be equipped to identify problematic responses.

LOCUS OF CONTROL

- Perception of control over personal behaviors
- Internal—personal control
- External—other's control

INTROVERSION

- Personality trait
- Self-focused
- Introspective
- Shy and quiet
- Quiet reflection
- Energy gained from quiet times
- Learns best in private environments
- Reflects first and acts thereafter

EXTROVERSION

- Personality trait
- Social and people-driven individual

- Learn in social and physically engaging environment
- Acts first and reflects thereafter

Quick fact Help injured athletes take control over components of their care.

RELAXATION

- Controlling muscle tension
- Use cue words to consciously relax
- Assists recovery from activity or injury
- Can be used with or without imagery
- Tension relaxation ratio: 10 to 15 seconds tense: 15 to 20 seconds relax

Quick fact Use humor as a coping strategy—having fun during treatment makes the process much easier.

IMAGERY

- Visualization
- Mental rehearsal of activity
- Used in rehabilitation or training
- Assists with coping of injury and skill mastery

Quick fact Trust, rapport, and empathy are key components to effectively treat injured athletes.

Quick fact The athletic trainer should use care and not overextend his or her training and comfort in areas of psychosocial care.

1. A starting forward on the football team has been injured and can only complete his rehabilitation program during practice in the athletic training room. What concern do you, as his athletic trainer, have for this arrangement?
   a. Athlete will become dependent on you with individual treatment
   b. Athlete will get poor care because you have too much to do
   c. Athlete's teammates will think of him as a malingerer
   d. Athlete will be alienated from his social support system
   e. Athlete will push himself to get better too quickly

2. Which is a major depressive disorder?
   a. General adaptation syndrome
   b. Paranoia
   c. Substance abuse
   d. Agoraphobia
   e. Post-traumatic stress disorder

3. Personality and mood state have been examined in the literature. Which of the following variables are not considered to relate to this concept?
   a. Pessimistic explanatory style
   b. Disproportionate optimism
   c. Hardiness
   d. Dispositional optimism
   e. All are related

4. Which psychotherapy professional has gone to medical school and completed 4-year residence?
   a. Counselor
   b. Psychologist
   c. Social worker
   d. Psychiatrist
   e. Sports psychiatrist

5. Adaptive response to adverse circumstances that requires an external incentive for being injured is termed:
   a. Boredom
   b. Malingering
   c. Self-perception
   d. Adherence
   e. Athletic identity

6. The combination of commitment, challenge, and control is called:
   a. Cognitive appraisal
   b. Adherence
   c. Hardiness
   d. Self-efficacy
   e. Disproportionate optimism

7. Style of nonverbal communication related to facial gestures and posture is called:
   a. Paralanguage
   b. Proxemics
   c. Kinesics
   d. Encoding
   e. Actions

8. A style of listening that reflects the ability to repeat what the athlete says using his words is termed:
   a. Active listening
   b. Parroting
   c. Paraphrasing
   d. Reflection of feeling
   e. Repertory

9. In order to help your athletes to create more options for outcomes, the rehabiliation professional should utilize all of the following skills except:
   a. Reframing
   b. Goal setting
   c. Reinforcement
   d. Directives
   e. Profile of mood states

10. In attempting to screen for suicide ideation, all of the following questions should be asked except?
    a. Is this the worst depression you have ever experienced?
    b. Has this depression prompted you to think that life is not worth living?
    c. Can you not see that this injury is not significant in the relative scheme of life?
    d. Is life worth living?
    e. Have you thought of a plan as to how you might end life?

11. All of the following are reasons to document counseling efforts with athletes except:
    a. Improved communications
    b. Professional standards

c. Memory aid
d. Referral processes
e. Legal protection

12. An ethical position that requires the sports medicine professional to refuse to divulge any aspect of the athlete's medical or psychological history except under very rare circumstances is called:
    a. Privilege
    b. Standard of care
    c. Standard of practice
    d. Confidentiality
    e. Informed consent

13. Jim is a 21-year-old athlete who has been injured for some time. You know that he has been partying quite a bit and may be drinking daily. In confronting him, he mentions that he needs to drink more frequently than he used to in order to be happy. You identify Jim as being at risk and exhibiting signs of:
    a. Withdrawal
    b. Tolerance
    c. Annoyance
    d. CAGE
    e. AUDIT

14. Which stage of general adaptation syndrome (GAS) is indicated by injury?
    a. Alarm stage
    b. Resistance stage
    c. Exhaustion stage
    d. Fatiguing stage
    e. Depression stage

15. When using an F-Q Max Screen, which statement(s) are true?
    a. Screen for alcohol abuse issues
    b. Screen for drug abuse
    c. Frequency times quantity exceeding 7 drinks for women or 14 for men in a single week may imply alcohol abuse
    d. Frequency times quantity exceeding four uses of drugs for women or seven uses of drugs for men in a single week may imply drug abuse
    e. A and C
    f. B and D

16. Substances that are taken for the purpose of enhancing athletic performance are called:
    a. Ergolytic aids
    b. Restorative drugs
    c. Ergogenic aids
    d. Hyperplasic drugs
    e. Hypertrophic drugs

17. All of the following are stages of change except:
    a. Maintenance
    b. Precontemplation
    c. Contemplation

d. Motivation
e. Action

18. DSM-IV criteria for anorexia nervosa includes all, except:
    a. Refusal to maintain body weight at or above a minimally normal weight for age and height
    b. Intense fear of gaining weight or becoming fat, even though underweight
    c. A sense of lack of control over eating during a specific episode
    d. In postmenarcheal females, amenorrhea for at least three consecutive cycles

19. Which is not an anxiety disorder?
    a. Dysthymia
    b. Agoraphobia
    c. Post-traumatic stress disorder
    d. Obsessive compulsive disorder
    e. Simple phobia

20. Which is the final stage in Kubler-Ross' stages of dying?
    a. Anger
    b. Bargaining
    c. Action
    d. Depression
    e. Acceptance

21. What is the highest level of Maslow's hierarchy of needs?
    a. Safety and security
    b. Belonging and love
    c. Self-actualization
    d. Esteem needs
    e. Exhaustion

22. Which is a sign of schizophrenia?
    a. Craving for carbohydrates
    b. Confusing thoughts
    c. Irritability
    d. Increased appetite
    e. Depressed mood

23. Which is not a form of nonverbal communications?
    a. Paralanguage
    b. Somatization
    c. Kinesics
    d. Proxemics
    e. Body language

24. Your athlete asks to talk with you in confidence starting by saying, "You have to promise that you will not tell anyone what I am telling you." Which is your biggest concern in this scenario?
    a. Athlete is concerned with confidentiality of information
    b. Your boss may want to know about the conversation

c. You discuss everything with your athletic training students
d. The athlete may share things outside your professional capability
e. The athlete is going to share traumatic event information with you

25. What term identifies the perception of control over personal behaviors?
a. Introversion
b. Goal setting
c. Linear control
d. Focused model
e. Locus of control

26. Which anxiety disorder is characterized as usually beginning in adults, sometimes leading to avoiding inescapable situations?
a. Specific phobia
b. Social phobia
c. Simple phobia
d. Agoraphobia
e. Panic disorder

27. Which component of Porchaska's stages of change identifies the desire to change?
a. Alarm
b. Action
c. Maintenance
d. Contemplation
e. Termination

28. The process by which a patient imagines their recovery from an injury or illness can best be described by which of the following terms?
a. Progressive relaxation
b. Mental relaxation
c. Imagery
d. Attention diversion
e. Parroting

29. Which is a form of progressive relaxation exercises?
a. Horschel's progressive relaxation
b. Cook's progressive relaxation
c. Kubler-Ross' progressive relaxation
d. Jacobson's progressive relaxation
e. Maxwell's progressive relaxation

30. Which of the following best describes when an athlete has a negative attitude toward their sport due to overtraining and exhaustion.
a. SAD
b. Depression
c. OCD
d. Burnout
e. Generalized anxiety disorder

31. Which personality type is characterized by reflecting and then acting?
a. Locus of control
b. Proxemics
c. Introversion
d. Extroversion
e. Judgmental

32. One of your athletes is struggling to achieve adequate range of motion (ROM) following knee surgery. What might be an effective way to improve her ROM?
a. Tell her to suck it up and work harder
b. Thought stoppage
c. Tension reduction
d. Attention diversion
e. Refuting irrational thoughts

33. Of these, which is the one most likely not to identify a reaction of an athlete to a season ending injury?
a. Fear
b. Anxiety
c. Hyperactivity
d. Apathy
e. Depression

34. Which disorder is characterized as disproportionate pain occurring often some time after the initial injury?
a. Somatization
b. Myofacial pain syndrome
c. Complex regional pain syndrome
d. Fibromyalgia
e. Dysphagia

35. Athletic trainers are considered:
a. First-level helpers
b. Second-level helpers
c. Third-level helpers
d. Fourth-level helpers
e. None of the above

36. All are considered warning signs associated with eating disorders, except:
a. Gastrointestinal complaints
b. Cuts on knuckles, blood shot eyes, and discolored teeth
c. Noticeable fluctuations in weight
d. Excessive concern with or self-deprecating comments about weight and shape
e. Frequent visits to the restroom following meals

37. Rapport is defined as:
a. A method of working with patients or clients to assist them in modifying or reducing factors that interfere with effective living
b. A goal-oriented act intended to benefit another person

c. A state of relationship between two or more people characterized by trust and confidence
d. The process of sending, receiving, and understanding information
e. The benefits to well-being that people derive through their relationships with others

38. Which of the following is not a counseling trap that sports medicine professionals should avoid?
    a. Conflict of interest
    b. Dependency
    c. Lack of resources
    d. Lack of training
    e. Short-term counseling

39. Which of the following are psychological factors of Andersen and Williams' stress response model of athletic injury?
    a. Personality, history of stressors, coping resources
    b. History of stressors, attentional changes, personality

c. Personality, coping resources, state of anxiety
d. Coping resources, social support, state of anxiety
e. Social support, attentional changes, coping resources

40. Which of the following is not an introverted personality trait?
    a. Shy
    b. Introspective
    c. Social
    d. First reflects, then acts
    e. Self-focused

 Use the DVD or visit the website at http://thePoint.lww.com/Long to take the *online examination.*

Nutritional Aspects of Injuries and Illnesses

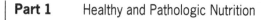

Part 1   Healthy and Pathologic Nutrition

Part 2   Nutrition and Athletic Performance

Part 3   Weight Management and Eating Disorders

Part 4   Dietary Supplements and Ergogenic Aids

Section 11 Examination

OVERVIEW

The nutritional component of a patient's lifestyle plays a large role in the activities of daily living, physical performance, and illness prevention. The athletic trainer will routinely be asked questions on topics such as weight control, healthy food choices, dietary supplements, and ergogenic aids, and therefore should be prepared to answer those types of inquiries. The athletic trainer must also possess the ability to use his or her knowledge of this content area to perform such tasks as designing precompetition meals, assessing body composition, and educating patients on healthy nutritional practices. Patient education plays a particularly important role in this content area because of the impact it can have on a person's life-long health.

CLINICAL PROFICIENCIES

- Demonstrate the ability to counsel a patient on proper nutrition. This may include providing basic nutritional information and/or an exercise and nutrition program for weight gain or weight loss. The student will demonstrate the ability to take measurements and figure calculations for a weight control plan (e.g., measurement of body composition and body mass index [BMI], calculation of energy expenditure, caloric intake, and basal metabolic rate [BMR]). Armed with basic nutritional data, the student will demonstrate the ability to develop and implement a preparticipation meal and an appropriate exercise and nutritional plan for an active individual. The student will develop an active listening relationship to effectively communicate with the patient and, as appropriate, refer the patient to other medical professionals (physician, nutritionist, counselor or psychologist) as needed.

- Demonstrate the ability to recognize disordered eating and eating disorders, establish a professional helping relationship with the patient, interact through support and education, and encourage vocal discussion and other support through referral to the appropriate medical professionals. (Reproduced with permission of the National Athletic Trainers' Association.)

Healthy and Pathologic Nutrition

KEY TERMS

- Amenorrhea
- Dietary reference intake (DRI)
- Amino acid (AA, aa)
- Calorie
- Cholesterol
- Fiber
- Malnutrition
- Recommended dietary allowance (RDA)
- Vegan

MACRONUTRIENTS

- Carbohydrates
- Fats
- Proteins

Carbohydrates

- Saccharides
- Abbreviation—CHO
- Energy-providing nutrient
- Most efficient energy source
- 4 Calories (kcal) per gram
- Liver breaks down into glucose (blood sugar)
- Primary function—supply energy

 Quick fact Athletes should consume a carbohydrate-rich diet to ensure maximization of muscle glycogen stores that are utilized during exercise.

Types of Carbohydrates

- Monosaccharides—single sugars
  - Basic unit of CHO
  - Glucose, fructose, galactose, and ribose
- Disaccharides—two monosaccharides (sugars)
  - Sucrose, lactose, and maltose
- Oligosaccharides—three to ten monosaccharides
  - Raffinose, stachyose, and verbacose
- Polysaccharides—11 or more monosaccharides
  - Starch, fiber, glycogen, and glycosaminoglycans (GAGs)

 Quick fact Monosaccharides and disaccharides are classified as simple sugars.

Monosaccharides

- Glucose
  - Dextrose or blood sugar
  - In blood—regulated by insulin and glucagon
  - Unused glucose (glycogen)—stored in liver and muscles
  - Not used or stored in liver/muscles—converted to fat for later energy use
  - Gluconeogenesis—glucose production in the body (liver primarily)
  - Food sources—honey, some fruits
- Fructose
  - Levulose or fruit sugar
  - Metabolized in liver—converted to glucose
  - Food sources—honey, some fruits
- Galactose
  - Brain sugar
  - Converted to glucose
  - Forms lactose—milk sugar
  - Food sources—dairy products
- Ribose
  - Role—formation of DNA and RNA
  - Synthesized from glucose

 Quick fact An instrument known as a *glucometer* can be used to measure an individual's blood glucose (sugar) level.

Disaccharides

- Sucrose
  - Table sugar
  - Glucose + fructose
  - Most common sweetener in food
  - Food sources—honey, maple syrup
- Lactose
  - Milk sugar
  - Glucose + galactose
  - Food sources—milk
- Maltose
  - Malt sugar
  - Glucose + glucose
  - Foods sources—barley, malted syrups

Quick fact Sucrose causes a rapid increase in an individual's blood glucose (sugar) level and is quickly utilized for energy during exercise.

Polysaccharides
- Starch
  - Found in plants
  - Long glucose chains
  - Converted to glucose for energy use
  - Food sources—potatoes, rice, pasta, peas
- Fiber
  - Structural part of plants
  - Poorly digested
  - Aids in bowel elimination
  - May reduce risk of some diseases—colon cancer, diabetes
  - Types: (i) soluble (e.g., pectins) and (ii) insoluble (e.g., cellulose)
  - Food sources—legumes, whole grains, avocado
- Glycogen
  - Animal polysaccharide
  - Branched glucose chains
  - Stored in liver and muscles
  - Liver glycogen—reconverted to glucose for energy use
  - Muscle glycogen—primary source of CHO energy for muscular function
- GAGs
  - Unbranched polysaccharides
  - Concentrated in joints
  - Examples—chondroitin sulfate, heparin sulfate

 Use the DVD or visit the website at http://thePoint.lww.com/Long for addition materials about *carbohydrate food sources*.

 Quick fact Excessive amounts of fiber in the diet can cause intestinal discomfort.

Quick fact Fiber binds to cholesterol, which can prevent the absorption of cholesterol.

Classes of Carbohydrates
- Simple CHO
  - Sugar
  - Food sources—fruits, honey, table sugar
- Complex CHO
  - Starch and fiber
  - Food sources—whole wheat breads, legumes, fruits, pasta

Quick fact The intake of complex carbohydrates are preferred for individuals engaged in athletic activities, versus the intake of simple carbohydrates, because they can provide a more sustained energy supply during exercise.

Table 11.1 Triglyceride Levels (American Heart Association)

Triglycerides	Level
<150 mg/dL	Normal
150–199 mg/dL	Borderline high
200–499 mg/dL	High
500 mg/dL	Very high

FATS

- Energy-providing nutrient
- Most concentrated source of energy
- 9 Calories (kcal) per gram
- Primary functions—provide energy, cell membrane formation, metabolism
- Lipids—organic compounds soluble in organic solvents, but insoluble in water
  - Fatty acids—long chains of carbon atoms
  - Triglycerides—primary fat in body and diet
  - Sterol—steroid alcohols (e.g., cholesterol)
- Types of fatty acids
  - Saturated fatty acids
  - Unsaturated fatty acids
- Triglycerides (see Table 11.1)
  - Three fatty acids + glycerol
  - Food sources—animal fats, vegetable oils

 Quick fact High triglyceride levels can increase an individual's risk of heart disease and stroke.

CHOLESTEROL

- Type of sterol
- Synthesized by body (liver primarily)
- Found in animal fats and plant foods (small amount)
- Essential for structural body function
- Food sources—beef, poultry, eggs, dairy products
- Transported in the blood by lipoproteins

TYPES OF LIPOPROTEINS

- Low-density lipoprotein (LDL)—"bad" cholesterol (see Table 11.2)
  - High intake—can increase risk of some diseases (e.g., coronary artery disease)
  - High-density lipoprotein (HDL)—"good" cholesterol (see Table 11.3)
  - Intake—can decrease risk of heart disease

Quick fact Cholesterol does not serve as an energy source for the body.

Table 11.2 Low-Density Lipoprotein (LDL) Cholesterol Levels (American Heart Association)

LDL Cholesterol	Level
<100 mg/dL	Optimal for people with heart disease or diabetes
100–129 mg/dL	Near or above optimal
130–159 mg/dL	Borderline high
160–189 mg/dL	High
190 mg/dL and above	Very high

 Hypercholesterolemia is the term for high blood cholesterol levels.

 The American Heart Association recommends that you limit your average daily cholesterol intake to <300 mg.

 Exercise can help increase an individual's level of high-density lipoprotein (HDL).

SATURATED FATTY ACIDS

- "Unhealthy" fats
- Can increase LDL blood cholesterol levels
- High intake—can increase risk of some diseases (e.g., atherosclerosis, stroke)
- Food sources—meat, dairy products, pastries

UNSATURATED FATTY ACIDS

- Monounsaturated fatty acids
  - "Healthy" fats
  - Food sources—avocados, nuts, canola oil, olive oil

Table 11.3 High-Density Lipoprotein (HDL) Cholesterol Levels and Risk (American Heart Association)

HDL Cholesterol	Level (Risk)
<40 mg/dL	Low (higher risk)
40 to 59 mg/dL	The higher, the better
60 mg/dL and above	High (lower risk)

Table 11.4 Total Cholesterol Levels and Risk (American Heart Association)

Total Cholesterol	Level (Risk)
<200 mg/dL	Desirable (lower risk)
200–239 mg/dL	Borderline high (higher risk)
240 mg/dL and above	High (more than twice the risk as desirable level)

- Polyunsaturated fatty acids
  - "Healthy" fats
  - Food sources—fish, soybean, corn oil
- Trans fatty acids
  - Made from partially hydrogenating plant oils
  - Can increase LDL blood cholesterol levels (see Table 11.4)
  - High intake—can increase risk of some diseases (e.g., coronary artery disease)
  - Should be consumed as little as possible
  - Food sources—margarine, fast foods, snack foods
- Omega-3 fatty acids
  - Type of polyunsaturated fatty acids
  - May reduce the risk of some diseases (e.g., heart disease, stroke)
  - Food sources—cold-water fish, kiwi, flax seed oil

 Oils such as olive oil and canola oil are a healthier alternative when cooking foods in comparison to using vegetable oils.

FAT SUBSTITUTES

- Taste and texture is similar to fat—fewer calories and less fat
- Examples—Olestra, Simplese
- Complications—gastrointestinal problems (e.g., abdominal cramps, diarrhea)

 Use the DVD or visit the website at http://thePoint.lww.com/Long for additional materials about *high-fat food sources*.

PROTEINS

- Energy providing nutrient
- 4 Calories (kcal) per gram
- Primary functions—supply energy, metabolism, body tissue formation
- Amino acids (20)—"building blocks" of protein
- Produced in body and supplied by dietary intake
- Food sources—animal foods (e.g., meat, poultry, eggs, fish) and plant sources

Types of Amino Acids

- Essential amino acids
  - Supplemented by diet
- Nonessential amino acids
  - Created by body

Classes of Proteins

- Complete proteins
  - Contain all essential amino acids
  - Animal products
- Incomplete proteins
  - Do not contain all essential amino acids
  - Plant products

Effects of Excessive Protein Intake

- Dehydration
- High level of ketone production
- Liver and kidney stress (may lead to organ disease/damage)
- Increased calcium excretion in urine (may lead to decrease in bone density = osteoporosis)

Use the DVD or visit the website at http://thePoint.lww.com/Long for additional materials about *protein food sources.*

Quick fact Excess protein in the diet may be converted into fat.

Quick fact Most athletes are able to meet their protein needs with little difficulty through their diet; therefore, protein supplements are seldom necessary.

MICRONUTRIENTS

- Vitamins
- Minerals
- Water

Vitamins

- Organic substances essential for optimal body functions
- Roles—hormones, antioxidants, coenzymes, neuromuscular
- Not an energy source
- Types of vitamins
  - Fat-soluble—dissolved in fat and stored in body
  - Water-soluble—dissolved in water and not stored (excreted in urine)

  - Antioxidants—protect cells from destructive effects of oxidation

Quick fact Vitamins A, C, and E are considered to be antioxidants and may reduce the risk of some diseases such as cancer and heart disease.

Quick fact Excessive vitamin intake can have a toxic effect on the body.

Fat-Soluble Vitamins

- Vitamins A, D, E, and K
- Food sources—meat, cheese, asparagus, soybeans

Quick fact A deficiency of vitamin K can impair blood coagulation.

Use the DVD or visit the website at http://thePoint.lww.com/Long for additional materials about the *roles and deficiencies of fat-soluble vitamins.*

Water-Soluble Vitamins

- Vitamin C (ascorbic acid)
- B complex vitamins
- Food sources—legumes, dairy products, poultry, citrus fruits

Use the DVD or visit the website at http://thePoint.lww.com/Long for additional materials about the *roles and deficiencies of water-soluble vitamins.*

Minerals

- Inorganic substances essential for growth and normal body function
- Roles—body tissue formation, metabolism
- Not an energy source
- Macrominerals (7)
  - Examples—calcium, potassium, sodium, phosphorus, and so on
- Microminerals (14)
  - Examples—chromium, fluoride, iron, zinc, and so on

Quick fact Calcium is the most abundant mineral in the body, and its deficiency can lead to osteoporosis.

Quick fact Vitamin D assists in increasing calcium absorption in the body.

 Use the DVD or visit the website at http://thePoint.lww.com/Long for additional materials about the *roles and deficiencies of macrominerals and microminerals.*

WATER

- Most essential nutrient
- Not an energy source
- Approximately 60% of body weight
- Roles—regulation of body temperature, transports nutrients, excretion of waste
- Water loss—increases risk of exertional heat illnesses (e.g., heat exhaustion, heat stroke)
- Excessive water intake in conjunction with low blood sodium levels can lead to hyponatremia (water intoxication)

ELECTROLYTES

- Minerals in body fluids that carry an electrical charge
- Not an energy source
- Roles—water balance, muscle function, joint lubrication
- Sodium, potassium, calcium, chloride, and magnesium
  - Sodium—concentrated in extracellular fluid
  - Potassium—concentrated in intracellular fluid
- During exercise—lost primarily through sweating
- Replenished through diet and sports drinks

 Quick fact Thirst is not a good indicator of hydration—when a person is thirsty he or she is already dehydrated.

Quick fact An individual's hydration level can be assessed using an instrument known as a *refractometer.*

NUTRITIONAL RECOMMENDATIONS

Selected and Summarized Recommendations from the Dietary Guidelines for Americans 2005 (United States Department of Agriculture)

- Meet recommended dietary intakes—based on personal energy needs
- Balance caloric intake with caloric expenditure—maintains a healthy body weight

- Regular physical activity—include cardiovascular conditioning, stretching, and resistive exercises/calisthenics
- Variety of fruits and vegetables
- Whole-grain and enriched-grain products
- Fat-free or low-fat milk products
- Potassium-rich products
- Fiber-rich fruits, vegetables, and whole-grains
- Meat, poultry, and so on—fat-free, low-fat, or lean
- Foods/beverages—little added sugar or caloric sweeteners
- Fats—20% to 35% of daily caloric intake (primarily polyunsaturated and monounsaturated fats)
- Saturated fats—<10% of daily caloric intake
- Trans fat—limit as much as possible
- Cholesterol—<300 mg per day
- Sodium—<2,300 mg per day
- Alcohol—limit consumption

 Use the DVD or visit the website at http://thePoint.lww.com/Long for additional materials about the *organizations that develop nutritional recommendations.*

Dietary Reference Intakes

- Developed by the Food and Nutrition Board of the Institute of Medicine, National Academy of Sciences
- Established standards for nutrient intake
- Updated the Recommended Dietary Allowances (RDAs)
- Four types of reference values
  - Estimated Average Requirement (EAR)
  - RDA
  - Adequate Intake (AI)
  - Tolerable Upper Intake Level (UL)

Food Pyramid (United States Department of Agriculture)

- Grains
- Vegetables
- Fruits
- Milk
- Meat and beans
- Oils
- Discretionary calories

 Use the DVD or visit the website at http://thePoint.lww.com/Long for additional materials about the *food pyramid categories and food sources.*

Food Labels

- Required by the U.S. Food and Drug Administration (FDA) under the Federal Food Drug and Cosmetic Act (see Fig. 11.1)
- Required for most prepared foods (raw produce and fish are voluntary)

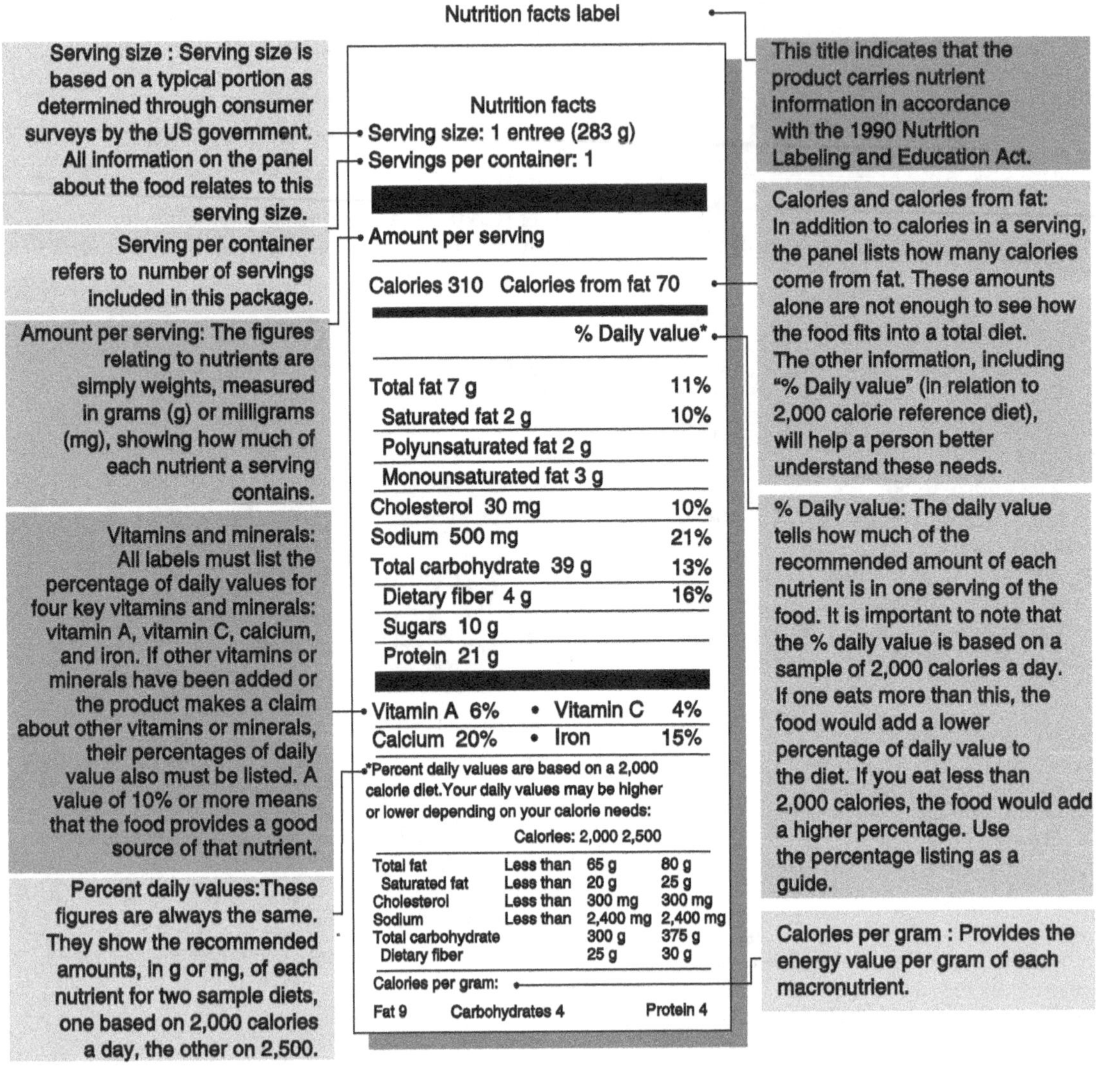

Serving size : Serving size is based on a typical portion as determined through consumer surveys by the US government. All information on the panel about the food relates to this serving size.

Nutrition facts
Serving size: 1 entree (283 g)
Servings per container: 1

Serving per container refers to number of servings included in this package.

Amount per serving

Amount per serving: The figures relating to nutrients are simply weights, measured in grams (g) or milligrams (mg), showing how much of each nutrient a serving contains.

Calories 310   Calories from fat 70

% Daily value*

Total fat 7 g	11%
Saturated fat 2 g	10%
Polyunsaturated fat 2 g	
Monounsaturated fat 3 g	
Cholesterol 30 mg	10%
Sodium 500 mg	21%
Total carbohydrate 39 g	13%
Dietary fiber 4 g	16%
Sugars 10 g	
Protein 21 g	

Vitamins and minerals: All labels must list the percentage of daily values for four key vitamins and minerals: vitamin A, vitamin C, calcium, and iron. If other vitamins or minerals have been added or the product makes a claim about other vitamins or minerals, their percentages of daily value also must be listed. A value of 10% or more means that the food provides a good source of that nutrient.

Vitamin A 6%	•	Vitamin C	4%
Calcium 20%	•	Iron	15%

*Percent daily values are based on a 2,000 calorie diet. Your daily values may be higher or lower depending on your calorie needs:

Calories: 2,000 2,500

Total fat	Less than	65 g	80 g
Saturated fat	Less than	20 g	25 g
Cholesterol	Less than	300 mg	300 mg
Sodium	Less than	2,400 mg	2,400 mg
Total carbohydrate		300 g	375 g
Dietary fiber		25 g	30 g

Percent daily values: These figures are always the same. They show the recommended amounts, in g or mg, of each nutrient for two sample diets, one based on 2,000 calories a day, the other on 2,500.

Calories per gram:

Fat 9	Carbohydrates 4	Protein 4

This title indicates that the product carries nutrient information in accordance with the 1990 Nutrition Labeling and Education Act.

Calories and calories from fat: In addition to calories in a serving, the panel lists how many calories come from fat. These amounts alone are not enough to see how the food fits into a total diet. The other information, including "% Daily value" (in relation to 2,000 calorie reference diet), will help a person better understand these needs.

% Daily value: The daily value tells how much of the recommended amount of each nutrient is in one serving of the food. It is important to note that the % daily value is based on a sample of 2,000 calories a day. If one eats more than this, the food would add a lower percentage of daily value to the diet. If you eat less than 2,000 calories, the food would add a higher percentage. Use the percentage listing as a guide.

Calories per gram : Provides the energy value per gram of each macronutrient.

Figure 11.1 Food Label with Explanation of Food Panel Information.

PART 2 — Nutrition and Athletic Performance

NUTRIENT INTAKE FOR ATHLETES

Selected and Summarized Key Points from the 2000 Nutrition and Athletic Performance Position Stand (American Dietetics Association, Dieticians of Canada, and the American College of Sports Medicine)

- CHO intake
  - Maintains blood-glucose levels and glycogen stores
  - Fifty-five percent to 58% of daily caloric intake
  - Daily—6 to 10 g per kg body weight
- Fat intake
  - Twenty-five percent to 30% of daily caloric intake
  - No performance benefit when <15% of daily caloric intake
  - No evidence of recommending high-fat diets
- Protein intake
  - Appropriate intake can typically be met through the diet
  - Twelve percent to 15% of daily caloric intake

- Daily for endurance training—1.2 to 1.4 g per kg body weight
- Daily for resistance/strength training—as high as 1.6 to 1.7 g per kg body weight
- Vitamin and mineral intake
  - Can be met by well-balanced diet
  - Supplementation typically not needed
  - Supplementation may be needed if deficiency is present (e.g., iron for iron-deficiency anemia)
- Fluid intake
  - Essential for optimal athletic performance
  - Reduces risk of dehydration and heat illnesses
  - Forms—water and/or CHO/electrolyte drinks
  - Drinks with CHO concentration of 4% to 8%

> **Quick fact**
> Carbohydrates are the primary source of energy for athletes.

> **Quick fact**
> Protein intake for athletes can usually be achieved with an appropriate diet; therefore, protein supplements are typically unnecessary.

> **Quick fact**
> Vegetarian athletes may need to supplement protein and/or iron due to potential deficiencies in a vegetarian diet.

> **Quick fact**
> Carbohydrate loading, or glycogen supercompensation, is the practice of increasing the amount of carbohydrate intake when preparing for an endurance event with the intent of maximizing glycogen stores.

THE PRECOMPETITION (PRE-EXERCISE) MEAL

Selected and Summarized Key Points from the 2000 Nutrition and Athletic Performance Position Stand (American Dietetics Association, Dieticians of Canada, and the American College of Sports Medicine)

- CHO—high amount (maintains blood glucose levels and maximizes glycogen stores)
- Fiber—low amount (minimizes occurrence of gastrointestinal distress)
- Fat—low amount (minimizes occurrence of gastrointestinal distress)
- Protein—moderate amount
- Fluids—14 to 22 oz 2 hours before
- Avoid foods that are not typically consumed

- Closer to competition/exercise time—smaller meals preferred (allows time for gastric emptying and less likely to experience gastrointestinal distress)
- Further from competition/exercise time—larger meals possible

> **Quick fact**
> The consumption time for the precompetition meal can range from 1 to 4 hours.

> **Quick fact**
> Nutrients are emptied from the stomach in the following order: fluids, carbohydrates, proteins, and then fats.

> **Quick fact**
> Digestion time of the precompetition meal will be dependent on the meal size and nutrient content.

> **Quick fact**
> Athletes should avoid eating foods such as beans or broccoli that could potentially lead to gastrointestinal discomfort.

NUTRIENT INTAKE DURING EXERCISE

Selected and Summarized Key Points from the 2000 Nutrition and Athletic Performance Position Stand (American Dietetics Association, Dieticians of Canada, and the American College of Sports Medicine)

- CHO—consist primarily of glucose
- Endurance competition/exercise—0.7 g of CHO/kg of body weight/hour (approximately 30 to 60 g per hour)
- Endurance competition/exercise—appropriate fluid intake is essential
- Fluids—6 to 12 oz every 15 to 20 minutes

> **Quick fact**
> Competing or exercising on a full stomach can cause gastrointestinal problems such as nausea, indigestion, abdominal cramps, and diarrhea.

> **Quick fact**
> Athletes should avoid caffeinated drinks before and during exercise because of their diuretic effect, which can cause an increase in body fluid loss.

THE POSTCOMPETITION (POSTEXERCISE) MEAL

Selected and Summarized Key Points from the 2000 Nutrition and Athletic Performance Position Stand (American Dietetics Association, Dieticians of Canada, and the American College of Sports Medicine)

- Contains a mixture of CHO, proteins, and fats
- Timing and composition—depend on length/intensity of competition/exercise and time until next competition/exercise
- CHO—1.5 g per kg body weight within 30 minutes and repeated every 2 hours for 4 to 6 hours
- Fluids—16 to 24 oz for every pound of body weight lost during activity

---

PART 3

Weight Management and Eating Disorders

ENERGY MEASUREMENTS

Energy Balance

- Energy—capacity to perform work
  - Measured in calories. (see Fig. 11.2)
- Energy balance—energy intake = energy expenditure
  - Calories consumed = calories burned

Energy Intake Estimation

- Keep a daily food diary (types and amounts of food/beverages)
- Enter data into a diet analysis computer program—provides estimate of daily caloric intake and nutrient composition

Quick fact   Daily caloric intake for athletes will vary from person to person, and will depend on the level of activity among other factors.

Energy Expenditure Estimation

- Direct and indirect calorimetry
  - Direct—laboratory setting with a human calorimeter (metabolic chamber)
  - Indirect—oxygen consumption and carbon dioxide production (more practical method)
- Total daily energy expenditure (TDEE)—total amount of energy expended in a 24-hour period (determined by three factors)
  - Resting metabolic rate (RMR)—often used interchangeably with basal metabolic rate (BMR) but has slight differences
  - Thermogenic effect of food
  - Physical activity
- Estimating BMR—a variety of equations exist

- Harris and Benedict equation to estimate BMR
  - Men BMR = 66 + [13.7 × weight (kg)] + [5 × height (cm)] – [6.8 × age (yr)]
  - Women BMR = 655 + [9.6 × weight (kg)] + [1.8 × height (cm)] – [4.7 × age (yr)]

METHODS FOR MEASURING BODY COMPOSITION

Body Mass Index

- Height and weight—estimates amount of body fat (see Table 11.5)
- Calculating body mass index (BMI)
  - $BMI = weight (kg)/[height (m)]^2$
- Quick and easy to use
- Not as accurate as other methods

Quick fact   Because of the increased amount of muscle and bone mass of some athletes, the BMI may incorrectly classify these individuals as being overweight.

Table 11.5   Body Mass Index (BMI) and Weight Status (Centers for Disease Control and Prevention)

BMI	Weight Status
Below 18.5	Underweight
18.5–24.9	Normal
25.0–29.9	Overweight
30.0 and above	Obese

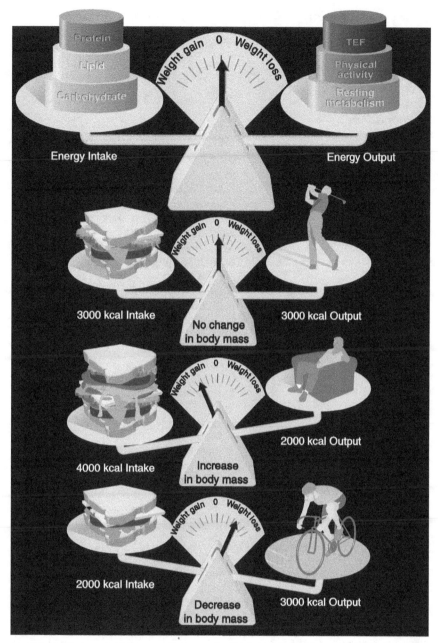

Figure 11.2 Concept of Energy Balance in Weight Management. TEF, thermic effect of food.

Waist-to-Hip Ratio

- Comparison of waist and hip circumferences to estimate amount of body fat
- Calculating waist-to-hip ratio (WHR)
  - WHR = waist circumference (cm)/hip circumference (cm)
- Measurements are relatively easy to obtain

Quick **fact** A high amount of body fat at the body's trunk region is associated with a greater risk of some diseases.

Skinfold Measurements

- Subcutaneous fat is measured using a skinfold caliper
- Very common and accurate method of assessing body fat percentage
- Accuracy of measurement—depends on properly calibrated equipment and correct technique
- Male skinfold sites (American College of Sports Medicine)
  - Three-site formula—chest, abdomen, and thigh
  - Three-site formula—chest, triceps, and subscapular
  - Seven-site formula—chest, midaxillary, triceps, subscapular, abdomen, suprailiac, and thigh

- Female skinfold sites (American College of Sports Medicine)
  - Three-site formula—triceps, suprailiac, and thigh
  - Three-site formula— triceps, suprailiac, and abdominal
  - Seven-site formula—chest, midaxillary, triceps, subscapular, abdomen, suprailiac, thigh

Bioelectrical Impedance Analysis

- Uses a painless electrical current that passes through body between two electrodes
- Speed of current travel estimates body fat percentage
  - Faster—lesser body fat
  - Slower—greater body fat
- Hydration status and electrolyte levels can result in an inaccurate measurement
- Handheld units—quick and easy method of assessing body fat percentage

> *Quick* **fact** Although handheld BIA units are a quick and easy way to assess body fat percentage, this method is not the most accurate of indirect measurements.

Hydrodensitometry

- Hydrostatic or underwater weighing
- Based on Archimedes' principle
  - Buoyant force on submerged object = weight of displaced liquid
- Uses underwater submersion on a scale to determine body composition
- Individual has to maximally exhale before being submerged
- Accurate, but may be uncomfortable for individual

> *Quick* **fact** Hydrodensitometry is considered to be the "gold standard" for assessing body composition.

Plethysmography

- Uses air displacement to estimate body composition
- Instrument is known as the *BOD POD* (Life Measurements Instruments)
- Individual is placed in a small chamber and breathes into an air apparatus

Dual-Energy X-ray Absorptiometry

- Uses a whole-body radiographic scanner to determine body composition
- Can also be used to assess for osteoporosis
- Accurate, but equipment is highly expensive

> *Quick* **fact** According to the American College of Sports Medicine, a healthy body fat percentage ranges from 10% to 22% for men and 20% to 32% for women.

HEALTHY WEIGHT LOSS AND GAIN

Healthy Weight Loss

- Identify healthy weight
- Assess current caloric and nutrient intake (e.g., diet analysis computer software)
- Develop a balanced dietary plan based on energy needs and weight loss goals
- Avoid "fad" diets and over-the-counter (OTC) weight-loss pills
- Weight loss goals—realistic and achievable
- Negative caloric balance—energy expenditure must be greater than energy intake
- Do not skip meals
- Keep healthy snacks available
- Substitute high-fat foods with low-fat food choices
- Avoid foods that contain trans fatty acids
- Reduce sugar intake
- Include more fruits and vegetables
- Drink appropriate amount of fluids—do not withhold fluid intake
- Engage in regular cardiovascular exercise
- Modify behaviors that contribute to weight gain
- Weight loss should be gradual: 1 to 2 lbs per week

> *Quick* **fact** There are 3,500 calories in 1 lb of body fat.

Healthy Weight Gain

- Assess current caloric and nutrient intake (e.g., diet analysis computer software)
- Develop a balanced dietary plan based on energy needs and weight gain goals
- Avoid the use of dietary supplements—not regulated by FDA
- Weight gain goals—realistic and achievable
- Positive caloric balance—energy intake must be greater than energy expenditure
- Ensure that protein intake is appropriate based on physical activity
- Engage in regular resistance training program—increases lean muscle mass

> *Quick* **fact** According to the American College of Sports Medicine, weight gain can be accomplished by increasing daily caloric intake by 500 to 1,000 calories.

EATING DISORDERS

Anorexia Nervosa

- Clinical eating disorder
- Engage in caloric restriction and exercise excessively (may also binge and purge at times)
- Excessive weight loss—refuses to maintain healthy body weight
- Obsessed with body weight
- Distorted body image
- Fear of gaining weight or being "fat"
- Can result in amenorrhea

Quick fact Even though anorexia nervosa is primarily identified in females, males can also suffer from this disorder.

Bulimia Nervosa

- Clinical eating disorder
- Engages in recurrent episodes of binge eating followed by compensatory behaviors (may also restrict caloric intake and exercise excessively)

- Compensatory behaviors—self-induced vomiting, laxatives, fasting
- Overly concerned about body weight and shape
- Appears as being of average body weight and size
- Feelings of guilt after binge eating

Anorexia Athletica

- Athletes engage in caloric restriction and/or exercise excessively
- Engages for performance enhancement rather than for body appearance
- May only engage in disordered eating habits during their athletic season

Binge Eating Disorder

- Engages in recurrent episodes of compulsive binge eating
- Do not purge body of excessively consumed calories

Quick fact The female athlete triad is a combination of an eating disorder, amenorrhea, and osteoporosis.

P A R T 4 **Dietary Supplements and Ergogenic Aids**

KEY TERMS

- Anabolic steroid
- Ergogenic aid
- Erythropoietin

DIETARY SUPPLEMENTS

Types of Dietary Supplements

- Vitamins
- Minerals
- Herbs
- Other organic substances

Reasons for Intake

- To supplement a deficiency in the diet
- To improve overall health
- To prevent and/or treat injury and illness
- To improve athletic performance

Quick fact Dietary supplements are usually not necessary if an individual consumes a well-balanced diet.

Potential Dangers

- Not regulated by the FDA
- Potential of unknown substances within supplement
- Lack of scientific research on effects

Commonly Used Supplements

- Calcium—prevents/treats osteoporosis (e.g., calcium citrate)
- Chondroitin sulfate—prevents/treats osteoarthritis (often used in conjunction with glucosamine)
- Glucosamine—prevents/treats osteoarthritis (often used in conjunction with chondroitin sulfate)
- Iron—treats iron-deficiency anemia

ERGOGENIC AIDS

Commonly Used Ergogenic Aids in Athletics

Ergogenic Aid	Intended Use	Comments
Anabolic steroids	Increase lean body mass Weight gain Decrease body fat Increase strength	Synthetic substances Mimic testosterone Anabolic and androgenic effects
Androstenedione	Increase lean body mass Increase strength	Testosterone precursor Androgenic and estrogenic effects
Amphetamines	Enhance mental alertness Decrease fatigue	CNS stimulants Sympathomimetic Mimic epinephrine and norepinephrine
β-Blockers	Improve steadiness	Used in sports such as archery, marksmanship, and fencing Adrenergic agent
Blood doping	Improves aerobic endurance	Reinfusion of stored blood plasma Increases hematocrit and hemoglobin levels
Creatine	Increases lean body mass Weight gain Decreases body fat Increases strength and power Decreases muscle fatigue and soreness	Phosphocreatine (PCr) is synthesized naturally in body (liver, kidneys, and pancreas) Stored in muscles Typically sold as creatine monohydrate
Caffeine	Enhances mental alertness Improves muscle function Improves aerobic endurance	CNS stimulant Increases fat metabolism which spares glycogen stores Example—Vivarin Food sources—coffee, tea, sodas
Erythropoietin (EPO)	Improves aerobic endurance	Hormone Stimulates RBC production Increases hematocrit and hemoglobin levels
Diuretics	Rapid weight loss Masking agent for drug testing	"Water pills" Increases water excretion
Ephedra	Weight loss Improves aerobic endurance	Ma Huang CNS stimulant Sympathomimetic
Human growth hormone (HGH)	Increases lean body mass Decreases body fat Increases strength	Produced by anterior pituitary gland Difficult to detect with drug testing

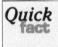 *Quick fact* An ergogenic aid is any method that is used (legally or illegally) in an attempt to enhance athletic performance.

 Quick fact "Stacking" is when an individual uses a combination of multiple types of anabolic steroids.

Quick fact Tetrahydrogestrinone (THG) is an illegal synthetic anabolic androgenic steroid.

 Quick fact Adderall, which is used to treat attention deficit hyperactivity disorder (ADHD), is an amphetamine.

1. Which is not a monosaccharide?
   a. Ribose
   b. Galactose
   c. Fructose
   d. Glucose
   e. Lactose

2. What is the scientific name for blood sugar?
   a. Lactose
   b. Maltose
   c. Glucose
   d. Glucagon
   e. Glycogen

3. What nutritional deficiency can be characterized by disorientation or irritability?
   a. Vitamin A
   b. Vitamin B_{12}
   c. Vitamin D
   d. Vitamin E
   e. Vitamin K

4. What nutritional deficiency can be characterized by hyporeflexia?
   a. Niacin
   b. Thiamine
   c. Beta-carotene
   d. Riboflavin
   e. Lactose

5. What nutritional deficiency can be characterized by peripheral neuropathy?
   a. Thiamine, vitamin B_6
   b. Riboflavin, vitamin B_3
   c. Choline, vitamin B_7
   d. Folate, vitamin B_9
   e. Niacin, vitamin B_6

6. What nutritional deficiency can be characterized by muscle wasting?
   a. Fiber, glucose, fat
   b. Starch, fiber, protein
   c. Protein, carbohydrate, fat
   d. Triglycerides, carbohydrate, fat
   e. Fruits, grains, vegetables

7. What nutritional deficiency can be characterized by joint pain?
   a. Vitamin A
   b. Vitamin B_{12}
   c. Vitamin B_9
   d. Vitamin C
   e. Vitamin D

8. What nutritional deficiency can be characterized by rickets?
   a. Vitamin A
   b. Vitamin B_6
   c. Vitamin B_9
   d. Vitamin C
   e. Vitamin D

9. What disorder is characterized by eating large amounts of food followed by purging?
   a. Binge-eating disorder
   b. Anorexia nervosa
   c. Anorexia athletica
   d. Bulimia nervosa
   e. Female athlete triad

10. What nutritional deficiency can be characterized by osteomalacia?
    a. Vitamin D, calcium
    b. Vitamin B_3, niacin
    c. Vitamin E, biotin
    d. Vitamin A, beta-carotene
    e. Vitamin C, ascorbic acid

11. What nutritional deficiency can be characterized by pain in the calves and thighs?
    a. Cobalamin
    b. Folate
    c. Biotin
    d. Thiamine
    e. Riboflavin

12. What nutritional deficiency can be characterized by splinter hemorrhages in the nails?
    a. Vitamin A
    b. Vitamin B
    c. Vitamin C
    d. Vitamin D
    e. Vitamin E

13. What nutritional deficiency can be characterized by koilonychias?
    a. Cobalt
    b. Iron
    c. Manganese
    d. Copper
    e. Iodine

14. Which of the following nutrients is an athlete's most efficient source of fuel for energy?
    a. Carbohydrates
    b. Fats
    c. Protein
    d. Vitamins
    e. Minerals

15. What nutritional deficiency can be characterized by bleeding gums?
    a. Vitamin A
    b. Vitamin B
    c. Vitamin C
    d. Vitamin D
    e. Vitamin E

16. What nutritional deficiency can be characterized by beefy-red tongue?
    a. Beta-carotene
    b. Vitamin B complex
    c. Fat soluble vitamins
    d. Electrolytes
    e. Microminerals

17. What nutritional deficiency can be characterized by pale tongue?
    a. Cobalt
    b. Iron
    c. Manganese
    d. Copper
    e. Iodine

18. What nutritional deficiency can be characterized by tongue papillary atrophy?
    a. Niacin
    b. Boron
    c. Folic acid
    d. Sulfur
    e. Calcium

19. What is the recommended amount of protein needed daily for a person who is involved in an intense strength-training program?
    a. 1.0 g per kg of body weight
    b. 1.7 g per kg of body weight
    c. 1.2 g per kg of body weight
    d. 3.0 g per kg of body weight
    e. 3.5 g per kg of body weight

20. What nutritional deficiency can be characterized by angular stomatitis (red cracks in the side of mouth)?
    a. Folic acid, protein
    b. Riboflavin, niacin, iron, vitamin B_6
    c. Vitamin C, fats, chloride
    d. Potassium, magnesium
    e. Fluoride, selenium, zinc

21. What nutritional deficiency can be characterized by cheilosis (vertical cracks in lips)?
    a. Folate, cobalamin
    b. Thiamine, choline
    c. Riboflavin, niacin
    d. Biotin, pyridoxine
    e. Ascorbic acid, folic acid

22. What nutritional deficiency can be characterized by red conjunctivae?
    a. Molybdenum
    b. Ascorbic acid
    c. Biotin
    d. Pantothenic acid
    e. Riboflavin

23. Which of the following vitamins are not considered to be fat soluble?
    a. Vitamin A
    b. Vitamin C
    c. Vitamin E
    d. Vitamin D
    e. Vitamin K

24. What nutritional deficiency can be characterized by pale conjunctivae?
    a. Iron, vitamins B_6 and B_{12}
    b. Iron
    c. Cobalamin, biotin, riboflavin
    d. Thiamine, riboflavin, B complex vitamins
    e. Biotin

25. What method of assessing body composition is the least accurate?
    a. Skinfold
    b. DEXA
    c. Plethysmography
    d. Hydrostatic weighing
    e. Body mass index

26. What nutritional deficiency can be characterized by xerophthalmia?
    a. Vitamin A
    b. Vitamin B
    c. Vitamin C
    d. Vitamin D
    e. Vitamin E

27. What nutritional deficiency can be characterized by keratomalacia?
    a. Niacin
    b. Vitamin A
    c. Pyridoxine
    d. Vitamin D
    e. Thiamine

28. What is the appropriate recommendation for daily carbohydrate consumption for athletes?
    a. 2 to 4 g per kg body weight
    b. 6 to 10 g per kg body weight
    c. 14 to 18 g per kg body weight
    d. 20 to 24 g per kg body weight
    e. 26 to 30 g per kg body weight

29. What nutritional deficiency can be characterized by blepharitis?
    a. B complex vitamins, biotin
    b. Vitamin D, niacin
    c. Vitamin E, ascorbic acid
    d. Vitamins A, D, and E
    e. Niacin, vitamin C

30. What nutritional deficiency can be characterized by corkscrew hair?
    a. Iron
    b. Magnesium
    c. Sulfur
    d. Potassium
    e. Copper

31. What is the appropriate recommendation for fluid consumption during exercise?
    a. 4 to 8 oz every 15 to 20 minutes
    b. 6 to 12 oz every 15 to 20 minutes
    c. 14 to 22 oz every 5 to 10 minutes
    d. 16 to 24 oz every 15 to 20 minutes
    e. 24 to 28 oz every 5 to 10 minutes

32. What nutritional deficiency can be characterized by dull, dry, and sparse hair?
    a. Water-soluble vitamins
    b. Antioxidants
    c. Chromium, sodium, fats
    d. Protein, zinc, linoleic acid
    e. B complex vitamins

33. What nutritional deficiency can be characterized by eczema?
    a. Ascorbic acid
    b. Linoleic acid
    c. Potassium
    d. Chloride
    e. Magnesium

34. What nutritional deficiency can be characterized by nasolabial seborrhea?
    a. Riboflavin, vitamin B_6
    b. Iodine
    c. Vanadium, molybdenum
    d. Phosphorus
    e. Potassium, sodium

35. Unused glucose units can be stored as glycogen in which of the following body parts?
    a. Stomach
    b. Blood
    c. Kidneys
    d. Bones
    e. None of the above

36. What nutritional deficiency can be characterized by pellagrous dermatosis?
    a. Riboflavin
    b. Niacin
    c. Iodine
    d. Thiamine
    e. Potassium

37. What nutritional deficiency can be characterized by cracks in the skin of hands, legs, face or neck?
    a. Biotin
    b. Riboflavin
    c. Niacin, tryptophan
    d. Linoleic acid
    e. Phosphorus

38. What nutritional deficiency can be characterized by acneiform forehead rash?
    a. Vitamin B_3
    b. Vitamin B_6
    c. Vitamin B_9
    d. Vitamin B_{12}
    e. Vitamin B_{16}

39. What nutritional deficiency can be characterized by petechiae/ecchymoses of the skin?
    a. Vitamins A and C
    b. Vitamins A and B
    c. Vitamins C and K
    d. Vitamins D and E
    e. Vitamins C and E

40. Which of the following foods is not a high source of trans fatty acids?
    a. Dairy products
    b. Crackers
    c. Meat
    d. Wheat bread
    e. French fries

41. What nutritional deficiency can be characterized by follicular hyperkeratosis?
   a. Vitamin A, linoleic acid
   b. B Complex vitamins
   c. Vitamins C and K
   d. Vitamins D and E
   e. Vitamins A and K

42. What nutritional deficiency can be characterized by dry, flaking skin?
   a. Vitamin A
   b. Vitamin B complex
   c. Linoleic acid
   d. Vitamin C
   e. All are characterized by dry, flaking skin

43. What nutritional deficiency can be characterized by color changes in hair?
   a. Iron and magnesium
   b. Selenium and manganese
   c. Copper or protein
   d. Iron and sodium
   e. Thiamine and pantothenic acid

44. What skin disorder is associated with a deficiency of vitamin A and/or linoleic acid and characterized by eczematous skin particularly in infants?
   a. Sebaceous keratosis
   b. Follicular hyperkeratosis
   c. Paget disease
   d. Beta-caratenosis
   e. Cobalamin reductase

45. What gum disorder is associated with a deficiency of vitamin C and characterized by swollen, ulcerated, and bleeding gums?
   a. Gingivitis
   b. Scorbutic gums
   c. Pellegra
   d. Bitot spots
   e. Cushing

46. What skin disorder is associated with a deficiency of niacin and characterized as lesions in areas exposed to the sun such as the extremities?
   a. Gingivitis
   b. Scorbutic gums
   c. Pellegra
   d. Bitot spots
   e. Cushing

47. Which abnormality occurs in people with high stress (surgery, illness); high carbohydrate little protein diet; and characterized as having decreased hair and skin pigmentation, scaling skin, and generalized edema?
   a. Kwashiorkor
   b. Cushing
   c. Paget disease

   d. Charcot-Marie-Tooth
   e. Guillain-Barré

48. Which abnormality is associated with vitamin A deficiency and characterized by foamy plaques of the cornea?
   a. Gingivitis
   b. Scorbutic gums
   c. Pellegra
   d. Bitot spots
   e. Cushing

49. Which statement is *false* regarding trans fatty acids?
   a. High amounts can be found in fast foods
   b. They can increase HDL blood cholesterol levels
   c. High intake can increase risk of coronary artery disease
   d. They are made from partially hydrogenating plant oils
   e. They provide no benefit to the body

50. Which abnormality is associated with vitamin D deficiency and characterized by osteomalacia or abnormal cartilage growth (in children)?
   a. Osteomalacia
   b. Rickets
   c. Osteoporosis
   d. Osteoblastoma
   e. Paget disease

51. Which statement is false regarding dietary supplements?
   a. There is little scientific evidence regarding their long-term effects
   b. Herbs are considered to be dietary supplements
   c. The FDA regulates their content
   d. They are typically not necessary if athletes eat a well-balanced diet
   e. They are used to improve injury recovery time

52. Caffeine is thought to do which of the following?
   a. Increase fat metabolism during endurance exercise
   b. Increase fatigue during endurance exercise
   c. Decrease glycogen stores
   d. Reduce anxiety
   e. Decrease muscle damage due to exercise

53. Where is phosphocreatine synthesized in the body?
   a. Kidneys
   b. Pancreas
   c. Thyroid gland
   d. Liver
   e. Adrenal gland

54. What abnormality is associated with riboflavin deficiency and characterized by a magenta-colored tongue?
   a. Roseola
   b. Rosacea

c. Magenta tongue

d. Madelung disease

e. Macrosis

55. Which of the following are signs of riboflavin deficiency?

a. Increased bleeding time

b. Cracked lips

c. Osteomalacia

d. Corneal degeneration

e. Muscle cramps

56. Which of the following nutrients provide energy for the body during exercise?

a. Fats

b. Water

c. Minerals

d. Vitamins

e. None of the above

57. Which of the following vitamins is not considered to be fat soluble?

a. Vitamin A

b. Vitamin C

c. Vitamin D

d. Vitamin E

e. Vitamin K

58. What do the letters DRI mean?

a. Daily Recommended Intake

b. Dietary Reference Intake

c. Dietary Research Institution

d. Daily Repetitive Ingestion

e. Dramatically Reduced Intake

59. Who developed the DRIs?

a. Food and Nutrition Board of the Institute of Medicine

b. Food and Drug Administration

c. Department of Agriculture

d. Department of Health and Human Services

e. Department of Nutritional Assessment

60. Which is not a goal of the precompetition meal?

a. Preventing fatigue

b. Minimizing hunger

c. Maintaining appropriate fluid levels

d. Preventing gastrointestinal discomfort

e. Decreasing the electrolyte uptake

61. Which is not a symptom of competing on a full stomach?

a. Nausea and/or vomiting

b. Gastrointestinal bleeding

c. Indigestion

d. Abdominal cramps

e. Diarrhea

62. What is the world's largest organization of food and nutritional professionals?

a. Center for Dietary Excellence

b. National Centers for Dietetics

c. Society for Dietary Examination

d. American Dietetic Association

e. Association of Nutritional Research

63. What is the premiere research society dedicated to improving quality of life through nutritional sciences?

a. National Institutes of Health

b. Centers for Disease Control

c. American Society for Nutritional Sciences

d. American Dietetic Association

e. Food and Drug Administration

64. What are the macronutrients?

a. Carbohydrates, proteins, fats

b. Sugars, fats

c. Triglycerides, carbohydrates, glycogen

d. Fats, electrolytes, protein

e. Water, carbohydrates, protein

65. Which is not a water-soluble vitamin?

a. Riboflavin

b. Vitamin C

c. Biotin

d. Vitamin A

e. Niacin

66. Which of the following is a water soluble vitamin?

a. Vitamin A

b. Vitamin K

c. Vitamin E

d. Vitamin C

e. Vitamin D

67. What mineral may cause hypertension in excess?

a. Magnesium

b. Chloride

c. Sodium

d. Potassium

e. Calcium

68. What mineral is added to water to prevent tooth decay?

a. Calcium

b. Fluorine

c. Chloride

d. Potassium

e. Sodium

69. What are charged ions dissolved in body water?

a. Oligosaccharides

b. Electrolytes

c. Phosphocreatine

d. Hyponatremia

e. Vanadium

70. Which is not an electrolyte within the body?
    a. Calcium
    b. Sodium
    c. Potassium
    d. Magnesium
    e. Chromium

71. What are good sources of thiamine?
    a. Lean pork, legumes, yeast
    b. Cooked dark green vegetables
    c. Chicken, legumes
    d. Beans (lima, green)
    e. Beans, pork, greens

72. What are good sources of vitamin K?
    a. Asparagus
    b. Cooked dark green vegetables
    c. Legumes
    d. Lima beans
    e. Carrots

73. Which vitamin is also known as *vitamin H*?
    a. Thiamine
    b. Riboflavin
    c. Folate
    d. Pantothenic acid
    e. Biotin

74. How many calories are in 1 g of carbohydrates?
    a. 2
    b. 4
    c. 6
    d. 9
    e. 12

75. How many calories are in 1 g of protein?
    a. 2
    b. 4
    c. 6
    d. 9
    e. 12

76. How many calories are in 1 g of fat?
    a. 2
    b. 4
    c. 6
    d. 9
    e. 12

77. Which is not a proposed effect of anabolic steroids?
    a. Weight gain
    b. Increased muscular strength
    c. Decreased body fat
    d. Lower HDL cholesterol levels
    e. Increased lean body mass

78. Which is not considered a health risk of obesity?
    a. Coronary artery disease
    b. Gynecomastia
    c. Dyslipidemia
    d. Stroke
    e. Osteoarthritis

79. Which is the gold standard for measuring body composition?
    a. Plethysmography
    b. Hydrostatic weighing
    c. BOD POD
    d. Skinfold thickness
    e. Body mass index

80. What is the acceptable minimal body fat for males?
    a. 5%
    b. 8%
    c. 10%
    d. 12%
    e. 18%

81. Safely losing weight requires decreasing daily caloric intake by:
    a. 5%
    b. 8%
    c. 10% to 20%
    d. 30% to 45%
    e. 50%

82. Which is a classification of ergogenic aids?
    a. Agonist
    b. Antagonist
    c. Mechanical
    d. Philosophical
    e. Synergistic

83. Which supplement increases red blood cell production?
    a. Anabolic steroids
    b. Erythropoietin
    c. Glutamine
    d. Human growth hormone
    e. Somatotropin

84. Which supplement is produced by the anterior pituitary gland?
    a. Testosterone
    b. Erythropoietin
    c. Human growth hormone
    d. Glutamine
    e. Glucosamine

85. What percentage of daily calories should come from fats?
    a. 5% to 10%
    b. 10% to 15%

c. 15% to 20%
d. 20% to 35%
e. 35% to 50%

86. How many calories would be in a steak with 20 g of protein?
   a. 180
   b. 120
   c. 90
   d. 80
   e. 40

87. How many calories would be in an ice cream with 10 g of fat and 20 g of sugar?
   a. 170
   b. 210
   c. 180
   d. 1,200
   e. 270

88. What policy exists with the NCAA regarding nutritional supplements?
   a. Athletic trainer is responsible for checking into all medications
   b. Medical release can assure safe participation
   c. Athlete is held responsible for whatever he or she ingests
   d. Athletes should never use prescribed nutriceuticals
   e. Moderate amounts of nutriceuticals are allowable without penalty

89. When should an athlete complete a pre-event meal?
   a. 30 Minutes
   b. 45 Minutes
   c. 1 to 4 Hours before
   d. 5 to 8 Hours before
   e. Never eat anything before a competition

90. In what order do nutrients empty from the stomach?
   a. Fats, carbohydrates, fluids, protein
   b. Carbohydrates, fluids, proteins, fats
   c. Fluids, carbohydrates, protein, fats
   d. Fluids, proteins, carbohydrates, fats
   e. Proteins, fluids, fats, carbohydrates

91. Which organization is not charged with developing nutritional recommendations?
   a. American Cancer Society
   b. National Institutes of Health
   c. U.S. Department of Health and Human Services
   d. American Heart Association
   e. American Dietetic Association

92. Which is not an adverse effect of human growth hormone?
   a. Acromegaly
   b. Hypotension
   c. Impotence
   d. Amenorrhea
   e. Arthritis

93. Which is not a high carbohydrate food?
   a. Yogurt
   b. Rice
   c. Potatoes
   d. Milk
   e. Cheese

94. Which is considered borderline high for triglyceride levels?
   a. 500 mg per dL
   b. 150 to 199 mg per dL
   c. <150 mg per dL
   d. 200 to 499 mg per dL
   e. <200 mg per dL

95. Which is not a side effect of Ma Huang?
   a. Bronchodilation
   b. Psychosis
   c. Tachycardia
   d. Arrhythmia
   e. Depression

96. Which is not an essential component of the food group?
   a. Breads and cereal
   b. Fruit and vegetables
   c. Meat and electrolytes
   d. Milk
   e. Fats

97. What should be the main content of pre-event meals?
   a. Fats
   b. Proteins
   c. Carbohydrates
   d. Fibers
   e. Electrolytes

98. What is the rate measure of calories required to sustain vital functions?
   a. Target metabolic rate
   b. Resting metabolic rate
   c. Sedentary metabolic rate
   d. Maximal metabolic rate
   e. Basal metabolic rate

99. What are the three processes of expending energy?
   a. Basal metabolic rate, glycolysis, oxidation
   b. Work, excretions, basal metabolic rate

c. Carbohydrate metabolism, work, power

d. Fat conversion, carbohydrate metabolism, glycolysis

e. Excretions, work, oxidation

100. How many calories are in 1 lb of fat?
    a. 2,400
    b. 3,200
    c. 3,500
    d. 3,800
    e. 4,200

Use the DVD or visit the website at http://thePoint.lww.com/Long to take the *online examination*.

✓ STUDY CHECKLIST

I have studied:
☐ Macronutrients
☐ Micronutrients
☐ Nutritional Recommendations
☐ Nutrient Intake for Athletes
☐ Pre-exercise Meal
☐ Nutrient Intake During Exercise
☐ Postexercise Meal
☐ Energy Measurements
☐ Body Compositions
☐ Health Weight Loss and Gain
☐ Eating Disorders
☐ Dietary Supplements
☐ Ergogenic Aids

SECTION 11

SUPPLEMENTAL READING

1. American Dietetic Association. www.eatright.org. 2008.
2. Dunford M, Doyle JA. *Nutrition for sport and exercise.* Belmont: Wadsworth/Thompson Learning; 2008.
3. McArdle WD, Katch FI, Katch VL. *Sports and exercise nutrition.* Philadelphia: Lippincott Williams & Wilkins; 2005.
4. National Athletic Trainers' Association. *Athletic training educational competencies,* 4th ed. Dallas: National Athletic Trainers' Association; 2006.
5. Prentice WE. *Arnheim's principles of athletic training: a competency-based approach.* New York: McGraw-Hill; 2006.
6. United States Department of Agriculture. www.uwda.gov. 2008.
7. Wildman REC, Miller BS. *Sports and fitness nutrition.* Belmont: Wadsworth/Thompson Learning; 2003.
8. Williams MH. *Nutrition for health, fitness, and sport,* 8th ed. New York: McGraw-Hill; 2007.

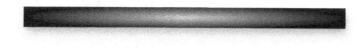

S E C T I O N

12

Health Care Administration

Part 1   Monitoring Systems

Part 2   Risk Management

Part 3   Resource Management

Part 4   Third-Party Reimbursement

Part 5   Federal Statutes

Part 6   Documentation

Part 7   Administrative Concepts

Section 12 Examination

OVERVIEW

The key to effective health care administration is found in appropriate communication and understanding of various health care concepts. A certified athletic trainer (ATC) is an administrator even if working as a single caregiver in the smallest school. Knowledge of the requirements expected of the allied health professional will assist the ATC in assuring professional protection for self and institution.

CLINICAL PROFICIENCIES

There are no proficiencies assigned by the *Athletic Training Competencies*, 4th edition for this section.

Monitoring Systems

NATIONAL ELECTRONIC INJURY SURVEILLANCE SYSTEM

- Origination: 1972
- Oversight: United States Consumer Product Safety Commission (CPSC)
- Information collection: Equipment manufacturers and distributors; sample of hospital emergency room monitoring
- Available data: Reported injuries related to consumer products; reports from manufacturers regarding equipment
- Actions: Seize products considered dangerous; create standards to decrease risk; provide data to the public

NATIONAL FOOTBALL HEAD AND NECK INJURY REGISTRY

- Origination: 1976 to 1991
- Oversight: Independent organization
- Information collection: Hospitals
- Available data: 72+ hour hospital admissions related to head and neck fractures, dislocations, permanent paralysis, surgery, or death
- Actions: Warehouse of data, no actions

NATIONAL COLLEGIATE ATHLETIC ASSOCIATION INJURY SURVEILLANCE SYSTEM

Origination: 1982

Oversight: National Collegiate Athletic Association (NCAA)

Information collection: Certified athletic trainers (ATCs)

Available data: Injury trends in intercollegiate sports

Actions: Report injury trends to the NCAA Committee on Competitive Safeguards and Medical Aspects of Sport; suggest changes to protective equipments, rules, and coaching techniques

NATIONAL HIGH SCHOOL SPORTS INJURIES REGISTRY

Origination: 1995 to 1998

Oversight: Med Sport Systems

Information collection: Secondary schools

Available data: Injuries related to ten high school sports

Actions: Warehouse of data, no actions

PART 2

Risk Management

KEY TERMS

- Material Safety Data Sheet (MSDS)
- National Library of Medicine (NLM)
- Negligence
- Outcomes management
- Peer review
- Population
- Practice
- Practice guidelines
- Principal diagnosis
- Public health
- Quality assurance (QA)
- Reciprocity
- Sequela, sequelae
- Standard of care
- Urgent care

RISK MANAGEMENT

- Process for loss protection
- Plans are critical to assure institutional and personal security
- Identify, evaluate, and manage risks

LIABILITY

- Legal responsibility for the harm caused to a person

- Superiors can be responsible for subordinate's negligence (vicarious liability or doctrine of *respondeat superior*)
- Diffuse liability
  - Writing good Standard Operating Procedures (policies and procedures)
  - Hiring professionals who remain current in their profession
  - Assuring employees understand roles within their jobs
  - Imploring employees to act reasonably and prudently

> *Quick* **fact** People are less likely to get sued, even with wrongdoing, if the patient has a positive relationship with the caregiver. Never underestimate good communications with patients.

NEGLIGENCE

- Type of legal tort (civil, not criminal wrong)
- Failure to act as a reasonably prudent professional would act under similar situations
- Requires four elements for trigger
  - Duty—defined by practices, duties, or job
  - Breach—failure to meet one's duty
  - Cause—reason for the event in question
  - Harm—injury occurring from negligence

Acts of Negligence

- Omission—not acting when required
- Commission—acting when should not have
- Nonfeasance—not doing what should have been done
- Misfeasance—acting inside legal boundaries in an incorrect fashion
- Malfeasance—acting outside legal boundaries

STANDARD OF CARE

- Legal duty
- Provide care to patients consistent with other professionals of the same training
- Circumstances must be similar

STATUTES OF LIMITATIONS

- Time limit on legal action for a wrongful act
- Usually begin at time of injury

- Differ by state
- Specific situations may have different statutes of limitations, for example, personal injury versus personal property injury
- A minor child's statute of limitations does not begin until 18 years of age

SOVEREIGN IMMUNITY

- Known as *governmental immunity*
- Doctrine where government cannot commit a legal wrong
- Civil and criminal prosecution not allowed
- Applies to federal, state, and local jurisdictions
- Can sue for negligence of governmental employees
- Public schools and employee actions may be protected under this doctrine

GOOD SAMARITAN LAWS

- Protections for aiding injured or ill persons
- Not a legal requirement to aid others in the United States
- Some countries require aid for injured and ill persons
- Does not apply if there is a caretaker relationship, for example, ATC–athlete
- Cannot gain financial reward for actions, for example, first aid as a result of employment
- Must act in good faith, rationally, and at level of training
- Must gain consent of patient (guardian of minors)
- Implied consent, for example, unconscious, intoxicated
- Required to stay at the scene unless calling emergency medical service (EMS), unsafe conditions, or other trained people take over

PRODUCT LIABILITY

- Express and implied warranty
- Design, construction, and defects, for example National Operating Committee on Standards for Athletic Equipment (NOCSAE)
- Understand and communicate; use directions
- Do not modify products

PARTICIPATION AGREEMENTS

- Waiver
- Release
- Agreement to participate
- Parental permission

Resource Management

BUDGET

- Operational plan
- Coordinates resources and expenses
- Equates mission statement into financial terms

Selected Types of Budgets

- Fixed
- Line item
- Lump sum
- Spending ceiling
- Spending reduction
- Variable
- Zero based

Fixed Budget

- Monthly projections dictate budget
- Allows program to estimate cash flow
- No variability of unforeseen expenses

Line-Item Budget

- Type of fixed budget
- Financial allocations based on program categories
- Cannot transfer money between categories
- No variability for unforeseen expenses in a given category
- Common categories
  - Capital equipment
  - Expendable supplies
  - Minor equipment

Lump-Sum Budget

- Type of fixed budget
- Program given a total amount of money for all needs
- Program administrator determines allotments within the services provided
- Allocations based on program needs

Spending Ceiling Budget

- Also known as the *incremental model*
- Must provide justification for expenses over previous spending cycle

Spending Reduction Budget

- Used when the program is experiencing financial distress
- Administrators require spending to reduce by a certain percentage to balance the budget

Variable Budget

- Based on monthly assessment of resources
- Expenses do not exceed revenue

Zero-Based Budget

- Type of performance budget
- Justification required for every expense
- Previous budget cycle has no impact on current budget cycle

PROGRAMMATIC NEEDS ASSESSMENT

- Sets program resource priorities
- Identifies differences between the current program and how it should exist

PROGRAM FUNDING OPPORTUNITIES

- Alumni
- Booster clubs
- Buying consortia
- Capital campaign
- Commercial loans
- Corporate sponsorship
- Endowment
- Fundraising
- Grants
- Institutional budget allocations

REQUEST FOR QUOTATION

- Also known as *bidding*
- Formalized request for price quote
- Includes specific requests for products, warranty, and shipping information
- Institutional requirements may dictate process

INVENTORY

- Recording in-stock expendable, nonexpendable, minor, and capital equipment
- Performed extensively annually
- Spot inventory often to avoid supply shortages
- Control process should be in place

PURCHASING

- Request for quotation (RFQ) (bid)
- Assess bid
- Determine vendor
- Request purchase order
- Place order—negotiate freight and warranties

PART 4

Third-Party Reimbursement

KEY TERMS

- Acute care hospital
- Capitation
- Case management
- Coinsurance
- Conflict of interest
- Coordination of Benefits (COB)
- Copayment
- Critical appraisal
- Current Procedural Terminology (CPT)
- Deductible
- Episode of care
- Evidence-based medicine
- Evidenced-based practice
- Exclusive provider organization (EPO)
- Explanation of Benefits (EOB)
- Gate-keeper
- Group model HMO
- Group practice
- Health care provider
- Health care system
- Health information management (HIM)
- Health information system
- Health insurance
- Health Insurance Portability and Accountability Act (HIPAA)
- Health maintenance organization (HMO)
- Health promotion
- Independent medical evaluation (IME)
- Inpatient
- Insurance
- International Classification of Diseases (ICD)
- Joint Commission on Accrediation of Healthcare Organizations (JCAHO)
- Managed care
- Medicaid
- Medicare
- Medicare Part A
- Medicare Part B
- Medigap insurance
- National Provider Identifier (NPI)
- Preauthorization
- Precertification
- Preferred provider organization (PPO)
- Primary care physician
- Workers compensation (WC)

INSURANCE IN ATHLETIC TRAINING

- Primary insurance
- Secondary insurance
- Liability insurance
- Catastrophic injury insurance

INDEMNITY PLAN

- Traditionally called *fee-for-service*
- Consumer can seek care with any provider
- Provider bills insurance company and insurer pays a portion
- Plan defined deductible before insurance company contributes total payment for services
- Not well controlled and some believe have contributed to rising health care costs

MANAGED CARE PLANS

- Health care plan
- Manage financial viability of programs
- Use designated providers of services
- Financial incentives to providers for cost-effective care
- Less choice for consumer
- Lower out-of-pocket cost for consumer

Types of Managed Care Plans

- Health Maintenance Organization (HMO)
- Preferred Provider Organization (PPO)
- Point-of-Service (POS) Plan
- Exclusive Provider Organization (EPO)

Health Maintenance Organization

- Contract between insurance company and providers
- Predefined service delivery
- Prepaid plan—expenses covered in advance of services
- Designated providers administer care
- Selected primary care physician manages care
- Care sought outside of HMO is at a cost to the patient

Preferred Provider Organization

- Insurance company has negotiated reduced rates with providers
- Care sought outside of PPO costs more to the patient

Point-of-Service Plan

- Covers treatment of an HMO provider as with an HMO plan
- Permits patient to seek care outside the HMO plan for higher copayment

Exclusive Provider Organization

- Providers have contract with insurance company, employer, or other entity
- Providers agree to fixed level of reimbursement
- Consumers must seek care from within the EPO
- EPO providers are often forbidden to deliver care to patients outside the plan

MEDICARE

- Formed by Title XVIII of the Social Security Act 1965
- Federal health insurance plan first postulated by President Harry S. Truman (1945)
- Insurance for people 65 years and older, qualified disabled people, and people with Social Security or Railroad Retirement
- Specific requirements for filing claims
- Hospital Insurance (Part A)—inpatient care
- Supplementary Medical Insurance (Part B)—outpatient charges
- Prescription medication plans
- Policies often dictate reimbursement of services by private insurers
- Managed by Centers for Medicare and Medicaid Services (CMS)

MEDICAID

- Formed by Title XIX of the Social Security Act 1965
- Joint venture between federal and state governments (CMS and state)
- Federal funds exist but states given authority to devise eligibility criteria
- Aids low-income families with children in getting medical care
- Assist with low-income disabled medical care

CURRENT PROCEDURAL TERMINOLOGY CODES

- Encourage standard descriptors and terms in documenting procedures in medical records

- Allow easy transmission of information to insurers
- Standardize outcomes research
- Published by the American Medical Association (AMA)
- 97005—Current Procedural Terminology (CPT) code for athletic training evaluation
- 97006—CPT code for athletic training reevaluation

> **Quick fact** The Health Care Financing Administration (HCFA) has been renamed the Centers for Medicare and Medicaid Services (CMS).

INTERNATIONAL CLASSIFICATION OF DISEASE

- Published by the World Health Organizations (WHO)
- Tenth edition is currently used
- International comparability of mortality statistics
- Format for cause of death reporting
- Medical coding
- Usually three to five digit codes, for example, 410.92—acute myocardial infarction

UB-92 (UNIVERSAL BILLING CODES)

- Universal billing form
- Required for billing Medicare Part A claims
- Criteria devised by CMS

ADVANCED BENEFICIARY NOTICE

- Medicare requires document of providers
- Form must be completed before rendering services
- Outlines payment responsibilities when Medicare may deny claim

EXPLANATION OF BENEFITS FORM

- Forms provided to patients and insurers
- Most insurers will not reimburse providers without an Explanation of Benefits (EOB)
- Identifies services, charges, date of service, provider, and claims denials/reductions
- Required to have contact information of provider and appeals information

Federal Statutes

- Health Care Financing Administration (HCFA)
- Patient's Bill of Rights
- U.S. Department of Health and Human Services (HHS)
- U.S. National Institutes of Health (NIH)
- WHO

AFFIRMATIVE ACTION

- Effective: 1965
- Entitlement: Assures minorities and women are treated equally in educational and employment setting
- Enforced: United States Department of Civil Rights

AMERICAN WITH DISABILITIES ACT

- Effective: 1990
- Entitlement: Reenforced Section 504 of the Rehabilitation Act
- Enforced: United States Department of Labor

EQUAL EMPLOYMENT OPPORTUNITY COMMISSION

- Part of Title VII of the Civil Rights Act
- Effective: 1964, administered 1965
- Enforces:
  - Title VII of the Civil Rights Act of 1964
  - Age Discrimination in Employment Act (ADEA)
  - Equal Pay Act
  - Title I and V of the Americans with Disabilities Act (ADA)
  - Section 501 and 505 of the Rehabilitation Act
  - Civil rights Act of 1991

FAIR LABOR STANDARDS ACT

- Effective: 1938
- Entitlement: Establishes minimum wage, overtime pay, record keeping, and child labor standards
- Enforced: Wage and Hour Division of United States Department of Labor

FAMILY MEDICAL LEAVE ACT

- Effective: 1993
- Entitlement: 12 weeks' unpaid job protection for family medical reasons
- Enforced: United States Department of Labor

FEDERAL EDUCATIONAL RIGHTS PRIVACY ACT

- Also known as the *Buckley Amendment*
- Effective 1974
- Entitlement: Protects privacy of student's educational records; parents have the right until student becomes 18 years old, then that right transfers to the student
- Enforced: United States Department of Education

HEALTH INSURANCE PORTABILITY AND ACCOUNTABILITY ACT

- Effective: 2001, with compliance by 2003
- Entitlement: Portability of insurance as jobs change; standardize procedural codes and billing; secure personal health care information
- Enforced: United States Department of Health and Human Services

OCCUPATIONAL SAFETY AND HEALTH ADMINISTRATION

- Effective: 1970
- Protection: Prevents work-related injuries, illnesses, and deaths
- Enforces: Workplace safety

SECTION 504 OF THE REHABILITATION ACT

- Effective: 1973
- Entitlement: Assures equal opportunities for qualified handicapped people
- Enforced: United States Office of Civil Rights
- Three elements required to trigger Section 504 of the Rehabilitation Act
  - Handicapped discrimination
  - Qualified individual
  - Federal funds

SEXUAL HARASSMENT

- Part of Title VII of the Civil Rights Act
- Effective: 1964
- Entitlement: Prevents intentional and perceived discriminatory practices on an individual basis; committed to discouraging a hostile work environment.
- Enforced: United States EEOC

TITLE IX OF THE EDUCATION AMENDMENT

- Effective: 1972
- Entitlement: Assures equitable participation in educational programs for both sexes
- Enforced: United States Office of Civil Rights

- Three elements required to trigger Title IX
  - Gender discrimination
  - Educational programs
  - Federal funds
- Impact on athletic programs participation

PART 6 Documentation

KEY TERMS

- Accreditation
- Adulteration
- Implied consent
- Informed consent
- POMR
- POR
- SOAP
- Subjective

DOCUMENTATION GUIDELINES

- Records must be neat
- Black ink (permanent)
- Patient name and identifying information, for example, medical records number, social security number (SSN) must be on each entry
- Every entry needs to be dated, signed, and professional abbreviations (some places require time as well)
- Describe care given and patient response

- Objective descriptions
- Entries are consecutive and in chronological order
- No skipped lines or gaps
- Write entries same day as care
- Be factual
- Include patient/family quotes if needed
- Document complaints (pain, etc.) and resolution
- Abbreviations must be from a facility-accepted list
- Chart what you do only, not what should have been done
- Document condition changes
- Comment on items taught to patient and the patient's response to that process
- Never erase errors and initial/date

TYPES OF PATIENT CHARTING OPTIONS

- SOAP—Subjective, Objective, Assessment, Plan
- POMR—Problem-Oriented Medical Records
- Focus charting
- Charting by exception
- Narrative charting
- Computerized systems
- HIPS—History, Inspection, Palpation, Special Tests
- HOPS—History, Observation, Palpation, Special Tests

MANAGEMENT CONCEPTS

- Scientific management
- Human relations management
- Behavioral management
- Modern management

Scientific Management

- Science determines model
- People prefer direction in the work environment
- People dislike work and only do what is required
- Money is the incentive for work
- Production most important
- No room for motivating factors like self-esteem or sense of achievement
- Maximize efficiency by identifying discrete job tasks
- Managers always respond the same way
- Theorist examples: Frederick Taylor and Harrington Emerson

Human Relations Management

- Incorporated behavioral sciences into management
- Managers can vary reactions based on situations
- Cooperation important
- Hawthorne studies from this era
- Proactive versus reactive
- Theorist examples: Mary Parker Follett and Elton Mayo

Behavioral Management

- Communication important
- Communications lines should be as short as possible
- People work for reasons other than money
- Defined autocratic, democratic, and laissez-faire leadership styles
- Defined formal organizational structure
- Theorist examples: Chester Barnard and Kurt Lewin

Modern Management

- Democratic in nature
- Believes that people prefer self-direction and project ownership
- Work is as natural as play
- Total quality management—customer is the major focus of the job
- Theorist examples: Edward Deming and Douglas McGregor

KEY MANAGEMENT STYLES

- Autocratic (authoritarian)
- Democratic (participative)
- Laissez-faire (anarchy)

Autocratic

- Decisions are made at the top of the organizations
- People including managers do as they are told
- Assumes people hate work and must be forced to work
- Chain of command, for example, military
- Fear motivates employees
- High absenteeism

Democratic

- Decisions are made at all levels
- People accept and seek greater responsibility
- Work can be a source of satisfaction
- Responsibilities are delegated
- Reward motivates employees

Laissez-Faire

- No real management style
- Lets employees do as they chose
- Employees have sense of responsibility
- Often seen as chaos

ORGANIZATIONAL STRUCTURE

- Model representation of organizational relationships
- Span of control
- Chain of command
- Organizational chart

STAFF MEETINGS

- Provide agenda in advance
- Do not waste time—discuss important issues
- Keep meeting on track

VISION STATEMENTS

- Concise statement
- State quality expectations of services
- Describe the perfect organizational state
- Comments ambitious and convincing
- Recognize business targets
- Expresses services offered
- Identify service providers

MISSION STATEMENTS

- Concise statement of the organization's characteristics, purposes, and philosophy
- Objective program goals
- Programmatic blueprint
- Simple statement yet complete
- Desired program image

STRATEGIC PLANNING

- Organizational decision-making process
- Upper management usually completes this process
- Assures mission and program are synchronized
- Occurs before action
- Maps organizational improvements
- Long-term activity planning
- Completed at least every 5 years

OPERATIONAL PLANNING

- Vision into workable plan
- Defines program activities
- Policy, processes, and procedures
- Short-term activity planning
- Completed at least every 2 years

POLICY

- Broad statements of expected actions
- No detailed explanations

PROCESSES

- Incremental steps
- Direct organizational tasks

PROCEDURE

- Specific directions for programs

WOTS UP

- **W**eaknesses, **O**pportunities, **T**hreats, **S**trengths and **U**nderlying **P**lanning

- Assessment technique to facilitate planning and improvements

SWOT

- **S**trengths, **W**eaknesses, **O**pportunities, and **T**hreats
- Assessment technique for organizational planning and improvements

ACCREDITATION

- Formal recognition of programs
- Programs meet minimal quality standards
- Specific accrediting organizations for education and health care organizations

JOINT COMMISSION ON ACCREDITATION OF HEALTHCARE ORGANIZATIONS

- Independent not-for-profit organization
- Set standards for health care in America
- Oldest and largest health care organization in the country
- Required to meet Medicare requirements
- Increase third-party reimbursement
- Required for facility requirements
- Improves community confidence
- Stimulates quality improvement

COMMISSION ON ACCREDITATION OF REHABILITATION FACILITIES

- Not-for-profit organization
- Integrated accreditation with Joint Commission on Accreditation of Healthcare Organizations (JCAHO)
- Specific to rehabilitation facilities

COMMISSION ON ACCREDITATION OF ATHLETIC TRAINING EDUCATION

- Accredits Athletic Training Education Programs
- Assures efficacy and standards for education of athletic training students
- Established in 2006

1. Which budget category houses expensive, durable equipment with 3-5 year lifespan?
   a. Minor equipment
   b. Expendable equipment
   c. Capital equipment
   d. Modality equipment
   e. Billable equipment

2. What state credentialing process protects the public and regulates specific professions by mandating what duties can and cannot be performed?
   a. Registration
   b. Certification
   c. Exemplification
   d. Licensure
   e. Standard of practice

3. Who must sign for medical record release in patients 18 years old?
   a. The patients themselves
   b. The parent or legal guardian
   c. No signature required
   d. A medical doctor must agree and sign

4. What term identifies the responsibilities for which a new employee is held accountable?
   a. Job specification
   b. Role delineation
   c. Job description
   d. Employment contract
   e. Position description

5. What federal act reenforces Section 504 of the Rehabilitation Act?
   a. Title IX
   b. Amendment XIV
   c. American with Disabilities Act
   d. Handicapped Hiring Act
   e. Disabilities Distress Act

6. What legal defense claims the plaintiff understood activity hazards?
   a. Cause of action
   b. Assumption of risks
   c. Informed consent
   d. Compulsory nonsuit
   e. Contributory negligence

7. What is unpermitted contact with another individual?
   a. Assault
   b. Cause of action
   c. Compulsory nonsuit
   d. Battery
   e. Adversarial contact

8. What condition represents a violation in standard of care?
   a. Liability
   b. Breach of duty
   c. Hold harmless clause
   d. Catastrophic professionalism
   e. Battery

9. What is the organizational responsibility delineation?
   a. Chain of command
   b. Matrix charting
   c. Operational plan
   d. Administrative hierarchy
   e. Facility charting

10. What type of negligence occurs when the plaintiff's actions add to the injury?
    a. Contributory liability
    b. Comparative negligence
    c. Commissionable liability
    d. Code of harm
    e. Breach of duty

11. What managed care program provides a set fee per member?
    a. Capitation
    b. Indemnity
    c. Beneficiary
    d. Tort
    e. Exemplification

12. What other name identifies a traditional indemnity insurance plan?
    a. Blue Cross/Blue Shield
    b. Price-per-exposure
    c. Insurance servicing program
    d. Point-of-service
    e. Fee-for-service

13. What health care organization provides defined services to enrolled patients for a specific sum of money during a specific time period?
    a. Capitation organization
    b. Health maintenance organization
    c. Not-for-profit organization
    d. Indemnity organization
    e. Exclusive provider organization

14. What situation exists when a health care worker commits a negligent act while providing care?
    a. Liability
    b. Malpractice
    c. Omission
    d. Commission
    e. Remission

15. What document contains a person's medical history including all health care interventions?
    a. Insurance records
    b. Assessment records
    c. Medical records
    d. Evaluation records
    e. Health materials

16. What negligent tort exists when a person performs an intervention within the professional boundaries but does the intervention incorrectly?
    a. Malfeasance
    b. Misfeasance
    c. Nonfeasance
    d. Unfeasance
    e. Nulfeasance

17. What written statement defines an organization's philosophy, purposes, and characteristics?
    a. Vision statement
    b. Mission statement
    c. Procedural statement
    d. Operational statement
    e. Performance statement

18. What procedure determines an organization's priorities and identified desires?
    a. Prioritization assessment
    b. Evaluative process
    c. Operational process
    d. Needs assessment
    e. Performance evaluation

19. What reimbursement codes do all health care workers use to describe the services provided?
    a. International Classification of Disease
    b. Universal Billing
    c. Current Procedural Terminology
    d. Indemnity Classification of Billing
    e. Request for Reimbursement

20. How should a manager communicate effectively with and extravert?
    a. Variety, action, discussion
    b. Reading, reflection, no interruptions
    c. Write notes
    d. None of the above is effective

21. What name is given to individuals who are unsupportive of a program or plan and untrustworthy?
    a. Opponents
    b. Adversaries
    c. Enemies
    d. Bedfellows
    e. Allies

22. What is a graphic representation of an organizational structure?
    a. Organizational chart
    b. Chain of command orientation
    c. Bubble charting
    d. Gantt chart
    e. Integrative charting

23. What federal act protects a patient's medical records?
    a. Health Information Privacy and Accountability Act
    b. Medical Records Portability and Accessibility Act
    c. Medical Information Privilege and Convenience Act
    d. Health Information Portability and Accountability Act
    e. None of the above ensures patient protection

24. What are the four types of managed health care organizations?
    a. HMO, POC, PPO, and IOP
    b. HMO, PPO, POS, and EPO
    c. HMO, POP, PSO, and IOP
    d. HMO, IOP, PPO, and ROP
    e. HMO, PCO, EOP, and POS

25. What is the difference between the current status and which is desired?
    a. Program goals
    b. Objectives
    c. Needs
    d. Operational goals
    e. Programmatic objectives

26. What is FERPA?
    a. Familiarized Employment Reparations Privilege Act
    b. Formation of Employment Rights and Privacy Act
    c. Financer Eligible Rights and Privilege Act
    d. Family Educational Rights and Privacy Act
    e. Formation of Educational Reparations and Punishment Act

27. What is JCAHO?
    a. Judgment Committee on Assurance of Healthcare Organizations
    b. Judgment Committee on Accreditation of Human Operations
    c. Joint Commission on Accreditation of Healthcare Organizations
    d. Judicial Contacts on Assurance of Hiring Operations
    e. Joint Commission on Acceptance of Hiring Operations

28. What federal act is infringed when a coworker makes an unwelcome sexual advance?
    a. Title VII of the Civil Rights Act
    b. Title IX of the Civil Rights Act
    c. Title XIV of the Civil Rights Act
    d. Fair Labor Standards Act
    e. Buckley Amendment

29. Who is considered the "gatekeeper" of managed health care systems?
    a. The patient
    b. Primary care physician
    c. Insurance provider
    d. Specialty physicians
    e. Employer

30. Who comprises the joint venture for Medicaid benefits?
    a. Individual and federal government
    b. Federal and state government
    c. Private insurance and tax payer
    d. Tax payer and federal government
    e. Insurer and tax payer

31. What should one do first if planning a new program?
    a. Devise a marketing plan
    b. Begin public relations procedures
    c. Devise a vision statement
    d. Write an operational plan
    e. Hire employees to run the program

32. What are CPT and ICD codes?
    a. Reimbursement codes
    b. Standardized care codes
    c. Usual and customary codes
    d. Universal billing codes
    e. Request for quotation codes

33. What management style did Mary Parker Follett propose?
    a. Employees are enticed by money
    b. Cooperation and democracy in the workplace
    c. Workers prefer not being bogged down with production details
    d. Workplace dynamics are changing so one should do a job without much input
    e. Work is as natural as leisure-time activities

34. What type of organizational chart accounts for services and functions?
    a. Matrix
    b. Function oriented
    c. Services oriented
    d. Multifunctional
    e. Integrated

35. What type of supplies generally needs to be purchased on a regular basis?
    a. Capital supplies
    b. Job-specific materials
    c. Minor equipment
    d. Expendable supplies

36. What term identifies the amount that a family agrees to pay out-of-pocket for medical expenses before an insurer pays any part?
    a. Cost allocations
    b. Copayment
    c. Deductible
    d. Margin
    e. Subscriber fee

37. What legal doctrine says that an employer may be responsible for the negligence caused by their employees?
    a. Doctrine of *certiorari*
    b. Doctrine of *respondeat superior*
    c. Doctrine of variable responsibility
    d. Doctrine of appellate responsibility
    e. Doctrine of *quid pro quo*

38. What are the three leadership roles of any administrator?
    a. Interpersonal, informational, and decisional
    b. Communicator, educator, and motivator
    c. Professionalism, communicator, and decisional
    d. Risk taking, realism, and market resource

39. What type of organizational chart delineates specific job tasks?
    a. Matrix
    b. Function oriented
    c. Services oriented
    d. Multifunctional
    e. Integrated

40. Which management style is defined as the absence of leadership?
    a. Capitalistic
    b. Anarchy
    c. Democratic
    d. Authoritarian
    e. Laissez-faire

41. What type of organizational culture is characterized by a consensus, teamwork atmosphere?
    a. Personalistic
    b. Formalistic

c. Collegial
d. Authoritarian
e. Anarchy

42. Which industrial studies were associated with Elton Mayo?
    a. Iowa studies
    b. Ohio State studies
    c. Hawthorne studies
    d. University of Michigan studies
    e. Behavioral studies

43. HIPAA is noted for protecting a patient's:
    a. Health rights
    b. Privacy
    c. Reimbursement ability
    d. Right to select health care options

44. Whose needs are paramount in total quality management?
    a. Administrators
    b. Employees
    c. Clients
    d. Future customers
    e. Every group

45. What tort exists when a health care worker fails to act as a reasonably and prudent professional under similar circumstances?
    a. Omission
    b. Negligence
    c. Harm
    d. Cause
    e. Commission

46. Which is not a component required for negligence?
    a. Duty
    b. Breach
    c. Malpractice
    d. Harm
    e. Cause

47. What negligent tort occurs when a person fails to perform his or her legal duty of care?
    a. Nonfeasance
    b. Negligence
    c. Misfeasance
    d. Malfeasance
    e. Liability

48. What specific statements define how an organization intends to accomplish a specific goal?
    a. Policy
    b. Objectives
    c. Goals
    d. Processes
    e. Procedures

49. What is a failure to act when there is some legal requirement to do so?
    a. Omission
    b. Negligence
    c. Harm
    d. Cause
    e. Commission

50. What organization does the letters OSHA represent?
    a. Organizational Specialty and Hospital Association
    b. Occupational Safety and Health Administration
    c. Organization of Superior Healthcare Association
    d. Occupations for Superior Health Administration
    e. Organizational Safety and Humanities Association

51. What is the federal government rule that requires employers to protect employees against accidental transmission of body fluid pathogens?
    a. Standards of Care
    b. Comparative Health Care Standards
    c. OSHA Bloodborne Pathogen Standards
    d. Vicarious Protection Program
    e. Buckley Amendment

52. What budget type requires allocation of funds for discrete activities?
    a. Zero-based budget
    b. Line-item budget
    c. Lump-sum budget
    d. Fixed budget
    e. Spending ceiling budget

53. What is the process of placing value on the work that an employee completes?
    a. Job specifications
    b. Job descriptions
    c. Performance evaluation
    d. Pay for performance
    e. Job qualifications

54. What type of insurance plan allows network participants the option of obtaining outside network care?
    a. Preferred Provider Organization (PPO)
    b. Point-of-Service (POS) Plan
    c. Health Maintenance Organization (HMO)
    d. Indemnity Plan
    e. Exclusive Provider Organization (EPO)

55. What is the basic framework of the rules and principles that govern and expedite the work environment?
    a. Policy
    b. Procedure
    c. Process
    d. Planning
    e. Profits

56. What team of health care workers are contracted to deliver health care to a specific population?
   a. Preferred Provider Organization (PPO)
   b. Point-of-Service (POS) Plan
   c. Health Maintenance Organization (HMO)
   d. Indemnity Plan
   e. Exclusive Provider Organization (EPO)

57. What is the description of the process by which a specific policy is completed?
   a. Policy
   b. Procedure
   c. Process
   d. Planning
   e. Profits

58. What are the incremental steps designed to direct an organization's most important tasks?
   a. Policy
   b. Procedure
   c. Process
   d. Planning
   e. Profits

59. What health care organization is a blending of health maintenance organizations (HMO) and preferred provider organizations (PPOs)?
   a. Preferred Provider Organization (PPO)
   b. Point-of-Service (POS) Plan
   c. Health Maintenance Organization (HMO)
   d. Indemnity Plan
   e. Exclusive Provider Organization (EPO)

60. What document is used by an organization to formalize the intention to purchase goods or services from a vendor?
   a. Sales receipt
   b. Needs assessment
   c. Purchase order
   d. Request for purchase
   e. Bid

61. What is the process of acquiring goods and services?
   a. Bidding
   b. Purchasing
   c. Requisitions
   d. Inventory
   e. Needs

62. What are CPT, UB, and ICD codes?
   a. Medicare codes
   b. Medicaid codes
   c. Insurance codes
   d. Reimbursement codes
   e. Healthcare codes

63. What reimbursement code do all health care workers use to describe the services provided?
   a. International Classification of Disease Codes
   b. Current Procedural Terminology Codes
   c. Universal Billing Codes
   d. Explanation of Benefits Codes
   e. Advanced Beneficiary Codes

64. What reimbursement code do hospitals use to describe the services provided?
   a. International Classification of Disease Codes
   b. Current Procedural Terminology Codes
   c. Universal Billing Codes
   d. Explanation of Benefits Codes
   e. Advanced Beneficiary Codes

65. What reimbursement code do all health care workers use to describe the patient's condition?
   a. International Classification of Disease Codes
   b. Current Procedural Terminology Codes
   c. Universal Billing Codes
   d. Explanation of Benefits Codes
   e. Advanced Beneficiary Codes

66. What document provides vendors specific information for bidding on goods and services?
   a. Bidding format
   b. Purchasing agreement
   c. Request for quotation
   d. Inventory request
   e. Needs assessment

67. What is the formal or informal authorization to purchase goods or services?
   a. Bidding
   b. Purchasing
   c. Requisitions
   d. Inventory
   e. Needs

68. What type of policies strives to eliminate, share, or modify the risks associated with a particular activity?
   a. Sovereign management
   b. Risk management
   c. Participation assessment
   d. Role assessment
   e. Loss protection

69. What document is used to construct the BOC certification examination?
   a. Educational Competencies
   b. Role Delineation Study
   c. Standard of Care
   d. Code of Participation
   e. Doctrine of Professional Competencies

70. What legal doctrine explains that neither governments nor their agents can be held liable for negligent actions?
   a. Good Samaritan law
   b. Sovereign immunity
   c. Doctrine of respondeat superior

d. Doctrine of appellate responsibility
e. Vicarious liability

71. What is the level of medical sophistication and competency required of a person who performs a health care role?
   a. Educational competencies
   b. Role delineation requirements
   c. Standard of care
   d. Code of participation
   e. Doctrine of professional competencies

72. What group of agreed-upon procedures are accumulated and used to define specific operations?
   a. Standard operating procedures
   b. Processes and procedures
   c. Operations delineations
   d. Organizational charting
   e. Comparative procedures and standards

73. What are the principles that guide professional activities of a health care provider?
   a. Principles of care
   b. Code of professionalism
   c. Professional conduct competencies
   d. Role delineation requirements
   e. Standards of practice

74. What is the length of time one has to file a claim against another?
   a. Legal limits
   b. Standard suit requirements
   c. Statute of limitations
   d. Compensatory limits
   e. Limited liability

75. What type of planning is used to critically examine an organization and bring about improvement?
   a. Operational planning
   b. Strategic planning
   c. Organizational planning
   d. Business plan
   e. Quality improvement program

76. What is a legal document that compels a person to provide testimony?
   a. Affidavit
   b. Subpoena
   c. Writ of testimony
   d. Appellate requirement
   e. Power of attorney

77. What are the legally binding statements offered as evidence in a legal proceeding?
   a. Exculpatory clause
   b. Testimony
   c. Defendant comments
   d. Appellate statement
   e. Prosecutors avowalment

78. What congressional act ensures employees are appropriately compensated for their duties within a workweek?
   a. Family Employment Act
   b. Fair Labor Standards Act
   c. Future Workers Amendment
   d. Fair Overtime Pay Amendment
   e. Employment Standards Amendment

79. What is a legal wrongdoing where the court system often provides remediation?
   a. Malfeasance
   b. Nonfeasance
   c. Breach
   d. Tort
   e. Harm

80. What budget system requires that monthly expenses be adjusted if revenue exceeds expenses?
   a. Zero-based budget
   b. Variable budget
   c. Lump-sum budget
   d. Fixed budget
   e. Spending ceiling budget

81. What federal law requires student authorization to release educational records to a third party?
   a. Student Educational Records Act
   b. Family Educational Rights and Privacy Act
   c. Fair Distribution of Educational Materials Act
   d. Student Educational Rights and Confidentiality Act
   e. Educational Records and Rights Act

82. What is another name for the Family Educational Rights and Privacy Act (FERPA)?
   a. Hawthorne Amendment
   b. Dickenson Amendment
   c. Buckley Amendment
   d. Maxwell Amendment
   e. Harrison Amendment

83. What concise statement describes the ideal state of an organization?
   a. Mission statement
   b. Strategic statement
   c. Operational statement
   d. Vision statement
   e. Procedural statement

84. What legal contract relieves a person of his or her right to sue for damages?
   a. Exculpatory clause
   b. Waiver
   c. Contributory permissions
   d. Release
   e. Parental permissions

85. What type of budget system constructs an annual budget without regard to past budget performance?
    a. Zero-based budget
    b. Line-item budget
    c. Lump-sum budget
    d. Fixed budget
    e. Spending ceiling budget

86. What technique is used to analyze an organization's weaknesses, strengths, threats, and opportunities?
    a. POMR Charting
    b. Matrix organizational Charting
    c. WOTS UP Analysis
    d. Integrated weaknesses and strengths analysis

87. What determines the length of time medical records must be retained?
    a. Doctrine of *respondeat superior*
    b. Statute of limitations
    c. Standard of care
    d. Standards of practice
    e. Standards of prudence

88. Where must an athlete's medical record be housed?
    a. Athletic training room
    b. Athletic training office
    c. File cabinet
    d. Confidential and secure location
    e. On a computer

89. What document must be signed by the patient explaining the risk, anticipated outcome, and alternatives of rehabilitation treatment?
    a. Waiver
    b. Release
    c. Informed consent
    d. Permission for care
    e. Agreement

90. What document gives a collegiate or scholastic high school athletic training staff permission to treat an injured athlete?
    a. Informed consent or authorization/permission to treat
    b. Waiver
    c. Parental exculpatory note
    d. Release
    e. Exculpatory clause

91. What medical record keeping dictates notation only when process deviates from norms?
    a. Narrative
    b. Charting by exception
    c. Progress oriented charting
    d. SOAP Note
    e. HIP Note

92. What standards are determined by a set of principles and moral values?
    a. Code of ethics
    b. Standard of care
    c. Code of participation
    d. Doctrine of professional competencies
    e. Code of professional practice

93. What occurs when interests of one individual/group is in competition with another?
    a. Competing interests
    b. Comparative interest
    c. Questionable interests
    d. Contributable interests
    e. Conflict of interest

94. What type of negligence occurs when the plaintiff's actions add to an injury?
    a. Cause of action
    b. Compulsory nonsuit
    c. Contributory negligence
    d. Comparative risk
    e. Commisionary negligence

95. What is the scientific study of human work?
    a. Ergonomics
    b. Capitation
    c. Ergogenics
    d. Ergolytics
    e. Ergology

96. What term identifies the reasonable care used to avoid unreasonable risk?
    a. Damage
    b. Breach
    c. Duty
    d. Cause
    e. Liability

97. What component of negligence indicates injury caused to another?
    a. Duty
    b. Cause
    c. Breach
    d. Damage
    e. Malfeasance

98. What written document specifies standard of care during an emergency?
    a. Emergency operational plan
    b. Emergency health plan
    c. Emergency action plan
    d. Emergency management plan
    e. Emergency risk management plan

99. What signed release from a patient waives all future legal claims against a health care worker or institution?
    a. Permanent waiver
    b. Exculpatory clause

c. Contributory clause
d. Comparative waiver
e. Informed consent

100. What statement defines specific conditions through which a vendor will replace or repair a faulty product?
  a. Implied warranty
  b. Expected warranty

c. Express warranty
d. Product warranty
e. Purchase warranty

Use the DVD or visit the website at http://thePoint.lww.com/Long to take the *online examination*.

Professional Development and Responsibility

Part 1   Professional History, Governance, and Standards

Part 2   Research and Evidence-Based Practice

Section 13 Examination

OVERVIEW

Athletic trainers are often charged with educating and motivating their athletes while simultaneously using knowledge to help within the domains of their field. Understanding the profession at national, regional, and state levels ensures a continually evolving and growing professional. Assuring that professional stagnation does not occur through attendance at career-long learning is crucial to any health care professional.

CLINICAL PROFICIENCIES

There are no proficiencies assigned by the *Athletic Training Educational Competencies*, 4th edition for this section.

PART 1

Professional History, Governance, and Standards

NATIONAL ATHLETIC TRAINERS' ASSOCIATION

- National Athletic Trainers' Association—1950
- 200 People in Kansas City, Missouri
- Approximately 30,000 members
- Dallas, Texas
- 10 Districts
- >30 Committees
- Board of directors

BOARD OF CERTIFICATION

- Established in 1989 as National Athletic Trainers' Association Board of Certification (NATABOC)
- Based in Omaha, NE
- Provides entry-level certification program
- Continuing education requirements
- Only accredited certification program for athletic trainers in the United States
- Castle Worldwide, Inc—administers/grades examination
- Online registration for test and report continuing education units (CEUs)
- Role Delineation Study 5th edition

NATIONAL ATHLETIC TRAINING RESEARCH AND EDUCATION FOUNDATION

- Scholarship program
- Grant and awards program
- Education program

NATIONAL ATHLETIC TRAINERS' ASSOCIATION EDUCATION COUNCIL

- Formed in 1996
- Involved in policy, development, and delivery of athletic training education
- Works with the Board of Certification (BOC), the Commission on Accreditation of Athletic Training Education (CAATE), and the National Athletic Training Research and Education Foundation (NATAREF)
- Author of the National Athletic Trainers' Association (NATA) Educational Competencies, 4th edition.

DOMAINS OF ATHLETIC TRAINING

- I: Prevention
- II: Clinical evaluation and diagnosis
- III: Immediate care
- IV: Treatment, rehabilitation, and reconditioning
- V: Organization and administration
- VI: Professional responsibility

BOARD OF CERTIFICATION CONTINUING EDUCATION UNITS

- Category A: Approved Provider Program (75 allowable CEUs)
- Category B: Professional Development (50 allowable CEUs)
- Category C: College/University Course (75 allowable CEUs)
- Category D: Individualized Option (20 allowable CEUs)
- 1 Contact hour equals one CEU
- 75 CEUs plus Emergency Cardiac Care every 3 years

PROFESSIONAL STANDARDS

Credentialing

- Licensure—highest level of state regulation
- Certification—national and/or state form of regulation
- Registration—submitting biographical information for state practice
- Exemption—professional not required to have state regulation

Standard of Care

- Required level of medical sophistication and competency
- Compared to professionals with same experience, background, and training
- Standard of care may differ from state to state

Scope of Practice

- Limited scope of practice
- Subordinate to physicians
- Delineates freedom to apply their knowledge, but within specific components

Role Differentiation of Health Care Professionals

- Roles that different health care professionals play in the market
- Each health care profession has specific delineated roles in patient care
- Athletic trainer's role, duties, and scope of practice differ from other health care professionals

Health Care as it Relates to the Community

- Community impact of services
- Health care delivery through prevention, education, intervention, consultation, and treatment

PART 2

Research and Evidence-Based Practice

KEY TERMS

- Cohort
- Continuing education units
- Histogram
- Impedance
- Independent variable
- Institutional Review Board (IRB)
- Interobserver error
- Likert scale
- Locus of control
- Mean
- Median
- MEDLINE
- MEDLINEplus
- Mode
- Null hypothesis
- Procedure
- Professional code
- Qualitative analysis
- Quantitative analysis
- Random sampling
- Randomization
- Sample
- Sampling
- Sampling bias
- Standard deviation
- Standard error of difference
- Variance

BLINDED STUDY

- Being unaware or masked to the research parameters

CASE STUDY

- Detailed analysis of a specific injury or illness

CLINICAL TRIALS

- Involvement in testing a new treatment procedure before commonly approved or accepted protocol

COHORT

- People with commonalities engaged in an activity for a period of time

DEPENDENT VARIABLES

- Observed variable for judgment on treatment effect

DOUBLE-BLIND STUDY

- Both participant and clinician unaware of research parameters

HYPOTHESIS

- Proposed correlation between phenomena
- Unproven concept

IMPLEMENTATION

- Conducting scientific research methods

INDEPENDENT VARIABLE

- Manipulated variable (treatment)
- Look for independent variable to cause changes

LITERATURE REVIEW

- Written summary of totality of published research on a topic
- Included in a research report, case study, or thesis
- Directly related to the topic or research question
- Summarize what is known and not known on a topic
- Identify controversy within the literature
- Determine unanswered questions

MEAN

- Average
- Data sum divided by sample size

MEDIAN

- Middle value in a sample

MODE

- Most popular point of distribution
- Peak on curve

NULL HYPOTHESIS

- Refutable hypothesis
- Alternative hypothesis

OUTCOME MEASUREMENT

- Data that is used to identify, measure, and evaluate the research results

QUALITATIVE RESEARCH

- Formulative or explorative studies

QUANTITATIVE RESEARCH

- Collection and analysis of numerical data

PROBABILITY

- Probability that the outcome could have occurred by chance
- $p < 0.05$ = <5% occurred by chance; 95% a result of studied variables

RELIABILITY

- Consistency of results

RESEARCH DESIGN

- Scientific research method to control or observe an independent variable

SIGNIFICANCE

- Difference in mean
- Determine what is attributed to chance

- $p < 0.05$—null hypothesis rejected
- $p > 0.05$—null hypothesis not rejected

STANDARD DEVIATION

- Spread of distribution around mean

STATISTICAL INTERPRETATION

- Graphical or narrative assessment of research statistics

VALIDITY

- Statistical instrument's ability to truly measure
- True assessment of the variable

VARIABLES

- Changeable measurements

EVIDENCE-BASED PRACTICE

- Clinical decision making with treatment efficacy at the forefront
- Scientific evidence required for good clinical problem solving
- Improvement of quality and effectiveness of health care

Steps to Evidence-Based Practice

- Form a clinical question
- Collect relevant evidence
- Assess quantitative evidence
- Coordinate clinical practice experience with scientific evidence
- Evaluate clinical application efficacy

1. An audiologist would be most qualified to treat which of the following types of medical conditions?
   a. Partial hearing loss
   b. Stuttering disorder
   c. Stroke
   d. Malnutrition
   e. Viral infection

2. What is the maximum number of continuing education units that can be submitted into Category B: Professional development?
   a. 15
   b. 25
   c. 30
   d. 50
   e. 75

3. What type of research involves the collection and analysis of numerical data?
   a. Quantitative
   b. Qualitative
   c. Applied
   d. Basic
   e. Experimental

4. Which of the following play the primary role in the development of the Athletic Training Educational Competencies?
   a. BOC
   b. NATAEC
   c. NOCA
   d. JRC-AT
   e. CAATE

5. What entity would need to grant permission to a person who is planning to conduct research on human subjects?
   a. Ethics and morals committee
   b. Institutional review board
   c. Committee on human rights
   d. Human research board
   e. Committee on research subjects

6. Which of the following health care professionals dispense drugs, and are the most qualified to educate patients about their potential side effects?
   a. A pharmacist
   b. A registered nurse
   c. A pharmacologist

d. A substance abuse counselor
e. A health educator

7. What document was created for the purpose of maintaining a high standard of professionalism for athletic trainers?
   a. Athletic Training Educational Competencies
   b. Role Delineation Study
   c. JRC-AT Standards and Guidelines
   d. Standards of Practice
   e. NATA Code of Ethics

8. How many continuing education units must an ATC complete in a 3-year period to maintain his or her certification?
   a. 25
   b. 50
   c. 75
   d. 80
   e. 100

9. The process of nonrandom selection of research subjects is best described by which of the following?
   a. Stratified random sampling
   b. Probability sampling
   c. Systemic sampling
   d. Nonprobability sampling
   e. Cluster sampling

10. What type of ATC employment setting would typically involve the least amount of travel responsibilities with an athletic team?
    a. Olympic games
    b. Physician extender
    c. High school
    d. College/University
    e. Professional team

11. When was the NATA established?
    a. 1945
    b. 1950
    c. 1967
    d. 1973
    e. 1983

12. Which health care professional would have the most appropriate training to assist physicians and/or

perform many of the duties that a physician does?
a. Physical therapist
b. Nurse practitioner
c. Registered nurse
d. Medical technologist
e. Prosthetist

13. Which is *not* a role of the certified athletic trainer?
a. Monitoring for hazardous environmental conditions
b. Evaluating athletic illnesses
c. Dispensing prescription medications to athletes
d. Implementing rehabilitation programs for injured athletes
e. Providing emergency care for injured or ill athletes

14. Which of the following is responsible for the development of the Role Delineation Study?
a. NOCA
b. NCCA
c. JRC-AT
d. BOC
e. CAATE

15. What would *not* fall under the ATC's role of prevention of athletic injuries?
a. Referring athletes to appropriate medical specialists
b. Being able to properly fit a football helmet
c. Monitoring environmental heat and humidity levels
d. Being knowledgeable in the effects of common over-the-counter medications
e. Being knowledgeable in appropriate precompetition meal content

16. Which of the following is *true* regarding the BOC examination?
a. It is delivered at testing centers using a computer format
b. It is divided into three different sections
c. The practical section of the examination takes the longest to complete
d. You have a total of 4 hours to complete the written examination
e. The national first-time pass rate is approximately 50%

17. What is the term used to describe when an athletic trainer performs their duties as another athletic trainer would in a similar situation?
a. Privilege
b. Assumption of risk
c. Scope of care
d. Standard of reasonable care
e. Scope of practice

18. Which organization is responsible for setting standards and guidelines for athletic training educational programs?

a. BOC
b. NCCA
c. NATAEC
d. NOCA
e. NCAA

19. Which health care professional would have the most training to treat and perform rehabilitation for a patient who has lost partial function of one of the hands due to a stroke, and wants to improve activities of daily living?
a. Physical therapist
b. Athletic trainer
c. Registered nurse
d. Physical therapy assistant
e. Occupational therapist

20. In regard to statistics, which of the terms is synonymous with the term average standard deviation?
a. Percentile
b. Frequency
c. Deviation
d. Median
e. Mean

21. The BOC is a member of what organization?
a. NATA
b. CAAHEP
c. NOCA
d. JRC-AT
e. CAATE

22. Which of the following health professionals is most qualified to measure, fit, and/or fabricate artificial limbs for persons with an amputated extremity?
a. Physical therapist
b. Medical technologist
c. Occupational therapist
d. Prosthetist
e. Physician assistant

23. What is the primary purpose of state athletic training practice acts?
a. To protect the public from harm
b. To assure minimal competency
c. To meet Board of Certification standards
d. To meet NATA standards of practice
e. To fulfill federal government requirements

24. Which of the following serves as the "blueprint" for the BOC certification examination?
a. Role Delineation Study
b. Standards of Practice
c. Athletic Training Clinical Proficiencies
d. Athletic Training Educational Competencies
e. NATA Code of Ethics

25. Which health care professional would be most qualified to work in a cardiac rehabilitation center?
    a. Exercise physiologist
    b. Respiratory therapist
    c. Physical therapist
    d. Fitness instructor
    e. Athletic trainer

26. What organization is responsible for accrediting entry-level athletic training education programs?
    a. NATA
    b. CAAHEP
    c. NOCA
    d. NCCA
    e. CAATE

27. What computer software program is designed to perform statistical tests?
    a. RSP
    b. OIS
    c. SOS
    d. SPSS
    e. SIM

28. Which health professional is skilled in performing musculoskeletal adjustments?
    a. Physician assistant
    b. Massage therapist
    c. Chiropractor
    d. Occupational therapist
    e. Prosthetist

29. The skill to assess heat and humidity with a sling psychrometer would fall under which performance domain of athletic training?
    a. Treatment, rehabilitation, and reconditioning
    b. Clinical evaluation and diagnosis
    c. Professional responsibility
    d. Immediate care
    e. Prevention

30. How would you describe a double-blind study when performing research?
    a. Both the independent and dependant variables are unknown to the subject
    b. Both the independent and dependant variables are known to the subject
    c. Both the subject and researcher are unaware of the research parameters
    d. Both the subject and researcher are unaware of the inherent risks of a study
    e. Both the hypothesis and null hypothesis are examined in the study

31. Which of the following is *not* a requirement for being a candidate for the BOC certification exam?
    a. Complete 800 athletic training experience hours
    b. Program Director endorsement from a CAATE Accredited Program
    c. Provide proof of current Emergency Cardiac Care certification
    d. Have completed, or will complete in their final semester, all academic and clinical program requirements
    e. All of the above

32. Which of the following are members of the NATA Board of Directors?
    a. Public Relations Committee Chairpersons
    b. State Association Presidents
    c. District Directors
    d. Membership Director
    e. Executive Director

33. What is one of the objectives of the NATAPAC?
    a. Ensure that the Code of Ethics is enforced
    b. Provide direction for the public relations program
    c. Engage in governmental affair initiatives to advance the profession
    d. Assist in the development of the Standards of Practice
    e. Fund research in the field of athletic training

34. The NATA is composed of how many districts?
    a. 5
    b. 7
    c. 8
    d. 10
    e. 12

35. A null hypothesis is accepted if p is greater than which of the following?
    a. 0.005
    b. 0.05
    c. 1.005
    d. 1.05
    e. 5.01

36. What is the term for when a measuring instrument provides the same measurement during multiple uses by the same examiner?
    a. Dependability
    b. Consistency
    c. Validity
    d. Reliability
    e. Standard

37. After attending an athletic training symposium for continuing education credits an ATC receives documentation for 20 CEUs. They actually only attended 10 contact hours worth of educational seminars, but are planning to submit 20 CEUs to the BOC. If they submit those 20 CEUs, under what would they be in violation of?
    a. Role Delineation Study
    b. Standards of Practice
    c. NATA Code of Ethics

d. Standards of Accreditation

e. Athletic Training Educational Competencies

38. What is the highest level of state regulation that an ATC can attain?

a. Certification

b. Licensure

c. Authorization

d. Accreditation

e. Registration

39. What organization is responsible for administering the national certification exam for athletic training?

a. NATAEC

b. NOCA

c. CAATE

d. NATA

e. BOC

40. What type of physician specializes in the diagnosis and treatment of kidney diseases?

a. Nephrologist

b. Orthopedist

c. Neurologist

d. Oncologist

e. Internist

 Use the DVD or visit the website at http://thePoint.lww.com/Long to take the *online examination*.

14

Flash Boxes

Flash Box 1   The Hip

Flash Box 2   The Knee

Flash Box 3   The Ankle

Flash Box 4   The Shoulder

Flash Box 5   The Elbow

Flash Box 6   The Wrist

1
FLASH BOX

The Hip

Hip Facts
- Capsular Pattern: F→ABD→IR (may vary)
- Close Packed Position: E/IR/ABD
- Loose Packed Position: 30 degrees F; ABD; slight ER
- Joint Type: Multiaxial ball-and-socket (enarthrodial)
- Dermatomes: L1 Anterior hip; L2 anteromedial Thigh
- Myotomes: L1-L2 Flexion
- DTR: None
- Arteries: Internal/external iliac
- Nerves: Superior/inferior gluteal
- Bones: Femur (convex); ilium (concave)

Hip PNF
- D1 E: E/ABD/IR
- D1 F: F/ADD/ER
- D2 E: E/ADD/ER
- D2 F: F/ABD/IR

Hip Ligaments
- Inguinal
- Ligamentum teres
- Ischiofemoral
- Iliofemoral
- Pubofemoral

Hip Flexion
- Rectus femoris
- Psoas major
- Psoas minor
- Iliacus
- Gluteus medius
- Gluteus minimus
- Gracilis
- Sartorius
- Plane of motion: Sagittal
- Axis of rotation: Frontal
- Normal ROM: 100 to 120 degrees
- Normal End Feel: Soft

Hip Tests
- 90-90 Straight leg raise
- Craig
- Ely
- Noble compression
- Ober
- Patrick (FABER)
- Piriformis
- Scouring (quadrant)
- Thomas
- Trendelenburg
- True/apparent leg length

Hip Adduction
- Gluteus maximus
- Adductor magnus
- Gracilis
- Biceps femoris
- Plane of Motion: Frontal
- Axis of Rotation: Sagittal
- Normal ROM: 20 to 30 degrees
- Normal End Feel: Firm

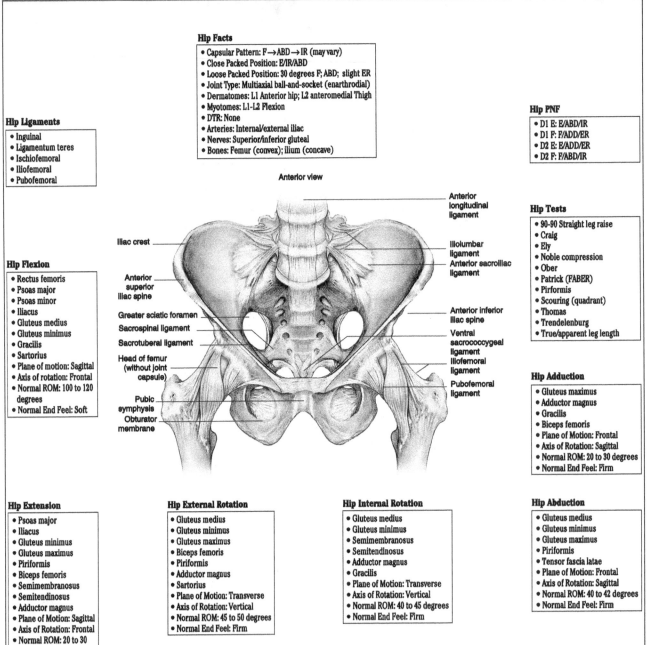

Anterior view

Anterior longitudinal ligament

Iliac crest

Iliolumbar ligament

Anterior sacroiliac ligament

Anterior superior iliac spine

Greater sciatic foramen

Sacrospinal ligament

Sacrotuberal ligament

Head of femur (without joint capsule)

Anterior inferior iliac spine

Ventral sacrococcygeal ligament

Iliofemoral ligament

Pubofemoral ligament

Pubic symphysis

Obturator membrane

Hip Extension
- Psoas major
- Iliacus
- Gluteus minimus
- Gluteus maximus
- Piriformis
- Biceps femoris
- Semimembranosus
- Semitendinosus
- Adductor magnus
- Plane of Motion: Sagittal
- Axis of Rotation: Frontal
- Normal ROM: 20 to 30 degrees
- Normal End Feel: Firm

Hip External Rotation
- Gluteus medius
- Gluteus minimus
- Gluteus maximus
- Biceps femoris
- Piriformis
- Adductor magnus
- Sartorius
- Plane of Motion: Transverse
- Axis of Rotation: Vertical
- Normal ROM: 45 to 50 degrees
- Normal End Feel: Firm

Hip Internal Rotation
- Gluteus medius
- Gluteus minimus
- Semimembranosus
- Semitendinosus
- Adductor magnus
- Gracilis
- Plane of Motion: Transverse
- Axis of Rotation: Vertical
- Normal ROM: 40 to 45 degrees
- Normal End Feel: Firm

Hip Abduction
- Gluteus medius
- Gluteus minimus
- Gluteus maximus
- Piriformis
- Tensor fascia latae
- Plane of Motion: Frontal
- Axis of Rotation: Sagittal
- Normal ROM: 40 to 42 degrees
- Normal End Feel: Firm

② FLASH BOX **The Knee**

Knee Facts (Tibiofemoral)

- Capsular pattern: F→E
- Close packed position: E→Tibial ER
- Loose packed position: 25 degrees F
- Joint type: Hinge (ginglymus)
- Dermatomes: L3 Medial knee
- Myotomes: L3 Knee E; S2 knee F
- DTR: L3-L4 Patellar tendon; L5 medial hamstring; S2 lateral hamstring
- Arteries: Femoral/popliteal
- Nerves: Femoral; saphenous; tibial; sural; common peroneal
- Bones: Femur (convex); tibia (concave); patella (both)

Knee PNF

- D1 E: E (Tibia ER)
- D1 F: F (Tibia IR)
- D2 E: E (Tibia IR)
- D2 F: F (Tibia ER)

Knee Ligaments

- Anterior cruciate
- Posterior cruciate
- Medial collateral
- Lateral collateral
- Transverse
- Coronary
- Patellomeniscal
- Wrisberg
- Humphrey
- Oblique
- Arcuate popliteal
- Posterior meniscofemoral
- Fibular head (posterior)

Knee Tests

- Apley compression
- Apley distraction
- Reverse pivot shift(Jakob)
- Varus
- Valgus
- Posterior Lachman
- Posterior sag (gravity drawer)
- Godfrey 90-90
- Posterior drawer
- Lateral pivot shift
- Slocum (ALRI)
- Slocum (AMRI)
- Jerk (Hughston)
- Anterior drawer
- Anterior Lachman
- McMurray
- Hughston plica
- Noble compression
- Renne
- Q-Angle
- Ballotable patella (tap)
- Bounce home
- Patella apprehension
- Patella grind
- Hughston posteromedial drawer
- Hughston posterolateral drawer

Knee Flexion

- Biceps femoris
- Semimembranosus
- Semitendinosus
- Gracilis
- Gastrocnemius
- Plane of Motion: Sagittal
- Axis of Rotation: Frontal
- Normal ROM: 135 to 150 degrees
- Normal End Feel: Soft

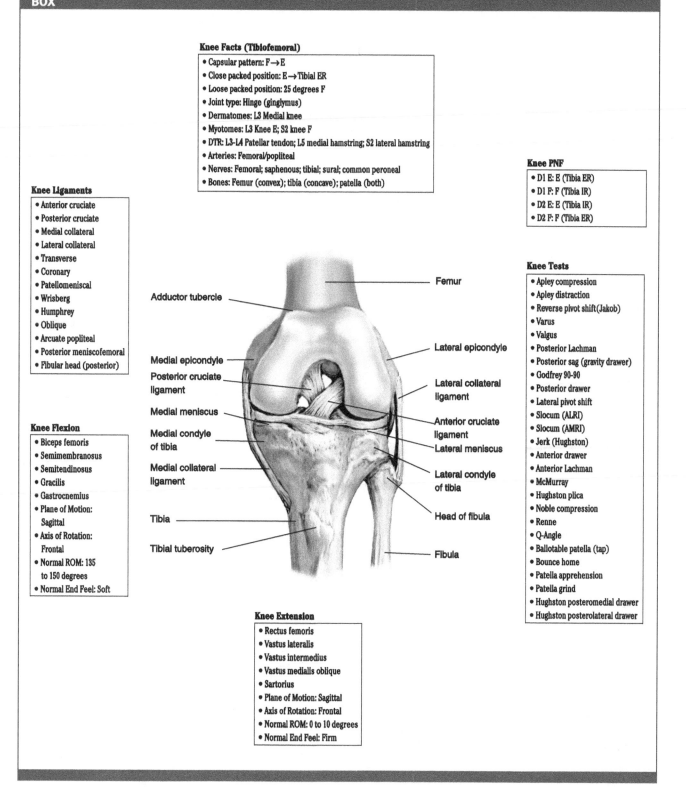

Adductor tubercle

Medial epicondyle

Posterior cruciate ligament

Medial meniscus

Medial condyle of tibia

Medial collateral ligament

Tibia

Tibial tuberosity

Femur

Lateral epicondyle

Lateral collateral ligament

Anterior cruciate ligament

Lateral meniscus

Lateral condyle of tibia

Head of fibula

Fibula

Knee Extension

- Rectus femoris
- Vastus lateralis
- Vastus intermedius
- Vastus medialis oblique
- Sartorius
- Plane of Motion: Sagittal
- Axis of Rotation: Frontal
- Normal ROM: 0 to 10 degrees
- Normal End Feel: Firm

3
FLASH BOX **Ankle (Talocrural)**

Ankle Facts

- Capsular Pattern: PF→DF
- Close Packed Position: DF
- Loose Packed Position: 10 degrees PF/mid INV/EV
- Joint Type: Hinge (ginglymus)
- Dermatomes: L4 Dorsum great toe; L5 dorsum 2-5 toes; S1 lateral 5th metatarsal; S2 heel
- Myotomes: L4 Ankle DF; L5 great toe E; S1 ankle PF
- DTR: S1 Achilles tendon
- Arteries: Anterior/posterior tibialis; dorsalis pedis
- Nerves: Deep peroneal; tibial; sural; common peroneal
- Bones: Talus (convex); tibia/fibula (concave)

Ankle Ligaments

- Anterior tibiofibular
- Posterior tibiofibular
- Crural interosseus
- Anterior talofibular
- Calcaneofibular
- Posterior talofibular
- Deltoid

Ankle PNF

- D1 E: PF (Tibia ER)
- D1 F: DF (Tibia IR)
- D2 E: PF (Tibia IR)
- D2 F: DF (Tibia ER)

Ankle Plantarflexion (Flexion)

- Gastrocnemius
- Soleus
- Tibialis posterior
- Peroneus longus
- Peroneus brevis
- Flexor digitorum longus
- Flexor hallucis longus
- Plane of Motion: Sagittal
- Axis of Rotation: Frontal
- Normal ROM: 20 degrees
- Normal End Feel: Firm

Ankle Tests

- Anterior drawer
- Talar tilt (inversion stress)
- Talar tilt (eversion stress)
- Kleiger (ER)
- Homan sign
- Thompson
- Percussion (bump)
- Squeeze (compression)
- Long bone compression

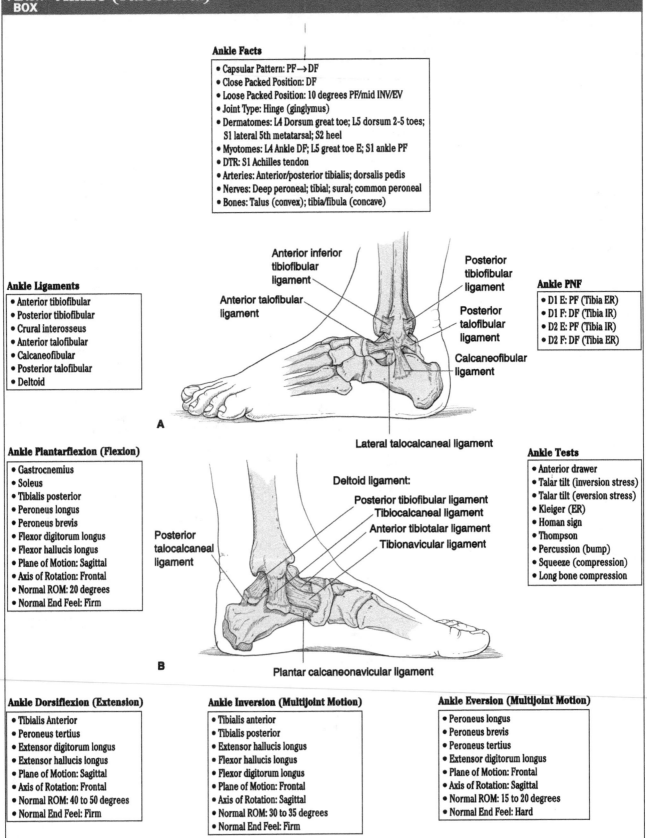

Anterior inferior tibiofibular ligament
Anterior talofibular ligament
Posterior tibiofibular ligament
Posterior talofibular ligament
Calcaneofibular ligament

A

Lateral talocalcaneal ligament

Deltoid ligament:
Posterior tibiofibular ligament
Tibiocalcaneal ligament
Anterior tibiotalar ligament
Tibionavicular ligament
Posterior talocalcaneal ligament

B

Plantar calcaneonavicular ligament

Ankle Dorsiflexion (Extension)

- Tibialis Anterior
- Peroneus tertius
- Extensor digitorum longus
- Extensor hallucis longus
- Plane of Motion: Sagittal
- Axis of Rotation: Frontal
- Normal ROM: 40 to 50 degrees
- Normal End Feel: Firm

Ankle Inversion (Multijoint Motion)

- Tibialis anterior
- Tibialis posterior
- Extensor hallucis longus
- Flexor hallucis longus
- Flexor digitorum longus
- Plane of Motion: Frontal
- Axis of Rotation: Sagittal
- Normal ROM: 30 to 35 degrees
- Normal End Feel: Firm

Ankle Eversion (Multijoint Motion)

- Peroneus longus
- Peroneus brevis
- Peroneus tertius
- Extensor digitorum longus
- Plane of Motion: Frontal
- Axis of Rotation: Sagittal
- Normal ROM: 15 to 20 degrees
- Normal End Feel: Hard

4
FLASH
BOX **Shoulder (Glenohumeral)**

Shoulder Facts

- Capsular Pattern: ER → ABD → IR
- Close Packed Position: ABD and ER
- Loose Packed Position: 55 degrees ABD and 30 degrees horizontal ADD
- Joint Type: Multiaxial ball-and-socket (enarthrodial)
- Dermatomes: C4 Clavicle; C5 lateral deltoid
- Myotomes: C4 Shoulder elevation; C5 shoulder abduction
- DTR: None
- Arteries: Subclavian; axillary; brachial; deep brachial
- Nerves: Brachial plexus; musculocutaneous; axillary
- Bones: Humerus (convex); scapular glenoid (concave)

Shoulder PNF

- D1 E: E/IR/ABD
- D1 F: F/ER/ADD
- D2 E: E/IR/ADD
- D2 F: F/ER/ABD

Shoulder Ligaments

- Transverse humeral (outside joint)
- Superior glenohumeral
- Middle glenohumeral
- Inferior glenohumeral
- Coracohumeral
- Coracoacromial
- Acromioclavicular
- Coracoclavicular (conoid/trapezoid)
- Anterior sternoclavicular
- Posterior sternoclavicular
- Interclavicular
- Costoclavicular

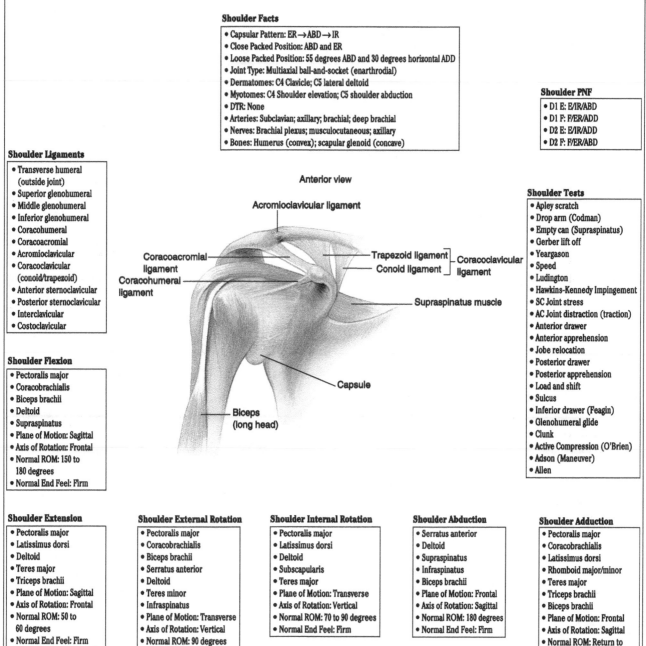

Anterior view

Acromioclavicular ligament

Coracoacromial ligament

Coracohumeral ligament

Trapezoid ligament

Conoid ligament

Coracoclavicular ligament

Supraspinatus muscle

Capsule

Biceps (long head)

Shoulder Tests

- Apley scratch
- Drop arm (Codman)
- Empty can (Supraspinatus)
- Gerber lift off
- Yeargason
- Speed
- Ludington
- Hawkins-Kennedy Impingement
- SC Joint stress
- AC Joint distraction (traction)
- Anterior drawer
- Anterior apprehension
- Jobe relocation
- Posterior drawer
- Posterior apprehension
- Load and shift
- Sulcus
- Inferior drawer (Feagin)
- Glenohumeral glide
- Clunk
- Active Compression (O'Brien)
- Adson (Maneuver)
- Allen

Shoulder Flexion

- Pectoralis major
- Coracobrachialis
- Biceps brachii
- Deltoid
- Supraspinatus
- Plane of Motion: Sagittal
- Axis of Rotation: Frontal
- Normal ROM: 150 to 180 degrees
- Normal End Feel: Firm

Shoulder Extension

- Pectoralis major
- Latissimus dorsi
- Deltoid
- Teres major
- Triceps brachii
- Plane of Motion: Sagittal
- Axis of Rotation: Frontal
- Normal ROM: 50 to 60 degrees
- Normal End Feel: Firm

Shoulder External Rotation

- Pectoralis major
- Coracobrachialis
- Biceps brachii
- Serratus anterior
- Deltoid
- Teres minor
- Infraspinatus
- Plane of Motion: Transverse
- Axis of Rotation: Vertical
- Normal ROM: 90 degrees
- Normal End Feel: Firm

Shoulder Internal Rotation

- Pectoralis major
- Latissimus dorsi
- Deltoid
- Subscapularis
- Teres major
- Plane of Motion: Transverse
- Axis of Rotation: Vertical
- Normal ROM: 70 to 90 degrees
- Normal End Feel: Firm

Shoulder Abduction

- Serratus anterior
- Deltoid
- Supraspinatus
- Infraspinatus
- Biceps brachii
- Plane of Motion: Frontal
- Axis of Rotation: Sagittal
- Normal ROM: 180 degrees
- Normal End Feel: Firm

Shoulder Adduction

- Pectoralis major
- Coracobrachialis
- Latissimus dorsi
- Rhomboid major/minor
- Teres major
- Triceps brachii
- Biceps brachii
- Plane of Motion: Frontal
- Axis of Rotation: Sagittal
- Normal ROM: Return to 0 degrees
- Normal End Feel: Firm

FLASH BOX 5 — Elbow (Humeroulnar)

Elbow Facts
- Capsular Pattern: F→E
- Close Packed Position: E/Supination
- Loose Packed Position: 70 degrees F/10 degrees supination
- Joint Type: Hinge (ginglymus)
- Dermatomes: T1 Medial epicondyle
- Myotomes: C6 Elbow F and wrist E; C7 elbow E and wrist F
- DTR: C5 Biceps brachii; C6 Brachioradialis; C7 triceps brachii
- Arteries: Brachial; ulnar; radial
- Nerves: Median; musculocutaneous
- Bones: Humerus (convex); ulna (concave)

Elbow PNF
- D1 E: Ulnar deviation
- D1 F: Radial deviation
- D2 E: Radial deviation
- D2 F: Ulnar deviation

Elbow Ligaments
- Ulnar collateral ligament complex
  - Anterior oblique
  - Posterior oblique
  - Transverse oblique
- Lateral ulnar collateral
- Radial collateral
- Annular
- Accessory lateral collateral

Elbow Tests
- Resistive tennis elbow (Cozen)
- Valgus
- Varus
- Pinch grip
- Golfer's elbow
- Hyperextension
- Elbow flexion
- Tinel sign

Elbow Flexion
- Biceps brachii
- Brachialis
- Brachioradialis
- Pronator teres
- Flexor carpi radialis
- Palmaris longus
- Flexor carpi ulnaris
- Flexor digitorum superficialis
- Plane of Motion: Sagittal
- Axis of Rotation: Frontal
- Normal ROM: Return to 140 to 150 degrees
- Normal End Feel: Soft

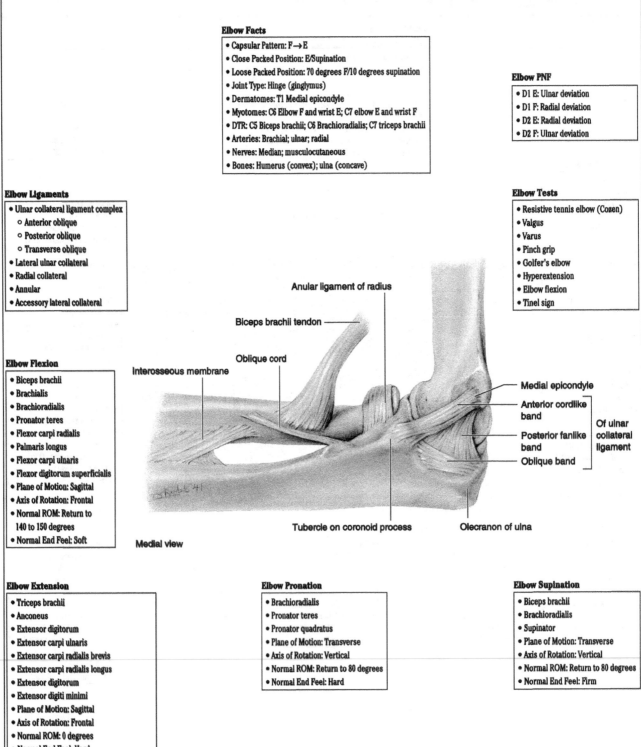

Anular ligament of radius

Biceps brachii tendon

Oblique cord

Interosseous membrane

Medial epicondyle

Anterior cordlike band

Posterior fanlike band — Of ulnar collateral ligament

Oblique band

Tubercle on coronoid process

Olecranon of ulna

Medial view

Elbow Extension
- Triceps brachii
- Anconeus
- Extensor digitorum
- Extensor carpi ulnaris
- Extensor carpi radialis brevis
- Extensor carpi radialis longus
- Extensor digitorum
- Extensor digiti minimi
- Plane of Motion: Sagittal
- Axis of Rotation: Frontal
- Normal ROM: 0 degrees
- Normal End Feel: Hard

Elbow Pronation
- Brachioradialis
- Pronator teres
- Pronator quadratus
- Plane of Motion: Transverse
- Axis of Rotation: Vertical
- Normal ROM: Return to 80 degrees
- Normal End Feel: Hard

Elbow Supination
- Biceps brachii
- Brachioradialis
- Supinator
- Plane of Motion: Transverse
- Axis of Rotation: Vertical
- Normal ROM: Return to 80 degrees
- Normal End Feel: Firm

6
FLASH BOX

Wrist (Radiocarpal)

Wrist Facts

- Capsular Pattern: F→E (equal)
- Close Packed Position: E/Radial deviation
- Loose Packed Position: Neutral/slight ulnar deviation
- Joint Type: Biaxial ball-and-socket (condyloidal)
- Dermatomes: C6 dorsal thumb; C7 dorsal third finger; C8 palmer fifth finger
- Myotomes: C6 Elbow F and wrist E; C7 elbow E and wrist F; C8 ulnar deviation and thumb E; T1 finger ADD/ABD
- DTR: C6 Brachioradialis
- Arteries: Ulnar; radial
- Nerves: Median; radial; ulnar
- Bones: Radius (concave); carpals (convex)

Wrist Ligaments

- Ulnar collateral
- Radial collateral

Wrist Tests

- Valgus
- Varus
- Phalen (wrist flexion)
- Finkelstein
- Tinel sign
- Digital Allen

Proximal palmar intercarpal ligaments

Palmar radiate carpal ligament

Pisohamate ligament

Distal palmar intercarpal ligaments

Pisometacarpal ligament

Capsule for meta-carpophalangeal joint of thumb

Palmar ligaments grooved for flexor tendons

Metacarpophalangeal joints

Deep transverse metacarpal ligaments

Collateral ligaments of metacarpo-phalangeal joints

Palmar ligaments of interphalangeal joints

Collateral ligaments of interphalangeal joints

Wrist Flexion

- Palmaris longus
- Flexor carpi ulnaris
- Flexor carpi radialis
- Flexor carpi superficialis
- Flexor digitorum profundus
- Flexor pollicis longus
- Plane of Motion: Sagittal
- Axis of Rotation: Frontal
- Normal ROM: Return to 60 to 80 degrees
- Normal End Feel: Firm

Wrist Ulnar Deviation

- Flexor carpi ulnaris
- Extensor carpi ulnaris
- Plane of Motion: Transverse
- Axis of Rotation: Vertical
- Normal ROM: Return to 30 degrees
- Normal End Feel: Firm

Wrist Extension

- Extensor digitorum
- Extensor carpi ulnaris
- Extensor carpi radialis brevis
- Extensor carpi radialis longus
- Extensor pollicis brevis
- Plane of Motion: Sagittal
- Axis of Rotation: Frontal
- Normal ROM: Return to 60 to 70 degrees
- Normal End Feel: Firm

Wrist Pronation

- Plamaris longus
- Pronator teres
- Flexor carpi radialis
- Plane of Motion: Transverse
- Axis of Rotation: Vertical
- Normal ROM: Return to 80 degrees
- Normal End Feel: Hard

Wrist Supination

- Supinator
- Brachioradialis
- Extensor pollicis longus
- Abductor pollicis longus
- Plane of Motion: Transverse
- Axis of Rotation: Vertical
- Normal ROM: Return to 80 degrees
- Normal End Feel: Firm

Wrist Radial Deviation

- Abductor pollicis longus
- Extensor pollicis brevis
- Flexor carpi radialis
- Flexor pollicis longus
- Extensor pollicis longus
- Extensor carpi radialis longus
- Plane of Motion: Transverse
- Axis of Rotation: Vertical
- Normal ROM: Return to 20 degrees
- Normal End Feel: Hard

Appendix:
Examination Answers

SECTION 1

1. C
2. C
3. B
4. C
5. A
6. E
7. E
8. E
9. E
10. D
11. C
12. B
13. C
14. B
15. A
16. C
17. E
18. B
19. C
20. D
21. E
22. B
23. C
24. D
25. B
26. E
27. A
28. E
29. C
30. C
31. D
32. E
33. E
34. D
35. C
36. E
37. E
38. C
39. E
40. B
41. A
42. C
43. D
44. B
45. B

46. B
47. A
48. E
49. B
50. E
51. A
52. D
53. C
54. C
55. C
56. B
57. D
58. E
59. C
60. C
61. E
62. D
63. C
64. C
65. A
66. E
67. C
68. C
69. E
70. D
71. B
72. B
73. A
74. E
75. A
76. A
77. D
78. A
79. C
80. B
81. A
82. C
83. E
84. D
85. C
86. B
87. E
88. A
89. D
90. A
91. E
92. E

93. B
94. B
95. E
96. D
97. E
98. C
99. C
100. A

SECTION 2

1. B
2. E
3. C
4. B
5. C
6. C
7. B
8. C
9. E
10. C
11. C
12. C
13. B
14. A
15. E
16. B
17. A
18. A
19. B
20. C
21. A
22. D
23. C
24. C
25. B
26. A
27. A
28. D
29. B
30. E
31. D
32. B
33. B
34. E
35. E

36. A
37. A
38. C
39. D
40. C
41. E
42. C
43. C
44. D
45. E
46. E
47. B
48. C
49. C
50. B
51. A
52. C
53. D
54. B
55. B
56. E
57. B
58. D
59. C
60. C
61. E
62. B
63. A
64. D
65. A
66. C
67. D
68. A
69. B
70. A
71. D
72. C
73. E
74. C
75. A
76. B
77. C
78. B
79. D
80. A
81. C
82. D
83. B
84. A
85. B
86. C
87. C
88. B
89. D
90. E
91. D
92. E
93. B
94. B
95. D
96. A
97. E

98. C
99. C
100. E

SECTION 3

1. C
2. C
3. C
4. D
5. E
6. B
7. E
8. B
9. C
10. B
11. B
12. C
13. A
14. A
15. E
16. B
17. B
18. B
19. A
20. C
21. D
22. E
23. B
24. G
25. C
26. D
27. C
28. C
29. C
30. A
31. B
32. D
33. D
34. B
35. A
36. C
37. B
38. C
39. E
40. C
41. B
42. C
43. D
44. C
45. A
46. C
47. C
48. C
49. B
50. D
51. B
52. B
53. D
54. C
55. C

56. B
57. C
58. B
59. B
60. D
61. D
62. B
63. B
64. A
65. B
66. D
67. B
68. B
69. D
70. C
71. B
72. D
73. C
74. B
75. A
76. C
77. B
78. B
79. B
80. B
81. A
82. D
83. E
84. D
85. B
86. B
87. D
88. D
89. B
90. C
91. B
92. D
93. B
94. E
95. C
96. C
97. D
98. C
99. B
100. A

SECTION 4

1. E
2. A
3. C
4. B
5. E
6. C
7. B
8. A
9. A
10. C
11. D
12. E
13. B

14. D	76. C	34. E
15. A	77. C	35. C
16. E	78. B	36. D
17. A	79. A	37. E
18. E	80. C	38. C
19. B	81. B	39. B
20. C	82. A	40. C
21. C	83. B	41. D
22. B	84. D	42. B
23. A	85. E	43. C
24. E	86. A	44. B
25. D	87. C	45. A
26. B	88. C	46. B
27. E	89. B	47. C
28. E	90. A	48. C
29. C	91. E	49. D
30. E	92. A	50. C
31. E	93. C	51. D
32. C	94. D	52. A
33. D	95. B	53. C
34. E	96. E	54. A
35. B	97. B	55. B
36. A	98. C	56. B
37. B	99. A	57. C
38. D	100. B	58. D
39. A		59. B
40. B		60. D
41. C	**SECTION 5**	61. E
42. A		62. B
43. D	1. A	63. D
44. E	2. B	64. B
45. B	3. C	65. B
46. C	4. B	66. D
47. E	5. D	67. A
48. D	6. B	68. C
49. A	7. C	69. B
50. C	8. D	70. E
51. B	9. A	71. B
52. A	10. E	72. B
53. B	11. A	73. A
54. B	12. A	74. C
55. D	13. C	75. C
56. A	14. D	76. C
57. E	15. C	77. B
58. C	16. D	78. A
59. E	17. B	79. E
60. C	18. B	80. A
61. E	19. A	81. A
62. B	20. C	82. C
63. A	21. A	83. A
64. D	22. E	84. B
65. B	23. C	85. C
66. D	24. E	86. B
67. E	25. A	87. A
68. B	26. B	88. A
69. C	27. D	89. A
70. A	28. B	90. A
71. C	29. C	91. C
72. B	30. D	92. E
73. C	31. D	93. D
74. A	32. C	94. C
75. E	33. B	95. B

96. C
97. C
98. D
99. B
100. B

SECTION 6

1. A
2. A
3. B
4. B
5. E
6. D
7. B
8. A
9. B
10. C
11. D
12. A
13. E
14. C
15. D
16. B
17. C
18. B
19. C
20. B
21. B
22. D
23. E
24. B
25. B
26. C
27. E
28. D
29. A
30. A
31. A
32. D
33. A
34. E
35. B
36. C
37. B
38. D
39. C
40. C
41. E
42. B
43. D
44. C
45. B
46. B
47. D
48. E
49. A
50. B
51. A
52. A
53. A

54. E
55. E
56. E
57. C
58. A
59. C
60. B
61. A
62. D
63. C
64. D
65. A
66. B
67. D
68. A
69. E
70. B
71. A
72. E
73. B
74. A
75. D
76. C
77. A
78. B
79. D
80. E
81. D
82. E
83. B
84. A
85. E
86. B
87. B
88. A
89. B
90. D
91. A
92. B
93. D
94. C
95. B
96. C
97. E
98. C
99. B
100. A

SECTION 7

1. C
2. A
3. B
4. E
5. A
6. A
7. B
8. A
9. C
10. E
11. B

12. A
13. C
14. A
15. B
16. B
17. C
18. A
19. A
20. C
21. E
22. D
23. C
24. B
25. E
26. A
27. B
28. E
29. B
30. A
31. A
32. C
33. E
34. E
35. D
36. A
37. B
38. D
39. E
40. B
41. B
42. C
43. C
44. A
45. C
46. A
47. B
48. A
49. B
50. C
51. B
52. C
53. C
54. E
55. A
56. B
57. A
58. E
59. A
60. B
61. A
62. C
63. B
64. E
65. C
66. C
67. D
68. C
69. D
70. B
71. A
72. C
73. D

74. D
75. D
76. B
77. C
78. B
79. D
80. A
81. C
82. E
83. E
84. C
85. D
86. A
87. A
88. D
89. C
90. E
91. A
92. C
93. C
94. A
95. C
96. E
97. C
98. E
99. C
100. C

SECTION 8

1. B
2. B
3. C
4. E
5. A
6. B
7. A
8. E
9. C
10. B
11. B
12. C
13. B
14. D
15. B
16. B
17. C
18. A
19. B
20. B
21. B
22. B
23. A
24. E
25. C
26. B
27. A
28. C
29. C
30. C
31. C

32. C
33. A
34. C
35. A
36. B
37. B
38. A
39. D
40. C
41. B
42. A
43. C
44. E
45. A
46. C
47. C
48. C
49. C
50. C
51. A
52. C
53. C
54. C
55. C
56. E
57. A
58. B
59. A
60. B
61. D
62. D
63. B
64. A
65. C
66. C
67. B
68. C
69. C
70. E
71. B
72. A
73. B
74. E
75. C
76. D
77. C
78. D
79. C
80. D
81. C
82. B
83. C
84. B
85. B
86. C
87. B
88. C
89. E
90. A
91. B
92. B
93. A

94. B
95. D
96. A
97. D
98. A
99. C
100. E

SECTION 9

1. C
2. C
3. C
4. B
5. E
6. B
7. D
8. C
9. B
10. A
11. D
12. D
13. D
14. D
15. D
16. B
17. D
18. D
19. C
20. E
21. B
22. A
23. C
24. C
25. D
26. C
27. B
28. C
29. C
30. E
31. A
32. C
33. C
34. B
35. C
36. D
37. C
38. E
39. B
40. C
41. C
42. D
43. D
44. E
45. A
46. D
47. C
48. C
49. B
50. A
51. C

52. B
53. B
54. C
55. C
56. E
57. D
58. A
59. A
60. C
61. E
62. B
63. A
64. B
65. B
66. C
67. B
68. B
69. D
70. D
71. C
72. E
73. A
74. C
75. E
76. D
77. C
78. A
79. C
80. B
81. A
82. B
83. B
84. A
85. C
86. E
87. D
88. C
89. B
90. B
91. B
92. D
93. D
94. D
95. C
96. B
97. A
98. B
99. D
100. D

SECTION 10

1. D
2. B
3. B
4. D
5. B
6. C
7. C
8. B
9. E

10. C
11. D
12. D
13. B
14. C
15. E
16. C
17. D
18. C
19. A
20. E
21. B
22. C
23. B
24. D
25. E
26. D
27. D
28. C
29. D
30. D
31. C
32. D
33. D
34. C
35. B
36. A
37. C
38. E
39. A
40. B

SECTION 11

1. E
2. C
3. B
4. B
5. A
6. C
7. D
8. E
9. D
10. A
11. D
12. C
13. B
14. A
15. C
16. B
17. B
18. A
19. B
20. B
21. C
22. E
23. B
24. A
25. E
26. A
27. B

28. B
29. A
30. E
31. B
32. D
33. B
34. A
35. E
36. B
37. C
38. B
39. C
40. D
41. A
42. D
43. C
44. B
45. B
46. C
47. A
48. D
49. B
50. B
51. C
52. A
53. D
54. C
55. B
56. A
57. B
58. B
59. A
60. E
61. B
62. D
63. C
64. A
65. D
66. D
67. C
68. B
69. B
70. E
71. A
72. B
73. E
74. B
75. B
76. D
77. D
78. B
79. B
80. A
81. C
82. C
83. B
84. C
85. D
86. D
87. A
88. C
89. C

90. C
91. B
92. B
93. E
94. B
95. A
96. C
97. C
98. E
99. B
100. B

SECTION 12

1. C
2. D
3. A
4. C
5. C
6. B
7. D
8. B
9. A
10. B
11. A
12. E
13. B
14. B
15. C
16. B
17. B
18. D
19. C
20. A
21. B
22. A
23. D
24. B
25. C
26. D
27. C
28. A
29. B
30. B
31. C
32. A
33. B
34. A
35. D
36. C
37. B
38. A
39. B

40. B
41. A
42. C
43. B
44. C
45. B
46. C
47. A
48. B
49. A
50. B
51. C
52. B
53. C
54. B
55. A
56. A
57. B
58. D
59. B
60. C
61. B
62. D
63. B
64. C
65. A
66. C
67. C
68. B
69. B
70. B
71. C
72. A
73. E
74. C
75. B
76. B
77. B
78. B
79. D
80. B
81. B
82. C
83. D
84. B
85. A
86. C
87. B
88. D
89. C
90. A
91. B
92. A

93. E
94. C
95. A
96. C
97. D
98. C
99. B
100. C

SECTION 13

1. A
2. D
3. A
4. B
5. B
6. A
7. E
8. C
9. D
10. B
11. B
12. B
13. C
14. D
15. A
16. A
17. D
18. C
19. E
20. E
21. C
22. D
23. A
24. A
25. A
26. E
27. D
28. C
29. E
30. C
31. A
32. C
33. C
34. D
35. A
36. D
37. C
38. B
39. E
40. A

Index

Abdominal aorta, 32, 48
Abdominal oblique, 42
Abducens nerve, 23
Abductor pollicis longus, 64
Abnormal respiratory rate, 235
ABO blood type groups, 131
Abrasion, 199
Absence seizure (Petit Mal), 201
Acetabular femoral joint, 95
Acetabular labrum, 6
Acetylcholine (ACh), 15, 260
Achilles bursitis, 141
Achilles tendinitis, 141
Achilles tendon rupture, 141
Achilles tenosynovitis, 141
Acne Vulgaris, 199
Acoustical media, 260
Acquired immunodeficiency syndrome (AIDS), 201
Acromioclavicular (AC) ligament, 7
Acromioclavicular joint distraction (traction) test, 169
Acromioclavicular joint sprain (shoulder pointer), 138
Acromion, 52
  process, 46, 47
Actin, 10
Active compression (O'Brien) test, 170
Active potential (AP), 15
Active range of motion (AROM), 154
Active transport, 120
Acute appendicitis, 227
Acute injuries, caring of
  abdomen and pelvis, 220
  ambulation and moving patients, 233–234
  asthma and allergic reactions, 232
  cardiac emergencies, 229
  clavicles and chest, 220
  clinical proficiencies, 214
  cold-related injuries and illnesses, 231
  diabetic emergencies, 232
  examination paper, 235–242
  eyes and ears, 219
  head and face, 223–226
  heat-related illnesses, 230–231
  lightning strikes, 231
  lower extremities, 220
  lungs, 220
  musculoskeletal, 221–222
  neck and cervical spine, 220
  nose, mouth, and jaw, 219
  overview, 213
  poisonings, 233
  preparing for emergencies, 215–216
  primary assessment, 216–217
  respiratory emergencies, 228
  scalp, skull, and face, 219
  secondary assessment, 217–219
  seizures, 233
  shock injuries, 231–232
  skin, 221
  spine and scapula, 221, 226–227
  thorax, 227
  upper extremities, 220
Acute mountain sickness, 201
Acute trauma, to the abdomen, 144
Adam apple, 27
Adderall, 336
Adductor magnus, 80

Adductor strain, 140
Adductor tendinitis, 140
Adenosine triphosphate (ATP), 10, 120
Adhesive capsulitis, 139
Adipose kidney, 32
ADME, 304
Adrenal cortex, 33, 34
Adrenal cortex hormones, 35
Adrenal gland, 33, 34–35, 147
Adrenaline, 15
Adrenal medulla hormones, 35
Adrenocorticotropic hormone (ACTH), 34
Adson (maneuver) test, 171
Adult blood pressure, 208
AED pads, 241
Aerobic exercise, 302
Aerobic respiration, 120
Afferent arteriole, 32
Afferent neuron, 17
Afferent peripheral nerves, 260
Afferent (sensory) neurons, 15
Aging, 132
Agonist muscle, 9–10, 284
AHA recommendations, for preparticipation evaluations for athletes, 109
Air pathway, 26
Airway obstructions, 228, 240
Albumins, 129
Aldosterone, 33
Alimentary (gastrointestinal or digestive) tract, 30
Allen test, 171
Allergic contact dermatitis, 199
Alopecia, 199
Alveoli, 27, 29
Ambien, 303
Amenorrhea, 201
American With Disabilities Act, 351
Amino acids, 33, 120
Amphetamines, 305, 336
Amputations, 132
Amyotrophic lateral sclerosis (Lou Gehrig disease), 201
Anabolic steroids, 336, 342
Anal sphincter, 31
Anconeus, 167
Andersen and Williams stress response model, of athletic injury, 321
Androstenedione, 336
Anemia, 130
Angina pectoris (chest pain) or heart attack, 229
Angle of inclination, 114
  of the femur, 95
Angle of mandible, 41
Angle of torsion, 174, 186
Anisocoria, 200
Ankle
  dislocation, 141
  dorsiflexion, 174, 185, 374
  eversion, 374
  facts about, 374
  inversion, 185, 374
  ligaments, 374
  plantar flexion, 95, 175
  plantarflexion (flexion), 374
  PNF, 374
  tests, 374
Annulus fibrosis, 94
Anorexia athletica, 335

Anorexia nervosa, 201, 335
Antagonistic muscle, 9, 90, 284
Anterior apprehension test, 169
Anterior capsulitis, 140
Anterior compartment syndrome, 141
Anterior Cruciate Ligament (ACL) sprain, 141
Anterior drawer test, 177
  for the ankle, 178
  for shoulder, 169
Anterior lachman test, 177
Anterior nasal spine, 40
Anterior pituitary hormones, 34
Anterior/posterior rib compression test, 163
Anterior scalene, 39, 160
Anterior talofibular ligament, tests for, 186
Anterior talofibular sprain, 141
Anterior tubercle, 41
Antidiuretic hormone, 33
Antidrug Abuse Act, 1988, 294
Antihelix, 23
Anus, 36, 38
Aortic arch, 25
Aortic valve, 25
Ape hand, 184
  deformity, 136
Apex, 25
  of lung, 28
Apley scratch test, 168
Apocrine, 13
Apophysitis, 138
Appendicitis, 199
Appendicular skeleton, 3
Appendix, 128
Aquatic exercise, 281–283, 286, 291
Aqueous humor, 21, 22
Arachnoid, 20, 21
Arachnoid villi, 20
Arch ligament, of the shoulder, 181
Arch of aorta, 48
Areola, 47
Arndt-Schultz principle, 247
Arteries, 6, 20, 131
  of head, neck, spine and thorax, 48
  of lower extremity, 75
Arterioles, 131
Arthritis, 132, 201
Articular cartilage, 4, 85, 186
Articular discs, 6
Articular facet, 52
Articular process, 42
Ascending aorta, 25
Ascending tracts—afferent (sensory), 17
Aspirin, 304
  syndrome associated with, 209
Asthma, 201
  and allergic reactions, 232
  attack, 232
Asthmatic athlete's peak expiratory volume, 112
Astigmatism, 200
Astrocytes (macroglia), 15
Athlete foot, 136
Athlete participation, conditions, 111
Athlete's agility, assessment of, 114
Athlete's foot, 199
Athlete with crutches, fitting, 110
Athletic footwear, 104
Athletic shoes, 113
Athletic trainers, 99
Athletic wrapping and taping, 104–105

Atlantooccipital joint, 94
Atria, 24–25
Atrial depolarization, 206
Atrioventricular node, 26
Atrium, 25
Atrophy, 121
Audiologist, 367
Auditory ossicles, 23
Auricular hematoma, 200, 224
Auricular nerve, great, 49
Auscultations, 148, 149, 191
Automated external defibrillator (AED), 101
Autonomic nervous system, 18, 206
   heart control, 26
AV bundle (bundle of His), 26
Avulsion fracture, of the epiphyseal plate, 182
Axial skeleton, 3
Axilla, 47
Axillary nerve contusion, 139
Axon, 14, 15, 121
   terminal, 16

Babinski reflex, 156
Bacterial vaginosis, 201
Baker cyst, 136
Balance, control of, 284
Bankart lesion, 136, 139
Barton fracture, 140
Basal nuclei (basal ganglia), 19
Baseball finger, 136
Base of support, 89
Battle sign, 136, 236
Beam nonuniformity ratio (BNR), 264–265
Bell clapper deformity, 150
Bench press, muscles in, 285
Benediction deformity, 136, 184
Bennett fracture, 136, 140
Biarticulate muscle, 95
Bicarbonate ion, 29
Bicarbonate production, 147
Biceps brachii, 47, 62, 167
Biceps femoris, 9, 76
Biceps tendon, 180
   rupture, 139
Bicipital tendinitis, 139
Bicipital tenosynovitis, 139
Bicuspid (mitral valve), 24
Bifid spinous process, 41
Bifurcated ligament sprain, 141
Bilateral straight leg raise test, 162
Binge eating disorder, 335
Bioelectrical impedance analysis, 334
Bipennate muscle, 9
Birth control, 196–197
Bishop deformity, 137
Blackheads, 14, 211
Bladder, 36, 38
   infections, 146
Bleeding, in the abdominal cavity, 240
Blister, 199
B–blockers, 336
Blocker's exostosis, 139
Blood analysis, 195–196
Blood circulation, systemic, 25, 144, 204
Blood clotting, 131, 204, 206
Blood doping, 336
Blood flow, local, temperature, 262
Blood formation, 204
Blood oxygen saturation (SpO$_2$) levels, 29
Blood pressure, 204, 235
   factors affecting, 26
Blood type group, 205
Blood vessels, 206
Blow-out fracture, 137
Blow-out injury, 137
Board of Certification, 364, 368–370
Board of Certification Continuing Education Units, 364, 369
Body composition assessment technique, underwater, 116
Body mass index, 332
Boils, group of, 205

Bone
   anatomy, 4
   classification, 4
   principles of physical stress, 6
   tissue, 4–6
Bony palpations
   of the lower extremity, 173
   of the upper extremity, 163–164
Bouchard nodes, 137
Bounce home test, 177
Boutonniere deformity, 137, 140
Bowler's thumb, 137, 140
Boxer's fracture, 137, 140
Brachial artery, 181
Brachialis, 9, 62, 167
Brachial plexus, 17
   injury, 185
Brachial plexus stretch, 138
   traction test, 161
Brachiocephalic artery, 25
Brachioradialis, 8, 63, 167
   muscle, 93
Bradycardia, 111, 149
Brain, 145
   basal nuclei (basal ganglia), 19
   cerebral cortex, 20
   cerebrospinal fluid, 20
   corpus callosum, 20
   hypothalamus, 21
   limbic system, 20
   lobes of the cerebrum (five), 19
   meninges, 20–21
   neural tube forms, 18–19
   reticular formation, 20
   rhombencephalon, 21
   thalamus, 21
Brainstem, 19
Brain tumors, 15
Breast cancer, 201
Breath sounds, normal, 147
Broca aphasia, 20
Brocca area, 20, 145
Bronchi, 27
Bronchioles, 27, 29
Bronchitis, 201
Bronchus, 27, 29
Bucket-handle tear, 137
Bulimia nervosa, 201, 335
Bulk transport, 120–121
Bundle, of muscle fibers, 91
Bunionette (Tailor's bunion), 141
Bunion (Hallus Valgus), 141
Bunnel Littler test, 184
Buoyancy, 282
Burn, 199
Bursae of knee, 7
Bursitis, 138

Caffeine, 336
Calcaneofibular ligament sprain, 141
Calcitonin, 35
Calcium ions, 10
Callus, 199
Calyces, 31
Cancellous bone, 4, 5
Cancer, 133, 145
Candidiasis, 199, 201
Cane fitting and instructions, 234
Capacity, to do work, 287
Capillaries, 29, 131
Capillary bed pressure, 263
Capillary exchange, 131
Capsular ligament, 45
Capsulitis, 138
Carbon dioxide transport, 29
Carbonic anhydrase, 29
Carbon monoxide, 29
Carbuncle, 150, 199
Cardiac arrest and automated external defibrillation, 229
Cardiac arrest and cardiopulmonary resuscitation (American Red Cross), 229
Cardiac cycle, 26, 207

Cardiac notch, 27, 28
Cardiac output, 206
Cardiac risk factors, associated with physical activity, 101
Cardiac tamponade, 199
Cardiomyopathy, 145
Cardiopulmonary resuscitation (CPR), 101
Cardiorespiratory fitness, assessment, 109
Cardiorespiratory training, 115
Cardiovascular system
   atrioventricular node, 26
   autonomic nervous system heart control, 26
   blood pressure, 26
   blood volume, total, 26
   cardiac cycle, 26
   conduction pathway of the heart, 26
   coronary arteries, 25
   heart sounds, 26
   layers of heart, 24
   pericardium, 24
   pulmonary circuit, 26
   regulation of stroke volume, 26
   sinoatrial node, 25–26
   structures of heart, 24–25
   systemic circuit, 26
   systemic circulation, 25
Cariocca drill, 286
Carotid artery, 25
Carpal bones, of the hand, 163
Carpals. *See* short bone
Carpal tunnel syndrome, 184
Carpometacarpal joint, 92
Carpometacarpal joint, of the thumb, 91
Carrying angle, of the elbow, 93
   for females, 109, 182
Cartilage, 6
Cartilage cells, 6
Cartilage matrix, 6
Catecholamines, 33, 147
Cauda equina, 15
Cauliflower ear, 200
Celiac trunk, 48
Cecum, 31
Celiac plexus syndrome (solar plexus contusion), 199
Cell body, 14, 16
Cells, 120
Acells, 35
Cellulitis, 199
Center of gravity, 89
Central artery, 22
Central biasing theory, 250
Central canal, 15, 16
Central nervous system (CNS), 14
Centrioles, 120, 121, 123
Cerebellum, 18, 19
Cerebral contusion, 200
Cerebral cortex, 19, 20, 29
Cerebral hemispheres, 18
Cerebral palsy, 133, 201
Cerebral vascular accident (CVA), 145, 201
Cerebral vein, 20
Cerebrospinal fluid (CSF), 15, 20
Cerebrum, 19
Ceruminous glands, 13, 23
Cervical cancer, 146
Cervical compression test, 161
Cervical extension, 159
Cervical flexion, 159
Cervical lateral flexion, 159–160
Cervical nerve root compression, test for, 186
Cervical nerve root impingement, 187
Cervical plexus, 17
   nerves of, 49
Cervical rotation, 160
Cervical strain, 138
Cervical traction energy, 261
Cervical vertebrae, 46, 93
Cervix, 36
Chalazion, 200
Chamber divisions, 24–25
Charcot marie tooth disease, 201
Chemical (gap) synapse, 15
Chest compression depth, 238

Chest compressions per cycle, 236
Chest-thrust technique, 228
Cheyne-stokes respiration, 137
Chickenpox, 201
Chilblains, 111, 199
Chlamydia, 201, 210
Chondral ankle fracture, 141
Chondral fracture, 138
Chondroblasts, 6
Chondrocytes, 6
Chondroitin sulfate, 6
Chondromalacia, 138
  patella, 141
Choroid, 22
Choroid plexus, 19
Chromatin, 121
Chronic fatigue syndrome, 201
Chronic obstructive pulmonary disease (COPD),
  201
Ciliary glands, 13
Ciliary muscle, 22
Ciliary process, 22
Circadian rhythms, 35
Circulation and homeostasis
  arteries, 131
  blood clotting, 131
  blood groups, 131
  blood pressure, 131
  blood vessels, 131
  capillary exchange, 131
  components of blood, 129–130
  functions of circulatory system, 129
  portal systems, 131
  veins, 131
Clap, 210
Clarke sign, 177
Claudication, 201
  symptom, 149
Clavicle, 3, 43, 49
  contusion, 199
  fracture, 199
Claw hand deformity, 137
Claw toe, 137
Clean and jerk test, 111
Clunk test, 170, 181
Coach finger, 137
Coccidioidomycosis (San Juan or Valley fever),
  201
Coccyx, of the spinal column, 4
Cochlea, 23, 24
Cochlear nerve, 23
Cold injuries and illnesses, 106
Cold Urticaria, 199
Cold whirlpools (convection), 251
Colitis, 201
Collagen, 6
Collateral fiber, 14
Colle fracture, 137, 140
Common cold, 201, 209
Commotio cordis, 201, 236
Compact bone, 6
Compartment syndrome, 140
Complex partial seizure, 201
Complex regional pain syndrome (reflex
  sympathetic dystrophy), 201
Compression, 259
Conchae, 27
Concussion, 187, 200, 223
Conduction, 246, 264
Conduction pathway, of the heart, 26
Condylar process, 41
Cones, 22
Confrontation tests, 194
Congestive heart failure, 201
Conjunctivitis, 200
Connective tissue, 6
Consent, for treatment, 215–216
Constipation, 201
Contractions, of muscles, 9–10
  initiation of, 12
Contrast whirlpool (convection), 251
Controlled Substances Act, 1970, 294
Contusion, 138
Convection, 246
Conversion, 246

Coracobrachialis, 62, 167
Coracoclavicular joint, 93
Corn, 199
Coronary artery disease (CAD), 25
Cornea, 21, 22
Corneal abrasions, 200, 224
Corneal laceration, 200, 224
Corneal light test (Hirschberg test), 194
Corn—hard (callus durum), 141
Corn—soft (callus molle), 141
Coronal suture, 40
Coronary arteries, 25
  right, 145
Coronary artery disease (CAD), 101, 201
Coronoid process, 41
Corpus callosum, 19, 20
Corpus cavernosum, 38
Corpus spongiosum, 38
Corticosteroids, 33, 304
Corticotropin, 34
Cortisol, 147
Coryza, 200, 201
Cosine law, 247, 265
Costal cartilage, 43, 148
Costal facet, 41, 94
Costochondral fracture, 199
Costochondral joint, 43
Costochondral sprain, 200
Costovertebral sprain, 200
Counseling trap, 321
Cover test, 194
Cozen test, 183
Cranial nerves (CNs), 18, 21, 154
  assessment, 155
  function, 18
Cranial nerve XII function, assessment of, 113
Creatine, 336
Crescent-shaped fibrocartilage, 6–7
Cricoid cartilage, 27, 28
Crutch fitting and instructions, 233–234
Cryostretch, 251, 263
Cryotherapy, 261
Cryptorchidism (Cryptorchism), 201
C-shaped cartilage, 27
Cubital fossa, 183
Cubital tunnel syndrome (Ulnar Neuropathy),
  140, 183
Cubitus recurvatum, 93
Cubitus valgus, 93
Cushing syndrome, 201
Cuticle, 13
Cyclist's nipples, 137
Cyclist's palsy, 137
Cystic artery, 32
Cystic fibrosis, 133, 201
Cytoplasm, 120, 121
Cytoskeleton, 121, 123
Cytosol, 120, 123

DAPRE techniques, 285
Dead arm syndrome, 137
Decorticate posture, 239
Deep external rotators, of the hip, 95
Deep (late) frostbite, 231
Deep nerve branches, 17
Deep pressure massage, 259
Deep Tendon Reflex (DTR) Grading Scale,
  156
Deep tendon reflexes (DTRs), 155
Deep vein thrombophlebitis (DVT), 179
Deep vein thrombosis (DVT), 201
Defecation, 31
Dehydration, 113, 230
DeLorme strength progression, 290
Deltoid, 9, 47, 51, 166–167
Deltoid ligament sprain, 141
Deltoid muscle, 46
Dendrites, 14, 121
Dental caries, 200
Deoxygenated blood, 29
Depolarization, 15
  of nerve, 259
De Quervain syndrome, 137, 140

De Quervain tenosynovitis, 185
Dermal papillae, 12
Dermal projections, 204
Dermatitis, 199
Dermatomes, 154–155
  distribution for the spinal and peripheral
    nerve roots, 157
Dermis, 12, 205
Descending tracts—efferent (motor), 17
Detached retina, 200, 225
Deviated septum, 200, 235
Diabetes mellitus, 133, 201
Diabetic athletes, snacks for, 148
Diabetic coma, 232
Diagnostic positions and test, 194
Diaphysis (shaft), 4, 6
Diarrhea, 201
Diarthrotic joint, 90
Diastolic blood pressure, 206
Diencephalon, 18, 19
Dietary Supplement Health And Education Act,
  1994, 295
Dietary supplements, 335
Differentiation, 121
Diffusion, 120
Digestive accessory organs, 31
Digestive system
  alimentary (gastrointestinal or digestive)
    tract, 30–31
  digestive accessory organs, 31
  functions, 29
  walls of the digestive tract, 30
Dilated pupils, in an unconscious patient,
  242
Diopter, 194
Diphtheria, 201
Diploic vein, 20
Diplopia, 200
Dislocation, 138
Disqualification, of an athlete, 111, 143
Distal convoluted tubule, 32
Distal epiphysis, 6
Distal femur epiphyseal plate injury, 141
Diuretics, 336
Division bronchus, 28
DOMS, 284
Donjoy Playmaker, 109
Dopamine, 260
Dorsal horn, 16
Dorsal root, 16
Dorsal root ganglion, 16
"Doughnut" pad, 110
Down syndrome, 133, 201
Drop arm (codman) test, 168
Dual-energy X-ray absorptiometry, 334
Ductus deferens, 36, 38
Duodenum, 32
Dupuytren contracture, 137, 140
Dural sheath, of optic nerve, 22
Dura mater, 20
Dynamic contractions, of a muscle, 289
Dysmenorrhea, 201

Ear guards, 111
Ears, 23–24
Eating disorders, 335, 337
Ecchymosis color change, 197
Eccrine, 13
Eczema, 199
Effector, 14, 16
Efferent arteriole, 32
Efferent (motor) neurons, 15, 17
Ejaculatory duct, 36, 38
Elastic cartilage, 6
Elastic wraps, 110, 114
Elastin, 6
Elbow
  dislocation, 140
  extension, 93, 376
  facts about, 376
  flexion, 376
  ligaments, 376
  PNF, 376

Elbow (*continued.*)
  pronation, 376
  subluxation, 140
  supination, 376
  tests, 376
Electrical simulation, 251–255
Electrical synapse, 15
Electrocardiogram, 195, 204, 205
Electron transport chain, 123
Ely test, 176
Emergency action plan, 215
Emergency information of athletes, 216
Empty can (supraspinatus) test, 168, 181
Encephalitis, 201
Endocardium, 24, 25
Endochondral ossification, 4
Endocrine functions, 147
Endocrine system
  adrenal glands, 34–35
  categories of hormones, 33–34
  endocrine gland and gland functions, 33
  female reproductive system, 36
  male reproductive system, 36–38
  pancreas, 35
  parathyroid gland, 35
  pineal gland, 35
  pituitary gland (hypophysis), 34
  sex glands, 36
  thymus, 35
  thyroid gland, 35
Endogenous opioid theory, 250
Endometriosis, 36, 201
Endometrium, 36
Endophthalmos, 200
Endoplasmic reticulum, 120, 121, 123
ß-endorphin and dynorphin theory,
  250
Endosteum, 4, 6
Energy measurements, 332
Energy transport, 120
Enthesitis, 138
Ephedra, 336
Epicardium, 24, 25
Epicondylitis, 138
Epidermis, 11–12, 205, 206
Epididymis, 36, 38
Epidural hematoma, 200
Epiglottis, 6, 28
Epilepsy, 201
Epimysium, 10
Epinephrine, 15, 33, 260
Epinephrine (adrenaline), 35
EpiPen, 237
Epiphyseal (growth) plates, 4
Epiphyseal plate injury, 138
Epiphyses bone, 4, 5
Epiphysitis, 138
Epistaxis, 200, 225, 238
Epithelial cells, 11
Equilibrium (vestibule and semicircular canals),
  24
Erb point, 163
Erector (arrector) pili, 13
Erector spinae, 160
Ergogenic aids, in athletics, 336, 342
Erythrocytes (RBCs), 129, 130, 205
Erythropoietin (EPO), 33, 336
Esophageal hiatus, 30
Esophageal reflux, 201
Esophagus, 28, 30
Estrogen, 36
Eustachian tube, 23, 28
Evaporation, 246
Eversion of the ankle, 97
Eversion stress (talar tilt) test, 179
Exercise-induced bronchospasm, 201
Exercise-induced urticaria, 199
Exercise program, components of, 290
Exercise-related cardiac deaths, prevention of,
  101
Exertional heat exhaustion, 230
Exertional heatstroke, 230
Exertional hyponatremia, 231
Exertional rhabdomyolysis, 144
Exhalation (expiration), 29

Exit order, for food, 147
Exocytosis, 16
Exophthalmos, 200
Exostosis, 138
Extensor carpi radialis longus, 64, 168
Extensor carpi ulnaris, 64, 168
Extensor digitorum, 63, 167–168
Extensor digitorum longus, 83
Extensor hallucis longus, 84
Extensor pollicis brevis, 64, 168
Extensor pollicis longus, 64, 168
External acoustic meatus, 23
External auditory canal, 23, 210
External bleeding, management, 221
External gas exchange, 26
Extracapsular ligaments, 7
Extrinsic eye muscles, 22
Eye
  medical field for treating, 113
  nerves of, 23
  structure, 22
  tests, 193–194

Facet joint pathology, 261
Facet of superior articular process, 41
Facial laceration, 138, 239
Facilitated diffusion, 120
Fairbank apprehension test, 186
Fair Labor Standards Act, 351
Falciform ligament, 32
Fallopian tubes, 36
False motion, 153
Falx cerebri, 20
Family Educational Rights and Privacy Act
  (FERPA), 360
Family Medical Leave Act, 351
Fasciitis, 138
Fat, calories in, 344
Fat pad contusion, 141
Faun beard, 137
Feces, 31
Federal Educational Rights Privacy Act, 351
Federal Food, Drug, And Cosmetic Act, 1938, 294
Feiss line assess, 113
Feldenkrais, 258
Felon, 140
Female reproductive system, 36
Femoral artery, 154
Femoral nerve, 50
Femoral stress fracture, 140
Femoral triangle, 95
Femur fracture, 140, 241
Fever, 146
Fibrinogen, 130
Fibrocartilage, 6
Fibromyalgia, 201
Fibrous fascia, 8
Fibula, 7
  fracture, 141
Fibular collateral ligament, 7
  sprain, 141
Fibular nerve, 50
Fibular stress fracture, 141
Finger dislocations, 140
Finger fracture, 140
Finger subluxations, 140
Finkelstein test, 171
Fixtors, 9
Flail chest injury, 227
Flash-to-bang method, 107
Flat bone, 4, 5
Flexor carpi radialis, 63, 167
Flexor carpi ulnaris, 63, 167
Flexor digitorum longus, 80
Flexor digitorum profundus, 63, 167
  tendon, 184
Flexor digitorum superficialis, 63, 167
Flexor hallucis longus, 80
Flexor pollicis brevis, 168
Flexor pollicis longus, 63, 168
Fluidotherapy, 251, 264
Fluorescein dye, 242
Fluoroquinolone, 307

Focalization, of a beam or wave, 262
Follicle-stimulating hormone, 146
Follicular phase, 36
Folliculitis, 199
Folliculotrophin, 34
Food poisoning, 201
Football helmet certification, standards, 113
Football helmet fitting, 103–104, 115
Football helmet removal, for spine injured
  athlete, 226, 237
Football shoulder pad fitting, 104, 110
Foraminal compression (spurling) test, 161
Foraminal distraction test, 161
Forearm pronation, 165
Forearm splints, 137
Forearm supination, 165
Foreign bodies, in eye, 225
Foreign material, removal of, 238
Four-Point Pitting Edema Scale, 197
Fractures, 138, 222
Freiberg disease, 137
Frontal bone, 40
Frontal lobe, 19, 20
Frontal sinus, 28
Frontozygomatic suture, 40
Frostbite, 199, 201
Frozen shoulder, 137
FSH, 38
Full-body hot whirlpool, 262
Fundus, 30
Furrow, over spinous process of thoracic
  vertebrae, 46
Furuncle, 150, 199
Furunculosis, 199

Gaenslen test, 186
Galeazzi fracture, 140
Gallbladder, 31, 32
Gamekeeper's thumb, 137, 140, 185
Gastritis, 201
Gastrocnemius, 80
Gastroenteritis (food poisoning/stomach flu),
  201
Gastroesophageal reflux disease (GERD), 149,
  201
Gate control theory, 249–250, 260
Geniohyoid muscle, 49
Genital herpes, 201
Genital warts, 146, 201
Genitofemoral nerve, 50
Genu valgum, 112, 174
Gerber lift-off test, 168, 181
Gerdy tubercle, 96, 173
Gingivitis, 200
Ginglymus joint, 91
Glabella, 40
Glans, 38
Glenohumeral dislocation, 139
Glenohumeral glide test, 170
Glenohumeral injuries, 92
Glenohumeral joint, 6, 284
Glenohumeral joint capsule, 7
Glenohumeral joint dislocation, 180
Glenohumeral joint instability, 180
Glenohumeral joint sprain, 139
Glenoid labrum, 6
  tear, 139
Glial cells, 15, 97, 148
Glioma, 207
Globulins, 129–130
Glomerular filtration, 33
Glomerulus, 32
Glottis, 27
Glucagon, 35
Glucocorticoids, 35
Glucosamine, 6
Gluteal muscle, 95
Gluteal nerve, superior and inferior, 50
Gluteus maximus, 65
Gluteus medius, 65
Gluteus minimus, 65
Glycerol, 120
Glycogen, 286

Glycolysis, 120, 122
Glycoproteins, 33
Godfrey 90–90 test, 178
Golfer's elbow, 137
Golgi apparatus, 120, 121, 123
Gonads (testes), 36
Goniometry, 86, 154, 159–160
Gonorrhea, 201, 210
Good samaritan laws, 347
Gout, 201
Gracilis, 80
Gray commissure, 15
Gray matter, 15, 16, 20
Great toe sprain (Turf Toe), 141
Grip strength, measurement tool for, 289
Ground substance, 6
Group A Streptococcus (GAS), 201
Growth hormone (GH), 34
Growth lines, 6
Guillian-Barré syndrome, 201
Gunstock deformity, 137
Guyon canal, 184
Gynecomastia, 201
Gyrus, 19

Haemophilis influenza type B (Hib), 201
Hair, 11, 13
Hair follicle, 13, 148, 204
Hair root, 13
Hallux rigidus, 141
Hamate fracture, 140
Hammer toe, 137, 141
    deformity, 113
Hamstrings, 79
    muscle group, 97
    strain, 140
    tendinitis, 140
Hard cast, 112
Harvard step test, 115
Hawkins-Kennedy impingement test, 169
Hay fever, 201
HBV live, 237
Head
    arteries, 48
    bones, 38–39
    ligaments, 38
    muscles, 38–42, 46–47
    nerves, 49–50
Health care administration
    administrative concepts, 353–354
    advanced beneficiary notice, 350
    agreed-upon procedures, 360
    BOC certification examination, 359
    budgeting, 348
    clinical proficiencies, 345
    documentation, 352, 356, 360, 361
    examination paper, 355–362
    federal statutes, 351–352, 354, 355–356
    healthcare policies, 349, 358–359
    indemnity insurance plan, 349, 355
    international classification of disease, 350
    JCAHO, 354, 357
    managed care plans, 349–350, 356–357
    management style, 357
    Mary Parker Follett management style, 357
    medicaid, 350, 357
    medicare, 350
    monitoring systems, 346
    overview, 345
    procedural codes, 350
    reimbursement codes, 356, 359
    resource management, 348, 359–361, 360–361
    risk management, 346–347
    signing authority for medical record release, 355
    third-party reimbursement, 349
    UB-92 (universal billing codes), 350
Health Insurance Portability And Accountability Act, 351
Healthy weight gain, 334
Healthy weight loss, 334
Hearing impairment, 133
Hearing process, 24

Hearing tests, 191–192
Heart
    autonomic nervous system heart control, 26
    cardiac cycle, 26
    conduction pathway of, 26
    contusion, 227
    factors that affect blood pressure, 26
    failure, 148
    murmur, 201
    muscle, thickening of, 109
    regulation of stroke volume, 26
    sounds, 26, 145
    structure of, 24–25
Heat cramps, 230
Heat exhaustion, 202, 240
    sign of, 110
Heat illness, 111
    prevention, 105
    signs and symptoms of, 107
    treatment, 106
    types, 106
Heat stroke, 202
Heat syncope, 202, 230
Heat transfer, 262
Heberden nodes, 137
Heel spur, 141
Hematuria, 200
Hemoglobin, 29, 130, 263
Hemophilia, 202
Hemopoiesis, 130–131
Hemorrhoids, 200, 202
Hemostasis, 131
Hemothorax, 200, 227
Hepatic artery, 31, 32
Hepatic duct, 32
Hepatitis, 210
Hepatitis A, 202
Hepatitis B, 202
Hepatitis C, 202
Hepatitis D, 202
Hepatitis E, 202
Hepatomegaly, 113
Hernia, 200
Herpes gladiatorum, 199
Herpes simplex, 199
Herpes Zoster (Shingles), 199, 202
Hill-Sachs lesion, 137, 139
Hilum, 31
Hindbrain, 21
Hip, 90
    abduction, 95, 372
    dislocation, 140, 242
    extension, 173, 372
    external rotation, 174, 372
    facts about, 372
    flexion, 173, 372
    flexors, flexibility of the, 110
    internal rotation, 174, 372
    ligaments, 372
    PNF, 372
    pointer, 137
    sprain, 140
    tests, 372
Hippocampus, 20
HIV, 202
Hives, 199
Hodgkin disease, 202
Homan sign, 179
Hoover test, 162
Hordeolum, 200
Horizontal fissure, 28
Hormone thymosin, 35
Hot whirlpool (convection), 251
Human cell function and dysfunction, 120–124
Human growth hormone (HGH), 336, 343
Human papillomavirus, 148
Humeral fracture, 139
Humeroulnar joint, 92
Humerus. *See* long bone
Hump back, 137
Hyaline (articular) cartilage, 6
Hydration status assessment, 106
Hydrocele, 200
Hydrodensitometry, 334

Hyoid bone, 28
Hyperactive deep tendon reflexes, 149
Hyperextension, of the knees, 96
Hyperglycemia, 202, 232
Hyperhidrosis, 199
Hyperopia, 200
Hyperplasia, 121
Hyperpnea, 149
Hypertension, 134, 208
    moderate, 144
Hyperthyroidism (Grave disease), 202
Hypertrophic cardiomyopathy, 202
Hypertrophy, 121
Hyperventilation, 29, 200, 202, 227
Hyphema, 200, 225, 238, 240
Hypoglossal nerve, 49
Hypoglycemia, 202, 232, 237
Hyporeflexive patellar tendon reflex, 112
Hypotension, 202, 207, 208
Hypothalamus, 18, 19, 21, 34
Hypothermia, 111, 114, 202, 231
    prevention, 106
Hypothyroidism, 202
Hypoventilation, 29

Ibuprofen, 304
Ice cream, calories in, 343
Ice immersion (convection), 251
Ice massage, 250, 261
Ileocecal valve, 31
Iliac crest, 46
Iliac crest contusion (hip pointer), 140
Iliacus, 65
Iliohypogastric nerve, 50
Ilioinguinal nerve, 50
Iliopectineal bursitis, 140
Iliotibial (IT) "band" syndrome, 141
Ilium, 3. *See* flat bone
Impacted Cerumen, 200
Impetigo, 199
Impingement syndrome, 139
Incision, 199
Incus, 23
Index finger dislocation, 239
Indigestion, 202
Infection diagnosis, 143
Infectious mononucleosis, 202
Inferior drawer (Feagin) test, 170
Inferior glenohumeral instability, assessment of, 181
Inferior orbital fissure, 40
Inferior vena cava, 25
Inflamed lymph node, 207
Inflammation and infection
    acute inflammatory process, 125
    attenuated vaccine, 129
    body's defense system, 127–128
    chain of infection, 126
    colonization *versus* infection, 126
    healing factors, 125
    immune defense mechanisms, 128–129
    immune serum (antiserum), 129
    inflammatory phase, 125
    injury process, 124
    lymphatic system and infection, 128
    portal of entry, 126
    proliferation/repair/
        revascularization/rebuilding/ fibroblastic phase, 126
    remodeling/maturation phase, 126
    signs of inflammation, 126
    tissue recovery process, 125
    transmission, 126
    Wolff law, 125
Influenza, 202, 209
Infraorbital foramen, 40
Infrapatellar bursitis, 141
Infrared lamps (radiant), 254, 257
Infraspinatus, 46, 62
Ingrown toenail, 141
Inhalation (inspiration), 27
Inion, 159
Inner ear (labyrinth), 23
Innominate bones, 95

Inoculation schedule, 197
Insertion, of a muscle, 91
Insula, 19
Insulin, 35, 210, 237
   shock, 202
Integrity of noncontractile tissues, test, 114
Integumentary (skin) system, 205
   skin color, 13
   skin functions, 11
   skin structure, 11–13
   system components, 11, 13
Interatrial septum, 24
Intermediary suture, 40
Intermittent compression, 257
Internal foam padding, 110
Internal gas exchange, 26
Interneurons (central or association neurons), 15, 16
Interpubic disc, 6
Interspinous ligament, 45
Intertransverse ligament, 45
Intertrigo, 199
Intertubercular groove, 163
Interventricular septum, 24, 25
Intervertebral disc herniation, 138
Intervertebral disc rupture, 138
Intervertebral foramen, 45
Intervertebral sprain, 138
Intestinal herniation, 144
Intracapsular ligaments, 6
Intracranial hematoma, 200
Intracranial pressure, 239
Intramembranous ossification, 4
Intraparenchymal hematoma (intracerebral hematoma), 200
Intrinsic eye muscles, 22
Intrinsic muscle, 97
Introitus, 36
Inverse square law, 247, 249
Inversion stress (talar tilt) test, 179
Iris, 22
Iron-deficiency anemia, 202
Irregular bone, 4
Irritable bowel syndrome, 202
Irritant contact dermatitis, 199
Ischium, 3
Islets of Langerhans, 34, 35
Isokinetic activities, 288–289
Isometric exercises, 288
Isometric (static) contraction, 9
Isotonic activities, 288
Isotonic (dynamic) contraction, 9–10
IT band friction syndrome, 141

Jersey finger, 137, 140
Jobe relocation test, 170
Jock itch, 137
Joint arthrokinematics, 86
Joint capsules, 7
Joint mice, 137
Joint mobilization and manual therapy techniques, 276–279, 287
Joints, 92
   anatomy, synovial, 84–85
   classification, 84
   motion, 85–86
   roles of, 84
Jones fracture, 137, 141
Juxtaglomerular apparatus, 32

Kaltenborn's mobilization grades, 277
Kaposi sarcoma, 207
Kehr sign, 137, 240
Keratin, 13
Keratitis, 109, 200
Kernig-Brudzinski (Brudzinksi-Kernig) test, 161–162
Key terms, 2–3
Kidney, 31–32, 32, 33, 242
   contusion, 200
   laceration, 200

stones, 200
Kienböck disease, 137, 140
Kinesiology
   biomechanical principles, 88–89
   joints, 84–88
   reference terms, 84
Kinetic chain activity, with distal segment, 289
Kleiger test (external rotation test), 179
Kneading, 259
Knee
   extension, 174, 373
   external rotation, range of motion for, 96
   facts about, 373
   flexion, 174, 373
   ligaments, 373
   PNF, 373
   tests, 373
Korotkoff sounds, 149, 194

Labrum, 6
Laceration, 199
Lachman test, 186
Lacrimal bone, 40
Lacrosse player, diagnosis of, 143
Lacteal, 31
Lambdoid suture, 40
Lamina, 41, 42
Language comprehension, 145
Large intestine, 31
Larsen-Johansson disease, 137
Laryngitis, 202
Laryngopharynx, 27
Larynx, 27
LASER (Light Amplification by the Stimulation of Emitted Radiation), 257
Lesser wing of sphenoid bone, 40
Lateral collateral ligament sprain, 140
Lateral cord, 17
Lateral curvature, of the thoracic spine, 115
Lateral epicondylitis (extensor tendonitis), 140
Lateral femoral cutaneous nerve, 50
Lateral meniscus, 7
Lateral pivot shift test, 178
Lateral rib compression test, 163
Latissimus dorsi, 9, 46, 47, 160
Law of Grotthus-Draper, 247
Legg-Calvés-Perthes disease, 137, 141
Lens, 21, 22
Leukemia, 146
Leukocytes (WBCs), 129, 130
Levator scapulae, 46, 160
Lever systems, in the body, 88, 92
Ligamentous and special tests, 161–163
Ligamentous tests, 112, 154, 168–172
Ligaments, 6–7, 85
   anterior longitudinal, 45
   of the Spine, 45
Ligamentum flavum, 45
Lightning hazard prevention, 106
   suspension of game, 116
Lightning monitoring and detection, 107
Lightning safety recommendations, 107
Limb girth, 110
Limbic system, 20
Linea alba, 47
Line of gravity, 89
Lingula, 28, 41
Lipid metabolism, 120
Lipid profile blood test, 112
Lisfranc injury, 137
Little Leaguer elbow, 137
Little League shoulder, 137
Liver, 31
   contusion, 200
   laceration, 200
Load and shift test, 170
Lobar bronchus, 28
Lobes, 28
Lobule of auricle, 23
Lock jaw, 113
Lockjaw symptoms, 143

Long bone, 4, 5, 6
Long bone compression test, 179
Longissimus dorsi muscle, 94
Longitudinal arch sprain, 141
Long-term memory (LTM), 20
Long thoracic nerve contusion, 139
Loop of Henle, 32
Lower extremities, 3
   arteries, 75
   bones, 64, 69–70
   ligaments, 64, 68, 71–74
   mobilizations, 278, 280–281
   muscles, 65, 76–84
   muscle tests, manual, 175–176
   nerves, 75
Lower extremity
   soft tissue palpations of, 173–175
Ludington test, 169, 182
Lumbar plexus, 17
   nerves of, 50
Lumbar spine, 94
Lumbar vertebra, 42
Lumbosacral sprain, 138
Lumbosacral strain, 138
Lumbosacral trunk, 50
Lunala ("little moon"), 13
Lung auscultation, 146, 235
Lungs, 27
Luteal phase, 36
Luteinizing hormone (LH), 34, 38
Lyme disease, 202
Lymphatic capillaries, 128
Lymphatic tissue tumor, 207
Lymph flow, cessation of, 207
Lymph node location, 128
Lymphoid organs, 145
Lysosome, 120, 121

MacIntosh test, 178
Macula lutea, 22
Ma Huang, 343
Maisonneuve fracture, 137
Maitland's mobilization grades, 277
Male reproductive system, 36–38
Malignant brain edema syndrome, 200
Malignant tumors, 210
Mallet finger, 137, 140, 184
Mallet toe, 137
Malleus, 23
Mammary glands, 13
Mammillary process, 42
Mandible, 40, 41
   fracture, 200, 224
   notch, 41
Manual Muscle Test Grading Scale, 154
Manual muscle tests (MMTs), 154
Manubrium, 43
Marathon runner, efficient energy system for a, 90
Marfan syndrome, 137, 202
Master gland, 34
Mastoid foramen, 40
Mastoid process, 40
Maxilla, 40
Maxillary fracture, 200, 223–224
Maximum expiration, 143
McBurney point, 137, 146, 159, 187
MCL sprain, 140
McMurray test, 154, 177
Meal blood sugar values, 147
Measles, 209
Medial collateral ligament (MCL), 6–7, 97
Medialcord, 17
Medial epicondylitis, 140
   of elbow, test, 183
Medial epiphysis, 182
Medial meniscus, 6
Medial rectus muscle, 22
Medial tibial stress syndrome, 141
Medial (ulnar) collateral ligament, 92
Median nerve palsy, 140
Median nerve pathology, 184
Mediastinum, 27

Medical disorders
  clinical proficiencies, 189
  examination, 204–211
  general assessment, 190–197
  medical conditions, 199–203
  overview, 189
Medulla oblongata, 18, 21
Medullary (marrow) cavity, 4, 6
Megahertz (MHz), 264, 265
Meibomian glands, 11, 12
Melanin, 13
Melanocytes, 13
Melanomas, 146
Meninges, 20
Meningitis, 109, 202
Meniscal tear, 141
Menisci, 6, 7
Menstrual cycle, 36, 37, 146
Menstruation, 146
Mental foramen, 40, 41
Mental protuberance, 40, 41
Mesencephalon (midbrain), 18
Mesentery, 30
Mesentric vein, 32
Mesocolon, 30
Mesomorph body build, 113
Metabolic disorder, 210
Metabolic pathways energy production, 124
Metacarpophalangeal joints, of the fingers, 185
Metaplasia, 121
Metatarsal arch sprain, 141
Metatarsal fracture, 141
Metatarsal stress fracture, 141
Metencephalon, 18, 21
Methicillin-resistant *Staphylococcus Aureus*
  (MRSA), 202
Microglia, 15
Midbrain, 19
Middle ear ossicles, 23
Migraine headache, 202
Miliaria profunda, 199
Miliaria rubra, 199
Military brace position, 180
Mineralocorticoids, 35
Minimal erythemal dose (MED), 261
Mitochondria, 16, 120, 121, 123
Mitral valve, 25
  prolapse, 202
MMR immunization, 143
Mnemonic ABCDE, 208
Moist heat packs (conduction), 251
Mole, changes in, 116
Molluscum contagiosum, 199
Mononucleosis, 148
Monorchidism, 202
Monosaccharide, 337
Monteggia fracture, 140, 182
Morphine, 304
Motion tests, 154
Motor aphasia, 20
Motor level pain control, 265
Motor nerves, 23
Motor neuron, 16
  axon, 10
Mottling, 263
Mouth, 30
Mouth guards, 103, 110, 111
Mover, 10
Mucosa, 30
Mucous membrane, 27
Mucus, 31
Multipennate muscle, 9
Multiple sclerosis, 202
Mumps, 202, 209
Murphy sign, 171, 184
Muscular dystrophy, 202
Muscular system, 90, 206, 207, 284
  contractions, 9–10, 289
  contractions, downhill, 285
  energy technique, 258
  fiber, 14
  of head, neck, spine and thorax, 46–47
  longest, 95
  of posterior hip and buttock, 76
  reeducation, 265

  role in moving the knee, 97
  roles of, 9
  skeletal tissue, 8–9
  sliding filament (mechanism) theory, 10–11
  soreness, 284
  structure and location of, 8, 9
  structure surrounding muscular
    compartments of leg, 96
  tests, manual, 160–161, 175–176, 185
  of upper limb, 60–61
Myasthenia gravis, 202
Myelencephalon, 18, 21
Myelinated fiber, 14
Myelin sheath, 10, 14
Myocardial infarction, 208
Myocardium, 24, 25
Myofascial release techniques, 258
Myofibrils, 10
  loss of, 284
Myoglobin, 9
Myometrium, 36
Myopia, 200
Myosin, 10
Myositis, 138, 207
Myotomes, 155
  assessment, of athlete, 113

Nail bed infection, 206
Nails, 11, 13
  matrix, 13
  root, 13
Na^+/K^+ pump, 15
Narcotic prescription, 303
Nares (nostrils), 27
Nasal bone, 40
Nasal cavities, 27
Nasal concha, 28, 40
Nasal fracture, 200, 225
Nasal septum, 27
Nasion, 40
Nasolacrimal canal, 40
Nasopharynx, 27, 28
NATAPAC, 369
National Athletic Trainers' Association, 364, 369
National Athletic Trainers' Association
  Education Council, 364
National Athletic Training Research And
  Education Foundation, 364
National Collegiate Athletic Association Injury
  Surveillance System, 346
National Electronic Injury Surveillance System,
  346
National Football Head And Neck Injury
  Registry, 346
National High School Sports Injuries Registry,
  346
National Operating Committee on Standards for
  Athletic Equipment (NOCSAE), 347
NCAA Sports Medicine Handbook, 107
Neck
  arteries, 48
  bones, 38–39
  ligaments, 38
  muscles, 38–42, 46–47
  nerves, 49–50
  rolls, 114
Negligence, 347, 361
Nephron, 32
Nerve cells, 259
Nerve impulses, 15, 121
Nerve root compression (radiculopathy), 138
Neurilemma cells, 15
Neuritis, 138
Neuroglia, 15, 145
Neurolemma cell, 10, 14
Neurologic hammer, 156
Neurologic system
  autonomic nervous system, 18
  cranial nerves, 18
  functional divisions, 14
  nerve impulse, 15
  neuroglia, 15
  neuron structure, 14–15

  neurotransmitters, 15
  parasympathetic nervous system, 18
  primary plexuses in the body (four), 17–18
  reflex arc, 17
  simplest reflex, 17
  somatic, 14
  spinal cord, 15–17
  spinal nerves, 17
  structural divisions, 14
  sympathetic nervous system, 18
  synapses, 15
Neurologic tests, 154
Neuromuscular junction, 10, 14
Neuron, 121
  fusion of, 16
  structure, 14–15
Neurotransmitter, 260
Neutralizers, 9
Newton laws, 88–89, 89, 282–283
Nightstick fracture, 137
Nipple, 47
Nissi bodies, 14
Nitrogen dioxide, 115
Noble compression test, 177
Nociceptors, 260
Node of ranvier, 14, 15
Nonaxial (gliding, sliding, or linear) motion, 86
Noradrenaline, 15
Norepinephrine, 15, 33, 35
Nosebleed. *See* epistaxis
NSAIDs, 302, 304
Nucleolus, 14, 121, 123
Nucleus, 10, 14, 120, 121, 123
Nucleus pulposus, 45
Numbness, 186
Nutritional aspects, of injuries and illnesses
  and athletic performance, 330–332
  carbohydrates, 325–326
  cholestrol, 326
  clinical proficiencies, 323–324
  dietary supplements and ergogenic aids,
    335–336, 342
  disaccharides, 325
  electrolytes, 329, 342
  examination paper, 337–344
  fats, 326
  fat substitutes, 327
  fatty acids, 327
  food label with explanation of food panel
    information, 330
  healthy and pathologic nutrition, 325–330
  lipoproteins, 326–327
  micronutrients, 328–329, 341
  monosaccharides, 325
  niacin deficiency, 340
  nutrient intake during exercise, 331
  nutrient intake for athletes, 330–331, 338
  nutritional deficiency, 337–340
  nutritional recommendations, 329
  overview, 323
  polysaccharides, 326
  postcompetition (postexercise) meal, 332
  precompetition (pre-exercise) meal, 331, 341,
    343
  process of expending energy, 343
  proteins, 327–328
  riboflavin deficiency, 340–341
  sources of vitamins, 328, 342
  for tooth decay, 341
  water, 329
  weight management, 332–335
Nutritional Labeling And Education Act, 1990,
  294

Ober test, 176
Obesity, 134
Oblique, internal and external, 47, 160
Oblique fissure, 28
Oblique line, 41
Obturator nerve, 50
Occipital bone, 40
Occipital lobe, 19
Occipital nerve, lesser, 49
Occipitomastoid suture, 40

Ocular fundus, 193
Oculomotor nerve, 23
Olecranon bursa, 7
Olecranon bursitis, 140
Olfaction (smell), 24
Oligodendrocytes (oligodendroglia), 15
Oligomenorrhea, 202
Omentums, 30
Omohyoid muscle, 49
One-way valves, 24–25
Onset (disorders), 147
Onychia, 199
Open wounds, management of, 221
Ophthalmoscope, 192–193
Oppenheim reflex, 156
Optic canal, 40
Optic disc, 22
Optic nerve, 22, 23
Optic retina, 22
Oral cavity, 28
Ora serrata, 22
Orbicularis occuli, 9
Orbital "blowout" fracture, 200
Orbital blowout fracture or globe rupture, 225
Orbital fissure, superior, 40
Organ of corti, 24
Oropharynx, 27, 28
Orthopaedic examination and diagnosis
    clinical examination process, 152–155
    clinical proficiency, 151
    documentation procedure, 155–158
    examination of head, neck, spine and thorax,
        158–163
    examination of lower extremity, 172–179
    examination of upper extremity, 163–172
    examination paper, 180–187
    principles, 152–158
Orthopaedic special test, 112
Osgood-Schlatter disease, 137, 141
Osmosis, 120, 124
Osteitis pubis, 141
Osteoblasts, 4
Osteochondral ankle fracture, 141
Osteochondral fracture, 138
Osteochondritis, 138
Osteochondritis dissecans, 138, 141
Osteoclasts, 4
Osteocytes, 4
Osteokinematic motion, 86
Osteomyelitis, 138
Osteons, 5
Osteoporosis, 134, 202
Otitis externa, 200
Otitis media, 200
Outer ear, 6
Ovarian cancer, 202
Ovaries, 33, 34, 36
Overload principle, 115, 116
Ovulation, 36
Oxford technique, of strength progression, 290
Oxygenated blood, 29
Oxygen transport, 29

Pain, right upper quadrant, 149
Painful urination, with pus discharge, diagnosis,
    144
Palmar crease, 184
Palmaris longus, 63, 167
    muscle, 63
Palpable pulses, 195
    location, 149
Palpation, 153
    bony, 158–159
    of the hamstring tendons, 177
    of lower extremity, 173–175
    soft tissue, 159
Pancreas, 31, 32, 33, 34, 35
Pancreatic cells, 147
Pancreatitis, 202
Panner disease, 183
Paraffin bath, 251, 263–264
Parallel (longitudinal) muscles, 8–9
Paraplegia, 134

Parasites, 205
Parasympathetic nervous system, 18, 26
Parathyroid gland, 33, 34, 35
Parathyroid hormone, 33
Pareitomastoid suture, 40
Parietal bone, 40
Parietal lobe, 19
Parietal peritoneum, 30
Parietal pleura, 27
Parkinson disease, 202
Paronychia, 199
Parotid glands, 31
Paroxysmal contractions, 145
Parrot-Break tear, 137
Participation agreements, 347
Passive range of motion (PROM), 154
Patella, 7, 95. See Sesamoid bone
Patella apprehension test, 177
Patella fracture, 141
Patellar dislocation, 141
Patellar grind test, 177
Patellar tendon, 7
Patellar tendon rupture, 141
Patella subluxation, 141
Patella tendinitis (Jumper's Knee), 141
Patella tendon length test, 186
Pathological hardening, of muscle, 207
Pathological reflexes, 156
Pathologic softening, of muscle, 207
Patrick (FABER) test, 163
Peak flow meter, 196
Pectoral girdle, 3
Pectoralis major, 47, 51
    lower, 161
    upper, 160–161
Pectoralis minor, 166
Pectus carinatum, 149
Pectus excavatum, 111
Pedicle, 41, 42
Pediculosis, 143, 199
Pelvic fracture, 141
Pelvic girdle, 3, 4
Pelvic inflammatory disease, 202
Pelvic stress fracture, 141
Pennate muscles, 9
Peptic ulcers, 150
Percussion (bump) test, 179
Pericardium, 24, 204
Pericoronitis, 200
Peridontitis, 200
Perimetrium, 36
Perimysium, 10
Periorbital ecchymosis, 200
Periosteum, 4, 6
Periostitis, 138
Peripheral nerve assessment, 158
Peripheral nervous system (PNS), 14
Peristalsis, 30
Peritoneum, 30
Peritoneum portions, 30
Peritonitis, 200
Perivascular subarachnoid space, 20
Pernio, 199
Peroneal nerve contusion, 141
Peroneal tendinitis, 141
Peroneal tendon dislocation, 141
Peroneal tendon subluxation, 141
Peroneus brevis, 83
Peroneus longus, 83
Peroneus tertius, 84
Peroxisomes, 120, 121
Pertussis, 146, 202
Pes anserine bursitis, 141
Pes anserine muscular movements, 96
Pes cavus, 141
Pes planus, 141
Petechiae, 199
Petit mal seizures, 145
PH, of blood plasma, 130, 206
Phagocytes, 15, 261
Phalen (wrist flexion) test, 171
Pharmacology
    administered medication, 299
    administrative and legal issues, 294–296, 304,
        306

adverse drug effect (side effect), 301, 303, 306,
    309
antibacterial medication, 304
basic medication information, 296
bioavailability, 299
bioequivalence, 299
biotransformation, 305
blue index, 305
brand names, 297
categories of adverse drug effects, 301
cause of tinnitus secondary, 305
chemical names, 297
classification, 308
clinical proficiencies, 293
common medication abbreviations, 294
controlled substances schedules, 295, 302
dispensed medications, 299–300
documentation, 296
dose–response curve, 300
drug approval time frame, 295
drug dependency, 301
drug dosage terminology, 299, 300, 302
drug interactions, 301, 303–305, 305
drug pH level, 305
drug potency, 300
drug's absorption, 302, 304
drug's molecular configuration, 303
drug standards, 300
drug storage, 296
drug storage sites, 300
drug tolerance, 301
examination paper, 302–309
first-pass effect, 297
generic drugs, 297
generic names, 297
injection routes, 303
intraspinal injections, 303
levels of controlled substances, 307–308
medication release, 296, 302
narcotic analgesic medication, 308
needle angles for injections, 300
needle gauge, 300
oral drug forms, 300
oral liquids, 303
over-the-counter medications, 300
overview, 293
pharmacodynamics, 299
pharmacotherapeutics, 301
pharmakinetics, 298
physicians' desk reference, 295
poison control centers, 295
prescription medications, 300
receptor theory, 299
requirements for over-the-counter medication
    labels, 295–296
requirements for prescription labels, 295
resource list, 295
science of chemical agents, 296–301
therapeutic index, 301
topical drugs, 300
traveling with medications, 296
variables affecting drug processing, 299
Pharyngitis, 202
Pharynx, 27
Phonophoresis, 257
Phrenic nerve, 49
Physiological and pathological response, to
    injury and illness
    circulation and homeostasis, 129–131
    clinical proficiencies, 119
    common injuries, 136–138
    due to exercise, 132–136
    examination, 143–150
    general injury conditions, 138–142
    human cell function and dysfunction, 120–124
    inflammation and infection, 124–129
    overview, 119
Physiological movement, 86
Piamater, 21
Pia matter, 20
Piano key sign, 181
Pigmentation, 13
Pigmented lesions, 197
Pinch grip test, 171, 182
Pineal gland, 19, 33, 34, 35

Pinna, 23
Pinocytic vesicle, 121
Piriformis syndrome, 65, 141
Piriformis test, 177
Pituitary gland, 33, 34
Pityriasis rosea, 199
Plane of motion, of knee, 96
Plantar fasciitis, 141
Plantaris muscle rupture, 142
Plantar neuroma, 142
Plantar warts, 137, 142
Plasma, 129
Plasma membrane, 120, 123
Plasma proteins, 205
Plasma volume, 130
Plethysmography, 334
Pleural space, 27
Plica syndrome, 141
Plyometrics, 272, 286
PMH, 116
Pneumonia, 202
Pneumothorax, 112, 200, 227
Poisonings, caring of, 232–233, 236, 241
Policies and procedures manual, 114
Poliomyelitis, 134, 202
Polypeptides, 33
Polyuria, 147
Pons, 18, 21
Popliteal bursae, 7
Popliteal cyst (Baker's Cyst), 141
Popliteus tendinitis, 141
Portal vein, 31, 32
Postconcussion syndrome, 200
Posterior apprehension test, 170
Posterior cord, 17
Posterior cruciate ligament (PCL) sprain, 141
Posterior displacement, of the eyes, 187
Posterior drawer test, 178
  for shoulder, 170
Posterior glenohumeral dislocation, test for, 182
Posterior pituitary hormones, 34
Posterior sag (gravity drawer) test, 178
Posterolateral rotary instability test, 183
Post polio syndrome, 202
Postsynaptic dendrite, 16
Postsynaptic neuron, 121
PPE echocardiography (ECG), 101
Pregnancy, 134, 202
Preparticipation examination
  assessment of ACL for laxity, 112
  associations and organizations associated with, 102
  components, 103
  diagnosis of basketball player, 143
  documentation, 102, 116
  examination frequency, 102–103
  for incoming athletes, 116
  personnel for, 112
  primary care physician examination format, 102
  station examination format, 102, 112
Prepatellar bursa, 7
Prepuce, 38
Presbyopia, 23, 200
Presynaptic neuron, 121
Prevertebral muscle group, 94
Prickly heat, 114, 137, 199
Primary care physician (PCP), 102
Professional development and responsibility
  ATC employment, 367–368, 370
  clinical proficiencies, 363
  continuing education, 363, 367, 369
  examination paper, 367
  governance, 363, 367, 369
  overview, 363
  research and evidence-based practice, 365–366, 367, 369
  Role Delineation Study, 368
  role of the certified athletic trainer, 368
  skills for diagnosis and treatment of kidney diseases, 370
  skills for health professional, 369
Profuse perspiration, 209
Progesterone, 36

Prolactin, 34
Pronator quadratus, 167
Pronator syndrome, 137
Pronator teres, 63, 167
Pronator teres syndrome test, 183
Prosencephalon (forebrain), 18
Prostate, 38
Protective braces, 104
Protective devices, 104, 115
Protective eyewear, 116
Protein metabolism, 120
Proteinuria, 200
Proteoglycans, 6
Proximal carpal row, 93
Proximal convoluted tubule, 32
Proximal epiphysis, 6
Proximal interphalangeal (PIP) joint, 92
Proximal joints of knee, 96
Proximal radioulnar joint, 92
Psoas major, 65
Psoriasis, 199
Psychosocial intervention and referral
  adjustment disorder, 314
  adjustment to injury, 316
  agoraphobia, 314
  anorexia athletica, 315
  anorexia nervosa, 315, 319
  anxiety disorders, 313–314, 319, 320
  binge eating disorder, 315
  bipolar disorder, 314
  bulimia nervosa, 315
  clinical proficiencies, 311–312
  communications, 315–316, 318, 319
  complex regional pain syndrome, 316
  coping strategy, 317
  depression, 314–315, 318
  dysthymia, 314
  eating disorders, 315
  examination paper, 318–321
  extroversion, 316–317
  general adaptation syndrome (GAS), 313, 319
  generalized anxiety disorder, 313
  goal setting, 316
  imagery, 317
  introversion, 316
  Kubler-Ross' stages of dying, 313, 319
  listening skills, 315, 318
  locus of control, 316
  major depressive disorders, 314
  Maslow's hierarchy of needs, 313, 319
  mental health and illnesses, 313–315
  myofascial pain syndrome, 316
  obsessive compulsive disorder, 314
  overview, 311
  panic disorder, 314
  personality and mood state, 318
  postpartum depression, 315
  post-traumatic stress disorder, 314
  premenstrual dysphoric disorder, 315
  Prochaska stages of change, 313, 320
  progressive relaxation exercises, 320
  psychological health, 313
  psychosocial interactions, 315–317
  psychotherapy professionals, 315
  for range of motion (ROM), 320
  relaxation, 317
  schizophrenia, 314
  seasonal affective disorder, 314
  self-esteem, 313
  situational factor, 321
  social phobia, 313, 314
  somatization, 316
  specific hormonal-induced depression, 315
  substance abuse, 315
  suicide ideation, 318
Pterygoid fossa, 41
Pubic lice (crabs), 202
Pubic symphysis, 6
Pubis, 3
Pull-up test, for upper body endurance, 116
Pulmonary arteriole, 29
Pulmonary artery, 25, 29
Pulmonary circulation, 205

Pulmonary contusion, 200, 227
Pulmonary disease, 135
Pulmonary veins, 25, 29
Pulmonary ventilation, 26
Pulmonary venule, 29
Pulmonic valve, 25
Pulse duration, 265
Pulse oximeter, 29
Puncture, 199
Pupil, 22
Pure Food And Drug Act, 1906, 294
P wave, 145
Pylorus, 32

Q-angle, in a female, 113
QT syndrome, treatment, 149
Quadratus lumborum, 39, 160
Quadriceps contusion, 141, 239
Quadriceps strain, 141
Quadriceps tendinitis, 141

Raccoon eyes, 137
Radial artery, 183
Radial nerve contusion, 140
Radial nerve palsy (wrist drop), 140
Radial tunnel syndrome, 183
Radiation, 246
Radiculitis, 138
Radiocapitellar chondromalacia, 183
Radiocarpal joint, 93
Ramus, 41
Rapport, 320
Ratchet theory. *See* sliding filament (mechanism) theory
Raynaud disease, 137
Raynaud syndrome (Raynaud phenomenon), 202
Receptors, 16
Reciprocal inhibition, 90
Rectum, 36, 38
Rectus abdominis, 8, 39, 47, 160
Rectus femoris, 65
Reddish discoloration, of the skin, 235
Reflex, of skeletal muscle, 97
Reflex arc, 16, 17
  impulse pathway of, 16
Reflex muscle contraction, 287
Reflex sympathetic dystrophy, 202
Refractory period, 121–122
Rehabilitation and conditioning, of athletes
  abnormal joint end-feels, 276
  aerobic endurance, 271–272
  agility, 272, 275
  anthropometric measurements, 273
  approximation, 280
  aquatic exercise, 281–283
  balance and proprioception, 275
  body weight activities, 271
  buoyancy, 282
  capsular pattern, 276
  cardiorespiratory endurance, 274–275
  categories of accessory motion, 276
  clinical proficiencies, 267–268
  closed *versus* open kinetic chain, 272
  close-packed position, 276
  close-packed position for selected joints, 276
  concave–convex principle, 276, 277
  core stability, 272
  energy systems for exercise, 270–271
  examination paper, 284–291
  exercise prescription, 270
  fitness examination components, 273
  flexibility, 273
  free weights, 271
  hydrostatic pressure, 282
  inhibition, 280
  isokinetic machine, 271
  isometrics, 271
  isotonic machines, 271
  joint mobilization and manual therapy techniques, 276–279
  Kaltenborn's mobilization grades, 277

Rehabilitation and conditioning, of athletes
    (continued.)
  lever arms, 277
  limits of mobility, 269–270
  loose-packed position, 276
  loose-packed position for selected joints, 277
  lower extremity mobilizations, 278, 280–281
  Maitland's mobilization grades, 277
  manual resistance, 271
  muscular endurance, 273–274
  muscular power, 274
  muscular strength, 274
  neuromuscular control, 272
  Newton law, 282–283
  normal joint end-feels, 276
  overview, 267
  patient positioning considerations, 283
  plyometrics, 272
  principle of overload, 270
  proprioceptive neuromuscular facilitation
    (PNF), 279–281
  range of motion and flexibility, 270
  recovery between isotonic sets, 270
  resistance training, 273
  rubber bands/tubing, 271
  specificity, 270
  speed, 275
  strength training in rehabilitation settings, 271
  stretching techniques, 270
  stretch reflex, 280
  swiss balls and foam rollers, 273
  target heart rate (THR), 270
  traction, 280
  upper extremity mobilizations, 278–279, 280
  viscosity, 282
Renal artery, 32
Renal capsule, 32
Renal cortex, 31
Renal medulla, 31–32
Renal pyramids, 31
Renal vein, 32
Renin-angiotensin pathway, 33
Repolarization, 15
Rescue breathing, for a child, 237
Resistance, to fluid flow, 260
Resistance, to tearing, 260
Resistive range of motion (RROM), 154
Resistive tennis elbow (Cozen) test, 171
Respirations, 195
Respiratory arrest and rescue breathing, 228
Respiratory distress, 228
Respiratory regulation, 29
Respiratory system
  air pathway, 26
  bicarbonate ion, 29
  carbon dioxide transport, 29
  exhalation (expiration), 29
  hyperventilation, 29
  hypoventilation, 29
  inhalation (inspiration), 27–29
  oxygen transport, 29
  phases of respiration, 26
  respiratory regulation, 29
  structures of, 27
Response law, 90
Resting nerve cells, 259
Resting state, 15
Reticular formation, 20
Retina, 21
Retinaculum, 8
Retrocalcaneal bursitis, 142
Retroperitoneal space, 31
Reye syndrome, 137, 202
Rhabdomyolysis, 135, 202
Rh factor (D antigen), 131, 205
Rhinencephalon, 20
Rhinitis, 202
Rhombencephalon, 18, 21
Rhomboid, major and minor, 166
Rhomboideus major, 46
Rhomboideus minor, 46
Rhomboid major, 62
Rhomboid minor, 62
Rib contusion, 200
Rib fracture, 200

Ribosomes, 120, 121, 123
Ribs, 3, 43, 44, 94, 148
Right cervical rotation movement, 94
Ringworm, 199
Rinne test, 192
Risk management and injury prevention
  cardiac risk factors, 101
  clinical proficiencies, 99–100
  environmental factors, 105–108
  examination section, 109–116
  overview, 99
  preparticipation examination, 101–103
  protective devices and procedures, 103–105
Ritalin, 304
Rocky mountain spotted fever, 202
Rods, 22
Rootnerves, 17
Rosacea, 199
Rotator cuff muscles, 180
Rotator cuff tear, 139
Rotator cuff tendinitis, 139, 181
Round ligament, 32
Rubella (German measles), 202, 209
Rubeola (measles), 202, 209
30–30 rule, 107
Runner's nipples, 137
Ruptured globe, 200

Sacral plexus, 17
  nerves of, 50
Sacroiliac joint compression test, 162
Sacroiliac joint distraction test, 162
Sacroiliac sprain, 138
Sacrospinalis muscle group, 94
Sacrum, 4, 36
Sagittal suture, 40
SAID, 285
Salivary glands, 31
Salter Harris epiphyseal plate injuries,
  138
Saphenous nerve, 50
Sarcolemma, 10
Sarcomere, 10
Sartorius, 8, 80
"Saw tooth" appearance, 240
Scabies, 199, 202
Scalp laceration, 138
Scaphoid fracture, 140
Scapula, 3, 43
  inferior angle of, 46
  superior angle of, 46
Scapular fracture, 139
Scheuermann disease, 137
Schwann cells, 10, 15
  nucleus, 14
Sciatic nerve, 17, 50
  pain, 177
Sclera, 22
Scleral trauma, 200
Scleral venous sinus, 22
Scoop stretcher, 238
Screw home mechanism, of the knee, 96
Scrotum, 38
Seasonal affective disorder, 202
Seated military press, muscles in, 285
Sebaceous cysts, 13, 199
Sebaceous (oil) glands, 11, 12
Second impact syndrome, 200, 202
Secretory granules, 16
Section 504, of Rehabilitation Act, 351, 354
Seizures, 233
Semen, 38
Semicircular canals, 24
Semilunar valves, 24
Semimembranosus, 79
Seminal vessicle, 38
Semispinalis capitis, 46
Semitendinosus, 79
Senses
  ears, 23–24
  eyes, 21–23
  general, 21
  sensory receptors, 21

  special, 21
  taste (gustation), 24
Sensory nerves, 23
Sensory neuron, 16
Sensory receptors, 21, 286
Septal deviation, 225
Serosa, 30
Serratus anterior, 46, 47, 62, 160
Serratus posterior interior, 46
Sesamoid bone, 4, 5, 91
Sever disease, 137
Sex glands, 33, 36
Sex hormones, 35
Sexually transmitted disease, 148, 210
Sharpey fibers, 8
Shingles, 113
Shin splints, 142
Shock, 202, 231–232, 236
Short bone, 4, 5
Shortwave diathermy (conversion), 251
Shoulder, 3
  abduction, 165, 375
  adduction, 375
  anterior apprehension test, 181
  complex internal rotation, 180
  extension, 375
  external rotation, 165, 375
  facts about, 375
  flexion, 91, 375
  girdle, 94
  girdle movement, 91
  impingement syndrome, 182
  internal rotation, 165, 375
  ligaments, 375
  pad removal, for spine injured athlete, 226
  pads, 112, 115
  tests, 375
Sickle cell anemia, 202
Sickle cell trait, 135, 202
Silver Fork deformity, 137
Simple partial seizure, 202
Simplest reflex, 17
Sinding-Larsen-Johansson disease, 141
Sinoatrial node, 25–26
Sinusitis, 202
Sitting root test, 162
Skeletal formation, 4
Skeletal muscles, 288
  fibers, 9
Skeletal system
  bone classification by shape, 4
  bone tissue, 4–6
  bursae, 7
  cartilage, 6
  divisions, 3
  joint capsules, 7
  ligaments, 6–7
  long bones, 4, 6
  muscle contractions (actions), 9–10
  principles of physical stress on bone, 6
  properties of skeletal connective tissues, 8
  roles, 4
  roles of muscle, 9
  skeleton formation, 4
  sliding filament (mechanism) theory, 10–11
  structure of skeletal muscle, 9
  tendons, 7–8
  types of muscle tissue, 8–9
Skier thumb, 137
Skin accessory structure, 205
Skin conditions, 150
Skinfold measurements, 333–334
Skin system. See integumentary (skin) system
  tinea versicolor, 110
Skipped heartbeat, 145
Skull, 3
  fracture, 200, 223
SLAP lesion, 140
  tests for, 180
Sliding filament (mechanism) theory, 10–11, 12
Slipped capital femoral epiphysis, 141
Slit lamp, 242
Slocum anterolateral rotary instability test, 178
Slocum anteromedial rotary instability test, 178
Slow-twitch muscle fibers, 91

Slump test, 162
Small intestine, 31
Smell brain, 20
Smith fracture, 140
Smooth muscles, of digestive wall, 30
Snapping Hip syndrome, 137
Snellen chart, 116
Snowball crepitation, 137
SOAP note format, 157
Soft palate, 28
Soft tissue palpations
  of the lower extremity, 173–175
  of the upper extremity, 164
Solar (celiac) plexus contusion, 227
Solar plexus contusion (celiac plexus
  syndrome), 200
Soleus, 80
Sovereign immunity, 347
Spear Tackler's spine, 138
Speech comprehension center, 20
Speed test, 169
Spermatic cord, 36, 38
  torsion, 200
Sphenoid bone, 40
Sphenoid sinus, 28
Spina bifida, 135, 202
Spinal accessory nerve, 49
Spinal column, 3
Spinal cord, 15–16
  concussion, 138
  contusion, 138
  injury, 206
Spinal nerve, 16, 17
Spinal nerve root, 97
  assessment, 155
  damages, 181
Spine
  arteries, 48
  bones, 38–39
  injuries, 238–239, 241
  ligaments, 38
  muscles, 38–42, 46–47
  nerves, 49–50
  of scapula, 44
Spinous process, 41, 42, 45
Spleen, 32
  contusion, 200
  enlarged, 207
  functions, 128
  injury, sign, 148
  laceration, 200
Splenic artery, 32
Splenic vein, 32
Splenius capitis, 39, 46
Splenius cervicis, 39
Splint, 237, 240
Spondylitis, 138
Spondylolisthesis, 138
Spondylolysis, 138
Spondylosis, 138
Spongy bone, 6
Sprain, 138
Sprengel deformity, 138, 181
Spring ligament, 138
  of the foot, 186
Spring test, 161
Squamous suture, 40
Squat, motion of, 90
  muscles in, 285
Squeeze (compression) test, 179
Stacking, 336
Stadiometer, 109
Standardized assessment of concussion (SAC)
  tool, 111, 187
Stapes, 23
Static contractions, of a muscle, 289
Statistical tests, 369
Steak, calories, 343
Stener lesion, 138
Sternal angle, 43
Sternal contusion, 200
Sternal fracture, 200
Sternoclavicular joint, 6, 93
Sternoclavicular joint sprain, 140
Sternoclavicular joint stress test, 169

Sternocleidomastoid, 39, 46
Sternocleidomastoid muscle, 47
Sternocleidomastoid scalene, 160
Sternocostal synchondrosis, 43
Sternum, 3, 4, 43, 47
  body of, 47
  manubrium of, 47
  superior, 146
Steroids, 33
Stethoscope, 206, 236
Stomach, 30, 32
  functions, 31
Stork standing (one-leg standing lumbar
  extension) test, 162
90–90 straight leg raise test, 177
Strain, 138
Strain–counterstrain, 258
Stratum basale (stratum germinativum), 12
Stratum corneum, 12
Stratum lucidum, 12
Stretches, 285
Stretching technique, 110, 115, 285
Stretch reflex, 286
Striae distensae, 199
Stroke volume, regulation of, 26
Stroking, 259
Stye, 200
Styloid process, 40
Subacromial bursitis, 140
Subarachnoid hematoma, 200
Subclavian artery, 25
Subconjunctival hemorrhage, 200
Subcutaneous edema, 146
Subcutaneous layer (hypodermis), 12
Subcutaneous prepatellar bursae, 7
Subdeltoid bursitis, 140
Subdural hematoma, 200
Subfascial prepatellar bursae, 7
Sublingual glands, 31
Subluxation, 138
Submaxillary (submandibular) glands, 31
Submucosa, 30
Subscapularis, 62, 166
  muscle, 92
Subtalar joint, 185
Subungual hematoma, 140, 142
Sudoriferous glands, 204
Sudoriferous (sweat) glands, 11, 13
Sulcus, 19
Sulcus sign test, 170
Sunburn, 199
Sunburn prevention, 108
  dosage of sunscreen lotions, 115
Superficial (early) frostbite, 231
Superficial nerve branches, 17
Superior articular process, 41, 45
Superior Labral Anterior Posterior (SLAP)
  lesion, 137
Superior nasal concha, 28
Superior rectus muscle, 22
Superior sagittal sinus, 20
Superior vena cava, 25
Supernumerary bones, 3
Supination, motion of, 96
Supinator, 63, 167
Supraclavicular nerves, 49
Supraorbital margin, 40
Supraorbital notch, 40
Suprapatellar bursae, 7
Suprapatellar bursitis, 141
Supraspinatus, 62, 166
Supraspinatus, 46
  muscle, 92
Suprasternal notch, 47
Surfactant, 27
Swan neck deformity, 138, 140
Sway back, 138
Sweat glands, 13
Swimmer's ear, 114
Swing phase, of the walking gait cycle,
  95
Swiss ball, selection criteria, 285
Sympathetic chains, 18
Sympathetic nervous system, 18, 26
Symphysis pubis, 36

Symptoms diagnosis, 143–144
Synapses, 15–16
Synaptic cleft, 16
Synaptic junctions, 121
Synaptic vesicles, 16
Syncope, 202
Syndesmosis sprain, 142
Synergistic hormones, 34, 147
Synergist muscle, 9
Synovial fluid, 84
Synovial fluid-filled sacs, 7
Synovial joints, 7, 84–85
Synovial membrane, 7
Synovitis, 138
Syphilis, 202
Systemic anatomy and physiology
  brain, 18–21
  cardiovascular system, 24–26
  digestive system, 29–31
  endocrine system, 33–38
  integumentary (skin) system, 11–13
  neurologic system, 14–18
  respiratory system, 27–29
  senses, 21–24
  skeletal system, 3–11

Tachypnea, 235
Tackler's exostosis, 138
Talar dome fracture, 142
Talotibial exostosis, 142
Talus bone, 96
Taping, principles, 105, 114
Taping procedure for sprains, 113
Tap (percussion) test, 172
Tarsal fracture, 142
Tarsal tunnel syndrome, 142
Taste (gustation), 24
T-drill shuffle test, 286
Telencephalon, 18
Temperature-Humidity Activity Index,
  105, 115
Temporal bone, 40
Temporal lobe, 19
Temporomandibular dislocation, 200
Temporomandibular dysfunction, 200
Tendinitis, 138
Tendon of popliteal muscle, 7
Tendon of quadriceps femoris muscle, 7
Tendons, 7–8, 10, 96, 184
Tennis elbow, 138, 182
Tenosynovitis, 138
Tension, development of, within a muscle,
  114
Tension pneumothorax, 200
TENS units, 261
Teres major, 46, 62, 166
Teres minor, 62
Testes, 33, 34, 36
Testicular cancer, 202
Testicular contusion, 200
Testis, 38
Testosterone, 33, 38
Tests, to identify motion deficits, 182
Tetanus, 202
Tetrahydrogestrinone (THG), 336
Tetraplegia (quadraplegia), 135
Thalamus, 18, 19, 21
Therapeutic massage, 257
Therapeutic modalities, 260
  acoustic, 247
  clinical proficiencies, 245
  cold, 250–251, 262
  electrical stimulation, 251–255
  electromagnetic radiation, 247
  frequency, 247
  heat, 251, 263
  indications, 255–256
  infrared lamps, 254, 257
  intermittent compression, 257
  LASER, 257
  manual therapy techniques, 257–258
  methods of heat transfer, 246
  overview, 245

Therapeutic modalities, *(continued.)*
  pain, 248–250
  shortwave diathermy (conversion), 251
  therapeutic massage, 257
  traction, 258
  ultrasound, 257
  ultraviolet, 257
  wavelength, 246–247
Thermometer, 149
Thermotherapy, 261
Thomas test, 176
Thompson test, 179
Thoracic aorta, 48
Thoracic duct, 128
Thoracic injuries, 237
Thoracic outlet compression syndrome, 140
Thoracic skeleton, 43
Thoracic vertebra, 41
Thoracolumbar fascia, 46
Thorax
  arteries, 48
  bones, 38–39
  ligaments, 38
  muscles, 38–42, 46–47
  nerves, 49–50
Throat infection, diagnosis, 144
Throat injuries, 236
Thrombocytes (platelets), 129, 130
Throwing motion, follow-through phase of the, 182
Thumb ulnar collateral ligament test, 172
Thymus, 33, 34, 35, 128, 147
Thyrohyoid muscle, 49
Thyroid cartilage, 27, 28
Thyroid gland, 33, 34, 35
Thyroid-stimulating hormone (TSH), 33
Thyroxine (T_4), 34
Thytrophin (TSH), 34
Tibia, 7
Tibial collateral ligament (MCL) Sprain, 141
Tibial fracture, 141, 142
Tibialis anterior, 83
Tibialis posterior, 80
Tibial nerve, 50
Tibial stress fracture, 142
Tibiofemoral dislocation (knee), 141
Tibiofemoral joint movement, 95
Tinea barbae, 199
Tinea capitis, 199
Tinea corporis, 199
Tinea cruris, 199
Tinea pedis, 199
Tinea unguium, 199
Tinea versicolor, 199, 211
Tinnitus, 239
Title IX of the Education Amendment, 352
Tongue blade test, 187, 237
Tongue taste map, 24
Tonic clonic seizure, 202
Tonsilitis, 202
Tonsils, 128
Tooth abscess, 201
Tooth avulsion (luxation), 226
Tooth extrusion, 201, 225
Tooth fracture, 201, 226
Tooth intrusion, 201, 226, 239
Tooth luxation, 201
Torticollis (Wry Neck), 138
Trachea, 27, 28
Traction treatment, 258
Transportation, of patients, 237
Transport mechanism, 120–121
Transverse abdominis, 39
Transverse arch sprain, 142
Transverse cervical nerve, 49
Transverse foramen, 41
Transverse process, 42, 45
Trapezius, 8, 39, 46, 160, 166
  muscle, 46
Trauma, to the radial nerve, 183

Traumatic asphyxia, 200, 227
Traumatic brain injury, 146
Trendelenburg test, 176
Triangular fibrocartilage complex tear, 140
Triceps brachii, 46, 62–63, 167
Triceps surae muscle group, 96
Trichomoniasis, 202
Tricuspid, 24
Tricuspid valve, 25
Trigeminal nerve, 23
Trigger finger, 138, 140
Triglyceride, 343
Trochanteric bursitis, 141
Trochlear nerve, 23
Troponin, 10
Trunk nerves, 17
Tubular portions of nephron, 32
Tubular reabsorption, 33
Tubular secretions, 33
Tumors, 121
Tuning fork tests, 192
Tunnel of Guyon, 163
Turf Toe, 138
T wave, 145
Tylenol, 305
Tympanic cavity, 23
Tympanic membrane (eardrum), 23
  rupture, 201, 224
Tympanic thermometer readings, 149
Type III acromioclavicular joint sprain, 180
Type III acromion shape, 181

UCL sprain, of the elbow, 183
Ulcer, 200
Ulcerative colitis, 203
Ulnar nerve contusion, 140
Ulnar nerve palsy, 140
Ulnar stress fracture, 140
Ultrasound (conversion), 257, 264, 265
Ultraviolet (radiant), 257
Umbilicus, 47
Unconscious adult patient, pulse in, 238
Unconscious spine-injured athlete, 239
Unhappy triad, 138
Unilateral scapular winging, 181
Unilateral straight leg raise (lasegue) test, 162
Unipennate muscle, 9
Unmyelinated fiber, 14
Unpermitted contact, 354
Upper body muscular strength, of an athlete, assessment, 109
Upper extremities, 3
  arteries, 51, 58
  bones, 51
  ligaments, 51, 56–58
  mobilizations, 278–279, 280
  muscles, 51, 60–64
  nerves, 51, 59
  soft tissue palpations of, 164
Upper motor neuron lesion, tests for, 187, 241
Upper respiratory infection, 203
Upper respiratory viral infection, 209
Urethra, 33, 36, 38
Urethritis, 203
Urinalysis, 195
Urinary system, 31–33
Urinary tract infection, 203
Urine formation, 33
Uterus, 36

Vascularity, 6
Vagina, 36
Vaginitis, 203
Valgus stress test, 178, 182
  of elbow, 171
  of the fingers, 172
  of the wrist, 172
Valium, 303

Valsalva effect, 138
Valsalva (maneuver) test, 161
Vancomycin resistant enterococci (VRE), 203
Varicella, 203
Varicocele, 200
Varus stress test, 178
  of elbow, 171
  of the fingers, 172
  of the wrist, 172
Vascular integrity assessment, 153
Vas deferens, 38
Vastus intermedius, 76
Vastus lateralis, 76
Vastus medialis, 65
Vein of retina, 22
Veins, 131
Ventral horn, 16
Ventral root, 16
Ventricles, 24–25, 25
Ventricular depolarization, 147, 205
Venules, 131
Vermiform (appendix), 31
Verruca plantaris, 199
Verruca vulgaris, 199
Vertebrae, of the spine, 94
Vertebral artery test, 154, 161
Vertebral dislocation, 138
Vertebral facet joints, 94
Vertebral foramen, 38, 41, 42
Vertebral fracture, 138
Vertebral subluxation, 138
Vertebra prominens, 46
Vesicles, 120
Vestibular ocular response, 286
Vestibule, 23
  of nose, 28
Vestibulocochlear nerve, 155
Viral infection, 114
Visceral peritoneum, 30
Visceral pleura, 27
Visceral system, 18
Viscosity, 282
20/20 vision, 111
Vision, normal values, 149
Visual acuity, 193–194
Visual impairment, 136
Visual process, 23
Vitiligo, 199
Vitreous body, 21, 22
Vocal cords, 27
Voice box, 27
Voice test, 192
Volkmann contractures, 138
Volkmann ischemic contracture, 140
Volumeter, 153
Vomer, 40
Vorticose vein, 22

Waist-to-hip ratio (WHR), 333
Water, body weight in, 286
Watson test, 184
Weber test, 187, 192
Wedge fracture, 138
Weight loss, diagnosis, 144
Wernicke aphasia, 20
Wernicke area, 20, 145
Wet Bulb Globe Temperature (WBGT) index, 105, 109
  globe thermometer temperature reading, 110
White color. *See* myelin sheath
White fiber. *See* myelin sheath
White matter, 16, 20. *See* myelin sheath
Whooping cough, 203
Wolff law, 125
Wolf-Parkinson-White Syndrome, 203
Work done, 287
Wormian bone, 4
Wrist
  drop, 138
  extension, 165, 377
  facts about, 377
  flexion, 165, 377
  ganglion, 140

ligaments, 377
pronation, 377
radial deviation, 165, 377
supination, 377
tests, 377
ulnar deviation, 165, 377
Written guarantee, of product, 110

Xerophthalmia, 338
Xerotic skin, 199
Xiphoid process, 43, 47

Yellow marrow, 6
Yergason test, 169

Zithromax, 302
Zonular fibers, of suspensory ligament of lens, 22
Zygomatic arch, 40
Zygomatic bone, 40
Zygomatic fractures, 201, 223
Zygomaticomaxillary suture, 40